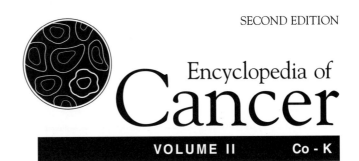

SECOND EDITION

Encyclopedia of
Cancer

VOLUME II   Co - K

SECOND EDITION

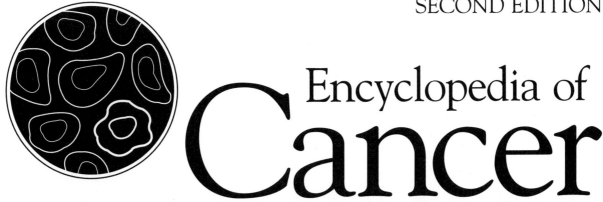

Encyclopedia of
Cancer

VOLUME II   Co - K

Editor-in-Chief

Joseph R. Bertino
The Cancer Institute of New Jersey
Robert Wood Johnson Medical School
New Brunswick, New Jersey

ACADEMIC PRESS
An imprint of Elsevier Science

Amsterdam   Boston   London   New York   Oxford   Paris   San Diego   San Francisco   Singapore   Sydney   Tokyo

Copyright © 2002, 1997, Elsevier Science (USA).

Academic Press
An imprint of Elsevier Science
525 B Street, Suite 1900, San Diego, California 92101-4495, USA
http://www.academicpress.com

Academic Press
84 Theobalds Road, London WC1X 8RR, UK
http://www.academicpress.com

Library of Congress Catalog Card Number: 2002102352

International Standard Book Number: 0-12-227555-1 (set)
International Standard Book Number: 0 12-227556-X (Volume 1)
International Standard Book Number: 0-12-227557-8 (Volume 2)
International Standard Book Number: 0-12-227558-6 (Volume 3)
International Standard Book Number: 0-12-227559-4 (Volume 4)

PRINTED IN THE UNITED STATES OF AMERICA
02   03   04   05   06   07   MM   9   8   7   6   5   4   3   2   1

Contents

I

J

K

VOLUME I

A

VOLUME III

L

Contents by Subject Area

VIRAL CARCINOGENESIS

Contributors

Sanjiv S. Agarwala
University of Pittsburgh Cancer Institute
Melanoma: Epidemiology

Siamak Agha-Mohammadi
University of Pittsburgh
Cytokine Gene Therapy

Jaffer A. Ajani
University of Texas M. D. Anderson Cancer
Center
Gastric Cancer: Epidemiology and Therapy

Anthony P. Albino
The American Health Foundation
Multistage Carcinogenesis

Jeffry R. Alger
University of California, Los Angeles Medical
Center
Brain Cancer and Magnetic Resonance Spectroscopy

Robert Amato
Baylor College of Medicine
Testicular Cancer

Howard Amols
Memorial Sloan-Kettering Cancer Center
*Dosimetry and Treatment Planning for
Three-Dimensional Radiation Therapy*

Darrell E. Anderson
Scientific Consulting Group, Inc., Gaithersburg,
Maryland
*Cancer Risk Reduction (Diet/Smoking
Cessation/Lifestyle Changes)*

Cristina R. Antonescu
Memorial Sloan-Kettering Cancer Center
TLS-CHOP in Myxoid Liposarcoma

Wadih Arap
University of Texas M. D. Anderson Cancer Center
Vascular Targeting

Ralph B. Arlinghaus
University of Texas M. D. Anderson Cancer
Center
BCR/ABL

Georg Aue
University of Pennsylvania School of Medicine
Antisense Nucleic Acids: Clinical Applications

Nicholas R. Bachur
University of Maryland Cancer Center
Anthracyclines

Richard Barakat
Memorial Sloan-Kettering Cancer Center
Endometrial Cancer

Fred G. Barker II
Massachusetts General Hospital
*Brain Tumors: Epidemiology and Molecular and
Cellular Abnormalities*

Frederic G. Barr
University of Pennsylvania School of Medicine
*PAX3–FKHR and PAX7–FKHR Gene Fusions in
Alveolar Rhabdomyosarcoma*

Michael T. Barrett
Fred Hutchinson Cancer Research Center
*Esophageal Cancer: Risk Factors and
Somatic Genetics*

P. Leif Bergsagel
Weill Medical College of Cornell University
Multiple Myeloma

Leslie Bernstein
University of Southern California Keck School of
Medicine
*Non-Hodgkin's Lymphoma and Multiple Myeloma:
Incidence and Risk Factors*

Sandra H. Bigner
Duke University Medical Center
Genetic Alterations in Brain Tumors

R. Michael Blaese
ValiGen, Inc., Newtown, Pennsylvania
Suicide Genes

Eda T. Bloom
U.S. Food and Drug Administration
Gene Therapy Vectors, Safety Considerations

Clara D. Bloomfield
Roswell Park Cancer Institute
Chromosome Aberrations

Peter Blume-Jensen
Serono Reproductive Biology Institute
Kinase-Regulated Signal Transduction Pathways
*Signal Transduction Mechanisms Initiated by Receptor
Tyrosine Kinases*

Paolo Boffetta
International Agency for Research on Cancer,
Lyon, France
Lung, Larynx, Oral Cavity, and Pharynx

Melissa Bondy
University of Texas M. D. Anderson Cancer
Center
Brain and Central Nervous System Cancer

David Boothman
University of Wisconsin–Madison
Radiation Resistance

Ernest C. Borden
Taussig Cancer Center
*Interferons: Cellular and Molecular Biology of
Their Actions*

George J. Bosl
Memorial Sloan-Kettering Cancer Center
Germ Cell Tumors

Marc E. Bracke
Ghent University Hospital
Molecular Mechanisms of Cancer Invasion

Patrick J. Brennan
University of Pennsylvania School of Medicine
Her2/neu

Ricardo R. Brentani
Ludwig Institute for Cancer Research,
Sao Paulo
Cell–Matrix Interactions

Norman E. Breslow
University of Washington, Seattle
Wilms Tumor: Epidemiology

Ronald Breslow
Columbia University
*Differentiation and the Role of Differentiation
Inducers in Cancer Treatment*

Jacqueline F. Bromberg
Memorial Sloan-Kettering Cancer Center
STAT Proteins in Growth Control

Steven J. Burakoff
Dana-Farber Cancer Institute
T Cells and Their Effector Functions

Barbara Burtness
Yale Univesity School of Medicine
Head and Neck Cancer

Anna Butturini
Children's Hospital of Los Angeles
BCR/ABL

Blake Cady
Brown University School of Medicine
Endocrine Tumors

José Campione-Piccardo
National Laboratory for Viral Oncology, Canada
Viral Agents

Judith Campisi
Lawrence Berkeley National Laboratory
Senescence, Cellular

Eli Canaani
Kimmel Cancer Center
ALL-1

France Carrier
University of Maryland
Ataxia Telangiectasia Syndrome

JoAnn C. Castelli
University of California, San Francisco
HIV (Human Immunodeficiency Virus)

Webster K. Cavenee
University of California, San Diego
PTEN

R. S. K. Chaganti
Memorial Sloan-Kettering Cancer Center
Germ Cell Tumors

Roger Chammas
Ludwig Institute for Cancer Research,
Sao Paulo
Cell–Matrix Interactions

Paul B. Chapman
Memorial Sloan-Kettering Cancer Center
Anti-idiotypic Antibody Vaccines

Irvin S. Y. Chen
University of California, Los Angeles School of
Medicine
Human T-Cell Leukemia/Lymphotropic Virus

Seng H. Cheng
Genzyme Corporation, Framingham,
Massachusetts
Cationic Lipid-Mediated Gene Therapy

David A. Cheresh
The Scripps Research Institute
Integrin-Targeted Angiostatics

Rajas Chodankar
University of Southern California Keck School
of Medicine
Ovarian Cancer: Molecular and Cellular Abnormalities

Ting-Chao Chou
Memorial Sloan-Kettering Cancer Center
Chemotherapy: Synergism and Antagonism

Edward Chu
Yale University School of Medicine
*Resistance to Inhibitor Compounds of
Thymidylate Synthase*

John A. Cidlowski
National Institute of Environmental Health Sciences
Corticosteroids

Lena Claesson-Welsh
Uppsala University
*Anti-Vascular Endothelial Growth
Factor-Based Angiostatics*

Bayard Clarkson
Memorial Sloan-Kettering Cancer Center
*Chronic Myelogenous Leukemia: Etiology, Incidence,
and Clincal Features*
*Chronic Myelogenous Leukemia: Prognosis and
Current Status of Treatment*

Jack S. Cohen
The Hebrew University
*Magnetic Resonance Spectroscopy and Magnetic
Resonance Imaging, Introduction*

Peter Cole
Cancer Institute of New Jersey
Folate Antagonists

Susan P. C. Cole
Queen's University, Canada
Multidrug Resistance II: MRP and Related Proteins

Jerry M. Collins
U.S. Food and Drug Administration
PET Imaging and Cancer

O. Michael Colvin
Duke University
Akylating Agents

Raymond L. Comenzo
Memorial Sloan-Kettering Cancer Center
Stem Cell Transplantation

Abigail A. Conley
The Mayo Clinic
*Pancreatic Cancer: Cellular and
Molecular Mechanisms*

Louis Constine
University of Rochester Medical Center
Late Effects of Radiation Therapy

Leslie C. Costello
University of Maryland, Baltimore
*Metabolic Diagnosis of Prostate Cancer by Magnetic
Resonance Spectroscopy*

Wendy Cozen
University of Southern California Keck School of
Medicine
*Non-Hodgkin's Lymphoma and Multiple Myeloma:
Incidence and Risk Factors*

Carlo M. Croce
Kimmel Cancer Center
ALL-1

Stanley T. Crooke
Isis Pharmaceuticals, Inc.
*Antisense: Progress toward Gene-Directed
Cancer Therapy*

Lloyd A. Culp
Case Western Reserve University School
of Medicine
*Extracellular Matrix and Matrix Receptors:
Alterations during Tumor Progression*

Thomas J. Cummings
Duke University Medical Center
Genetic Alterations in Brain Tumors

David T. Curiel
University of Alabama at Birmingham
Targeted Vectors for Cancer Gene Therapy

Tom Curran
St. Jude Children's Research Hospital
fos Oncogene

George Q. Daley
Whitehead Institute
Cytokines: Hematopoietic Growth Factors

Chi V. Dang
The Johns Hopkins University School of
Medicine
c-myc Protooncogene

James E. Darnell, Jr.
Rockefeller University
STAT Proteins in Growth Control

Michael David
University of California, San Diego
Jak/STAT Pathway

Roger G. Deeley
Queen's University, Canada
*Multidrug Resistance II: MRP and
Related Proteins*

Samuel R. Denmeade
Johns Hopkins University School of Medicine
Hormone Resistance in Prostate Cancer

Christopher T. Denny
University of California, Los Angeles School
of Medicine
EWS/ETS Fusion Genes

Channing J. Der
University of North Carolina at Chapel Hill
Ras Proteins

Mark W. Dewhirst
Duke University Medical Center
Hyperthermia

Frederick A. Dick
Massachusetts General Hospital Cancer Center
Retinoblastoma Tumor Suppressor Gene

John P. Dileo
University of Pittsburgh
Liposome-Mediated Gene Therapy

Eugene P. DiMagno
The Mayo Clinic
Pancreatic Cancer: Cellular and Molecular Mechanisms

Clark W. Distelhorst
Case Western Reserve University
Steroid Hormones and Hormone Receptors

Ethan Dmitrovsky
Dartmouth Medical School
Chemoprevention, Pharmacology of

M. Eileen Dolan
University of Chicago
Resistance to DNA-Damaging Agents

Alessia Donadio
Memorial Sloan-Kettering Cancer Center
Germ Cell Tumors

Zhongyun Dong
University of Texas M. D. Anderson Cancer
Center
Macrophages

Harold O. Douglass, Jr.
Roswell Park Cancer Institute
Pancreas and Periampullary Tumors

Louis Dubeau
University of Southern California Keck School
of Medicine
*Ovarian Cancer: Molecular and
Cellular Abnormalities*

Anita K. Dunbier
University of Otago
Gastric Cancer: Inherited Predisposition

Nicholas J. Dyson
Massachusetts General Hospital Cancer Center
Retinoblastoma Tumor Suppressor Gene

Timothy J. Eberlein
Washington University School of Medicine,
St. Louis
T Cells against Tumors

Randa El-Zein
University of Texas M. D. Anderson Cancer
Center
Brain and Central Nervous System Cancer

Elaine A. Elion
Harvard Medical School
MAP Kinase Modules in Signaling

Volker Ellenreider
The Mayo Clinic
Pancreatic Cancer: Cellular and Molecular Mechanisms

Paul F. Engstrom
Fox Chase Cancer Center
Hepatocellular Carcinoma (HCC)

Zelig Eshhar
Weizmann Institute of Science
Antibodies in the Gene Therapy of Cancer

Conrad B. Falkson
McMaster University
Malignant Mesothelioma

Geoffrey Falkson
University of Pretoria
Malignant Mesothelioma

Gerold Feuer
State University of New York Upstate
Medical University
Human T-Cell Leukemia/Lymphotropic Virus

Isaiah J. Fidler
University of Texas M. D. Anderson Cancer
Center
Macrophages

Mary E. Fidler
The Mayo Foundation
Renal Cell Cancer

Richard Fishel
Thomas Jefferson University
*Hereditary Colon Cancer and DNA
Mismatch Repair*

David FitzGerald
National Cancer Institute
*Antibody–Toxin and Growth Factor–Toxin
Fusion Proteins*

Hernan Flores-Rozas
Ludwig Institute for Cancer Research
Mismatch Repair: Biochemistry and Genetics

Albert J. Fornace Jr.
National Cancer Institute
Ataxia Telangiectasia Syndrome

Ruben C. Fragoso
Dana-Farber Cancer Institute
T Cells and Their Effector Functions

Thomas S. Frank
Myriad Genetic Laboratories, Salt Lake City
*Hereditary Risk of Breast and Ovarian
Cancer: BRCA1 and BRCA2*

R. B. Franklin
University of Maryland, Baltimore
*Metabolic Diagnosis of Prostate Cancer by Magnetic
Resonance Spectroscopy*

Eric O. Freed
National Institute of Allergy and Infectious
Diseases
Retroviruses

Michael L. Freeman
Vanderbilt University School of Medicine
Hyperthermia

Krystyna Frenkel
New York University School of Medicine
*Carcinogenesis: Role of Active Oxygen and Nitrogen
Species*

Frank B. Furnari
University of California, San Diego
PTEN

Robert Peter Gale
Center for Advanced Studies in Leukemia,
Los Angeles
BCR/ABL

Susan Gapstur
Arizona Cancer Center and Southern Arizona
VA Health Care System
*Nutritional Supplements and Diet as
Chemoprevention Agents*

Lawrence B. Gardner
The Johns Hopkins University School of
Medicine
c-myc Protooncogene

Harinder Garewal
Arizona Cancer Center and Southern Arizona
VA Health Care System
*Nutritional Supplements and Diet as
Chemoprevention Agents*

James E. Gervasoni, Jr.
Robert Wood Johnson Medical School
Endocrine Tumors

Pär Gerwins
Uppsala University
*Anti-Vascular Endothelial Growth
Factor-Based Angiostatics*

Alan M. Gewirtz
University of Pennsylvania School
of Medicine
Antisense Nucleic Acids: Clinical Applications

John F. Gibbs
Roswell Park Cancer Institute
Pancreas and Periampullary Tumors

Anna Giuliano
Arizona Cancer Center and Southern Arizona
    VA Health Care System
*Nutritional Supplements and Diet as
    Chemoprevention Agents*

R. A. Gjerset
Sidney Kimmel Cancer Center
p53 Gene Therapy

Peter S. Goedegebuure
Washington University School of Medicine,
    St. Louis
T Cells against Tumors

Jason S. Gold
Memorial Sloan-Kettering Cancer Center
Cell-Mediated Immunity to Cancer

Ashwin Gollerkeri
Yale University School of Medicine
*Resistance to Inhibitor Compounds of
    Thymidylate Synthase*

Jesús Gómez-Navarro
University of Alabama at Birmingham
Targeted Vectors for Cancer Gene Therapy

Ellen L. Goode
University of Washington
Genetic Predisposition to Prostate Cancer

Richard Gorlick
Memorial Sloan-Kettering Cancer Center
Bone Tumors

Kathleen Heppner Goss
University of Cincinnati College of Medicine
*APC (Adenomatous Polyposis Coli) Tumor
    Suppressor*

Michael M. Gottesman
National Cancer Institute
Multidrug Resistance I: P-Glycoprotein

Joseph P. Grande
The Mayo Foundation
*Kidney, Epidemiology
Renal Cell Cancer*

Ellen Graver
Arizona Cancer Center and Southern Arizona
    VA Health Care System
*Nutritional Supplements and Diet as
    Chemoprevention Agents*

F. Anthony Greco
Sarah Cannon–Minnie Pearl Cancer Center
Neoplasms of Unknown Primary Site

Mark I. Greene
University of Pennsylvania
    School of Medicine
Her2/neu

Peter Greenwald
National Cancer Institute
*Cancer Risk Reduction (Diet/Smoking
    Cessation/Lifestyle Changes)*

John R. Griffiths
St. George's Hospital Medical School, London
*Magnetic Resonance Spectroscopy of Cancer: Clinical
    Overview*

Joanna Groden
University of Cincinnati College of Medicine
*APC (Adenomatous Polyposis Coli)
    Tumor Suppressor*

Jun-Lin Guan
Cornell University College of
    Veterinary Medicine
Integrin Receptor Signaling Pathways

Udayan Guha
Albert Einstein Cancer Center
Transgenic Mice in Cancer Research

Parry J. Guilford
University of Otago
Gastric Cancer: Inherited Predisposition

Anjali Gupta
University of Pennsylvania Hospital
Molecular Aspects of Radiation Biology

John D. Hainsworth
Sarah Cannon–Minnie Pearl Cancer Center
Neoplasms of Unknown Primary Site

Joshua W. Hamilton
Dartmouth Medical School
Chemical Mutagenesis and Carcinogenesis

Joyce L. Hamlin
University of Virginia School of Medicine
Drug Resistance: DNA Sequence Amplification

Kenneth R. Hande
Vanderbilt University School of Medicine
Purine Antimetabolites

J. Marie Hardwick
Johns Hopkins School of Public Health
Caspases in Programmed Cell Death

Louis B. Harrison
Beth Israel Medical Center
Brachytherapy

Lynda K. Hawkins
Genetic Therapy Institute, Gaithersburg, Maryland
Replication-Selective Viruses for Cancer Treatment

Lifeng He
Albert Einstein College of Medicine
Taxol and Other Molecules That Interact with Microtubules

Stephen S. Hecht
University of Minnesota Cancer Center
Tobacco Carcinogenesis

Ingegerd Hellström
Pacific Northwest Research Institute
Tumor Antigens

Karl Erik Hellström
Pacific Northwest Research Institute
Tumor Antigens

Kurt J. Henle
University of Arkansas for Medical Sciences
Hyperthermia

Meenhard Herlyn
The Wistar Institute
Melanoma: Biology

Masao Hirose
Nagoya City University Medical School
Antioxidants: Carcinogenic and Chemopreventive Properties

Dah H. Ho
University of Texas M. D. Anderson Cancer Center
L-Asparaginase

Samuel B. Ho
University of Minnesota Medical School
Glycoproteins and Glycosylation Changes in Cancer

F. Stephen Hodi
Dana-Farber Cancer Institute
Interleukins

Kyle Holen
Memorial Sloan-Kettering Cancer Center
Colorectal Cancer: Epidemiology and Treatment

Julianne L. Holleran
Case Western Reserve University School of Medicine
Extracellular Matrix and Matrix Receptors: Alterations during Tumor Progression

Waun Ki Hong
University of Texas M. D. Anderson Cancer Center
Chemoprevention Trials

Susan Band Horwitz
Albert Einstein College of Medicine
Taxol and Other Molecules That Interact with Microtubules

Alan N. Houghton
Memorial Sloan-Kettering Cancer Center
Cell-Mediated Immunity to Cancer
DNA-Based Cancer Vaccines

Jane Houldsworth
Memorial Sloan-Kettering Cancer Center
Germ Cell Tumors

Franklyn A. Howe
St. George's Hospital Medical School, London
Magnetic Resonance Spectroscopy of Cancer: Clinical Overview

H.-J. Su Huang
University of California, San Diego
PTEN

Leaf Huang
University of Pittsburgh
Liposome-Mediated Gene Therapy

James Hulit
Albert Einstein Cancer Center
Transgenic Mice in Cancer Research

Tony Hunter
The Salk Institute
Kinase-Regulated Signal Transduction Pathways
Signal Transduction Mechanisms Initiated by Receptor Tyrosine Kinases

Mark D. Hurwitz
Harvard Medical School
Bladder Cancer: Assessment and Management

David H. Ilson
Memorial Sloan-Kettering Cancer Center
Esophageal Cancer: Treatment

Katsumi Imaida
Nagoya City University Medical School
Antioxidants: Carcinogenic and Chemopreventive Properties

Harry L. Ioachim
Lenox Hill Hospital
Immune Deficiency: Opportunistic Tumors

John T. Isaacs
Johns Hopkins University School of Medicine
Hormone Resistance in Prostate Cancer

Mark A. Israel
University of California, San Francisco
Brain Tumors: Epidemiology and Molecular and Cellular Abnormalities

Nobuyuki Ito
Nagoya City University Medical School
Antioxidants: Carcinogenic and Chemopreventive Properties

Helen A. James
University of East Anglia
Ribozymes and Their Applications

Gail P. Jarvik
University of Washington Medical Center
Genetic Predisposition to Prostate Cancer

Alan M. Jeffrey
Columbia University
Carcinogen–DNA Adducts

D. Joseph Jerry
University of Massachusetts, Amherst
TP53 Tumor Suppressor Gene: Structure and Function

Eric Johannsen
Harvard Medical School
Epstein–Barr Virus and Associated Malignancies

Ricky W. Johnstone
Peter MacCallum Cancer Institute, East Melbourne
P-Glycoprotein as a General Antiapoptotic Protein
Wilms Tumor Suppressor WT1

Douglas J. Jolly
Chiron Viagene, Inc., San Diego, California
Retroviral Vectors

Peter A. Jones
University of Southern California
DNA Methylation and Cancer

V. Craig Jordan
Northwestern University Medical School
Estrogens and Antiestrogens

Ellen D. Jorgensen
The American Health Foundation
Multistage Carcinogenesis

Jacqueline Jouanneau
Institut Curie
Tumor Cell Motility and Invasion

Raymond Judware
Case Western Reserve University School of Medicine
Extracellular Matrix and Matrix Receptors: Alterations during Tumor Progression

Joseph G. Jurcic
Memorial Sloan-Kettering Cancer Center
Monoclonal Antibodies: Leukemia and Lymphoma

Joanna Kaczynski
The Mayo Clinic
Pancreatic Cancer: Cellular and Molecular Mechanisms

William G. Kaelin, Jr.
Harvard Medical School
von Hippel–Lindau Disease

Dhananjaya V. Kalvakolanu
Greenebaum Cancer Center
Interferons: Cellular and Molecular Biology of Their Actions

Barton A. Kamen
Cancer Institute of New Jersey
Folate Antagonists

Mark P. Kamps
University of California, San Diego School of Medicine
Differentiation and Cancer: Basic Research

Gary D. Kao
University of Pennsylvania Hospital
Molecular Aspects of Radiation Biology

Johanne M. Kaplan
Genzyme Corporation, Framingham, Massachusetts
Cationic Lipid-Mediated Gene Therapy

Emmanuel Katsanis
University of Arizona
Neuroblastoma

Frederic J. Kaye
National Cancer Institute
Lung Cancer: Molecular and Cellular Abnormalities

Michael J. Keating
University of Texas M. D. Anderson Cancer Center
Chronic Lymphocytic Leukemia

David Kelsen
Cornell University Medical College
Esophageal Cancer: Treatment

Nancy Kemeny
Memorial Sloan-Kettering Cancer Center
Colorectal Cancer: Epidemiology and Treatment

Fadlo R. Khuri
University of Texas M. D. Anderson Cancer
Center
Chemoprevention Trials

Se Won Ki
University of California, San Diego
Cellular Responses to DNA Damage

Edward S. Kim
University of Texas M. D. Anderson Cancer
Center
Chemoprevention Trials

Young S. Kim
University of California, San Francisco
*Glycoproteins and Glycosylation Changes
in Cancer*

Sol Kimel
Sheba Medical Center, Israel
*Photodynamic Therapy: Basic Principles and
Applications to Skin Cancer*

Timothy Kinsella
University of Wisconsin–Madison
Radiation Resistance

John M. Kirkwood
University of Pittsburgh Cancer Institute
Melanoma: Epidemiology

David Kirn
Kirn Biopharmaceutical Consulting
*Replication-Selective Viruses for
Cancer Treatment*

Jan Kitajewski
Columbia University
Wnt Signaling

George Klein
Karolinska Institute
Tumor Suppressor Genes: Specific Classes

Priit Kogerman
Case Western Reserve University School
of Medicine
*Extracellular Matrix and Matrix Receptors:
Alterations during Tumor Progression*

Richard D. Kolodner
Ludwig Institute for Cancer Research
*Mismatch Repair: Biochemistry
and Genetics*

Genady Kostenich
Sheba Medical Center, Israel
*Photodynamic Therapy: Basic Principles and
Applications to Skin Cancer*

Robert J. Kreitman
National Cancer Institute
*Antibody–Toxin and Growth Factor–Toxin
Fusion Proteins*

J. Kurhanewicz
University of California, San Francisco
*Metabolic Diagnosis of Prostate Cancer by Magnetic
Resonance Spectroscopy*

Alexander E. Kuta
U.S. Food and Drug Administration
Gene Therapy Vectors, Safety Considerations

Mark Ladanyi
Memorial Sloan-Kettering Cancer Center
TLS-CHOP in Myxoid Liposarcoma

Michael M. C. Lai
University of Southern California Keck School
of Medicine
Hepatitis C Virus (HCV)

Wayne D. Lancaster
Wayne State University School of Medicine
Viral Agents

Jean-Baptiste Latouche
Memorial Sloan-Kettering Cancer Center
*Cancer Vaccines: Gene Therapy and Dendritic
Cell-Based Vaccines*

John S. Lazo
University of Pittsburgh
Bleomycin

Derek Le Roith
National Institutes of Health
Insulin-like Growth Factors

Jane S. Lebkowski
Applied Immune Sciences, Inc.,
Santa Clara, California
*Adeno-Associated Virus: A Vector for
High-Efficiency Gene Transduction*

Linda A. Lee
The Johns Hopkins University School
of Medicine
c-myc Protooncogene

Loïc Le Marchand
Cancer Research Center of Hawaii
Lung, Larynx, Oral Cavity, and Pharynx

Alexandra M. Levine
University of Southern California Keck School
of Medicine
*Neoplasms in Acquired
Immunodeficiency Syndrome*

Alexander Levitzki
The Hebrew University of Jerusalem
Protein Kinase Inhibitors

Jay A. Levy
University of California, San Francisco
HIV (Human Immunodeficiency Virus)

Runzhao Li
Medical University of South Carolina
ETS Family of Transcription Factors

Nicole T. Liberati
Duke University Medical Center
TGFβ Signaling Mechanisms

David C. Linehan
Washington University School of Medicine,
St. Louis
T Cells against Tumors

Stephen J. Lippard
Massachusetts Institute of Technology
Cisplatin and Related Drugs

Philip O. Livingston
Memorial Sloan-Kettering Cancer Center
Carbohydrate-Based Vaccines

Jay S. Loeffler
Harvard Medical School
Proton Beam Radiation Therapy

W. Thomas London
Fox Chase Cancer Center
Liver Cancer: Etiology and Prevention

Dan L. Longo
National Institute on Aging
Lymphoma, Non-Hodgkin's

Ti Li Loo
George Washington University Medical Center
L-Asparaginase

Michael T. Lotze
University of Pittsburgh
Cytokine Gene Therapy

Henry T. Lynch
Creighton University School of Medicine
*Colorectal Cancer: Molecular and
Cellular Abnormalities*

Wendy J. Mack
University of Southern California
Thyroid Cancer

Robert G. Maki
Memorial Sloan-Kettering Cancer Center
Sarcomas of Soft Tissue

David Malkin
University of Toronto School of Medicine
Li-Fraumeni Syndrome

Yael Mardor
Sheba Medical Center, Israel
*Magnetic Resonance Spectroscopy and Magnetic
Resonance Imaging, Introduction*

Marc M. Mareel
Ghent University Hospital
Molecular Mechanisms of Cancer Invasion

Paul A. Marks
Memorial Sloan-Kettering Cancer Center
*Differentiation and the Role of Differentiation
Inducers in Cancer Treatment*

Peter M. Mauch
Harvard Medical School
Lymphoma, Hodgkin's Disease

Harold M. Maurer
University of Nebraska Medical Center
Rhabdomyosarcoma, Early Onset

George Mavrothalassitis
University of Crete
ETS Family of Transcription Factors

William H. McBride
University of California, Los Angeles
Radiobiology, Principles of

Thomas S. McCormick
Case Western Reserve University
Steroid Hormones and Hormone Receptors

Charles J. McDonald
Brown University Medical School
Skin Cancer, Non-Melanoma

Sharon S. McDonald
Scientific Consulting Group, Inc.,
Gaithersburg, Maryland
*Cancer Risk Reduction (Diet/Smoking
Cessation/Lifestyle Changes)*

Clare H. McGowan
The Scripps Research Institute
Cell Cycle Checkpoints

Melissa S. McGrath
Memorial Sloan-Kettering Cancer Center
Resistance to Antibody Therapy

W. Gillies McKenna
University of Pennsylvania Hospital
Molecular Aspects of Radiation Biology

Paul M. J. McSheehy
St. George's Hospital Medical School, London
Magnetic Resonance Spectroscopy of Cancer: Clinical Overview

Peter W. Melera
University of Maryland School of Medicine
Resistance to Inhibitors of Dihydrofolate Reductase

Richard A. Messmann
National Cancer Institute
Targeted Toxins

Paul A. Meyers
Memorial Sloan-Kettering Cancer Center
Bone Tumors

Carson J. Miller
Case Western Reserve University School of Medicine
Extracellular Matrix and Matrix Receptors: Alterations during Tumor Progression

Amin Mirhadi
University of California, Los Angeles
Radiobiology, Principles of

Elizabeth Moran
Temple University School of Medicine
DNA Tumor Viruses: Adenovirus

Thomas Moritz
University of Essen Medical School
Transfer of Drug Resistance Genes to Hematopoietic Precursors

John C. Morris
National Cancer Institute
Suicide Genes

Krzysztof Mrózek
Roswell Park Cancer Institute
Chromosome Aberrations

Bijay Mukherji
University of Connecticut Health Center
Molecular Basis for Tumor Immunity

Annegret Müller
Thomas Jefferson University
Hereditary Colon Cancer and DNA Mismatch Repair

Karl Münger
Harvard Medical School
Papillomaviruses

Tatsuya Nakamura
Kimmel Cancer Center
ALL-1

Hector R. Nava
Roswell Park Cancer Institute
Pancreas and Periampullary Tumors

Andrea K. Ng
Harvard Medical School
Lymphoma, Hodgkin's Disease

Jac A. Nickoloff
University of New Mexico School of Medicine
Recombination: Mechanisms and Roles in Tumorigenesis

Garth L. Nicolson
Institute for Molecular Medicine
Autocrine and Paracrine Growth Mechanisms in Cancer Progression and Metastasis

John L. Nitiss
St. Jude Children's Research Hospital
Resistance to Topoisomerase-Targeting Agents

Karin C. Nitiss
St. Jude Children's Research Hospital
Resistance to Topoisomerase-Targeting Agents

Philip D. Noguchi
U.S. Food and Drug Administration
Gene Therapy Vectors, Safety Considerations

Shoichiro Ohta
University of California, San Francisco
Brain Tumors: Epidemiology and Molecular and Cellular Abnormalities

Arie Orenstein
Sheba Medical Center, Israel
Photodynamic Therapy: Basic Principles and Applications to Skin Cancer

George A. Orr
Albert Einstein College of Medicine
Taxol and Other Molecules That Interact with Microtubules

Keren Osman
Memorial Sloan-Kettering Cancer Center
Stem Cell Transplantation

Michelle A. Ozbun
University of New Mexico School of Medicine
TP53 Tumor Suppressor Gene: Structure and Function

Robert F. Ozols
Fox Chase Cancer Center
Ovarian Cancer: Epidemiology

Kevin W. Page
Applied Immune Sciences, Inc.,
Santa Clara, California
*Adeno-Associated Virus: A Vector for
High-Efficiency Gene Transduction*

Tej Krishan Pandita
Columbia University
Telomeres and Telomerase

Renata Pasqualini
University of Texas M. D. Anderson Cancer
Center
Vascular Targeting

Ira Pastan
National Cancer Institute
*Antibody–Toxin and Growth Factor–Toxin
Fusion Proteins*

Frederica P. Perera
Mailman School of Public Health at Columbia
University
Molecular Epidemiology and Cancer Risk

Richard G. Pestell
Albert Einstein Cancer Center
Transgenic Mice in Cancer Research

Anusch Peyman
Avetis Pharma Deutschland GmbH
Antisense: Medicinal Chemistry

Pieter Pil
Massachusetts Institute of Technology
Cisplatin and Related Drugs

Giuseppe Pizzorno
Yale University School of Medicine
Pyrimidine Antimetabolites

Miriam C. Poirier
National Cancer Institute
DNA Damage, DNA Repair, and Mutagenesis

Pamela M. Pollock
National Human Genome Research Institute
Melanoma: Molecular and Cellular Abnormalities

Randy Y. C. Poon
Hong Kong University of Science and Technology
Cell Cycle Control

Susan Preston-Martin
University of Southern California
Thyroid Cancer

Wendy Morse Pruitt
University of North Carolina at Chapel Hill
Ras Proteins

Amanda Psyrri
Yale University School of Medicine
Pyrimidine Antimetabolites

Harry Quon
Beth Israel Medical Center
Brachytherapy

Govindaswami Ragupathi
Memorial Sloan-Kettering Cancer Center
Carbohydrate-Based Vaccines

R. Beverly Raney
University of Texas M. D. Anderson Cancer
Center
Rhabdomyosarcoma, Early Onset

Ritesh Rathore
Boston University School of Medicine
Vinca Alkaloids and Epipodophyllotoxins

Bandaru S. Reddy
American Health Foundation
Animal Models for Colon Cancer Chemoprevention

E. Premkumar Reddy
Fels Institute for Cancer Research and Molecular
Biology
myb

John C. Reed
The Burnham Institute
*Bcl-2 Family Proteins and the Dysregulation of
Programmed Cell Death*

Heinz R. Reiske
Cornell University College of Veterinary Medicine
Integrin Receptor Signaling Pathways

Victoria Richon
Memorial Sloan-Kettering Cancer Center
*Differentiation and the Role of Differentiation
Inducers in Cancer Treatment*

Richard A. Rifkind
Memorial Sloan-Kettering Cancer Center
*Differentiation and the Role of Differentiation
Inducers in Cancer Treatment*

Gert Rijksen
University Hospital, Utrecht, The Netherlands
Pyruvate Kinases

Paul F. Robbins
National Cancer Institute
Cancer Vaccines: Peptide- and Protein-Based Vaccines

Leslie Robinson-Bostom
Brown University Medical School
Skin Cancer, Non-Melanoma

Sara Rockwell
Yale University School of Medicine
Hypoxia and Drug Resistance

Charles E. Rogler
Albert Einstein College of Medicine
Hepatitis B Viruses

Ronald K. Ross
University of Southern California/Norris
Comprehensive Cancer Center
Bladder Cancer: Epidemiology

Astrid A. Ruefli
Peter MacCallum Cancer Institute,
East Melbourne
P-Glycoprotein as a General Antiapoptotic Protein

N. Saadatmandi
Sidney Kimmel Cancer Center
p53 Gene Therapy

Michel Sadelain
Memorial Sloan-Kettering Cancer Center
*Cancer Vaccines: Gene Therapy and Dendritic
Cell-Based Vaccines*

Ajay Sandhu
Eastern Virginia Medical School
Late Effects of Radiation Therapy

Kapaettu Satyamoorthy
Manipal Academy of Higher Education, India
Melanoma: Biology

Edward A. Sausville
National Cancer Institute
Targeted Toxins

David A. Scheinberg
Memorial Sloan-Kettering Cancer Center
*Monoclonal Antibodies: Leukemia and Lymphoma
Resistance to Antibody Therapy*

Charles A. Schiffer
Barbara Ann Karmanos Cancer Institute
Acute Lymphoblastic Leukemia in Adults

Cornelius Schmaltz
Memorial Sloan-Kettering Cancer Center
Graft versus Leukemia and Graft versus Tumor Activity

John D. Schuetz
St. Jude Children's Research Hospital
*Genetic Basis for Quantitative and Qualitative
Changes in Drug Targets*

Nicholas T. Schulz
University of Pittsburgh School of Medicine
c-mos Protooncogene

Shelley Schwarzbaum
Weizmann Institute of Science
Antibodies in the Gene Therapy of Cancer

Andrew D. Seidman
Memorial Sloan-Kettering Cancer Center
Breast Cancer

Victor Sementchenko
Medical University of South Carolina
ETS Family of Transcription Factors

Arun Seth
University of Toronto
ETS Family of Transcription Factors

George Sgouros
Memorial Sloan-Kettering Cancer Center
Radiolabeled Antibodies, Overview

Brenda Shank
University of California, San Francisco
Total Body Irradiation

Navneet Sharda
University of Wisconsin–Madison
Radiation Resistance

Yang Shi
Harvard Medical School
Wilms Tumor Suppressor WT1

Kang Sup Shim
Thomas Jefferson University
*Hereditary Colon Cancer and DNA
Mismatch Repair*

James D. Shull
University of Nebraska Medical Center
Hormonal Carcinogenesis

William M. Siders
Genzyme Corporation, Framingham, Massachusetts
Cationic Lipid-Mediated Gene Therapy

Alfred R. Smith
Harvard Medical School
Proton Beam Radiation Therapy

Judy L. Smith
Roswell Park Cancer Institute
Pancreas and Periampullary Tumors

Thomas Smyrk
Creighton University School of Medicine
*Colorectal Cancer: Molecular and
Cellular Abnormalities*

Mark J. Smyth
Peter MacCallum Cancer Institute,
East Melbourne
P-Glycoprotein as a General Antiapoptotic Protein

Robert J. Soiffer
Dana-Farber Cancer Institute
Interleukins

Michael B. Sporn
Dartmouth Medical School
Chemoprevention, Pharmacology of

Gerard E. J. Staal
University Hospital, Utrecht, The Netherlands
Pyruvate Kinases

Patricia S. Steeg
National Cancer Institute
nm23 Metastasis Suppressor Gene

Peter G. Steinherz
Memorial Sloan-Kettering Cancer Center
Acute Lymphoblastic Leukemia in Children

M. I. Straub
Connecticut Veterans Administration
Medical Center
Carcinogen–DNA Adducts

Dwayne G. Stupack
The Scripps Research Institute
Integrin-Targeted Angiostatics

Michael Wei-Chih Su
Dana-Farber Cancer Institute
T Cells and Their Effector Functions

Hubert Szelényi
Weill Medical College of Cornell University
Multiple Myeloma

Chris H. Takimoto
University of Texas Health Science Center
Camptothecins

R. V. Tantravahi
Fels Institute for Cancer Research and Molecular
Biology
myb

Jean Paul Thiery
Institut Curie
Tumor Cell Motility and Invasion

Gian Paolo Tonini
National Institute for Cancer
Research, Genoa
Pediatric Cancers, Molecular Features

Timothy J. Triche
Keck School of Medicine at the University of
Southern California
Ewing's Sarcoma (Ewing's Family Tumors)

Donald L. Trump
University of Pittsburgh Medical Center
Prostate Cancer

Shigeki Tsuchida
Hirosaki University School of Medicine
Glutathione Transferases

Eugen Uhlmann
Aventis Pharma Deutschland GmbH
Antisense: Medicinal Chemistry

Raul Urrutia
The Mayo Clinic
*Pancreatic Cancer: Cellular and
Molecular Mechanisms*

Marcel R. M. van den Brink
Memorial Sloan-Kettering Cancer Center
*Graft versus Leukemia and Graft versus
Tumor Activity*

Catherine Van Poznak
Memorial Sloan-Kettering Cancer Center
Breast Cancer

Amelia M. Wall
St. Jude Children's Research Hospital
*Genetic Basis for Quantitative and Qualitative
Changes in Drug Targets*

Andrew D. Wallace
National Institute of Environmental Health Sciences
Corticosteroids

Fred Wang
Harvard Medical School
Epstein–Barr Virus and Associated Malignancies

Hwei-Gene Heidi Wang
Bristol Myers Squibb, Wallingford, Connecticut
DNA Tumor Viruses: Adenovirus

Jean Y. J. Wang
University of California, San Diego
Cellular Responses to DNA Damage

Xiao-Fan Wang
Duke University Medical Center
TGFβ Signaling Mechanisms

Carl F. Ware
La Jolla Institute for Allergy and Immunology
Tumor Necrosis Factors

Dennis K. Watson
Medical University of South Carolina
ETS Family of Transcription Factors

Pascal A. Oude Weernink
University Hospital, Utrecht,
The Netherlands
Pyruvate Kinases

Alan B. Weitberg
Boston University School of Medicine
Vinca Alkaloids and Epipodophyllotoxins

Haim Werner
Tel Aviv University, Israel
Insulin-like Growth Factors

Ainsley Weston
National Institute for Occupational Safety and
Health
DNA Damage, DNA Repair, and Mutagenesis

Luke Whitesell
University of Arizona
Neuroblastoma

Peter H. Wiernik
New York Medical College
Acute Myelocytic Leukemia

David W. Will
Avetis Pharma Deutschland GmbH
Antisense: Medicinal Chemistry

David A. Williams
Children's Hospital Medical Center
*Transfer of Drug Resistance Genes to
Hematopoietic Precursors*

Jacqueline Williams
University of Rochester Medical Center
Late Effects of Radiation Therapy

Brian C. Wilson
Ontario Cancer Institute
Photodynamic Therapy: Clinical Applications

D. R. Wilson
Introgen Therapeutics, Inc.
p53 Gene Therapy

Jedd D. Wolchok
Memorial Sloan-Kettering Cancer Center
DNA-Based Cancer Vaccines

Margaret Wrensch
University of California, San Francisco
Brain and Central Nervous System Cancer

Yue Xiong
University of North Carolina at Chapel Hill
p16 and ARF: Crossroads of Tumorigenesis

Yoshiya Yamada
Memorial Sloan-Kettering Cancer Center
Stereotactic Radiosurgery of Intracranial Neoplasms

Chin-Rang Yang
University of Wisconsin–Madison
Radiation Resistance

Wendell G. Yarbrough
University of North Carolina at Chapel Hill
p16 and ARF: Crossroads of Tumorigenesis

James W. Young
Memorial Sloan-Kettering Cancer Center
*Cancer Vaccines: Gene Therapy and Dendritic
Cell-Based Vaccines*

Mimi C. Yu
University of Southern California/Norris
Comprehensive Cancer Center
Bladder Cancer: Epidemiology

Brad Zerler
Locus Discovery Inc., Blue Bell,
Pennsylvania
DNA Tumor Viruses: Adenovirus

Dong-Er Zhang
The Scripps Research Institute
RUNX/CBF Transcription Factors

Foreword

Cancer, a most feared and morbid disease, is the second most common cause of mortality in the United States after cardiovascular disease. Clinical and research information with respect to cancer is expanding at an extraordinary rate. Keeping abreast of information relative to one's field, whether a clinician, researcher, student, or patient, is an increasing challenge. The *Encyclopedia of Cancer, Second Edition* organizes such information in a style that is highly effective and remarkably useful. The encyclopedia will be a source of great assistance to general practitioners, cancer specialists, and researchers and should be available in all institutional and private libraries. The editors and the contributors have been carefully selected for their outstanding credentials and should be congratulated for the excellence of the encyclopedia they produced.

Emil Frei
Director and Physician-in-Chief, Emeritus
Dana-Farber Cancer Institute
Professor of Medicine, Emeritus
Harvard Medical School

Preface

Since the last edition of the *Encyclopedia of Cancer*, there has been an amazing amount of new information published in the cancer research field. This second edition has attempted to capture these advances that have occurred in the etiology, prevention, and treatment of this disease. Accordingly, we have increased the coverage of topics, and the encyclopedia now requires four volumes instead of three volumes to accommodate the increase in articles.

Feedback about and reviews of the first edition have been positive, and this second edition builds on the format of the first edition. Our goal was to cover all aspects of cancer, from basic science to clinical application. A distinguished group of associate editors has provided topics to be covered, suggested authors for those topics, and reviewed the submitted manuscripts. Without them, this compendium would not have been possible. The authors chosen to write the articles are experts in their fields, and we are indebted to them for their contributions.

A major problem in organizing this effort was to avoid overlap of the material presented. While some redundancy is unavoidable, it also may be of interest to the reader to have a subject covered from more than one vantage point. We have limited references to a few key ones listed at the end of each article as a guide for further reading. The intent of the encyclopedia is not to provide a comprehensive, detailed review of each subject, but a concise exposition of the topic, directed toward the reader who would like information on topics outside of his or her expertise. Thus the encyclopedia should be especially useful as a reference for students, fellows in training, and educators.

I thank the many authors who made this second edition possible and the associate editors for their invaluable input. I also thank Craig Panner, Hilary Rowe, and Cindy Minor of Academic Press, who have been instrumental in bringing this effort to fruition.

Joseph R. Bertino

Guide to the Use of the Encyclopedia

The *Encyclopedia of Cancer, Second Edition* is a comprehensive summary of the field of cancer research. This reference work consists of four separate volumes and 220 different articles on various aspects of the disease of cancer, including its epidemiology, its treatment, and its molecular and genetic processes. Each article provides a comprehensive overview of the selected topic to inform a wide range of readers, from research professionals to students.

This *Encyclopedia of Cancer* is the second edition of an award-winning, widely used reference work first published six years ago. Dr. Joseph Bertino has served as Editor-in-Chief for both editions, and the Editorial Board has remained largely the same.

This new version provides a substantial revision of the first edition, reflecting the dynamic nature of cancer research. Of the 220 articles appearing here, more than 60% have been newly commissioned for this edition, and virtually all the others have been significantly rewritten, making this in effect more of an original work than a revision.

ORGANIZATION

The *Encyclopedia of Cancer* is organized to provide the maximum ease of use for its readers. All of the articles are arranged in a single alphabetical sequence by title. Articles whose titles begin with the letters A to Cm are in Volume 1, articles with titles from Co to K are in Volume 2, articles from L to Q to in Volume 3, and R to Z in Volume 4.

So that they can be easily located, article titles generally begin with the key word or phrase indicating the topic, with any descriptive terms following (e.g., "Radiobiology, Principles of" is the article title rather than "Principles of Radiobiology").

TABLE OF CONTENTS

A complete table of contents for the entire encyclopedia appears in the front of each volume. This list of article titles represents topics that have been carefully selected by Dr. Bertino and the members of the Editorial Board (see p. ii for a list of editors).

Following this list of articles by title is a second complete table of contents, in which the articles are listed alphabetically according to subject area. The *Encyclopedia of Cancer* provides coverage of twenty specific subject areas within the overall field of cancer, such as cell proliferation, drug resistance, gene therapy, oncogenes, tumor suppressor genes, and viral carcinogenesis.

INDEX

A subject index is located at the end of Volume 4. Consisting of more than 7,500 entries, this index is the most convenient way to locate a desired topic within the encyclopedia. The subjects in the index are listed alphabetically and indicate the volume and page number where information on this topic can be found.

ARTICLE FORMAT

Each new article in the *Encyclopedia of Cancer* begins at the top of a right-hand page so that it may be quickly located by the reader. The author's name and affiliation are displayed at the beginning of the article.

Each article in the encyclopedia is organized according to a standard format, as follows:

- Title and author
- Outline
- Glossary
- Defining paragraph
- Body of the article
- Cross-references
- Bibliography

OUTLINE

Each article begins with an outline indicating the content of the article to come. This outline provides a brief overview of the article so that the reader can get a sense of what is contained there without having to leaf through the pages. It also serves to highlight

important subtopics that will be discussed within the article (for example, risk factors in the article "Thyroid Cancer"). The outline is intended as an overview and thus it lists only the major headings of the article. In addition, extensive second-level and third-level headings will be found within the article.

GLOSSARY

The glossary contains terms that are important to an understanding of the article and that may be unfamiliar to the reader. Each term is defined in the context of the particular article in which it is used. Thus the same term may be defined in two or more articles, with the details of the definition varying slightly from one article to another. The encyclopedia includes approximately 1,700 glossary entries.

DEFINING PARAGRAPH

The text of each article begins with a single introductory paragraph that defines the topic under discussion and summarizes the content of the article. For example, the article "Camptothecins" begins with the following defining paragraph:

C amptothecin derivatives are a novel group of antitumor agents with clinical utility in the treatment of human malignancies, including colorectal, lung, and ovarian tumors. Camptothecins uniquely target target topoisomerase I, an enzyme that catalyzes the relaxation of torsionally strained double-stranded DNA. Camptothecins stabilize the binding of topoisomerase I to DNA and, in the presence of ongoing DNA synthesis, can generate potentially lethal DNA damage.

CROSS-REFERENCES

Many of the articles in the encyclopedia have cross-references to other articles. These cross-references appear at the end of the article, following the article text and preceding the bibliography. The cross-references indicate related articles that can be consulted for further information on the same topic, or for other information on a related topic.

BIBLIOGRAPHY

The bibliography appears as the last element in an article. It lists recent secondary sources to aid the reader in locating more detailed or technical information. Review articles and research papers that are important to an understanding of the topic are also listed.

The bibliographies in this encyclopedia are for the benefit of the reader, to provide references for further research on the given topic. Thus they typically consist of a half-dozen to a dozen entries. They are not intended to represent a complete listing of all materials consulted by the author in preparing the article.

COMPANION WORKS

The *Encyclopedia of Cancer* is one of a series of multivolume references in the life sciences published by Academic Press/Elsevier Science. Other such works include the *Encyclopedia of Human Biology, Encyclopedia of Virology, Encyclopedia of Immunology, Encyclopedia of Microbiology, Encyclopedia of Reproduction, Encyclopedia of Stress, and Encyclopedia of Genetics*.

Colorectal Cancer: Epidemiology and Treatment

Kyle Holen
Nancy Kemeny
Memorial Sloan-Kettering Cancer Center

I. Colon Cancer
II. Rectal Cancer

GLOSSARY

carcinoembryonic antigen A protein found on the surface of colonic and rectal neoplasms that also is secreted into the bloodstream. It is used as a marker for disease and may also be useful for risk stratification preoperatively.

colonoscopy A procedure that involves passing a colonoscope, a specialized camera, into the colon. It can reach as far as the cecum and sometimes further. It requires mild sedation of the patient and adequate cleansing of the bowel.

digital rectal exam A procedure where the clinician examines the rectum with his or her finger, reaching approximately 7–8 cm.

edrocolomab A murine monoclonal antibody that targets the 17-1A glycoprotein on the surface of the colon and rectal cancer tumors.

familial adenomatous polyposis A syndrome characterized by hundreds or thousands of small polyps throughout the large intestine. It has been linked to a mutation on chromosome 5q, the APC gene.

fecal occult blood testing This test detects small amounts of blood in the stool. It is not specific for cancer and not particularly sensitive.

floxuridine A fluorouracil analog that is most commonly administered through a hepatic artery infusion pump.

fluorouracil An antimetabolite chemotherapeutic medicine that works by inhibiting thymine synthesis.

hereditary nonpolyposis colorectal cancer A syndrome of aggregations of colon cancers among families not associated with hyperpolyposis. It has been linked to multiple genes that are responsible for DNA repair.

intrahepatic chemotherapy A route of administration of chemotherapy designed to give high doses of chemotherapy directly into the liver with lower doses seen systemically. Most commonly, an infusion pump is placed internally over the abdominal muscles and connected to a catheter placed inside the hepatic artery.

irinotecan (CPT-11) The 11th derivative of camptothecin, a derivative of an Asian tree. It works by inhibiting topoisomerase I, an enzyme important in DNA replication.

leucovorin An antimetabolite that works synergistically with fluorouracil in inhibiting thymine synthesis.

levamisole An antihelminthic agent with nonspecific immunostimulating properties used in combination with fluorouracil for adjuvant therapy.

sigmoidoscopy Similar to colonoscopy, where a specialized camera is placed into the sigmoid colon to visualize possible abnormalities. In this case, the sigmoidoscope is shorter than the colonoscope, does not require sedation, but can only visualize sigmoid and right-sided colonic neoplasms.

I t was 1932 when Sir Cuthbert Dukes first described a staging system for colorectal cancer. As a testament to his work in this disease, his staging system has undergone only slight modifications in the past 70 years. However, there have been tremendous advances in the field, from the initial studies with fluorouracil to the latest new chemotherapeutics for metastatic disease. Still, about 56,600 people in the United States died of colorectal cancers in the year 2000, necessitating improvements in screening methods and compliance, preventive efforts, and, ultimately, surgical, radiation, and medical treatments.

I. COLON CANCER

A. Epidemiology

1. Incidence and Mortality

There are approximately 110,000 new cases of colon cancer diagnosed in the United States each year; these are approximately 15% of all cancer cases. The overall incidence is nearly identical in men and women. The mean age is between 60 and 65 years with over 90% of cases diagnosed in people over the age of 50.

The mortality from colorectal cancers has shown a slight decline for women since about 1950 and for men since about 1985. Many factors have been attributed to this decline, such as improvements in surgical resections, adjuvant chemotherapies, and dietary changes in the population as a whole. Unfortunately, African-Americans have not enjoyed the same decline in mortality as whites. The death rates among African-American men have increased and now surpass rates for white men and white women.

The death rates for African-American women have been stable.

2. Etiology and Risk Factors

a. Diet There has been a long debate as to the role of fat and fiber in one's diet and the risk of colorectal cancer. Across the world, countries in Asia, Africa, and Latin America that have a low-fat, high-fiber diet have a much lower incidence of colon cancer as compared to countries in North America and Europe that have a high-fat, low-fiber diet. Those who adhere to a vegetarian diet have also been documented to have a lower incidence of colon cancer. Interestingly, immigrants from Japan to the United States have a colon cancer rate 2.5 times that of their native Japan counterparts. The mechanisms of high fiber aiding in preventing colon cancer is thought to be secondary to a decreased amount of time the stool is in the colon and the general diluting and absorption of possible carcinogens. A high-fat diet results in changes in the gut microflora and increases the concentration of fecal bile acids.

Beyond this correlative evidence, however, prospective trials have yet to show any relation between diet and colon cancer risk. Four large studies from Japan, Israel, and the United States have failed to show a relationship between neither meat nor fat intake and colonic malignancy. Controversy continues regarding fiber and its role in causing colorectal cancers. Several studies have shown inverse relationships between fiber intake and colon cancer incidence. However, a study by Fuchs and colleagues found no association between the intake of dietary fiber and the risk of colorectal cancer.

b. Genetic Factors There are clear genetic susceptibilities associated with colon cancer. However, even without detectable genetic abnormalities, children and siblings of those diagnosed with colon cancer remain at increased risk. The general concept of all inherited colon cancers follows the multistep model created by Fearon and Vogelstein. The model outlines the multiple genetic mutations that need to occur when normal colonic mucosa progresses to adenomas, carcinomas, and eventually metastatic disease. In such a model, those who inherit mutations would need fewer acquired mutations in order to progress to colon cancer. Two examples of colon cancer syndromes associated with genetic mutations include familial adenomatous polyposis (FAP), a germline mutation in the APC gene on chromosome 5q, and hereditary nonpolyposis colorectal cancer (HNPCC), associated with defects in mismatch repair enzymes. These defects can lead to microsatellite instability, an instability at short, tandemly repeated DNA sequences. Those with colon cancer secondary to microsatellite instability have been shown to have favorable outcomes and a decreased likelihood of metastases.

c. Inflammatory Bowel Disease Patients with inflammatory bowel disease have a higher than normal incidence of colon cancer. This is true for both ulcerative colitis and Crohn's disease. The risk of colon cancer increases with the duration of disease, from 3% in the first decade of disease to upward of 30% in the third decade.

d. Other Associated Risk Factors Other epidemiological and environmental factors have also been suggested as contributors in the development of colon cancer; these include decreased physical activity, increased degree of parity, and occupational exposure to various materials, including asbestos and organic solvents.

3. Prevention and Screening

a. Chemoprevention Agents that have been implicated in preventing colorectal cancer include aspirin, cyclooxygenase-2 inhibitors, folate, calcium, and estrogens. A randomized trial from the Nurses' Health Study showed a reduction in colon cancer in those who had regular aspirin use (two or more tablets per week) and an even greater reduction in those who took four to six tablets per week. Celecoxib (a cyclooxygenase-2 inhibitor) has been shown to decrease the number of colonic polyps in those with familial adenomatous polyposis.

b. Digital Rectal Exam (DRE) The digital rectal exam is of little value if used alone as a screening method for colon cancer in that it can only detect tumors 7–8 cm from the anal verge. It is estimated that fewer than 10% of colorectal cancers can be palpated by the examining finger, with all of these being rectal cancers. It is easy to do and can be done as part of the fecal occult blood test (FOBT), a test recommended by many physician organizations.

c. Fecal Occult Blood Testing The U.S. Preventive Services Task Force recommends annual FOBT for those over age 50 based on a randomized controlled trial showing decreased mortality from colorectal cancer in those who underwent FOBT screening. The American Cancer Society, the American Gastroenterological Association, and the American College of Obstetricians and Gynecologists have also recommended annual FOBT.

d. Sigmoidoscopy Sigmoidoscopy has also been shown to reduce colorectal cancer mortality from cancers detectable within the reach of the sigmoidoscope. Because of this, the U.S. Preventive Services Task Force has recommended the procedure for those people over 50 with or without FOBT. The American Cancer Society recommends the procedure every 3–5 years, again starting at the age of 50. The major limitation of sigmoidoscopy is the inability to visualize the transverse and right colon, missing upward of 40% of all colon cancers.

e. Colonoscopy Of course, the better way to visualize the entire colon is with a colonoscopy. Its sensitivity is extremely high and is generally recommended for those with a prior diagnosis of colon cancer, those with inflammatory bowel disease, those with a strong family history of colon cancers, and those with multiple polyps noted on prior enteroscopies. Screening colonoscopies for asymptomatic adults are also becoming more widely accepted, based on evidence from recent studies suggesting that many colonic neoplasms are missed with sigmoidoscopy alone.

f. Barium Enema Another method to visual the colon is with a barium enema. A barium enema should be viewed as complementary to colonoscopy; however, it is not as routinely recommended. Its limitation is the inability to resect or biopsy suspicious lesions, requiring follow-up colonoscopies.

g. Virtual Colonoscopy   A relatively new method of screening for colon cancer is called virtual colonoscopy. It is done by first taking high-resolution, two-dimensional computed tomography images. A radiologist then examines a reconstructed three-dimensional image to evaluate any suspicious polyps. In a comparison of conventional colonoscopy and virtual colonoscopy, virtual colonoscopy detected all colonic neoplasms and 71% of polyps. Large trials proving this to be a accepted screening tool have yet to be done, and like barium enemas, the procedure is limited in its ability to resect or biopsy suspicious lesions.

B. Staging and Prognosis

Staging systems are devised to separate patients with high probability of relapse from those with low probability in order to guide further therapy and provide information to the patient regarding prognosis. The most widely used staging systems are the Dukes staging system, modified by Astler-Coller in 1954, and the TNM staging system, proposed by the American Joint Committee. The Dukes staging system was most recently modified by the Gastrointestinal Tumor Study Group (GITSG) in order to better prognosticate those with multiple involved lymph nodes, thereby breaking stage C into C1 and C2 (Table I).

The survival rates correlate well with the staging system. For stage I there is a 90–100% 5-year survival, stage II disease has a 60–80% 5-year survival, stage III

disease has a 42% 5-year survival, and stage IV only a 8.5% survival. Survival worsens, however, with the associated poor risk factors: histologic grade, lymphatic or blood vessel invasion, elevated CEA, increased number of lymph nodes involved, bowel obstruction or perforation at presentation, African-American race, and expression of thymidylate synthase in the tumor.

In those who present with metastatic disease, an elevated LDH, WBC greater than 10,000, and a Karnofsky performance status of less than 60 all correlate with a decreased survival.

C. Treatment

1. Stages I and II

Curative therapy for localized disease consists of surgical removal of the tumor and involved lymph nodes. The type of resection depends on the location of the tumor, requiring a right, transverse, or left partial hemicolectomy. In most cases, a reanastomosis of the bowel can be done at the time of surgery; however, there are some cases that require a colostomy. Evidence suggests that a more extensive lymph node dissection improves local control and that high-volume centers may have improved survival rates as compared to low-volume centers.

There is no clear benefit to adjuvant chemotherapy in stage II disease, and therefore it is not recommended. Most trials show no change in overall sur-

TABLE I
TNM/Dukes Staging

Stage	Definition	TNM stage	Dukes modified stage
T			
Tis	Carcinoma in situ	0	A
T1	Tumor invades submucosa	I	
T2	Tumor invades muscularis propria		B1
T3	Tumor invades into the subserosa		B2
T4	Tumor invades other organs or structures	II	B3
N			
N0	No lymph node metastasis		
N1	Metastases in one to three pericolic lymph nodes	IIIA	C1
N2	Metastases in four or more pericolic lymph nodes	IIIB	C2
N3	Metastases in any lymph node along the course of a named vascular trunk		
M			
M0	No distant metastases		
M1	Distant metastases	IV	D

vival despite a possible decreased relapse rate. Most clinicians therefore choose to treat only high-risk Dukes' B patients or those presenting with bowel obstruction or perforation. Other factors that predict high risk include an elevated CEA preoperatively and a high-grade tumor.

The disease recurrence for Dukes' B colon cancer is approximately 20%; thus further trials to find improved adjuvant therapies are needed.

2. Stage III

When lymph nodes are involved with tumor, it is generally accepted that most people will have residual disease even with adequate primary tumor resection and extensive surrounding lymph node dissection due to the fact that approximately 60% of those with stage III disease recur.

Fluorouracil (5FU) and leucovorin or fluorouracil and levamisole are the combinations used most commonly. Flourouracil and leucovorin work by modulating the folic acid pathway. They inhibit thymine synthesis and thus prevent the tumor from replicating DNA and disabling cell division. Levamisole is an antihelminthic agent with nonspecific immunostimulating properties. These agents are well tolerated; however, some of the more common side effects are mucositis, diarrhea, bone marrow suppression, and mild nausea. Levamisole has been associated with memory loss, disorientation, fatty liver, and rare cases of progressive multifocal leukoencephalopathy.

Initial studies have shown as high as 30% reduction in tumor recurrence with adjuvant fluorouracil and levamisole, as well as an increased overall survival. Further studies have clarified that 12 months of treatment confer no additional advantage over 6 months of treatment with fluorouracil and leucovorin.

Accepted regimens for adjuvant therapy include:

a. Fluorouracil and leucovorin weekly. This regimen consists of weekly treatments of fluorouracil at 500 mg/m^2 combined with leucovorin at 500 or 50 mg/m^2 for 6 weeks in an 8-week cycle repeated for four cycles. Data from the QUASAR collaborative group suggest that low-dose leucovorin may be equivalent to high dose leucovorin.

b. Fluorouracil and leucovorin daily. This regimen uses daily injections of fluorouracil at 425 mg/m^2 with leucovorin at 20 mg/m^2 for five days given in 4-week cycles for six cycles. This regimen has been studied extensively at the Mayo Clinic and is therefore sometimes referred to as the Mayo Clinic regimen.

c. Fluorouracil and levamisole. Fluorouracil is given at 450 mg/m^2 daily for 5 days and then weekly for 48 weeks. Levamisole is given concurrently at a dose of 50 mg orally three times a day for 3 days every 2 weeks for 1 year. This regimen is not as favorable as the fluorouracil and leucovorin regimen due to results from a large, randomized trial from the National Surgical Adjuvant Breast and Bowel Project (NSABP). This trial showed a slight yet statistically significant prolongation in disease-free survival in favor of those treated with fluorouracil and leucovorin (65% vs 60%; $P = 0.04$).

In Europe, antibody therapy with edrocolomab has also been used as adjuvant treatment. It is a murine monoclonal antibody that binds to 17-1A, a glycoprotein on the surface of colorectal cancer cells. The antibody participates in antibody-dependent, cell-mediated cytotoxicity in the presence of effector cells of murine and human origin. A European multicenter randomized placebo-controlled trial demonstrated improved survival and decreased mortality for those with stage III disease who were given edrocolomab. Further studies evaluating its role in combination with fluorouracil are ongoing.

Other studies hoping to improve adjuvant therapy are ongoing. They add newer agents such as irinotecan or oxaliplatin to fluorouracil and leucovorin.

3. Stage IV

Please see Section I.E.

D. Surveillance

The American Society of Clinical Oncology formed a colorectal cancer surveillance expert panel to form guidelines as to the most cost effective ways to detect recurrent colon and rectal cancer, and the results were published in the *Journal of Clinical Oncology*, April 1999. To summarize, the expert panel reviewed the data and recommended carcinoembryonic antigen testing every 2–3 months for about 2 years postdiagnosis for those with resected stage II or III disease, a history and physical exam every 3–6 months, and a colonoscopy perioperatively and every 3–5 years thereafter. They recommended against liver function tests, fecal occult blood testing, computed tomography scans, chest x-ray, pelvic imaging, or complete blood counts (see Table II for some of their recommendations).

A. Metastatic Disease

1. Solitary Nodules

Solitary nodules in the liver, lung, abdominal cavity, or head can usually be safely resected with improved long-term survival. Five-year survival rates for those with resected solitary liver nodules are about 25–30%. Recommendations for chemotherapy postoperatively in these cases need to be made on a case-by-case basis.

2. Liver Metastases

a. Resectable Disease As mentioned earlier, solitary nodules in the liver can be safely resected with improved long-term survival. Occasionally, multiple nodules can be resected as well. After resection, chemotherapy administered through a hepatic artery infusion (HAI) pump with systemic chemotherapy has shown an improved median survival compared to systemic chemotherapy alone (72 months vs 60 months). Fluorouracil is administered daily for 5 days as an intravenous bolus of 325 mg/m^2, preceded each day by a half-hour infusion of leucovorin at a dose of 200 mg/m^2. Two weeks later, floxuridine (FUDR) plus dexamethasone is administered for 14 days alternating with heparinized saline. This chemotherapy is given on 5-week cycles for six cycles.

b. Unresectable Disease Studies with FUDR via HAI in those with unresectable disease have shown higher response rates as well as longer times to progression. A meta-analysis of these trials has shown a clear survival benefit. Therefore, those with liver metastases should be evaluated for possible HAI therapy. Studies with floxuridine combined with irinotecan are ongoing and presently produce high response rates (71%) even in previously treated patients. It is hoped that new combinations of systemic chemotherapy and hepatic artery infusion pump treatments will improve the overall survival times even further.

3. Diffuse Metastases

a. Fluorouracil Fluorouracil is the most active single agent in metastatic colorectal carcinoma. Traditional schedules include iv bolus (500 mg/m^2 per day for 5 days every 5 weeks) and short-term infusions (1000 mg/m^2 per day for 5 days every 4 weeks), with response rates averaging around 20%. Newer studies with protracted infusion 5FU (300 mg/m^2 per day for up to 6 weeks) have yielded eligibly higher response rates and, in some studies, an increase in survival.

b. Irinotecan Irinotecan (CPT-11) is a camptothecin synthesized from *Camptotheca acuminata*, a tree that is native to China. It works by inhibiting topoisomerase I and has significant activity in metastatic colorectal cancer. It was first noted in patients with colorectal cancer refractory to fluorouracil that it has a 15–20% response rate. Next, irinotecan was compared to best supportive care in patients who have received fluorouracil as first-line therapy in metastatic colorectal cancer. Irinotecan increased median survival by 27 and 41%, respectively.

TABLE II
ASCO Screening Guidelines

Test	ASCO guidelines
History and physical exam	Although there is no clear evidence to suggest improved survival and detection of recurrent disease, it is recommended to be done every 3–6 months
Carcinoembryonic antigen (CEA)	It is recommended to test CEA every 2–3 months for 2 years postdiagnosis
Fecal occult blood tests (FOBTs)	There are sufficient data to recommend against routine FOBTs
Computed tomography (CT)	There are sufficient data to recommend against routine CT scans
Colonoscopy	All patients should have a colonoscopy perioperatively to document a cancer and polyp-free colon. It is then recommended to have a colonoscopy every 3–5 years to detect new cancers and polyps

As first-line therapy in metastatic disease, it is being used in combination with fluorouracil and leucovorin. In two randomized phase III trials, irinotecan, fluorouracil, and leucovorin therapy was compared to fluorouracil and leucovorin alone. The combination with CPT-11 improved time to progression and significantly improved overall survival as compared to fluorouracil and leucovorin alone.

c. Oxaliplatin   Oxaliplatin is a new diaminocyclohexane platinum compound that is undergoing clinical investigation in Europe and the United States. When given to patients who have fluorouracil-resistant metastatic disease, it has little activity alone (about 10%) but significant activity in combination with fluorouracil (45%). Untreated patients have response rates even higher, 27% alone and 57% when used with fluorouracil. It is only available in the United States on a compassionate use basis until FDA approval.

d. Raltitrexed   Raltitrexed is a potent inhibitor of thymidylate synthase and has been approved in Europe due to equivalent response rates and survival data when compared to fluorouracil in metastatic disease. New trials are underway evaluating raltitrexed in combination with fluorouracil, irinotecan, and oxaliplatin.

e. Oral Fluoropyrimidines   UFT (a combination of uracil and tegafur) and capecitabine are new oral fluoropyrimidines. Tegafur is metabolized by the liver to fluorouracil, whereas uracil increases blood levels of fluorouracil by inhibiting its degradation. UFT in combination with leucovorin has had similar response rates and overall survival compared to fluorouracil and leucovorin with significantly lower rates of neutropenia. Capecitabine is also metabolized by the liver, but undergoes a second transformation at the tumor site to the active fluorouracil. Again, it has comparable efficacy to infusional fluorouracil in otherwise fluorouracil refractory patients.

II. RECTAL CANCER

A. Epidemiology

There are approximately 45,000 new cases of rectal cancer diagnosed in the United States each year, representing about 30% of all colorectal cancers. Mortality will be about 7300. Rectal cancer is very uncommon below the age of 20; the median age is about 60 years old.

B. Staging

The staging system used for rectal cancer is similar to that used in colon cancer (see Table I).

C. Treatment

The mainstay of treatment for rectal cancer is surgical excision. Stage B2 and C rectal neoplasms are best treated with adjuvant chemotherapy, which can be given preoperatively or postoperatively.

1. Stage I

The rate of local recurrence for those with stage I disease is only 5–10% and therefore adjuvant therapy after local excision is not indicated.

2. Stages II and III

There are high rates of recurrence in this staging group. Stage II disease recurs approximately 20–25% and stage III tumors recur at rates as high as 50%. There are higher rates of local recurrent disease in rectal cancer as compared to colon cancer; however, metastatic disease can often appear in the liver, lungs, bones, and other sites.

GITSG trials have shown that postsurgical fluorouracil-based chemotherapy combined with pelvic radiation is superior to either modality alone in reducing locoregional failures and improving disease-free and overall survival. Mortality from cancer was reduced by 36%.

There is experience giving chemotherapy and radiation prior to surgery. In this way, patients are selected for presurgical therapy based on staging done via transrectal ultrasound. For stage II and III patients, chemotherapy with fluorouracil and pelvic radiation is given prior to surgery, followed by chemotherapy postsurgery. In this way, T3 and T4 tumors may benefit by enhanced resectability, and those tumors that are close to the anal verge may benefit from greater rates of anal sphincter preservation. Randomized trials comparing pre- and postsurgical treatments are ongoing.

3. Stage IV

For local control, radiation therapy to the pelvis should be maximized. Pain is decreased in 80% of patients treated with palliative radiation, whereas bleeding is stopped in 70% of those treated. Chemoradiation at times can convert fixed, unresectable local lesions into resectable lesions.

Metastatic disease in rectal cancer is treated similarly to colon cancer with a multimodality approach. Isolated tumors outside the rectum can be surgically resected if there is good local control. Lesions in the liver can be treated with FUDR adjuvantly. Those with widespread metastatic disease require systemic control with chemotherapy. Again, similar to colon cancer, fluorouracil has been the mainstay of therapy for metastatic disease. For those who fail fluorouracil, irinotecan, oxaliplatin, and capecitabine have also been used.

See Also the Following Articles

ANIMAL MODELS FOR COLON CANCER CHEMOPREVENTION • CANCER RISK REDUCTION (DIET/SMOKING CESSATION/LIFESTYLE CHANGES) • COLORECTAL CANCER: MOLECULAR AND CELLULAR ABNORMALITIES • ESOPHAGEAL CANCER • GASTRIC CANCER

Bibliography

American Cancer Society (1999). "Cancer Facts and Figures 1999: Special Section: Colorectal Cancer." American Cancer Society, New York.

Cancer M-AG (1996). Reappraisal of hepatic arterial infusion in the treatment of nonresectable liver metastases from colorectal cancer. *Natl. Cancer Inst.* **88**, 252–258.

Douillard J. Y., Cunningham, D., Roth, A. D., *et al.* (2000). *Lancet* **355**, 1041–1047.

Fenlon, H. M., Nunes, D. P., Schroy, P. C., *et al.* (1999). A comparison of virtual and conventional colonoscopy for the detection of colorectal polyps. *N. Engl. J. Med.* **341**, 1496–1503.

Giovannucci, E., Egan, K. M., Hunter, D. J., *et al.* (1995). Aspirin and the risk of colorectal cancer in women. *N. Engl. J. Med.* **333**, 609–614.

Gryfe, R., Kim, H., Hsieh, E., *et al.* (2000). Tumor microsatellite instability and clinical outcome in young patients with colorectal cancer. *N. Engl. J. Med.* **342**, 69–77.

Imperiale, T., Wagner, D., Lin, C., *et al.* (2000). Risk of advanced proximal neoplasms in asymptomatic adults according to the distal colorectal findings. *N. Engl. J. Med.* **343**, 169–174.

International Multicentre Pooled Analysis of Colon Cancer Trials (IMPACT) investigators. (1995). Efficacy of adjuvant fluorouracil and folinic acid in colon cancer. *Lancet* **345** (8955), 939–944.

Janne, P., and Mayer, R. (2000). Chemoprevention of colorectal cancer. *N. Engl. J. Med.* **342**, 1960–1968.

Kemeny, N., and Braun, D. (1983). Prognostic factors in advanced colorectal carcinoma. *Am. J. Med.* **74**, 786–794.

Kemeny, N., Huang, Y., Cohen, A., *et al.* (1999). Hepatic arterial infusion of chemotherapy after resection of hepatic metastases from colorectal cancer. *N. Engl. J. Med.* **341**, 2039–2048.

Lieberman, D., Weiss, D., Bond, J., *et al.* (2000). Use of colonoscopy to screen asymptomatic adults for colorectal cancer. *N. Engl. J. Med.* **343**, 162–168.

Mamounas, E., Wieand, S., Wolmark, N., *et al.* (1999). Comparative efficacy of adjuvant chemotherapy in patients with Dukes' B versus Dukes' C colon cancer: Results from four national surgical adjuvant breast and bowel project adjuvant studies (C-01, C-02, C-03, and C-04). *J. Clin. Oncol.* **17**(5), 1349–1355.

Mandel, J. S., Bond, J. H., Church, T. R., *et al.* (1993). Reducing mortality from colorectal cancer by screening for fecal occult blood. *N. Engl. J. Med.* **328**, 1365–1371.

Pazdur, R., (1999). *Proc. Am. Soc. Clin. Oncol.* **1009.** [Abstract].

QUASAR Colloborative Group (2000). Comparison of flourouracil with additional levamisole, higher-dose folinic acid, or both, as adjuvant chemotherapy for colorectal cancer: A randomized trial. *Lancet* **6**, 1588–1596.

Ries, L., Kosary, C., Hankey, B., Miller, B., Edwards, B. (eds.). (1998). SEER Cancer Statistics Review, 1973–1995. National Cancer Institute, Bethesda, MD.

Saltz, L., Locker, P., Pirotta, N., et al. (1999). *Proc. Am. Soc. Clin. Oncol.* **18**:233a. [Abstract].

Steinbach, G., Lynch, P. M., Phillips, R. K. S., *et al.* (2000). The effect of celecoxib, a cyclooxygenase-2 inhibitor, in familial adenomatous polyposis. *N. Engl. J. Med.* **342**, 1946–1952.

Twelves, C. (1999). *Proc. Am. Soc. Clin. Oncol.* **1010.** [Abstract].

U.S. Preventive Services Task Force (1996). Screening for colorectal cancer. In "Preventive Services Task Force: Guide to Clinical Preventive Services." 2nd Ed. Williams & Wilkins, Baltimore.

Wolmark, N., Rockette, H., Mamounas, E., et al. (1999). Clinical trial to assess the relative efficacy of flourouracil and leucovorin, flourouracil and levamisole, and flourouracil, leucovorin, and levamisole in patients with Dukes' B and C carcinoma of the colon: Results from National Surgical Adjuvant Breast and Bowel Project C-04. *J. Clin. Oncol.* **17**(11), 3553–3559.

Colorectal Cancer: Molecular and Cellular Abnormalities

Thomas Smyrk
Henry T. Lynch
Creighton University School of Medicine, Omaha, Nebraska

GLOSSARY

adenoma–carcinoma sequence A series of morphologic changes representing stages in the malignant transformation of benign mucosa.

allelic loss The deletion of specific chromosomal regions, leaving the cell with unpaired alleles for the genes in that region.

apoptosis The process of genetically programmed cell death that helps control the size of continuously renewing cell populations.

gene penetrance The proportion of family members with a specific genotype who manifest the expected phenotype characteristic of a particular disease (in the case of hereditary nonpolyposis colorectal cancer, it is cancer).

loss of heterozygosity The absence of paired alleles for a given chromosome or portion of a chromosome. In somatic cells, this indicates that allelic loss has occurred.

microsatellite instability A difference in the length of DNA microsatellites between normal tissue and tumor tissue from the same patient, implying that mutations have occurred in the tumor tissue.

tumor suppressor gene A gene, usually with a growth suppressive effect, that requires mutation or loss of both alleles in order for the abnormal phenotype to occur.

wild-type allele (gene) The allele which is most commonly found in nature and which arbitrarily may be designated as "normal."

Cancer results from genetic changes at the cellular level. Malignant transformation is a multistep process driven by the accumulation of mutations in genes responsible for normal cell growth, differentiation, and function. The colorectum has been an excellent source of insights into this multistep process for two reasons: First, the genetic changes have an anatomic correlate in the adenoma–carcinoma sequence, and connections between histologic features and genetic alterations have helped flesh out the multistep model. Second, there are several hereditary syndromes with a very high risk for colorectal carcinoma, and discoveries about genetic abnormalities in hereditary cancers have proved applicable to the general population. Familial adenomatous polyposis (FAP), for example, results from germline mutations in the adenomatous polyposis coli (APC) gene. The recognition that APC mutations also occur in sporadic colon cancers and their precursors was instrumental in formulating the multistep model of carcinogenesis. A second syndrome, hereditary nonpolyposis colorectal cancer (HNPCC), results from germline mutations in genes responsible for the repair of DNA mismatch errors. The concept of ineffective DNA mismatch repair has been applied to the general population to great effect, introducing a novel method of carcinogenesis that complements and expands the multistep model.

I. INTRODUCTION

Approximately 133,500 new cases of colorectal cancer were diagnosed in the United States in 1996, and 54,900 patients will die of the disease. This common malignancy results from a complex interaction between environmental and host factors. This article describes the molecular changes detected in colorectal cancers and their precursor lesions. Particular emphasis will be given to the hereditary syndromes FAP and HNPCC. Although hereditary conditions account for a minority of the total colorectal cancer burden (1% for FAP and about 5% for HNPCC), these syndromes have provided invaluable information about the molecular basis for all colorectal cancers.

II. MULTISTEP MODEL OF COLORECTAL CARCINOGENESIS

"Every dogma must have its day," wrote H. G. Wells, and the reigning dogma in colorectal carcinogenesis

since the late 1980s has been the multistep model created by Fearon and Vogelstein. As shown in Fig. 1, the model posits the acquisition of mutations in a series of genes critical to cell function; some of the candidate genes are oncogenes whereas others are tumor suppressor genes. The progressive accumulation of mutations is accompanied by changes in the gross and microscopic appearance of the colonic mucosa, culminating in the development of a tumor with the capacity for local invasion and distant spread.

Before discussing the molecular changes in more detail, we will review the adenoma–carcinoma sequence from a histologic perspective. Premalignant changes in colonic mucosa appear to the microscopist as "dysplasia," a term used in this setting to signify a neoplastic transformation with the potential to proceed to malignancy. Dysplasia takes the form of cells with enlarged, dark nuclei, often with decreased amounts of cytoplasmic mucin, that pile up in the colonic crypt. Even small neoplasms are clonal, indicating that the mutation(s) that causes dysplasia

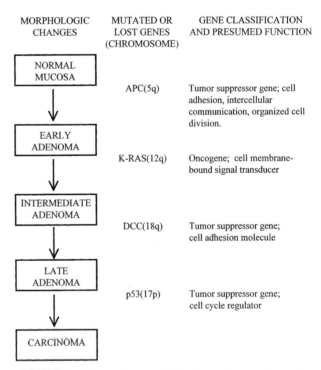

FIGURE 1 The multistep model of colorectal cancer. Progressive morphologic changes are accompanied by increasing numbers of genetic alterations. The key genetic changes are listed in their approximate order of appearance (see text), but the net accumulation of mutations is more important than the order in which they are acquired.

occurs in one or a few stem cells and confers a proliferation/survival advantage that allows the neoplastic clone to replace first one crypt, then several adjacent crypts (Fig. 2A). Eventually, the proliferating cells produce a mass visible to the naked eye, the adenoma (Fig. 2B). An adenoma, then, is a mass of cells showing low-grade dysplasia. A subset of adenomas will develop areas of high-grade dysplasia (sometimes called carcinoma *in situ*), with loss of normal architecture and significant variation in nuclear size and shape (Fig. 2C). Experience has shown that adenomas are more likely to harbor high-grade dysplasia when they are larger and when they have villous architecture (finger-like growths on the surface). In the genetic model shown in Fig. 1, "early adenoma" corresponds to a small adenoma without villous architecture, "intermediate adenoma" corresponds to a larger adenoma with villous architecture, and "late adenoma" corresponds to an adenoma with high-grade dysplasia.

Several asides are necessary here. First, a "preadenomatous" lesion has been proposed: the aberrant crypt focus (ACF). ACF were originally described in carcinogen-treated mice and rats, but have since been found in humans. They are collections of enlarged crypts with a thickened epithelial lining. ACF are slightly elevated above the surrounding mucosa and can be seen grossly with the aid of a magnifying lens. The epithelial lining varies; some ACF have a serrated lining similar to that of hyperplastic (nonneoplastic) polyps, others have a dysplastic (adenomatous) lining, and still others have a lining not unlike that of normal colon. This variety has led some to conclude that ACF represent a nonhomogeneous collection of small hyperplastic polyps, small adenomas, and incidental, nonspecific mucosal irregularities. ACF may well be morphologically and biologically heterogeneous—not all ACF progress to malignancy in animal models—but it is intriguing that immunohistochemical stains for carcinoembryonic antigen (CEA) are consistently and diffusely positive in human ACF. CEA is an oncofetal protein highly expressed during fetal development, but much less so in adult colon. It plays a role in cell–cell and cell–substrate adhesion, and may help regulate cell migration from crypt base to mucosal surface. Thus, abnormal CEA expression in ACF correlates with the histologic impression of abnormal crypt architecture. In addition, K-ras mutations have been found in about half of ACF; because K-ras mutations are also found in adenomas and carcinomas (see later), but not in normal mucosa, the case for ACF as early cancer precursors is further strengthened.

Next, we introduce another candidate preadenomatous lesion, this one even more controversial than aberrant crypt foci: transitional mucosa (TM). There is no doubt that mucosa immediately adjacent to colorectal carcinoma (within 2–3 cm of the tumor) is different from mucosa elsewhere. The differences are morphologic (colonic crypts tend to be longer and the cells lining them larger), biochemical (increased production of sialomucins), and functional (expansion of the proliferative compartment). Upregulation of some cell cycle genes has also been described in TM. The unresolved question is: are these changes secondary to the tumor or do they precede it? If the latter is true, it suggests that the carcinogenic process begins in a field of abnormal mucosa rather than as a discrete focus. This is a minority view, but, as shown in Section IV, fields of abnormal mucosa do give rise to the subset of colorectal carcinomas that complicate inflammatory bowel disease, so it is not entirely unreasonable that other cancers have a similar origin.

Finally, we must emphasize that the "adenoma–carcinoma sequence" is not synonymous with the "polyp–carcinoma sequence"; a more accurate term for the process would be "dysplasia–carcinoma sequence," as the model does not insist that all carcinomas must develop from grossly visible masses of dysplastic tissue. It is quite possible that some lesions acquire the mutations necessary to move from low-grade dysplasia to high-grade dysplasia to carcinoma without ever forming a visible polyp. A too literal interpretation of the "adenoma–carcinoma sequence" has given rise to the unsatisfactory term *de novo* carcinoma to describe small carcinomas without recognizable residual adenoma. The *de novo* carcinoma vs adenoma–carcinoma dichotomy is really only a semantic disagreement; yes, the multistep model undoubtedly oversimplifies a complex process (that is what models are for, after all), and yes, in some malignancies carcinogenesis may be accelerated or achieved along alternate pathways, but there is no evidence that "*de novo*" carcinoma is the product of a

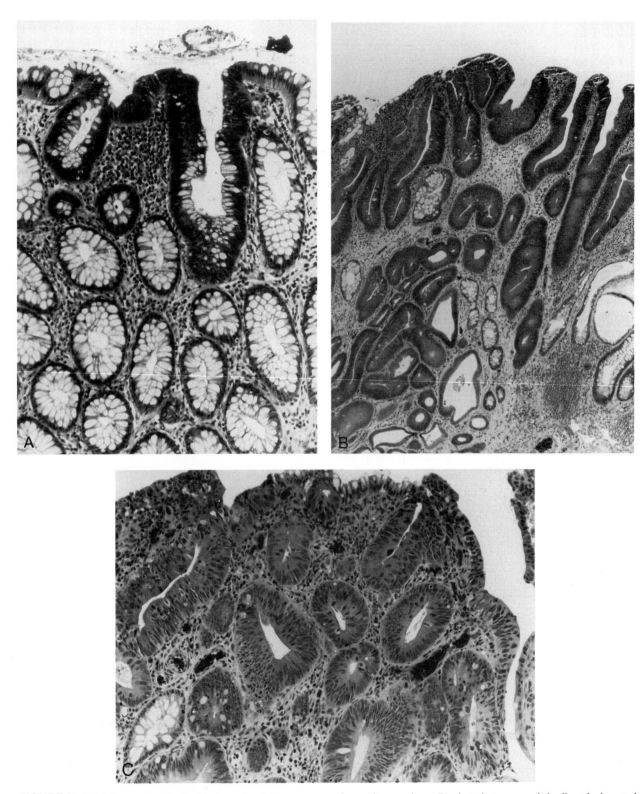

FIGURE 2 (A) Adenomatous (dysplastic) change involving one crypt and part of a second one. Dysplasia features crowded cells with elongated nuclei and decreased cytoplasmic mucin (×13.2). (B) More extensive dysplasia forming a mass, the adenoma (×13.2). (C) High-grade dysplasia in an adenoma. Nuclei are darker, more irregular, and more haphazardly arranged (×33).

one-step switch from normal mucosa to carcinoma; the general framework of the multistep model probably applies in all cases.

This is not to downplay the potential for variability in the adenoma–carcinoma sequence. It is becoming clear that not all adenomas are created equal. One variant is the "flat adenoma." Flat adenomas are masses of dysplastic tissue that form slightly raised plaques rather than polyps in colonic mucosa. Histologically, flat adenomas have dysplastic tubules concentrated near the surface of the mucosa (Fig. 3). The importance of flat adenomas is that they seem to have a higher prevalence of high-grade dysplasia than polypoid adenomas of similar size, suggesting that they have an important role as cancer precursors. Molecular findings, discussed later, support the notion that flat adenomas are inherently different from polyploid adenomas.

A second example of variability in the adenoma–carcinoma sequence is the concept of the "aggressive adenoma." This term was coined to explain two observations about patients with HNPCC: (1) they have an 80 to 90% chance of developing colon cancer, de-

spite the fact that they form adenomas only about as often as the general population, and (2) they commonly develop carcinomas within 2 to 5 years of a normal colonoscopic screening examination, a very short interval compared to the general population. If the adenoma–carcinoma sequence applies in HNPCC, then the adenomas formed by affected patients must be more likely to progress to carcinoma and must do so more quickly than adenomas in the general population. There is strong clinical evidence for this idea: when HNPCC patients in a surveillance program are compared to those who refuse surveillance, it can be shown that one colorectal cancer is prevented for every 2.8 adenomas discovered and removed from those under surveillance. In contrast, it is estimated that 41–119 polypectomies are needed to prevent one cancer in the general population. The discovery that HNPCC results from defective DNA mismatch repair has provided a molecular mechanism for the aggressive adenoma: the relentlessly accumulating mutations in a repair-deficient cells probably accelerate the multistep transformation to malignancy.

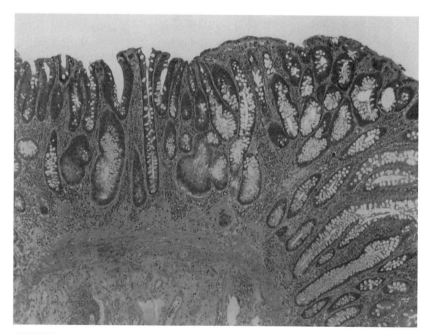

FIGURE 3 A flat adenoma. Adenomatous glands are grouped near the mucosal surface, forming a plaque. This is only slightly raised above adjacent mucosa (right) (×13.2).

Having reviewed the phenotypic manifestations of the multistep model, we can proceed to its genotype—the genetic abnormalities implicated in colonic carcinogenesis. Figure 1 shows the mutations most often detected in colorectal cancer. We will review the rationale for assigning each mutation its putative place in the model, but it must be emphasized that the order in which mutations are acquired is less important than the fact that multiple mutations accumulate in the transforming cells.

A. APC Gene

Individuals with FAP carry germline mutations in the APC gene on chromosome 5q. The gene product is a cytoplasmic protein that plays a role in cellular adhesion and intercellular communication. Mutations are inactivating. The gene is classified as a tumor suppressor gene, implying that mutations of both alleles are required for an effect, but in some cases, a mutant APC allele encodes a protein that can inactivate the wild-type protein by oligomerization (dominant negative effect) and, in other cases, inactivation of one allele may be sufficient to alter normal APC function (gene dosage).

Mutations in APC are common in sporadic colorectal neoplasms, being found in 65–70% of cancers and, more important, in a similar percentage of adenomas. APC mutations are found even in very small (>0.5 cm) adenomas, suggesting that they are an early event, perhaps even the initiating event, in the adenoma–carcinoma sequence.

B. K-*ras*

The *ras* gene family (H-*ras*, K-*ras*, N-*ras*) encodes for proteins that act as signal transducers across cell membranes. Point mutations at certain codons result in mutant proteins with transforming activity. About 50% of colorectal cancers have a mutation in the K-*ras* gene. The same frequency holds true for adenomas larger than 1 cm. Smaller adenomas, however, have a much lower prevalence of K-ras mutations (less than 10%). These findings have two possible explanations: K-ras mutations may occur in a subset of small adenomas and encourage progression to larger adenoma or K-ras mutations may be an early or initiating event

in some adenomas, and such adenomas progress to larger, more dysplastic adenomas faster and more often than adenomas without K-ras mutations. The observation that adenomas with K-ras mutation have those mutations in discrete areas of the polyp (unlike carcinomas in which K-ras mutations are diffuse) adds support to the first interpretation.

K-ras mutations have been detected in roughly half of aberrant crypt foci, indicating that at least some of those lesions are precursors to malignancy.

Flat adenomas have a relatively low frequency of K-ras mutations, and the frequency does not seem to increase with increasing degrees of dysplasia. The difference may mean that flat adenomas progress to carcinoma along a somewhat different pathway than polypoid adenomas.

C. DCC

The tumor suppressor gene DCC (deleted colon cancer) has its locus on chromosome 18q. The gene encodes a protein similar to the neural cell adhesion molecule (NCAM) family. The DCC protein is expressed in goblet cells of normal mucosa. As a cell surface molecule related to adhesion proteins, the DCC protein may regulate cell growth through the recognition of extracellular signals. Inactivation of DCC probably contributes to a loss of normal adhesion in colonic mucosa. DCC expression is absent or greatly reduced in 85% of colorectal cancer cell lines. Allelic loss of 18q is a common event in colorectal cancer (70%) and in "late" adenomas (50%), but uncommon in early adenomatous (10%).

D. *p53*

The *p53* gene on chromosome 17p is classified as a tumor suppressor gene. The gene product is a cell cycle regulator with growth suppressive activity. *p53* seems to regulate the G_1 checkpoint in the cell cycle, preventing cells with damaged DNA from entering into cell division. Mutations of p53 were first described in colon cancer, but have since been found in nearly every human malignancy.

Chromosome 17p is the region most frequently affected by allelic loss in colorectal cancer, being deleted in 75% of such tumors, and the region of 17p commonly lost includes the *p53* gene. Conversely, allelic loss of 17p is infrequent in adenomas, even large, late-stage adenomas. The vast majority of colon cancers with an allelic loss of 17p have missense mutations of p53 on the remaining allele. p53 mutations have not been detected in aberrant crypt foci. Allelic loss and point mutations of p53 are thought to be late events in colon carcinogenesis.

E. Other Genetic Alterations

Mutations and deletions of APC, K-ras, DCC, and p53 are the most commonly detected abnormalities in colorectal carcinoma, forming the backbone of the multistep model. But regulation of cell function and differentiation can be perturbed in many other ways, some of which may be critical. Some of the additional genetic changes detected in colorectal carcinoma are described next.

1. Cell Cycle Regulators

The interval between each cell division is defined as a cell cycle. Control of the cell cycle is critical to the preservation of normal cell function. Dysregulation leads to uncontrolled proliferation. Because checkpoints in the normal cycle allow time for detection and repair of errors in DNA, infidelity of DNA replication can result from loss of checkpoint control. We have already seen that abnormalities of the *p53* gene, an important cell cycle regulator, are found in a large percentage of colorectal carcinomas.

Cyclin D1 is another cell cycle regulator implicated in colon carcinogenesis. It belongs to the family of activating proteins that stimulate progression through the cell cycle. Immunohistochemical studies have shown increased nuclear expression of cyclin D1 protein in about 30% of adenomas and colorectal carcinomas. Nuclear accumulation in adenomas does not correlate with size or degree of dysplasia, making increased expression of cyclin D1 a candidate for an early event in colon carcinogenesis.

2. Growth Factors and Signal Transduction

Complex intercellular signaling networks, mediated by growth factors and their receptors, influence cell proliferation and differentiation. Genetic alterations that activate growth factor signaling pathways con-

tribute to the development and progression of most human malignancies.

In the colon, high levels of transforming growth factor-β1 (TGF-β1) have been associated with the progression of carcinoma. An increased expression of TGF-β1 correlates with an advanced stage of diagnosis. TGF-β1 is a multifunctional polypeptide that promotes angiogenesis, stimulates the accumulation of cell adhesion proteins, and inhibits the growth of epithelial cells and immune cells. Overexpression of TGF-β1 in colorectal carcinoma could contribute to tumor progression by enhancing the blood supply or by inhibiting immune responses. Interestingly, certain colon cancers have mutations in the TGF-β1 receptor gene that lead to absence of those receptors; such tumors may be able to escape the growth inhibitory effects of TGF-β1 while enjoying its angiogenesis-stimulating and immune-suppressing properties.

3. Programmed Cell Death

Our discussion so far has focused on mutations that deregulate cell proliferation, but continuously renewing cell populations have controls on both the rate of cell production and the rate of cell loss. The rate of cell loss is mediated by genetically programmed cell death (apoptosis). Inhibition of apoptosis results in expansion of a cell population; such inhibition may come from several sources, but the principal inhibitor of apoptosis is the bcl-2 protooncogene. In normal colon, bcl-2 expression is seen in the proliferative zone at the base of the crypts, but not in more mature cells near the mucosal surface. In tubular adenomas, bcl-2 expression is also limited to crypt bases, but expression is expanded in adenomas with villous architecture (the intermediate adenomas of the multistep model) and is markedly expanded in colorectal carcinomas. There is an inverse correlation between bcl-2 expression and apoptosis: apoptotic bodies are common in tubular adenomas, reduced in tubulovillous adenomas, and absent in colorectal carcinomas. Abnormal expression of bcl-2, with inhibition of apoptosis, may be an early event in the adenoma–carcinoma sequence.

4. Cell Adhesion Molecules

Cell–cell and cell–substrate interactions are mediated by adhesion molecules expressed on the cell surface and on the substrate, where they help maintain normal tissue homeostasis. Alterations in the expression of adhesion molecules are characteristic of tumors. As discussed earlier, DCC mutations are common in colorectal carcinoma, and dysregulation of CEA expression is seen in carcinomas, adenomas, and aberrant crypt foci. Other adhesion molecules of interest in colonic carcinogenesis include E-cadherin, integrins, and CD44. E-cadherin is a transmembrane glycoprotein found at adherens junctions, specialized areas of the cell membrane critical to cell–cell adhesion and cytoskeletal organization. Adult tissues are dependent on cadherins for maintenance of structural integrity and polarity. Alterations of cadherins could play a role in the progressive loss of cellular organization associated with carcinogenesis. In the colon, decreased E-cadherin expression is associated with progression and metastasis of carcinomas. Expression of integrins, transmembrane proteins that function in cell–substrate interactions, is also progressively lost in the course of the adenoma–carcinoma sequence. CD44, another transmembrane glycoprotein that mediates cell–cell and cell–substrate adhesion (in addition to functioning as a lymphocyte-homing receptor on circulating lymphocytes), may be altered early in the carcinogenic process. Variant forms of CD44, not detected in normal colonic mucosa, are found in carcinomas and in adenomas. There appears to be no correlation of variant CD44 expression with adenoma size or degree of dysplasia, suggesting that this change is another early event in the adenoma–carcinoma sequence.

III. FAMILIAL ADENOMATOUS POLYPOSIS

We now turn to two hereditary cancer syndromes for a more detailed look at specific genetic abnormalities and their clinical manifestations.

Familial adenomatous polyposis is the best known colon cancer syndrome; it accounts for about 1% of all colorectal carcinomas. Classic FAP features hundreds or thousands of adenomas distributed diffusely throughout the colon, presenting at the time of puberty. If prophylactic colectomy is not performed, carcinoma develops by the end of the fourth decade. Extracolonic manifestations are common and include adenomas and carcinomas of the duodenum, adenomas and fundic gland polyps of the stomach, epidermoid cysts, osteomas, and an abnormality of the retina known as congenital hypertrophy of the retinal pigment epithelium (CHRPE). Desmoid tumors, a nonneoplastic but locally aggressive fibromatosis, characterize the Gardner syndrome variant. There is also an attenuated variant (AFAP), in which affected individuals have fewer adenomas, generally limited to the proximal colon, and a somewhat lower risk for colorectal carcinoma. An aggressive variant has also been described in which very large numbers of adenomas develop even before puberty, with carcinomas often supervening in the third decade.

FAP results from a germline mutation of the APC gene on chromosome 5. The gene comprises 15 exons encoding a protein with 2843 amino acid residues. Exon 15 makes up 77% of the coding region. The gene product is a cytoplasmic protein expressed in epithelial cells. The APC protein may influence cellular adhesion and intercellular communication by interacting with elements essential to such functions, such as catenins and E-cadherin. APC protein also binds to microtubules, suggesting a role in organizing cell division.

A variety of APC mutations have been found in FAP families. All mutations discovered thus far inactive gene function. The inactivating mutations are usually deletions or insertions of short sequences that create stop codons, producing a premature signal to stop translation that results in a truncated protein product. There is some correlation between the location of the mutation and the clinical manifestations of the syndrome. Figure 4 shows the genotype–phenotype correlations as currently understood. Mutations nearest the 5′ end produce the attenuated phenotype, whereas mutations nearest the 3′ end produce the more aggressive phenotype. Desmoid tumors are associated with mutations between codons 1445 and 1578 of exon 15. Proximal mutations are generally CHRPE negative and distal mutations CHRPE positive, although mutations in the "desmoid-producing" region do not seem to induce CHRPE.

The correlation between genotype and phenotype may be explained by the fact that normal APC molecules function as dimers. Distal mutations, near the

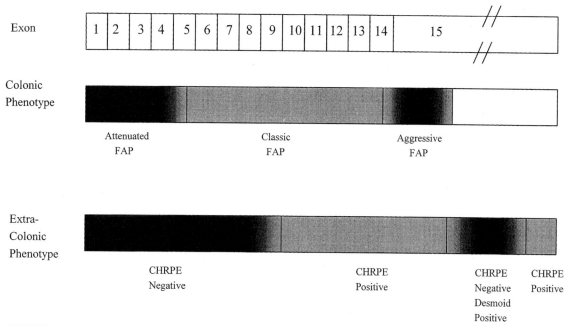

FIGURE 4 Genotype–phenotype correlations in FAP. Mutations near the proximal end of the large APC gene result in an attenuated phenotype (less than 100 adenomas, later age of cancer onset), whereas distal mutations result in an aggressive phenotype (thousands of adenomas, earlier cancer onset). Note: Identical mutations can produce varied clinical features, suggesting that there are environmental or clinical modifiers of phenotype.

3′ end, produce a less truncated protein that may bind to the wild-type APC protein and interfere with its function (a dominant-negative effect). A severely truncated protein, produced by a mutation near the 5′ end, may be unable to dimerize, leaving the wild-type protein free to function normally.

Genotype–phenotype correlations are not consistent. Identical APC mutations may produce diverse clinical features. In attenuated FAP, for example, the number of colonic adenomas in patients from a single family may range from two to hundreds. There are likely to be environmental modifiers, or other genetic factors, that account for these phenotypic variations. One candidate modifying gene is a locus on chromosome 1p that may influence the severity of duodenal polyposis.

IV. HEREDITARY NONPOLYPOSIS COLORECTAL CANCER

HNPCC is a syndrome that results from inherited mutations of genes responsible for the repair of DNA mismatches. There are at least 11 such genes in humans; so far, mutations in 4 of them have been linked to the syndrome of HNPCC. The disease was described almost 100 years before it was proven to be an inherited condition. In HNPCC, colorectal cancer develops at a fairly young age (average 44 years) and tends to involve the proximal colon (70% of tumors are proximal to the splenic flexure). Affected individuals frequently have multiple colon cancers. As the name implies, the syndrome is not a polyposis; HNPCC patients form colonic adenomas about as often as the general population. In some families, colon cancer is the only manifestation of the syndrome, whereas in others there may be a statistically significant excess of carcinoma involving the endometrium, stomach, small bowel, pancreas, biliary tract, renal pelvis, or ureter. The former situation is referred to as Lynch syndrome I, whereas families with a pattern of colonic and extracolonic cancers are said to have Lynch syndrome II. When stringent clinical criteria are used for the diagnosis [at least three first-degree relatives with colorectal cancer, involving at least two generations, and at least one person affected before age 50 (Amsterdam Criteria)], HNPCC is estimated to account for 1 to 5% of all colon cancers. However, the frequency may prove to be higher when the extracolonic syndrome cancers of HNPCC are included and genetic testing is employed for diagnosis.

In addition to preferentially involving the proximal colon, HNPCC cancers have some special histologic features. About a third of them are poorly differentiated, meaning that they tend to form solid sheets of malignant cells rather than producing glands as most sporadic colon cancers do. In addition, HNPCC cancers are more likely than sporadic ones to have abundant extracellular mucin. Mucinous histology and poor differentiation generally indicate poor prognosis, so the histologic features of HNPCC were difficult to reconcile with clinical evidence that HNPCC cancers actually have a somewhat better prognosis than sporadic cancer, with 5-year survivals of 65% vs 44% in one study. The paradox may be resolved by the molecular basis of the syndrome, as described later.

DNA mismatch repair was first recognized in yeast and bacteria. Briefly, mismatch repair is one of the mechanisms employed by cells to enhance replication fidelity, allowing accurate transmission of genetic information from a cell to its progeny. The mismatch repair system is capable of recognizing abnormal base pairs and correcting the sequence on one strand to restore the normal A–T and G–C pairings. Mismatch errors can arise either through the formation of abnormal base pairs (C–A, T–G, etc.) or by slippage of DNA polymerase on the template during the replication of long repetitive sequences. In bacteria, DNA mismatch repair involves the cooperation of several gene products. The mismatch is bound by MutS; a second protein (MutH) identifies the newly formed strand by virtue of differences in methylation between the old and the new strands. (This is a critical function. Without it, there would be a 50% change that correction of a mismatch base pair would result in removal of the correct base from the old strand.) A third protein (MutL) complexes with MutS and MutH, initiating excision of the mismatched base(s). An intact mismatch repair system increases the accuracy of DNA replication by 100- to 1000-fold.

A phenomenon known as microsatellite instability provided the crucial hint that mismatch repair genes

played a role in the development of human cancers, particularly those of HNPCC. Microsatellites are dispersed throughout the human genome; there are stable stretches of DNA with repetitive sequence that do not encode proteins. Their function is unknown, but they are useful in genetic linkage studies because of their high degree of polymorphism. Approximately 15–17% of sporadic colorectal cancers show microsatellite instability, i.e., the length of the microsatellites varies between tumor DNA and nontumor DNA from the same patient. In contrast, most cancers from HNPCC patients show microsatellite instability. The high frequency of microsatellite instability in HNPCC-related cancer pointed the way to the discovery that the HNPCC genes are human homologs of DNA mismatch repair genes of yeast and bacteria. Patients with HNPCC inherit a mutation in one of the genes responsible for the repair of DNA mismatch errors. Four such genes have been implicated in HNPCC: hMSH2 on chromosome 2p22-21; the mutL homolog (hMLH1) on chromosome 3p21, and two other mutL homologs (Table I).

How does a germline mutation of a DNA mismatch repair gene cause the colorectal and extracolonic cancers of HNPCC? The working hypothesis is that mismatch repair genes function like tumor suppressor genes, so that heterozygous cells have normal or nearly normal repair activity, but somatic loss or mutation of the wild-type allele results in cells with defective mismatch repair.

Cells deficient in DNA repair accumulate large numbers of mutations. Yeast with defective mismatch repair may have 700 times as many mutations as repair-proficient yeast, and the frequency of mutations in human cells may be increased 1000-fold. Studies with mice bred for homozygosity of a mutated

TABLE I
Genes Mutated in HNPCC

Gene	Chromosome	Approximate contribution to HNPCC (%)
hMSH2	2p21-22	30
hMLH1	3p21	30
hPMS1	2q31-33	<5
hPMS2	7p22	<5

mismatch repair gene (MSH2) offer evidence that defective mismatch repair is sufficient to produce malignancy; the MSH2-deficient mice develop malignant lymphoma beginning at 2 months of age. The lymphomas have microsatellite instability, thus establishing a link between MSH2 deficiency and malignancy. What are the crucial mutations that must be acquired and how do they encourage malignant transformation? It appears that cancers with microsatellite instability accumulate mutations in the same critical oncogenes and tumor suppressor genes (K-ras, p53) that sporadic cancers do. One potentially exciting difference is the finding that 90% of colorectal cancers with microsatellite instability have mutations of the TGF-β type II receptor gene. The specificity of this mutation for cells with defective mismatch repair may be due to the fact that the gene has a sequence of 10 consecutive A bases—the sort of structure particularly prone to mismatch errors. Because TGF-β inhibits the growth of colon epithelial cells, inactivation of the receptor may prevent growth inhibition.

Microsatellite instability is not limited to colon cancer. It is seen in 17% of sporadic endometrial carcinomas and in 75% of endometrial carcinoma from HNPCC kindreds. The prevalence of microsatellite instability in sporadic gastric carcinomas has ranged from 15 to 39%. Pancreatic carcinoma had a high prevalence of instability in one small study (6 of 9). The phenomenon was not seen in early surveys of tumors of the lung, breast, and testis, suggesting that tumors which are not part of the HNPCC syndrome had low rates of microsatellite instability. Later studies, however, reported instability in 65% of prostate cancers, 20% of breast cancers, and 45% of small cell lung cancers.

It appears that the presence of microsatellite instability does not necessarily imply mutations in the known mismatch repair genes. When sporadic endometrial carcinomas with numerous microsatellite alterations were analyzed for mutations in DNA mismatch repair genes, somatic mutations in hMSH2 were found in only two of the tumors. In addition, microsatellite instability without germline mutations in mismatch repair genes has been described in benign conditions known to be at risk for malignancy, such as ulcerative colitis and chronic pancreatitis. The significance of these findings is unknown.

V. CARCINOMA IN INFLAMMATORY BOWEL DISEASE

Inflammatory bowel disease (IBD) (ulcerative colitis and Crohn's disease) predisposes to the development of colorectal carcinoma. For ulcerative colitis, the risk is highest in patients with long-standing pancolitis. There is some debate about the magnitude of risk, but it is estimated to be six to eight times that of the general population, rising to 15–19 times for those with pancolitis of 25 to 30 years duration. The risk that carcinoma will complicate Crohn's disease is less well quantified, but it is certainly greater than for individuals without IBD.

As with sporadic colorectal cancer, the development of an IBD-associated carcinoma involves a multistep genetic process paralleled histologically by a dysplasia–carcinoma sequence. There are similarities in the molecular alterations associated with tumor development; allelic loss of p53, for example, is a common finding in both types of cancer, and the frequency of p53 allelic loss in ulcerative colitis increases with increasing degrees of dysplasia, just as it becomes more common in the later stages of adenoma.

Some important differences between the two conditions have been detected. Abnormalities of p53 generally occur at an earlier stage in the development of IBD-associated cancer; conversely, mutations of K-ras are distinctly infrequent in this setting, at least in some studies. When dysplasia develops, it often involves large fields rather than forming discrete masses (adenomas). There may be more than one abnormal field, each populated by its own clone of genetically deranged cells. Molecular abnormalities have been found in mucosa that is negative for dysplasia by histologic criteria. The most frequent change in such cells is abnormal DNA content (DNA aneuploidy), but p53 allelic loss is occasionally seen in nondysplastic mucosa.

VI. MULTISTEP MODEL REVISITED: NEW INSIGHTS, NEW COMPLEXITIES

A fully developed colon cancer probably has changes in about 1000 cellular genes, and the genetic alterations in precursor lesions are probably no less complex. Any effort to make colon carcinogenesis comprehensible by reducing it to a model will necessarily be a simplification, but if it provides a framework for further investigation, then it has been successful. The multistep model of Fearon and Vogelstein has served well in this regard.

The discovery that mutations in DNA mismatch repair genes form the basis for HNPCC and for a subset of sporadic colorectal carcinoma helps resolve a problem for the multistep model: How does a cell acquire the multiple mutations necessary for malignant transformation during its relatively short life span since the spontaneous mutation rate is insufficient to account for the large number of mutations found in colon cancer? Even before the discovery of defective mismatch repair in humans, it had been proposed that one solution would be a mutation conferring hypermutability on affected cells. HNPCC cancers and other malignancies with microsatellite instability exemplify this "mutator phenotype." The detection of microsatellite instability in certain chronic inflammatory conditions suggests that DNA repair mechanisms can also be subverted with altering the genes themselves.

In contrast to the simple linear construct of the multistep model, evidence of variability in the adenoma–carcinoma sequence suggests that there may be multiple pathways to malignancy. The flat adenoma has a different mutational profile than most polypoid adenomas, and adenomas in other settings (e.g., HNPCC) pursue a more "aggressive" course. In addition, small carcinomas without detectable residual adenoma, ("de novo" carcinoma) have a different mutational profile (less frequent allelic loss of chromosomes 5q, 18q, and 17p) than carcinomas associated with adenoma. Figure 5 illustrates some possible pathways from normal mucosa to colorectal cancer.

The multistep model may understate the extent to which colon cancer is a heterogeneous disease. One example of this heterogeneity is the difference between cancer of the proximal colon and cancer of the distal colon. Proximal cancers tend to occur in more elderly individuals and to affect women more often than men. Microsatellite instability, seen in 10–15% of sporadic cancers, is much more common in proximal cancers. Allelic deletions are more frequent in distal cancers, and tumor DNA is more often aneuploid, whereas proximal tumors tend to have diploid DNA content.

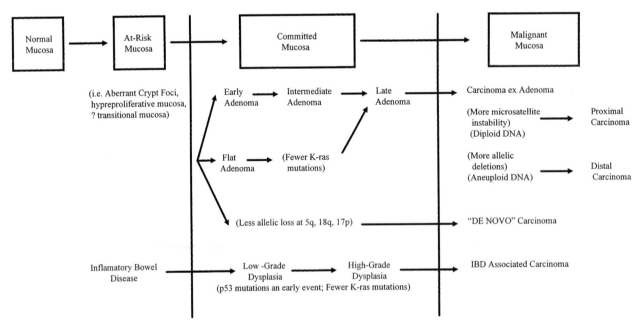

FIGURE 5   Colon cancer is a heterogeneous disease, and the lesions that precede it may be heterogeneous as well. Some possible pathways to malignancy within the overall framework of the multistep model are shown.

VII. SUMMARY

The multistep model of colon carcinogenesis has provided the framework to advance our understanding of the molecular basis of colon cancer. There is an ever-expanding list of genes that are candidates for inclusion in the process, some occurring early and some late. One challenge for the future will be to identify the key mutations and learn ways to prevent them, or ameliorate their effect.

The discovery of the molecular basis of HNPCC is exciting, not just because it promises the ability to identify gene carriers before malignant disease develops, but because it suggests a mechanism for cells to acquire multiple mutations. Cells that acquire mutations in mismatch repair genes possess the "mutator phenotype" that may be necessary to negotiate a multistep process of carcinogenesis.

The genetics of FAP has provided examples of correlation between genotype and phenotype. It may be that genotype–phenotype correlations can be extended to the sporadic setting, giving us some understanding of the molecular basis for the clinical heterogeneity of colon cancer.

See Also the Following Article

ANIMAL MODELS FOR COLON CANCER CHEMOPREVENTION • APC • BLADDER CANCER: EPIDEMIOLOGY • CAMPTOTHECINS • COLORECTAL CANCER: EPIDEMIOLOGY AND TREATMENT • GASTRIC CANCER: INHERITED PREDISPOSITION • HEREDITARY COLON CANCER AND DNA MISMATCH REPAIR • MULTISTAGE CARCINOGENESIS

Bibliography

Chung, D. C., and Rustgi, A. K. (1995). DNA mismatch repair and cancer. *Gastroenterology* **109,** 1685–1699.

Cunningham, C., and Dunlop, M. G. (1996). Molecular genetic basis of colorectal cancer susceptibility. *Br. J. Surg.* **83,** 321–329.

Fearon, E. B., and Vogelstein, B. (1990). A genetic model for colorectal tumorigenesis. *Cell* **61,** 759–767.

Lynch, H. T., Smyrk, T. C., Watson, P., Lanspa, S. J., Lynch, J. F., Lynch, P. M., Cavalieri, R. J., and Boland, C. R. (1993). Genetics, natural history, tumor spectrum, and pathology of hereditary nonpolyposis colorectal cancer: An updated review. *Gastroenterology* **104,** 1535–1549.

Rhyu, M. S. (1996). Molecular mechanisms underlying hereditary nonpolyposis colorectal carcinoma. *J. Natl. Cancer Inst.* **88,** 240–251.

Corticosteroids

Andrew D. Wallace
John A. Cidlowski

National Institute of Environmental Health Sciences
Research Triangle Park, North Carolina

GLOSSARY

apoptosis or programmed cell death An active genetically controlled process that normally removes unwanted or damaged cells characterized by internucleosomal DNA cleavage, caspase protease activation, blebbing of the plasma membrane, and loss of mitochondrial function.

corticosteroids A group of hormones, including cortisol and aldosterone, produced by the adrenal gland that includes a series of synthetic products—prednisone, prednisolone, methylprednisolone, and dexamethasone—used in the treatment of lymphocytic leukemias, lymphomas, and myeloma. Glucocorticoids effect metabolism and have both anti-inflammatory and immunosuppressive effects.

DNA regulatory element A specific sequence of DNA, such as a hormone responsive element, that is recognized by nuclear receptors that bind and effect transcription of mRNA of the target gene to elicit a biological response.

glucocorticoid receptor A glucocorticoid hormone-dependent transcription factor that resides in the cytoplasm. Upon glucocorticoid binding the receptor is activated to enter the nucleus where it can bind to specific DNA elements or interact with other transcription factors to activate or repress the transcription of target genes.

Corticosteroids are a class of steroid hormones produced by the cortex of the adrenal gland that primarily includes glucocorticoids and mineralocorticoids. In the treatment of cancer the corticosteroids that are mainly utilized include the synthetic forms of glucocorticoids. Glucocorticoids have been utilized in cancer treatments since the 1940s and are some of the most effective treatments for targeting cells of the immune system in leukemic and lymphoid malignancies. Therapeutic effects are due to their ability to bind and activate a type of nuclear hormone receptor known as the glucocorticoid receptor (GR). Hormone-bound activated receptors act as transcription factors in the nucleus of cells, causing selective increases and decreases in the expression of target genes. Therapeutically, potent glucocorticoids can act to inhibit cancer cell growth or, in some cases, kill cancer cells by a process of apoptosis or programmed cell death. Glucocorticoids are also included in cancer treatments in combination with chemotherapeutic drugs for their antiemetic effects, anti-inflammatory effects, and many other beneficial effects. This article discusses the clinical use of glucocorticoids to activate the corticosteroid signaling pathway in cancer treatment. Topics covered include the types of glucocorticoids, mechanism of action, and the types of cancer treated.

I. INTRODUCTION

Corticosteroids are steroid hormones produced by the adrenal cortex and include glucocorticoids and mineralocorticoids. Cholesterol is the precursor of these lipophilic hormones with cortisol (hydrocortisone) and aldosterone being the most prominently secreted in humans. Aldosterone functions to maintain levels of electrolytes by causing the retention of sodium and excretion of potassium in the kidney. In the treatment of cancer, glucocorticoids are the most important corticosteroids. The major glucocorticoid in humans is cortisol, which is secreted in a diurnal rhythm and after stress. Cortisol has effects upon virtually every organ and tissue in the body at the circulating levels of approximately 10^{-8}–10^{-7} M free cortisol. Continued production of cortisol is essential for life, and secretion is under the control of a negative feedback mechanism involving the hypothalamic–pituitary–adrenal axis.

The general effects of high levels of glucocorticoids on most tissue types are catabolic, and glucocorticoids received their name for their ability to inhibit glucose uptake in many tissue types. In muscle, skin, lymphoid, connective, and adipose tissue, effects include decreased synthesis and increased degradation of protein and RNA. In contrast, under normal physiological conditions, glucocorticoid actions are anabolic in the liver, causing activation of the gluconeogenesis pathways and storage of glycogen. A major physiological role proposed for circulating levels of glucocorticoids is as an endogenous anti-inflammatory agent that acts to appropriately limit the extent of immunological defense mechanisms from overshooting and damaging the organism. With the development of synthetic forms of glucocorticoids in the 1950s it became apparent that neoplastic cells of the immune system are exquisitely sensitive to glucocorticoids. These agents not only inhibit the proliferation of these neoplasms, but are also very cytotoxic, causing the cells to die by a process known as apoptosis or programmed cell death.

II. THE CORTICOSTEROID SIGNAL TRANSDUCTION PATHWAY

A. Natural and Synthetic Corticosteroids

Under normal physiological conditions, the adrenal cortex secretes cortisol under the control of the pituitary-produced adrenocorticotropic hormone (ACTH). Cortisol has weak mineralocorticoid actions, which limits its therapeutic value. In the 1950s, glucocorticoid analogs were synthesized that had enhanced glucocorticoid action and reduced mineralocorticoid action. Synthetic glucocorticoids that are widely used have differing glucocorticoid potency and differing durations of actions. Short-acting and low potency forms include cortisone and cortisol, whereas intermediate-acting forms include prednisone, prednisolone, and methylprednisolone (Table I). Dexamethasone is a long-acting glucocorticoid that is widely prescribed. Dexamethasone as one of the first synthesized corticosteroids in the 1950s, having 30 times the glucocorticoid activity of cortisol, little to no mineralocorticoid activity, and a much longer half-life than cortisol. Unfortunately, therapeutically relevant levels of glucocorticoids cause a number of side effects when administered for extended durations or at high doses. These include a susceptibility to infection, growth retardation in children, osteoporosis, dementia, gastrointestinal bleeding, myopathy, and hyperglycemia.

B. Molecular Mechanism of Corticosteroid Action, the Glucocorticoid Receptor

The therapeutic benefits of corticosteroid administration are due to its ability to (1) enhance the transcription of a number of primary target genes and

TABLE I
Glucocorticoid Potencies and Duration of Action[a]

Duration of action	Glucocorticoid potency	Equivalent dose	Mineralocorticoid activity
Short acting			
Cortisol	1	20	Yes
Cortisone	0.8	25	Yes
Immediate acting			
Methylprednisolone	4	4	No
Prednisone	4	5	No
Prednisolone	4	5	No
Triamcinolone	5	4	No
Long acting			
Betamethasone	25	0.60	No
Dexamethasone	30	0.75	No

[a]Short acting indicates 8–12 h, intermediate acting indicates 12–36 h, and long acting indicates 36–72 h for the biological half-life of the hormone. Adapted with permission from Alexrod, L. (1990). Corticosteroid therapy. *In* "Principles and Practice of Endocrinology and Metabolism" (K. L. Becker, ed.), p. 614. Lippincott, Philadelphia, PA.

(2) repress the transcription of numerous target genes by interfering with the function of other transcription factors, such as nuclear factor (NF)-κB or activator protein-1 (AP-1) (Fig. 1). These changes in gene expression are responsible for most known glucocorticoid actions, including therapeutic benefits, normal physiologic responses, and unfortunately toxic side effects. Glucocorticoid actions are dependent on high-affinity hormone binding to the cytoplasmic glucocorticoid receptor.

The glucocorticoid receptor is a member of a highly conserved family of nuclear hormone receptors that includes receptors for mineralocorticoids, estrogens, progestins, androgens, thyroid, retinoid, and many others, including a growing number of orphan receptors for which specific ligands have not yet been identified. Like the other members of the nuclear receptor superfamily, the glucocorticoid receptor can be divided into modular domains. The N-terminal region contains a transactivating domain termed tau 1 (τ1), which may interact with the basal transcriptional machinery. The central portion of the protein contains two zinc finger DNA-binding domains that are also important in dimerization and nuclear translocation. The C-terminal portion of the protein contains the ligand-binding domain and also has functions in dimerization and transactivation (τ2). Two forms of GR in humans, known as α and β, exist due to alternative mRNA splicing. The GR α form is expressed in most tissues and is the form that binds ligand-causing changes in gene expression. The GR β lacks 50 amino acids found in the C-terminal of the GR α form and contains a novel stretch of 15 amino acids. GRβ does not bind to hormone, resides in the nucleus, and seems to antagonize GR α functions. Hereafter, GR will refer to the GR α form. Ligand-bound GR enters the nucleus where it can interact with other transcription factors and/or bind to hormone response elements (HREs) with a DNA sequence similar to G/C/T G/T T/C/G A/T C A/C N N N T G T T/C C T. Once bound to DNA the GR interacts with other transcription factors, the basal transcriptional machinery, and a growing number of coactivators.

A number of genes coding for specific proteins have been described that are either positively or negatively regulated by glucocorticoids. Positive gene regulation occurs due to GR binding to glucocorticoid responsive element (GREs), causing an increase in the amount RNA transcript of the target gene. Alternatively, GR can bind to DNA sequences known as negative glucocorticoid responsive element (nGREs). More commonly, glucocorticoids negatively regulate the transcription of a number of target genes by GR interacting with other transcription factors. Hormone-activated GR can interfere with the functions of important transcription factors involved in inflammatory responses and tumor growth. Examples include NF-κB and the c-fos and c-jun components

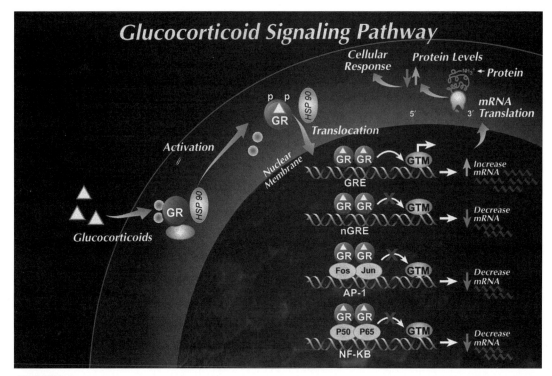

FIGURE 1 The glucocorticoid signaling pathway. Circulating glucocorticoids enter the cell passively and activate cytoplasmic GR by binding. The activated GR then translocates to the nucleus where it interacts with specific DNA elements and/or other transcription factors causing increases or decreases in the transcription of target gene mRNA. Regulated mRNAs are translated into protein, which mediate the cellular response to hormone, GR, glucocorticoid receptor; GRE, glucocorticoid responsive element; nGRE, negative glucocorticoid responsive element; HSP, heat shock protein; GTM, general transcriptional machinery; AP-1, activating protein-1 responsive element; NF-κB, NF-κB responsive element.

of AP-1. Glucocorticoids also have secondary effects on a number of genes where secondary transcription depends on RNA and protein synthesis of a *trans*-acting factor(s).

The glucocorticoid receptor is expressed in most tissue types, but the levels can be quite different. In any glucocorticoid therapeutic regime it is important to realize that the glucocorticoid responsiveness of any specific cell type can be correlated with the ability of the cell to bind hormone, and the sensitivity of cells to glucocorticoids has been shown to be dependent on the number of glucocorticoid receptors found within the cell. Following glucocorticoid treatment in most cell types, GR mRNA and protein levels decrease dramatically in a process known as homologous downregulation. The clinical significance of glucocorticoid receptor protein downregulation is evident when considering that without downregulation there exists the potential for overstimulation when circulating levels of hormone are high. Conversely, the ef-

fects of long-term glucocorticoid treatment could lead to GR downregulation, leaving cells unresponsive to hormone treatment.

C. Apoptosis of Immune Cells

The ability of glucocorticoids to affect cancer cells was discovered in the 1940s in rodent studies that demonstrated tumor regression after glucocorticoid administration. These studies led to the treatment of patients with lymphomas and leukemias with adrenocorticotropic hormone (ACTH) or cortisone, a precursor of the active form of the hormone, which resulted in tumor regression. Glucocorticoids have been extensively studied for their ability to cause tumor regression, which has been documented to be due to tumor cells dying. Tumor growth can occur when the balance between cell proliferation and normal cell death is altered. Cancers associated with immune cell proliferation were found to be exquisitely sensitive to glucocorticoids, which induce a type of controlled cell death known as programmed cell death or apoptosis. Apoptosis is thought of as a cell suicide program that causes the cell to self-destruct.

Cells typically die by either of two processes known as necrosis or apoptosis. Necrosis is a pathological process characterized by cellular swelling, rapid decreases in cellular energy levels, and rapid degradation of cellular protein, RNA, and DNA. Cellular membranes quickly rupture, causing the spillage of cellular contents with deleterious effects on surrounding cells, resulting in damage to surrounding tissues and an inflammatory response. In contrast, apoptosis is a normal physiological process that occurs in embryogenesis, differentiation, metamorphosis, and normal tissue turnover without harmful effects to surrounding cells and no inflammatory response. Disruption of the normal process of apoptosis has been linked to cancer formation, autoimmune diseases, and neurodegenerative diseases. Characteristics of cell death

by glucocorticoid-induced apoptosis that are readily observed include loss of cell volume by loss of water and ions, plasma membrane blebbing of apoptotic bodies containing intracellular components, and nuclear condensation (Fig. 2). A hallmark of apoptosis is that cellular DNA is degraded in an enzymatic manner that cleaves chromatin at the internucleosomal regions, creating a laddering of DNA. Other changes within the cell include loss of mitochondrial membrane potential, activation of specific cellular proteases known as caspases, and degradation of RNA and protein. After the cell dies, cellular components are phagocytosized by surrounding cells or macrophages without loss of tissue architecture.

The survival of cells or tissues is often dependent on the presence or absence of very specific regulatory factors. Alterations in the levels of specific mediators such as growth factors or hormones can trigger sensitive cells to undergo apoptosis. The classic model used to study glucocorticoid-induced apoptosis are

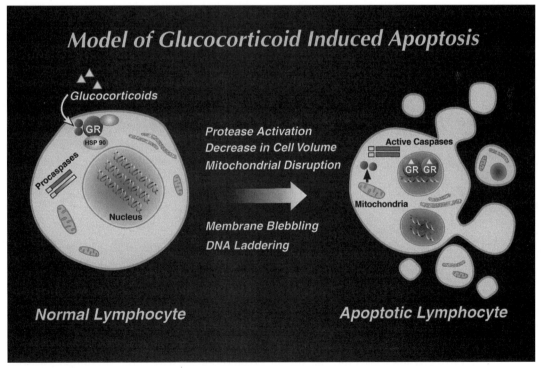

FIGURE 2 A model of glucocorticoid-induced apoptosis of lymphocytes. Glucocorticoids enter the cell and activate the cytoplasmic glucocorticoid receptor (GR), which translocates to the nucleus. *De novo* transcription and translation are necessary for the glucocorticoid induction of apoptosis. Hallmarks of lymphocyte apoptosis include a rapid loss of cell volume, proteases of the caspase family are activated, membrane blebbing or release of apoptotic bodies, mitochondrial disruption and release of proapoptotic proteins, and nuclease digestion of chromatin resulting in DNA laddering.

cells of the thymus gland, with immature thymocytes being sensitive to physiological levels of glucocorticoids. Cancer cells arising from the immune system are often extremely sensitive to glucocorticoids and are associated with a number of cancers, including acute lymphoblastic leukemia, chronic lymphocytic leukemia, acute myeloid leukemia, and multiple myeloma. Specific cell types of the hematopoietic lineage associated with these cancers have been identified that undergo apoptosis due to glucocorticoids include cortical and medullary thymus cells, mature Th cells, natural killer cells, cytotoxic T lymphocytes, and immature B cells. The mechanism(s) of glucocorticoid induction of apoptosis has been under investigation for many years in experimental models, such as mouse or rat thymocytes, and is known to be dependent on *de novo* RNA and protein synthesis following hormone treatment. The ability of glucocorticoids to induce apoptosis or programmed cell death in T lymphocytes has been proposed to be due to the induction of lysis genes or the repression of survival genes. However, researchers have failed to identify the critical induced lysis genes or repressed survival genes. Overall, there has been an inability to identify the specific mediators of the glucocorticoid-related apoptotic response in sensitive cells.

III. USE OF CORTICOSTEROIDS IN CANCER TREATMENT

Corticosteroids are widely used in the treatment of cancer. Therapeutic doses have been shown quite successful in treating cancers of lymphoid origin such as leukemia or lymphoma. In lymphoblastic leukemia there is an excessive accumulation of immature cells of the bone or blood. Glucocorticoids are exquisitely cytotoxic to these cell types, causing cells to die by the process known as programmed cell death or apoptosis. Solid tumor lymphomas are also responsive to glucocorticoids, and treatment leads to inhibition of cell growth and/or shrinkage of the tumor mass by cells undergoing apoptosis. Glucocorticoids are not often given by themselves, yet are included in chemotherapeutic regimes not only for their ability to induce apoptosis, but also for their antiemetic effects, anti-inflammatory actions, and pain management.

A. Leukemias

Glucocorticosteroids have been utilized in the treatments of acute lymphocytic leukemia (ALL) since the 1950s. ALL is characterized by the rapid proliferation of immature immune cells mainly of the B-cell lineage, but a T-cell lineage form also occurs. Extensive literature supports the efficacy of dexamethasone or prednisone as single agents or included in combination with other drugs. These glucocorticoids lead to a rapid decrease in malignant lymphoblasts by the process of apoptosis or programmed cell death. In cases of childhood ALL, single-agent glucocorticoid treatment results in high remission rates. When freshly isolated cells from the blood or bone marrow of children with ALL are treated with glucocorticoids *in vitro,* the cells die rapidly by apoptosis. More commonly, glucocorticoids are used in combination with antimitotic chemotherapeutic agents such as the vinca alkaloid vincristine.

Glucocorticoids are included in the chemotherapeutic treatment of chronic lymphoblastic leukemias, which are a slower progressing cancer typically of the immature B-cell lineage. Glucocorticoids have been shown to induce apoptosis of immature B cells found in this cancer type and display sensitivity similar to that of immature thymocytes. Cells of the B-cell lineage have been found to become resistant to glucocorticoids upon the chromosomal translocation of the protooncogenes B-cell leukemia/lymphoma-2 gene (Bcl-2) or c-myc. Glucocorticoids are also utilized, but less successfully, in the treatment of acute myeloid leukemia and chronic myeloid leukemia in combination therapies.

B. Lymphomas and Multiple Myeloma

Non-Hodgkin's lymphoma includes numerous cancers of lymphoid cells that develop in the lymphatic system. These include cells of the B and T lineage of varying differentiation, including B cell lymphoma, Burkitt's lymphoma, diffuse cell lymphoma, follicular lymphoma mantle cell lymphoma, posttransplantation lymphoproliferative disorder, and T-cell lymphoma. Glucocorticoids have been shown to produce an inhibitory response in tumor cell growth when used as single agents. For this reason, glucocorticoids are included in all chemotherapeutic regimes for non-Hodgkin's lymphomas. The success of chemotherapy depends on the stage and cell type of the cancer. Prednisone and dexamethasone are commonly used in most chemotherapeutic regimes for non-Hodgkin's lymphoma.

Hodgkin's lymphoma is a solid tumor cancer of the lymphatic system that is characterized by enlargement of the lymph nodes, spleen, or other lymphatic tissues. This uncommon cancer of the B-cell lineage often occurs in a single lymph node and spreads in an orderly fashion. It often arises in the lymph nodes in the neck, but can occur in any part of the body. Early in the disease state, it is highly curable when treated with radiotherapy and is often combined with chemotherapeutic treatments that include glucocorticoids. In later stages of Hodgkin's lymphoma progression, high doses of glucocorticoids are employed in combination with chemotherapy. Prednisone is most commonly utilized in these combination therapies.

Multiple myeloma is a neoplastic disease characterized by bone marrow infiltration by antibody-producing plasma cells of the immune system. Myeloma cells synthesize abnormal amount of immunoglobulins and tend to collect in the bone marrow or outer parts of bones where they can form tumor masses, causing bone pain and sometimes fractures. This is a malignancy of cells of the B lineage of varying maturity that have undergone antigenic selection. Studies have shown that treatment of multiple myeloma with the glucocorticoid dexamethasone as a single agent produces a sharp reduction in tumor mass that occurs by tumor cells undergoing apoptosis. More often glucocorticoids such as prednisone are included in combination chemotherapeutic treatments, with prednisone administered orally for 5 days a month for up to 6 months. Glucocorticoid resistance often arises after initial treatment and some mutations of the glucocorticoid receptor have been identified associated with resistance.

C. Other Uses: Antiemetic Action, Anti-inflammatory Action, and Pain Management

In most nonimmune cell malignancies, glucocorticoids may not actively inhibit tumor cell growth or kill cancer cells. Nevertheless, glucocorticoids are widely included in chemotherapeutic cancer treatments for their antiemetic effects, anti-inflammatory actions, ability to aid in pain management, and many other beneficial affects.

A major side effect of chemotherapeutic and radiation treatments for cancer is that they cause varying degrees of nausea and vomiting. Emesis, or vomiting, occurs soon after chemotherapeutic treatments and has a major impact on patient rehospitalization and quality of life. More and more interest has been focused on antiemetic therapies, but the underlying mechanisms of the physiology of emesis and nausea remain unknown. Glucocorticoids are commonly included in chemotherapeutic regimes for their ability to act as an antiemetic and are included with serotonin receptor antagonists as having the highest therapeutic index. Most commonly, dexamethasone or methylprednisolone is administered in single doses and with a high degree of success. Glucocorticoids have been used in combination with serotonin antagonists and have been found to be highly effective.

The ability of glucocorticoids to act as powerful anti-inflammatory agents is utilized after bone marrow transplantation in the treatment of leukemias and lymphomas. Glucocorticoids suppress the immune system, preventing graft-versus-host disease. In the 1940s, glucocorticoids were first reported to be effective drugs for rheumatoid arthritis and quickly were realized to be highly potent anti-inflammatory agents in the treatment of a wide variety of immune disorders. The major mechanism of glucocorticoid immunosuppression is thought to be able to due to their ability to inhibit the production of cytokines at transcriptional and posttranscriptional levels. Glucocorticoids downregulate a number of proinflammatory genes such as the interleukins, prostaglandin G/H synthase 2 (cyclooxygenase-2), inducible nitric oxide synthase (iNOS), tumor necrosis factor α (TNF-α), and interferon γ (IFN-γ). Due to the severe effects associated with long-term and high-dose treatment, glucocorticoids are often not administered until after other anti-inflammatory agents, such as nonsteroidal anti-inflammatory drugs, have been found ineffective. A major side effect of many other cancers and their treatments is activation of the immune system, resulting in severe side effects, necessitating the use of glucocorticoids.

Glucocorticoids have been used to lessen the symptoms of brain tumors and as treatments for brain tumors since the 1960s. Glucocorticoids reduce the immune response and edema around the tumor and lessen the adverse side affects of cranial irradiation and surgery of brain tumors. The decrease in edema may occur by reduction of blood flow by the anti-inflammatory actions of glucocorticoids. It should be noted that this might lessen the amount of drug that gets to the brain tumor in chemotherapeutic treatments. Some reports indicate that glucocorticoids are sometimes cytotoxic to certain brain tumor types. Dexamethasone and prednisolone are the most commonly prescribed glucocorticoid and are highly effective after several days of treatment.

In terminal patients, where concerns of long-term administration are not pertinent, glucocorticoids are commonly administered to alleviate symptoms of cancer. The ability of glucocorticoids, such as prednisone and dexamethasone, to alleviate symptoms is due to their ability to reduce tumor size in some cases, as well as lessen inflammation and edema. Treatment with glucocorticoids generally results in an increase in the patient's appetite, activity, and improved mood. Often with terminal cancer, patients' tumor metastasis can cause severe pain. Glucocorticoids are used to alleviate pain due to spinal cord tumors and bone metastases. Similarly, the growth of cancers may cause obstructions, which affect other organs, and glucocorticoids are utilized to treat tumors of the lung, thyroid, liver metastases, masses in pelvis, large bowel, and many others.

D. Glucocorticoid Resistance

Unfortunately, no discussion of the use of glucocorticoids in cancer treatment would be complete without mention of the development of glucocorticoid resistance seen after initial treatments. Resistance is a major limiting factor in the glucocorticoid therapy of lymphoid cancers and the mechanism(s) by which it occurs remains unclear. After initial treatment with glucocorticoids, there is a substantial decrease in tumor size and patients often go into remission. Subsequently, these patients relapse and the response of a

second glucocorticoid treatment is greatly reduced. Glucocorticoid resistance has been studied for many years using both human and rodent *in vitro* cell culture models. In these models, it has been demonstrated that resistance can be due to a decrease in glucocorticoid receptor levels, decreased receptor binding to hormone, lack of response downstream of the glucocorticoid receptor, or to a loss of receptor function by mutation of the receptor. Mutations of the glucocorticoid receptor gene or in the GR-coding region itself have also been shown to cause production of a defective receptor.

In vivo studies in humans have demonstrated higher levels of glucocorticoid receptors are associated with greater cancer remission rates. Studies of resistance have also identified genetic mutations of GR which lead to a defective receptor. More recently, a few reports indicated that elevated levels of the dominant-negative glucocorticoid receptor β isoform were seen in resistant patients with varying malignancies of the immune system. The mechanisms at work in human glucocorticoid resistance remain poorly understood, but the loss of glucocorticoid receptor function seems to be central and is thought to block the signaling pathway of glucocorticoid-induced apoptosis.

IV. SUMMARY AND CONCLUSIONS

Glucocorticoids have been utilized in cancer treatments since the early 1950s. They remain one of the most successful drugs for treatment of a number of cancers arising from the immune system, such as leukemias and lymphomas. The use of glucocorticoids in the treatment of a number of lymphomas and leukemia is due to the ability of these hormones to selectively inhibit tumor cell growth and/or kill tumor cells by the process of apoptosis or programmed cell death. Our understanding of the glucocorticoid signal transduction pathway and the importance of the glucocorticoid receptor have dramatically increased over the years, but the causes of glucocorticoid-induced apoptosis and the susceptibility of malignant lymphocytes remain unknown. Glucocorticoids continue to be widely used in the treatment of many other cancers for the ability to alleviate the side effects of cancer tumor formation as well as their ability to lessen the effects of cancer therapies. Glucocorticoids remain as some of the most successful drugs for the treatment of emesis and nausea associated with chemotherapeutic regimes. As potent anti-inflammatory agents, glucocorticoids are extensively utilized to alleviate many of the symptoms of cancer and its treatment. It is the long-term hope that a greater understanding of the mechanisms of glucocorticoid action will aid in the development of better drugs and improved therapeutic regimes in the treatment of cancer patients.

See Also the Following Articles

ACUTE LYMPHOBLASTIC LEUKEMIA • BRAIN TUMORS • CHRONIC LYMPHOCYTIC LEUKEMIA • HORMONAL CARCINOGENESIS • HORMONE RESISTANCE IN PROSTATE CANCER • NON-HODGKIN'S LYMPHOMA AND MULTIPLE MYELOMA • STEROID HORMONES AND HORMONE RECEPTORS

Bibliography

Ashwell, J. D., Vacchio, M. S., and Galon, J. (2000). Do glucocorticoids participate in thymocyte development? *Immunol Today* **21**(12), 644–646.

Barnes, P. J. (1998). Anti-inflammatory actions of glucocorticoids: Molecular mechanisms. *Clin. Sci. (Colch.)* **94**(6), 557–572.

Distelhorst, C. W. (1996). Basic and clinical studies of glucocorticosteroid receptors in lymphoid malignancies. *In* "Hormones and Cancer" (W. V. Vedeckis, ed.), p. 495. Birkhauser, Boston, MA.

Fauser, A. A., Fellhauer, M., Hoffmann, M., Link, H., Schlimok, G., and Gralla, R. J. (1999). Guidelines for anti-emetic therapy: Acute emesis. *Eur. J. Cancer* **35**(3), 361–370.

Gaynon, P. S., and Carrel, A. L. (1999). Glucocorticosteroid therapy in childhood acute lymphoblastic leukemia. *Adv. Exp. Med. Biol.* **457**, 593–605.

Gralla, R. J., Osoba, D., Kris, M. G., Kirkbride, P., Hesketh, P. J., Chinnery, L. W., Clark-Snow, R., Gill, D. P., Groshen, S., Grunberg, S., Koeller, J. M., Morrow, G. R., Perez, E. A., Silber, J. H., and Pfister, D. G. (1999). Recommendations for the use of antiemetics: Evidence-based, clinical practice guidelines. *J. Clin. Oncol.* **17**(9), 2971–2994.

McKay, L. I., and Cidlowski, J. A. (2000). Corticosteroids. *In* "Cancer Medicine" (R. C. Blast, D. W. Kufe, R. E. Pollock, R. R. Weichselbaum, J. F. Holland, and E. Frei, eds.), p. 730. Decker, Hamilton, Ontario, Canada.

Mihal, V., Hajduch, M., Noskova, V., Feketova, G., Jess, K., Gojova, L., Kasparek, I., Stary, J., Blazek, B., Pospisilova, D., and Novak, Z. (1999). Differential antileukemic activity of prednisolone and dexamethasone in freshly isolated leukemic cells. *Adv. Exp. Med. Biol.* **457**, 461–471.

Montague, J. W., and Cidlowski, J. A. (1996). Glucocorticoid actions on normal and neoplastic lymphocytes: Activation of apoptosis. *In* "Hormones and Cancer" (W. V. Vedeckis, ed.), p. 517. Birkhauser, Boston, MA.

Newton, R. (2000). Molecular mechanisms of glucocorticoid action: What is important? *Thorax* **55**(7), 603–613.

Schuler, D., and Szende, B. (1997). Apoptosis and acute lymphocytic leukemia in children. *Ann. N. Y. Acad. Sci.* **824**, 28–37.

Smets, L. A., Salomons, G., and van den Berg, J. (1999). Glucocorticoid induced apoptosis in leukemia. *Adv. Exp. Med. Biol.* **457**, 607–614.

Twycross, R. (1994). The risks and benefits of corticosteroids in advanced cancer. *Drug Saf.* **11**(3), 163–178.

Zoorob, R. J., and Cender, D. (1998). A different look at corticosteroids. *Am. Fam. Phys.* **58**(2), 443–450.

Cytokine Gene Therapy

Siamak Agha-Mohammadi
Michael T. Lotze
University of Pittsburgh Medical Center

GLOSSARY

allogenic Derived from another organism which is genetically dissimilar.

antigen-presenting cell A cell that carries on its surface antigen bound to major histocompatability complex class I or class II molecules and presents the antigen in this context to T lymphocytes. They include macrophages, endothelium, dendritic cells, and Langerhans cells of the skin.

autologous Derived from the same organism.

colony-stimulating factor A group of cytokines that induce the maturation and proliferation of white blood cells from the primitive cell types present in bone marrow such as the leukocyte, macrophage, and monocyte lines.

cytokines A group of proteins that are secreted by inflammatory leukocytes and some nonleukocytic cells. They act as intercellular mediators and play an important role in eliciting immune responses. They generally act locally in a paracrine or autocrine manner.

gene therapy Treatment of a disease caused by malfunction of a gene through delivery of a normal copy of the gene into cells of the organism.

interferons A group of cytokines that are secreted by vertebrate cells in response to a wide variety of inducers. They confer resistance against many different viruses, impede multiplication of intracellular parasites, inhibit proliferation of normal and malignant cells, and enhance macrophage, granulocyte, and natural killer cell activity.

interleukins A group of cytokines that affect functions of specific cell types. They are secreted as regulatory proteins produced by lymphocytes, monocytes, and various other cell types and are released by cells in response to antigenic and nonantigenic stimuli.

T lymphocytes A class of lymphocytes derived from the thymus and matured through thymic processing. They are primarily involved in controlling cell-mediated immune reactions and in the control of B-cell development. They also coordinate the immune system by secreting cytokines.

The fundamental basis of cancer immunotherapy relies on the ability of the immune system to identify and destroy tumor cells and to elicit a long-lasting memory of this interaction. In natural circumstances, however, the ability of tumor cells to trigger an effective immune response is limited. The nominal poor immunogenicity of tumor cells is a consequence of various cellular features, including (1) absent or decreased expression of major histocompatability complex (MHC) class I and/or class II antigens, (2) lack of expression of adhesion molecules or costimulatory signals required for complete T-cell activation, (3) local secretion of immunosuppressive molecules (IL-10, TGF-β, PGE$_2$) that impair the effector arm of the immune response, and (4) absence of appropriate local immunomodulatory cytokines. These immune response evasion strategies may be overcome by introducing immunomodulatory molecules/genes into the tumor milieu to increase the immunogenicity of tumor cells.

I. INTRODUCTION

The immediate goal of immunotherapy is to induce an effective antitumor reaction that primarily involves a cellular immune response (cytotoxic CD8$^+$ T and helper CD4$^+$ T lymphocytes). Indeed, it has been shown that rejection of transplanted tumors in murine models is primarily mediated by T cells. Moreover, the adoptive transfer of bulk populations of effector T cells derived from either tumor tissue or peripheral blood has been used to protect and even treat relevant tumor-bearing, syngeneic animals. These results demonstrated the importance of T cells in antitumor responses. To engage in an adaptive immune response, circulating naïve T cells must be induced to proliferate and differentiate into cells capable of responding to tumor cells. Naïve T cells are primed to specific antigens (Ags) by antigen-presenting cells (APCs), the most important of which are dendritic cells (DCs). This priming occurs in secondary lymphoid organs, where APCs migrate to present the Ag after it has been taken up at the tumor site and processed. Three different functional classes of effector T cells derive from this priming, leave the lymphoid organs, and reenter the bloodstream so that they can migrate to the tumor site. These are CD8 cytotoxic T cells that recognize Ags presented by MHC class I molecules on the cell surface, CD4 Th1 cells that activate macrophages and other resident cells at the site of inflammation, and CD4 Th2 cells, which activate specific B cells to produce antibodies. CD8 T cells mediate their killing through two predominant pathways, a membrane attack complex initiated with the formation of pores in target cell membranes by perforin, allowing delivery of apoptosis-inducing granzymes, and a nonsecretory one initiated by receptor-mediated triggering of apoptosis by factors such as the tumor necrosis factor (TNF), Fas ligand, and TNF-related apoptosis-inducing ligand. At the same time, immunologic memory is established with generation of memory cells that are long lived and will respond to Ags with an accelerated response.

The most promising approach to activate the cellular immune response has employed natural cytokines. Cytokines and chemokines regulate immune responses through maturation, activation, and migration of inflammatory cells. The identification of cytokines that modulate the immune response has led to an expanding research effort over the last two decades on the use of these proteins to stimulate antitumor immunity. Most work has been conducted in animals and results have been encouraging enough that several human trials have been initiated.

II. DIRECT INJECTION OF CYTOKINE TO BOOST IMMUNE RESPONSE

The concept that cytokines such as colony-stimulating factors, interferons, and interleukins can enhance immunogenicity and tumor regression has led to increasing interest in their study and clinical application. Clinical trials employing interferon or interleukin-2 have indicated that an objective antitumor response could be elicited by the systemic administration of exogenous cytokines. Of the cytokines originally screened, IL-2 appears to be the most active as an antineoplastic agent. Following administration of high doses of IL-2 to 283 consecutive patients between 1985 and 1992, a complete response was seen in 9% of patients with renal cell carcinoma and 7% of those with melanoma. Other studies have confirmed the observation that systemic and repeated administration of high doses of IL-2 can result in tumor regression. Systemic use of cytokines is, however, hampered by substantial toxicity, and their effectiveness is reduced by rapid degradation and elimination. To overcome these concerns, local delivery/expression of cytokines was proposed to mimic more closely the paracrine release of cytokines. Also, local expression is more likely to promote T-cell responses, to enhance tumor antigen presentation, or to activate nonspecific killing by natural killer (NK) cells, lymphokine-activated killer cells, and monocytes/macrophages. This notion was supported by observing rejection of tumors after repeated local administration of exogeneous cytokines. Forni and colleagues were the first to show that paracrine delivery rather than endocrine delivery of cytokines could induce immune-mediated tumoricidal responses. Repeated injections of IL-2 into an experimentally implanted tumor induced the intratumoral recruitment and activation of macrophages, neutrophils, lymphocytes, and NK cells, which resulted in rejection of the tumor. Furthermore, the local antitumor effect had systemic benefits, protecting against small doses of live tumor challenges. The precise site of paracrine delivery of cytokines also appeared to identify another important variable in the analysis of the effects of cytokines in eliciting antitumor immunity. Unlike IL-2, high doses of IL-4 and IL-1 induced greater antitumor immunity if injected in the draining lymph nodes rather than directly into the tumor. The pharmacology of paracrine delivery of cytokines around tumor cells was transformed into a gene therapy approach with the use of the tumor cells engineered to express cytokine genes. Since it appears that cytokines act through continuous secretion, injection of cytokine-engineered tumor cells whose proliferation results in both the provision of antigen and a continuous local

build-up of the cytokine is a more effective means of delivering the molecules to tumor milieu than repeated injections of the protein.

III. *EX VIVO* CYTOKINE GENE THERAPY

Introduction of cytokine genes directly into tumor cells by transfection or viral vectors, followed by inoculation of the genetically engineered cells into animal hosts, has been termed tumor–cytokine transplantation assay. This assay, which originally studied the role of IL-2 and IL-4, helped demonstrate that these cytokine-modified tumor vaccines are capable of reducing tumorigenicity of a cancer by stimulating localized inflammatory and/or immune responses. Other studies confirmed that the expression of IL-2 by weakly immunogenic tumor cells resulted in growth inhibition of the tumor mass. The inhibitory effect is dose dependent and the degree of suppression of growth correlated directly with the amount of IL-2 produced by the tumor cells. These original findings were extended to evaluate the role of other cytokines in immune system. Studies in various mouse and human tumor models have established that administration into syngeneic hosts of tumor cells engineered to secrete IL-1, IL-2, IL-4, IL-6, IL-7, IL-12, IL-18, TNF-α, G-CSF, GM-CSF (granulocyte–macrophage colony stimulating factor), or IFN-γ can lead to tumor rejection by stimulating both a specific and a nonspecific antitumor response. As most of these studies have shown, the *in vitro* growth of tumor cells is not affected by action of the transfected cytokine, suggesting that inhibition of tumor growth *in vivo* results from the stimulation of host immune effector cells by the activity of the secreted cytokine. Tumor rejection is dependent on a high level of cytokine production by the gene-modified cells and in part is due to stimulation of the host antitumor effector response. In some circumstances, the alteration of the immunological environment of the tumor allowed the complete rejection of the tumor inoculum and even protected the host against subsequent challenge with unmodified tumor cells. The tumor–cytokine transplantation assay also demonstrated the lack of activity of IL-5 in inducing antitumor killing. Among the most important features emphasized by all these studies is that the local sustained release of cytokines produces local inflammatory or immune-mediated effects without significant evidence of systemic toxicity. These cytokines have different mechanisms of action, and it is important to distinguish localized tumor killing and the desired generation of systemic T-cell-mediated antitumor immunity. This in turn allows for an effective antitumor response at a distal site.

The complexity of the action of cytokines and immune mechanisms and the features of individual tumors hamper analysis of the exact mechanisms of the induction of antitumor immunity, but it is likely that different cytokines selectively elicit recruitment of granulocytes, macrophages, DCs, NK, or T cells. Research over the last two decades has shown that T cells are the most potent effectors in the host antitumor response. Systemic antitumor immunity induced by cytokines has, for the most part, depended on $CD8^+$ or $CD4^+$ T cells or both. $CD8^+$ cytotoxic T lymphocytes characterized by specificity and memory appear most useful for human cancer therapy. T-cell-mediated tumor immunity is enhanced by several cytokines, including GM-CSF, IL-2, IL-6, IL-7, IL-12, and IL-18. However, cytokines can also stimulate nonspecific immune responses, which may be important for interaction of an effective adoptive immune response. The most common example of this is use of IL-2 to stimulate NK cells to become lymphokine-activated killer cells, which nonspecifically can lyse NK-resistant cell lines. Other cell types, such as eosinophils, have been shown to be important in IL-4- and IL-2 mediated tumor killing. Neutrophils play a role in the antitumor activity of G-CSF and macrophages in the antitumor activity of G-CSF, IL-2, INF-γ, TNF-α, IL-4, and IL-7. IL-4 has been shown to be more effective than IL-2, IL-18, and CSF or GM-CSF in increasing the influx of DCs into the tumor. Some cytokines may also have a direct action on the endothelium. In fact, INF-γ, INF-α, IL-1, and IL-4 have been shown to upregulate the expression of various adhesion molecules on endothelial cells. This action on endothelial cells could allow transmigration of specific inflammatory cells into tissue sites. It is still not clear from these models which cytokine is the most potent for generating antitumor responses,

and it is quite possible that different cytokines generate different types of responses against tumor types.

IV. CLINICAL TRIALS OF TUMOR VACCINES

Even though rejection of established disease was achieved only in some experimental systems, the promising results obtained in animal studies have established the basic biological value of gene therapy with cytokine-secreting cells and these approaches are increasingly used in clinical trials. Based on preclinical data, a number of phase I/II clinical trials using cytokine gene-modified cells have been initiated. Clinical vaccine trials can be divided into two general types depending on the cell type transfected, autologous tumor cells or allogenic tumor cell lines, with both having advantages and disadvantages. The use of autologous tumor cells require that the patient's tumor be surgically removed followed by the introduction of the gene *ex vivo*. Indisputably, this strategy has the advantage that the patient's own tumor cells have the greatest chance to vaccinate against the spectrum of relevant tumor antigens both shared and unique to the individual. However, isolation of primary autologous cells that stably express high levels of the therapeutic gene is cumbersome, often expensive, and labor-intensive. Also, this approach suffers from the considerable variation of individual batches of engineered cells, which complicates analysis of the biological effects observed in each patient. The use of allogenic vaccines avoids these two parameters by using a single standardized transduced cell line, but for this technique to be successful, it is critical that the transduced cells share antigens with the patient's tumor. Most studies use irradiated tumor cells over nonirradiated ones to prevent having the live vaccine tumor cells continue to multiply *in vivo*. Not only does the Ag dose increase, so does the introduced gene product in nonirradiated cells. Irradiation causes growth arrest, allowing a more accurate determination of the vaccine inoculum and better comparison of the relative efficacy between different transfectants.

Over 60% of recent clinical cytokine gene therapy trials use IL-2, whereas the others utilize IL-4, IL-7, IL-12, IFN-γ, GM-CSF, and TNF cytokines individually or in combination (Table I). The results gathered so far from the clinical trials are similar to those noted in murine models, confirming that even though the approach itself is safe, only about 10 to 20% of patients displayed an objective response.

V. LIMITATIONS OF *EX VIVO* CYTOKINE GENE THERAPY

Abrogation of the tumorgenicity of gene-transduced tumor cells and immunization of healthy animals against a challenge with tumor cells that they have not previously encountered do not demonstrate a true therapeutic effect. Also, the therapeutic efficacy of cytokine gene-transduced tumor cells is low. In most

TABLE I
Mechanism of Cytokine-Induced Antitumor Activity

Cytokine	Effector cells	Memory response	Effect on established tumor
GM-CSF	NK cells Macrophages Eosinophils CD8$^+$ T cells Neutrophils	Yes	+
TNF-α	CD4$^+$ and CD8$^+$ T cells Macrophages NK cells	Yes	+
IL-2	Neutrophils and NK cells CD4$^+$ and CD8$^+$ T cells Macrophages	Yes	+
IL-4	Macrophages Eosinophils CD8$^+$ T cells NK cells	Yes	+
IL-6	CD4$^+$ and CD8$^+$ T cells	Yes	+
IL-7	CD4$^+$ and CD8$^+$ T cells Macrophages NK cells	Yes	+/−
IL-12	CD4$^+$ and CD8$^+$ T cells NK cells Macrophages	Yes	+
IL-18	NK cells CD4$^+$ and CD8$^+$ T cells	Yes	+
INF-γ	CD8$^+$ T cells NK cells Macrophages		+

cases, only a minority of tumor-bearing mice were cured by administration of cytokine gene-transduced tumor cells. The limited efficacy of these vaccines was completely lost if they were not administered in the first few days after the implantation of tumor cells. In addition, therapeutic immunization has shown no consistent effect on the growth of established tumors beyond the period of concomitant immunity. The situation is slightly more encouraging in the case of micrometastases. A significant reduction in tumor metastasis has been documented with application of several cytokines. Once again, however, only a minority of the mice are cured.

VI. *IN VIVO* CYTOKINE GENE TRANSFER

Implantation into syngeneic hosts of mouse tumor cell lines only imperfectly mimics the biology of spontaneous human cancers. This and other related limitations of *ex vivo* gene therapy may be addressed by direct transduction of tumor cells *in vivo* by viral and nonviral vectors. Although this strategy appears attractive and simple, it requires extremely efficient gene transfer vectors that have limited immunogenicity and can transduce cells *in vivo*.

A few studies have demonstrated the effectiveness of directly transducing established tumors with cytokine genes using retrovial vectors. Retroviruses are an attractive *in vivo* vector, as they only transduce actively dividing cells and can be delivered by intravascular injections to target tumor cells, sparing adjacent normal parenchymal cells. Similarly, adenovirus-mediated *in vivo* transduction of tumors with cytokine genes has stimulated significant systemic antitumor responses. Delivery of IL-2, INF-γ, and GM-CSF genes via this vector is currently being examined in several clinical trials (Table II). The main disadvantages of this approach relate to the additive immune response elicited by the viral vector, as well as the variability of cytokine production upon *in vivo* transduction. Given the biosafety issues over injection of tumors with viral vectors, interest in nonviral gene transfer methods has been mounting. A number of animal models have demonstrated the efficient delivery of cytokine gene and other transgenes *in vivo* by

TABLE II
Current Cytokine Gene Therapy Clinical Trials

Cytokine	Tumor type	Primary investigator
IL-2		
Direct liposomal transfer of IL-2 gene	Prostate cancer	Belldegrun
Direct liposomal transfer of IL-2 gene		Hersh
Direct liposomal transfer of IL-2 gene	Metastatic renal cell CA	Figlin
IL-2-transduced tumor cells		Rosenberg
IL-2-transduced allogenic renal cells	Metastatic renal cell CA	Gansbacher
IL-2-transduced breast cells	Metastatic breast CA	Lyerly
IL-2-transduced small cell lung cancer cells	Small cell lung cancer	Cassileth
IL-2-transduced autologous glioblastoma cells	Glioblastoma	Sobol
IL-2-transduced fibroblasts and irradiated autologous colonic cells	Colon CA	Sobol
IL-2-transduced autologous melanoma cells	Melanoma	Stingl
IL-2-transduced autologous ovarian cells	Metastatic ovarian cancer	Berchuck
IL-2-transduced autologous prostate cells	Metastatic prostate cancer	Paulson
IL-2-transduced irradiated allogeneic melanoma cells	Melanoma	Das Gupta
IL-2-transduced melanoma cells	Melanoma	Osanto
IL-2-transduced autologous melanoma cells	Melanoma	Economou
Adenovirus-mediated IL-2 transfer	Metastatic breast cancer or melanoma	Stewart
Vaccinia-virus-MUC1-IL-2 gene transfer	Nonsmall cell lung cancer	Gitlitz
MVA-HPV-IL-2 gene transfer	Advanced cervical cancer	Goff
MVA-HPV-IL-2 gene transfer	Cervical intraepithelial neoplasia	Kaufman
Direct liposomal transfer of HLA-B7 and IL-2 genes	Metastatic melanoma	Gonzales
HLA-A2- and IL-2-transduced allogenic melanoma cells Prostate cells	Melanoma	Gansbacher
IL-2- and INF-γ-transduced MHC class I-matched allogenic prostate cells	Prostatic CA	Gansbacher
IL-4		
IL-4-transduced allogenic melanoma cells	Melanoma	Cascinelli
IL-4-transduced allogenic melanoma cells	Melanoma	Parmiani
IL-4-transduced autologous tumor cells		Lotze
IL-4-transduced fibroblasts admixed with autologous tumor cells		Lotze
IL-6		
Autologous tumor cells admixed with IL-6-/soluble IL-6 receptor-transduced allogenic melanoma cells	Melanoma	Mackiewicz
IL-7		
IL-7-transduced melanoma cells	Melanoma	Economou
IL-7 gene transfer	Metastatic colonic CA, renal CA, melanoma, lymphoma	Schmidt-Wolf
IL-12		
IL-12-transduced autologous fibroblasts		Lotze
Canarypox virus-mediated B7.1 and IL-12 transfer	Melanoma	Conry
GM-CSF		
GM-CSF-transduced autologous-irradiated melanoma cells	Melanoma	Dranoff
GM-CSF-transduced autologous tumor cells	Melanoma and sarcoma	Mahvi
GM-CSF-transduced irradiated allogenic prostate cells	Hormone-naïve prostate cancer	Small
GM-CSF-transduced irradiated allogenic prostate cells	Prostate cancer	Simons
GM-CSF-transduced nonreplicating autologous renal cells	Renal cell CA	Simons
Adenovirus-mediated GM-CSF *ex vivo* transduction of autologous, irradiated melanoma cells	Melanoma	Dranoff
Adenovirus-mediated GM-CSF *ex vivo* transduction of autologous, irradiated nonsmall cell lung cancer	Nonsmall cell lung cancer	Dranoff
Adenovirus-mediated GM-CSF *ex vivo* transduction of autologous, irradiated melanoma cells	Melanoma	Suzuki
Adenovirus-mediated GM-CSF *ex vivo* transduction of autologous, irradiated cancer cells	Breast, colon, head and neck, soft tissue	Suzuki

continues

TABLE II Continued

Cytokine	Tumor type	Primary investigator
Particle-mediated transfer of GP-100 and GM-CSF genes into normal skin	Melanoma	Albertini
TNF		
TNF-transduced autologous cancer cells		Rosenberg
INF-γ		
INF-γ-transduced neuroblastoma cells	Neuroblastoma	Walker
INF-γ-transduced autologous melanoma cells	Melanoma	Siegler
Adenovirus-INF-γ gene transfer	Malignant melanoma	Rosenblatt

liposome- and particle-mediated gene transfer techniques. Based on these initial observations, several clinical studies are examining the effect of IL-2 gene in tumor cells following direct liposomal delivery (Table II).

VII. COMBINATION CYTOKINE THERAPY

The order of production of cytokines in a physiological immune response signifies the importance of multiple cytokines in triggering an effective immune response. Several studies have reported greater therapeutic activity using vaccines consisting of tumor cells transduced with multiple cytokine genes when compared with single-gene vaccines. A combination of IL-12 and IL-18, GM-CSF and IFN-γ, IL-2 and IL-4, GM-CSF and IL-4, IFN-γ, IL-4, and IL-6, IL-2 and IL-12, pro-IL-18, and IL-1β-converting enzyme have been shown to significantly augment antitumor effects. The objective of such "multiple" gene therapies is to orchestrate an effective multicellular response. Hence the order, the type, the dose, and the duration of produced cytokines can have distinct biological effects in antitumor gene therapy, reflecting in part the complexities of the underlying immune response. Cytokine immunotherapy has also been evaluated in combination with other chemokines, costimulatory molecules, suicide genes, immunosuppressive genes, and tumor-specific and -nonspecific Ags. In general, combination therapy results in a more effective antitumor response than the single therapeutic agent.

VIII. CONCLUSION

The need for new innovative and effective antineoplastic strategies is clear and critical to the advancement of cancer treatment. The use of immunostimulatory agents to stimulate antitumor immunity has emerged as a potentially powerful and useful adjuvant to currently used anticancer strategies such as surgery, radiation, and chemotherapy. Cytokine gene transfer is a flexible technology that provides a new approach to fight cancer. Within the past decade, there has been increasing interest in the role of these proteins in the immune system and their application in an appropriate immune response against a desired antigen. Animal experiments have demonstrated that immunomodulatory genes can prevent tumor growth or significantly delay the relapse of naturally occurring tumors. Consequently, the median survival time of the treated animals are significantly prolonged compared to control animals. Even though the results of these investigations have been less than consistent, three facts have emerged from studies on local cytokines.

1. The oncogenic potential of tumors can be significantly hampered through the immune reaction elicited by cytokines injected at tumor sites, or locally released by engineered tumor cells.

2. The reaction elicited by engineered normal or neoplastic cells is sometimes strong enough to eradicate a tumor antigenically unrelated to the cytokine-releasing cells. This extended bystander effect displays a certain degree of selectivity, as surrounding normal tissue remains undamaged.

3. The prompt debulking of tumors engineered to release cytokines is often followed by the establishment

of a systemic, tumor-specific immune memory. If poorly immunogenic tumors can be rendered immunogenic enough to raise such a memory by the local presence of cytokines, a new form of vaccination against tumors would be intrinsically feasible.

Based on experiments in murine models, a number of clinical trials have been initiated to evaluate the role of these agents in eliciting an antitumor response in human subjects (Table II). Initial results of these trials suggest significant but temporary tumor regressions with use of certain cytokines in some patients. However, considering that only patients with advanced tumors have been treated so far, less substantial successes can be validly taken as evidence that vaccination and immunotherapy are alternative means of reviving the host response to a tumor. To date, most work has been conducted on gene-transduced tumor cells, but more recent studies have employed fibroblasts, xenografts, tumor infiltrating lymphocytes, dendritic cells, or direct *in vivo* gene transfer. Future protocols are expected to include combinations of immunogens, in particular using molecules that act at different phases of the immune response. Already, a triple combination of molecules that attract immune system cells to the tumor sites (e.g., lymphotactin), with costimulator molecules (e.g., CD40 ligand) that enhance a positive activation response, with amplification signals (e.g., cytokines), has shown enhanced responses relative to the single component.

See Also the Following Articles

CATIONIC LIPID-MEDIATED GENE THERAPY • CELL-MEDIATED IMMUNITY TO CANCER • INTERFERONS • INTERLEUKINS • MOLECULAR BASIS OF TUMOR IMMUNITY • RETROVIRAL VECTORS • T CELLS, FUNCTION OF

Bibliography

Borberg, H., Oettgen, H. F., Choudry, K., and Beattie, E. J. (1972). Inhibition of established transplants of chemically induced sarcomas in syngeneic mice by lymphocytes from immunized donors. *Int. J. Cancer* 10, 539.

Bosco, M., Giovarelli, M., Forni, M., Modesti, A., Scarpa, S., Masuelli, L., and Forni, G. (1990). Low doses of IL-4 injected perilymphatically in tumor-bearing mice inhibit the growth of poorly and apparently nonimmunogenic tumors and induce a tumor-specific immune memory. *J. Immunol.* 145, 3136.

Caux, C., Liu, Y. J., and Banchereau, J. (1995). Recent advances in the study of dendritic cells and follicular dendritic cells. *Immunol. Today* 16, 2.

Fraser, A., and Evan, G. (1996). A license to kill. *Cell* 85, 781.

Forni, G., Giovarelli, M., and Santoni, A. (1985). Lymphokine-activated tumor inhibition in vivo. I. The local administration of interleukin 2 triggers nonreactive lymphocytes from tumor-bearing mice to inhibit tumor growth. *J. Immunol* 134, 1305.

Gansbacher, B. (1994). Clinical application of immunostimulatory gene transfer. *Eur. J. Cancer* 30A, 1187.

Gilboa, E., Lyerly, H. K., Vieweg, J., and Saito, S. (1994). Immunotherapy of cancer using cytokine gene-modified tumor vaccines. *Semin. Cancer Biol.* 5, 409.

Grimm, E. A., Mazumder, A., Zhang, H. Z., and Rosenberg, S. A. (1982). Lymphokine-activated killer cell phenomenon: Lysis of natural killer resistant fresh solid tumor cells by interleukin 2-activated autologous human peripheral blood lymphocytes. *J. Exp. Med.* 155, 1823.

Human gene marker/therapy clinical protocols (1999). *Hum. Gene Ther.* 18, 3067.

Krueger-Krasagakes, S., Li, W., Richter, G., Diamantstein, T., and Blankestein, T. (1993). Eosinophils infiltrating interleukin-g gene-transfected tumors do not suppress tumor growth. *Eur. J. Immunol.* 23, 992.

Lotze, M. T., Grimm, E. A., Mazumder, A., Strausser, J. L., and Rosenberg, S. A. (1981). Lysis of fresh and cultured autologous tumor by human lymphocytes cultured in T-cell growth factor. *Cancer Res.* 1, 4420.

Melief, C. J., and Kast, W. M. (1991). Cytotoxic T lymphocyte therapy of cancer and tumor escape mechanisms. *Semin. Cancer Biol.* 2, 347.

Nagata, S. (1997). Apoptosis by death factor. *Cell* 88, 355.

Panelli, M. C., and Marincola, F. M. (1998). Immunotherapy update: From interleukin-2 to antigen-specific therapy. In "ASCO Educational Book, American Society of Clinical Oncology 34th Annual Meeting" (M. C. Perry, ed.), p. 467.

Peron, J.-M., Shurin, M. R., and Lotze, M. T. (1999). Cytokine gene therapy of cancer. In "Gene Therapy of Cancer" (E. C. Lattime and S. L. Gerson, eds.), p. 359. Academic Press, San Diego.

Rosenberg, S. A., Spiess, P., and Lafreniere, R. (1986). A new approach to the adoptive immunotherapy of cancer with tumor-infiltrating lymphocytes. *Science* 233, 1318.

Steinman, R. M. (1991). The dendritic cell system and its role in immunogenicity. *Annu. Rev. Immunol.* 9, 271.

Viret, C., and Lindemann, A. (1997). Tumor immunotherapy by vaccination with cytokine gene transfected cells. *Int. Rev. Immunol.* 14, 193.

Wiley, S. R., Schooley, K., Smolak, P. J., Din, W. S., Huang, C. P., Nicholl, J. K., Sutherland, G. R., Smith, T. D., Rauch, C., Smith, C. A., et al. (1995). Identification and characterization of a new member of the TNF family that induces apoptosis. *Immunity* 3, 673.

Cytokines: Hematopoietic Growth Factors

George Q. Daley
Whitehead Institute and Harvard Medical School

GLOSSARY

apheresis A process used to isolate hematopoietic stem cells, red blood cells, white blood cells, platelets, or plasma for transfusion from one individual to another or for therapeutic exchange of diseased components for healthy components in a given patient. Apheresis entails siphoning blood from a peripheral vein, separating it into its constituent parts by continuous centrifugation (spinning at high rates of speed to separate components by density), isolating specific components such as the white blood cells, and returning the remainder to the patient.

cell surface receptor Integral membrane protein docking site on the surface of cells that interacts with secreted proteins, such as cytokines, in the extracellular milieu. Binding of the appropriate ligand activates a conformational change in the receptor protein, leading to transmission of a signal from the extracellular space into the interior of the cell.

colony-forming cell A primitive cell of the hematopoietic system that gives rise to a colony of blood cells when it is cultured in semisolid growth media supplemented with cytokines and growth factors.

cytokines Secreted protein factors that act by binding to cell surface receptors on cells of the hematopoietic system to stimulate cell proliferation, survival, differentiation, and activity. Examples include the erythropoietin and granulocyte–colony stimulating factor.

gene cloning The process whereby one original copy of a gene is isolated and amplified into many millions of exact copies to allow for analysis of the gene's sequence composition, characterization of its biological function, and production of protein for therapeutic delivery.

hematopoietic stem cells The rare master cell of the bone marrow that generates all of the diverse cells of the blood and immune system. This cell represents <0.001% of all cells in the bone marrow and has properties of self-renewal, multilineage differentiation potential (pluripotency), and the capacity to reconstitute the entire blood forming system of an organism.

signal transduction The process whereby a signal from the extracellular milieu, typically carried by a secreted or matrix-associated protein or a membrane element of another cell, gets transmitted into the interior of a target cell in order to elicit a specific response, such as growth, differentiation, or apoptosis (programmed cell death). The first stage of signal transduction involves binding of the signaling protein (or small molecule) by a receptor, followed by a conformational change that elicits a cascade of intracellular protein–protein interactions and enzymatic activity that culminates in a change in cell behavior.

The blood is composed of no fewer than eight distinct cell types produced from a single versatile cell, the hematopoietic stem cell. During the lifetime of a healthy organism, the levels of red blood cells, white blood cells, and platelets in the circulating blood are regulated within a narrow range, but can vary dramatically in response to stress or disease. A trauma victim suffering from blood loss or a mountaineer confronting the thin air of Mount Everest will robustly increase their production of oxygen-carrying red blood cells. An infant suffering from an ear infection or the chicken pox will mobilize white blood cells to ward off the invading microorganisms. Blood cell populations are regulated by protein factors made locally in the bone marrow and at sites of inflammation and infection. These factors act on various blood cell precursors to modulate their production, maturation, and fate. These protein factors fall into one of several categories, including cytokines, interleukins, chemokines, lymphokines, and colony-stimulating factors (CSFs). Unraveling how these factors function has been critical to our understanding of the biology of blood cell regulation and response of the immune system to infection. The proteins themselves have also become powerful weapons in clinical medicine and among the most successful products of modern biotechnology. This article reviews the history of how these factors—collectively called cytokines—were discovered and how they function to regulate blood cell production, and concludes with a discussion of current and emerging clinical applications of cytokines in disease.

I. CYTOKINES FOR RED CELLS, WHITE CELLS, AND PLATELETS

Under the microscope, a variety of distinct cell types can be discerned in a smear of blood. Erythrocytes, or red blood cells, dominate the image and are notable for their small size, red color, biconcave shape, and lack of nucleus. The red hue derives from hemoglobin, the principal protein of the red blood cell that endows it with oxygen-carrying capacity. Also notable are the many small dark staining cell fragments, called platelets, that plug tiny holes in blood vessels, initiate blood clots, and promote the wound-healing process. Less frequent, but striking in appearance due to their large size and convoluted nuclei, are the granulocytes, which are specialized to migrate between the blood and the tissues, where they engulf invading pathogens and initiate a cascade of inflammation and repair. A host of other cell types that are critical to fighting infection or providing tissue repair also appear on the smear, including the T and B lymphocytes of the immune system and the various monocytic cells that constitute the remaining cells of the myeloid (white blood cell) series. Each of these cells has evolved its unique specialized functions in the blood, but all descend from a single ancestral cell that resides in the bone marrow, the pluripotent hematopoietic stem cell. This cell has the ability to divide and produce identical daughter stem cells, a property called self-renewal, or to differentiate, wherein the cell expresses a novel program of genes and becomes increasingly more specialized along the path to becoming a red cell, white cell, or platelet. Another key feature of the stem cell is its capacity to regenerate the bone marrow and blood-forming capacity of an organism that has been subjected to irradiation or chemotherapy. The powerful regenerative potential of hematopoietic stem cells has prompted their use in bone marrow transplantation, a curative therapy for genetic and malignant diseases of the blood and immune system. In bone marrow transplantion, patients are treated with high-dose chemotherapy and irradiation to destroy the diseased bone marrow and are infused with healthy stem cells from a donor to reconstitute normal blood formation.

A. Erythropoietin (EPO)

The first cytokine to be discovered was erythropoietin. EPO (pronounced "ee-poh") was first hypothesized to exist in the early 1900s, based on the observation that animals boosted their production of juvenile red blood cells (called reticulocytes) in response to anemia or low oxygen. Serum from anemic animals was shown to stimulate red blood cell production when injected into other animals, but the factor responsible was not isolated until decades later. The EPO protein was purified from the urine of anemic patients in 1977, and the EPO gene was isolated in 1985. EPO is made by the kidney and is lacking in patients with chronic kidney failure. Only 4 years after the gene was cloned, the Food and Drug Administration approved EPO for clinical use to treat anemia in kidney failure patients. Since initial approval, EPO has been used more widely to treat anemia due to a variety of causes, including the anemia that results from chemotherapy and AIDS therapy. EPO remains one of the most intensely studied cytokines, and insights into EPO regulation and its effects on target cells have provided paradigms for understanding the modes of action of a variety of hematopoietic growth factors.

B. Colony-Stimulating Factors

Discovery of a wide array of hematopoietic growth factors was greatly facilitated by experimental methods for growing blood cells in tissue culture. When individual bone marrow cells are dispersed in semisolid growth media, a small minority of primitive cells, called progenitors, proliferate and differentiate into a cluster of blood cells. Such colonies, visible to the naked eye, form only if the cultures are supplemented by extracts of spleen cells or media conditioned by the growth of cells taken from supportive elements of the bone marrow, called stroma. The protein growth factors in these supernatants, called colony stimulating factors, were discovered and characterized by Donald Metcalfe and Leo Sachs and their co-workers beginning in the 1960s. A number of such CSFs were initially identified by biochemical purification and later by gene cloning and were shown to stimulate primitive blood cells to develop into specific colony types. As their names suggest, granulocyte–colony-stimulating factor (G-CSF) stimulated colonies consisting of granulocytes, whereas granulocyte–macrophage (GM) CSF prompted the formation of colonies with both granulocytes and macrophages. Still other factors have been defined that promote colonies of macrophages (M-CSF, also called CSF-1),

megakaryocytes (megakaryocyte growth/differentiation factor or thrombopoietin), mast cells or colonies of multiple types (multi-CSF, also known as interleukin-3), and the list goes on. Although these CSFs were named based on their capacity to induce formation of specific blood cell colonies, it has become clear that these factors may influence a diversity of blood cell types in protean ways and have profound effects on cells outside of the blood system as well.

C. Interleukins and Other Mediators of Blood Cell Communication

A variety of bioassays have revealed numerous and varied effects of serum protein factors on blood cells of the immune system. Such factors are typically secreted by blood cells as a means of intercellular communication with other blood cells and are thus called interleukins. Interleukin-1 (IL-1) is a mediator of fever and inflammation; IL-2 activates T-cell proliferation; IL-4 and IL-7 promote B-cell responsiveness, whereas IL-8 induces chemotaxis of eosinophils. Another family of proteins called interferons have diverse effects on hematopoietic and nonhematopoietic cells. Often liberated by cells in response to stress, such as viral infection, interferons modulate cell reactivity in the immune system and have broad antiproliferative effects on primitive blood cells, thus serving to both activate and modulate the immune response to infection and inflammation. Interferons have become widely used agents for the treatment of malignancy, autommimmune disease, and chronic viral infection. Several cytokines, CSFs, interleukins, and interferons that have been approved for clinical use are listed in Table I. Unraveling the complex biology of these factors and finding appropriate disease targets remain active areas of research in hematology and medicine.

II. CYTOKINE ACTIONS

A. Signaling through Cytokine Receptors

Cytokines exert their influence by binding to a docking site, or receptor, on the surface of a target cell. Receptors are proteins that span the plasma membrane

TABLE I
Cytokines in Clinical Use

Cytokine	Mode of action	Approved clinical indications
Erythropoietin	Stimulates red blood cell production	Anemia of chronic renal failure Therapy-related anemia in HIV Chemotherapy-related anemia Pre-operative augmentation of hematocrit
Granulocyte–CSF	Stimulates granulocyte production, action	Chemotherapy-induced myelosuppression Bone marrow transplantation Peripheral stem cell harvest Chronic cyclic neutropenia
Granulocyte–Macrophage–CSF	Stimulates myeloid cell production	Chemotherapy-induced myelosuppression Bone marrow transplantation Peripheral stem cell harvest
Interleukin-2	Stimulates lymphoid cell proliferation	Renal cell carcinoma Melanoma
Interleukin-11	Stimulates megakaryocyte production	Chemotherapy-induced thrombocytopenia
Interferon-α (type I)	Biological response modifier	Chronic hepatitis C Genital warts Hairy cell leukemia Chronic myeloid leukemia AIDS-related Kaposi's Sarcoma Follicular lymphoma
Interferon-β (type I)	Biological response modifier	Multiple sclerosis
Interferon-γ (type II)	Biological response modifier	Chronic granulomatous disease

and provide a conduit for transducing signals from the exterior to the interior of the cell. Receptors typically contain an extracellular domain that binds the cytokine, a hydrophobic domain that spans the lipid milieu of the plasma membrane, and an intracellular domain. The intracellular, or cytoplasmic, domain of several cytokine receptors encodes an intrinsic enzyme activity that is activated by the binding of the cytokine to the extracellular domain of the receptor. The intracellular protein domain for the receptor for M-CSF, called c-FMS, encodes an enzyme function that modifies substrate proteins by adding phosphate groups to specific tyrosines. This tyrosine-specific protein kinase activity is a property of a number of cellular receptors and intracellular proteins linked to cell proliferation. The cytoplasmic domains of receptors for other cytokines, like EPO, lack an intrinsic enzymatic activity and instead bind to cytoplasmic enzymes that initiate a cascade of protein–protein interactions that change cell behavior. Still other receptors have only minimal intracellular domains and signal via association with distinct integral membrane proteins with enzymatic or adaptor properties as part of a multisubunit complex.

Cytokines influence blood cell fate by effects on cell proliferation, differentiation, and cell survival. Most cytokines are potent mitogens, stimulating cell division and increases in cell number. Treatment of anemic patients with EPO induces a marked expansion of red blood cell precursors in the bone marrow, which ultimately leads to the restoration of red cell counts in the circulation. The bone marrow is one of the most actively proliferating tissues in the body and is responsible for the production of billions of cells each day. Most blood cell types exist only transiently. While red blood cells survive in the circulation for around 100 days, granulocytes have a life span of less than a day in the blood. Blood cell populations undergo a natural cycle of cell proliferation, differentiation, and cell elimination. Therefore it follows that cytokines can have a profound impact on blood cell numbers by inhibiting cell death, and numerous cytokines promote cell survival. A lingering controversy in hematology is whether cytokines influence cell fate directly, through changing the gene expression patterns of target cells (the "instructive" hypothesis), or whether cell fate is determined probabilistically, with populations regulated by effects on cell survival (the "selective" hypothesis). The debate rages on after decades, although evidence is mounting that both phenomena may operate, depending on the particular context of the cytokine and its target cell.

The signaling pathways that emanate from cytokine receptors have a remarkable degree of redundancy. Numerous cytokines activate the same intracellular enzymes, such as the small GTP-binding protein Ras, phosphatidyl inositol-3 kinase, phospholipases, janus kinases, and STATs (signal transducer and activators of transcription), among many others. This begs the question of how individual receptors confer specific signals on the target cell. Unraveling the code of signaling specificity remains one of the great challenges of modern cell biology. Part of the specificity of cytokine receptor signaling derives from the unique, cell-specific patterns of receptor expression. Stated simply, the EPO receptor stimulates red blood cell production largely due to its expression on cells that are destined to become red blood cells. When expressed experimentally on primitive blood cell types that have not committed themselves to develop along any specific lineage, the EPO receptor stimulates proliferation of all hematopoietic cells but does not appear to bias cells to become erythrocytes. The EPO receptor thus sends generic signals for cell proliferation and survival and not specific signals unique to the program of red blood cell differentiation. This is illustrated by the fact that the prolactin receptor, a receptor unrelated to red blood cell function, can support complete differentiaton of red blood cells if introduced into blood precursors from mice with genetic deficiency in either EPO or the EPO receptor. Taken together, these data argue that the EPO receptor does not instruct the differentiation of red blood cells but facilitates erythrocyte development in cells already primed to become red cells. These data support the notion that cytokines influence target cells through selective effects on cell survival. While data seem particularly compelling for EPO, data are far less conclusive for cytokines that influence other hematopoietic lineages. In many experimental models, forced expression of one type of cytokine receptor appears to

bias or redirect cell fate toward the specificity dictated by the corresponding cytokine. Much remains to be learned about how cytokines, acting through cytokine receptor signal transduction, influence the differentiation program of hematopoietic cells.

B. Murine Models of Cytokine Excess and Deficiency

There is strong evidence that cytokines stimulate cell production in response to environmental stresses, such as hemorrhage, hypoxia, and infection. Genetically modified strains of mice that make too much or too little of a cytokine have shed light on the role of cytokines in the basal regulation of blood cell populations. Uncontrolled myeloid cell proliferation develops in mice whose bone marrow cells are engineered to express high levels of GM-CSF, IL-3, or EPO. These latter mice model certain forms of human kidney and brain cancer, which secrete EPO, and rare congenital syndromes with excess EPO production or a hyperactive EPO receptor, all of which lead to inappropriate erythrocytosis. Gene inactivation studies in mice have demonstrated the essential role of EPO in red blood cell production, as mutant mice lacking EPO or EPO receptor function die *in utero* due to fetal anemia. Gene disruption of the colony-stimulating factors and interleukins has revealed various degrees of redundancy in cytokine function on basal levels of hematopoiesis. Interestingly, lack of G-CSF results in only a modest deficiency of granulocytes (neutropenia), suggesting that other cytokines play redundant and partially overlapping roles in maintaining granulocyte populations. Perhaps surprisingly, deficiency of GM-CSF has only modest effects on granulocyte levels, but instead results in an excessive production of protein in the lungs and impaired resistance to lung infection, which reflects deficiencies in the function of critical granulocytic and macrophage populations. Deletion of M-CSF modestly depletes macrophage populations in mice, but results in a condition called osteopetrosis, which is characterized by a profound overgrowth of bone, reflecting the probable role of this cytokine in maintenance or maturation of osteoclast populations. Mice with cytokine deficiency model rare human conditions where a loss of action of particular cytokines through autoimmune antibody blockade has been associated with cytopenias, or inadequate cell counts, for both myeloid cells and platelets. Given the large numbers of cytokines, there is enormous combinatorial complexity in their actions on distinct target cells, necessitating continued research to sort out their overlapping and complementary functions in blood cell development.

III. CLINICAL APPLICATIONS OF CYTOKINES

The widespread use of EPO and G-CSF in clinical medicine represents one of the triumphs of modern medicine. These two multibillion dollar blockbuster products were largely responsible for ushering in the biotechnology revolution, as countless patients have had their lives saved or improved by delivering these proteins as therapeutic drugs. A number of other cytokines have found their way into more modest clinical use, and there is widespread promise that additional cytokines will be shown to have tremendous therapeutic value.

EPO was initially approved for the treatment of the anemia of chronic renal failure. Such patients typically have normal bone marrow cell populations, but because of kidney dysfunction fail to produce adequate quantities of EPO and hence suffer from a hypoproliferative anemia that readily responds to pharmaceutical protein replacement. Because of the specificity of EPO for the erythroid lineage, no other cells in the marrow show significant responses to the growth factor. EPO has also been approved for use in cancer patients undergoing chemotherapy. In these individuals, the production of red blood cells from the bone marrow is inadequate because of the chronic suppressive effects of chemotherapy. These patients have higher levels of EPO in the circulating blood than normal persons, but the levels are inadequate to compensate for the toxicity of the chemotherapy. In this case, providing excess EPO in the form of a subcutaneous injection can boost red blood cell production, allowing patients to avoid blood transfusions and enjoy an enhanced quality of life. EPO is also used to counteract the anemia associated with drug therapy for AIDS. Because of the blood-enhancing properties of EPO, it has become a drug of

abuse in athletes looking to improve performance by boosting the oxygen-carrying capacity of their blood. Unfortunately, this strategy of "blood doping" is highly risky, as chronic overdosing of EPO generates a condition of excess red blood cell production called polycythemia, which can greatly increase the risk of stroke and death by inducing high blood pressure and enhancing the tendency for blood clot formation.

The other cytokine in widespread clinical use, G-CSF, has been approved for patients undergoing chemotherapy to lessen the time spent with dangerously low levels of infection-fighting white blood cells (called neutropenia). Again, although chemotherapy patients have elevated levels of G-CSF in the circulation, the response does not adequately maintain granulocyte (neutrophil) production. While pharmaceutical delivery of G-CSF cannot eliminate the profound depletion of white blood cells that follows intensive chemotherapy, it accelerates the recovery of functional granulocytes, decreases the time patients need to remain in the hospital, and reduces the need for antibiotics to fight the inevitable infections sustained by neutropenic patients. Thus, G-CSF has been a remarkably valuable adjunct to clinical cancer care and has allowed patients to sustain much more aggressive forms of chemotherapy.

G-CSF has also been widely used to facilitate the isolation of hematopoietic stem cells for transplantation. Injection of G-CSF mobilizes blood cell progenitors, including hematopoietic stem cells from the bone marrow into the circulation, enabling them to be collected by a relatively noninvasive technique called therapeutic apheresis. This entails siphoning blood from a peripheral vein, separating it into its constituent parts, isolating the white blood cells, and returning the red blood cells and plasma to the patient. Therapeutic apheresis obviates the need for the more cumbersome and invasive bone marrow harvests that are routinely performed in the operating room under general anesthesia. In addition to enhancing granulocyte levels in the blood, G-CSF also enhances their infection-fighting function. Investigations are underway to determine whether G-CSF might enhance the body's ability to successfully counter severe infections and might ameliorate the severe mucosal injury sustained in the gastrointestinal tract when patients are treated with high-dose chemotherapy or irradiation. GM-CSF, which has a somewhat broader effect on blood cell populations and has been associated with modestly worse side effects than G-CSF, is approved for the enhancement of hematopoietic recovery following bone marrow transplantation. Because of its profound capacity to stimulate professional antigen-processing dendritic cells, GM-CSF is being actively investigated for its potential to enhance immune responses against tumors.

Although the megakaryocyte growth and differentiation factor thrombopoietin (TPO, pronounced "tee-poh") has been isolated and appears to stimulate platelet production in normal individuals, approval for clinical use has been delayed, in part because of the frustrating development of autoantibodies that neutralize TPO and induce low platelets in some patients. A minor regulator of platelet production, IL-11, has been approved based on its capacity to augment platelet counts in chemotherapy patients, again demonstrating the remarkable redundancy of cytokine action on hematopoietic cells.

Other cytokines have been approved for specific indications, chiefly to augment endogenous responses against cancer (interleukin-2 for renal cell carcinoma and melanoma) or as antileukemic agents (interferon-α). Interferon-α also acts to reduce viral load in some patients with hepatitis, whereas interferon-β has been used to suppress the autoimmunity associated with multiple sclerosis. A catalogue of cytokines in clinical use along with their approved clinical indications can be found in Table I.

Despite over a decade of clinical experience with cytokines, current therapeutic applications do not take full advantage of their enormous potential. *In vitro* data suggest that combinations of cytokines work best to synergistically augment blood cell production, and yet it has been difficult to determine the optimal combination strategies in clinical medicine. Only a small number of cytokines have found their way into clinical use, but testing combinations of even these few approved agents would represent an enormous number of different conditions and require expensive and time-consuming trials. With the ever-growing catalogue of secreted proteins emerging from human genome sequencing efforts, future clinical uses must be prioritized based on carefully designed preclinical studies. With the increasing appreciation of the diverse roles of extracellular communicators, more therapeutic applications of cytokines are certain to follow, promising profound benefits in health and medicine.

See Also the Following Articles

Cell–Matrix Interactions • Cytokine Gene Therapy • Interleukins • JAK/STAT Pathway • Signal Transduction Mechanisms Initiated by Receptor Tyrosine Kinases • Stem Cell Transplantation • T Cells, Function of

Bibliography

Crawford, J., Foote, M., and Morstyn, G. (1999). Hematopoietic growth factors in cancer chemotherapy. *Cancer Chemother. Biol. Response Modif.* **18,** 250–267.

Gabrilove, J. (2000). Overview: Erythropoiesis, anemia, and the impact of erythropoietin. *Semin. Hematol.* **37**(4 Suppl. 6), 1–3.

Mach, N., and Dranoff, G. (2000). Cytokine secreting tumor cell vaccines. *Curr. Opin. Immunol.* **12**(5), 571–575.

Metcalfe, D., and Nicola, N. A. (1995). "The Hematopoietic Colony-Stimulating Factors." Cambridge Univ. Press, Cambridge.

Socolovsky, M., Lodish, H. F., and Daley, G. Q. (1998). Control of hematopoietic differentiation: Lack of specificity in signaling by cytokine receptors. *Proc. Natl. Acad. Sci. USA* **95**(12), 5573–5575.

Uings, I. J., and Farrow, S. N. (2000). Cell receptors and cell signaling. *Mol. Pathol.* **53**(6), 295–299.

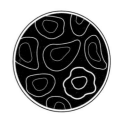

Differentiation and Cancer: Basic Research

Mark P. Kamps
University of California, San Diego School of Medicine

GLOSSARY

differentiation The process by which a cell or a number of cells that lack a specific function proliferate for a defined period and change their pattern of gene expression, creating a structure that performs a specialized function.

hematopoiesis The process by which all blood cells differentiate from a common progenitor through "proliferate—execute genetic differentiation program—stop proliferation" cascades.

homeodomain A DNA-binding domain approximately 60 residues in size that is contained within numerous transcription factors that regulate developmental genetic programs.

homeotic selector genes Genes whose expression selects a specific genetic response to extracellular stimuli.

leukemia Cancer of blood cells or their progenitors.

morphogen A factor that induces differentiation by activating signaling in a position- and time-dependent manner.

I. LINK BETWEEN PROLIFERATION AND DIFFERENTIATION IN CANCER

Differentiation is the process by which a cell or a number of cells that lack a specific function proliferate for a defined period and change their pattern of gene expression, creating a structure that performs a specialized function. During normal differentiation, each step in the "proliferate—execute genetic differentiation program—stop proliferation" cascade is highly regulated and precisely executed by transcription factors working in conjunction with extracellular signals. Embryogenesis is the most striking form of differentiation, during which all specialized functions of the adult arise from a single fertilized egg.

Differentiation continues in the adult life in specific cells that must be continually replenished in the body, such as intestinal brush boarder, blood, and skin. The failure of cells in leukemia, colon carcinoma, and skin cancer to fully differentiate prompted the hypothesis that mutations preventing differentiation are selected during tumorigenesis and are primary mediators of cancer. Three genetic systems dictate how cells differentiate (e.g., wing, leg, eye, liver, muscle, brain). Remarkably, genes within each system are oncogenes in human cancer. The first system "programs" cells to differentiate into specific structures in response to environmental morphogens. This step is accomplished by expressing transcription factor "selector" genes, master regulators of genetic cascades. Mutations in selector genes produce striking "homeotic" phenotypes in which the differentiation of one tissue shifts to that of another. Hox genes are classic examples of selector genes, and when expressed aberrantly, Hox genes become oncogenes that prevent completion of the "execute genetic differentiation program" step of the cascade, thus preventing the cell from arriving at "stop proliferation." The second system that controls differentiation uses concentration gradients of active extracellular signaling molecules (morphogens) to induce differentiation in a position-dependent manner. In *Drosophila*, these morphogens include Hedgehog (Hh), Decapentapleigic (Dpp), Wingless (Wg), and Notch ligands, which bind surface receptors and activate the function of preexisting, latent transcription factors. Components of these signaling cascades are present in cells, awaiting activation. Humans have families of proteins homologous to these factors, and mutations that activate signaling through the Hh, Wg, or Notch pathways or prevent signaling through the Dpp pathway are oncogenes in human cancer. By maintaining chronic activation of "proliferate—execute genetic program—stop proliferation" cascades, the oncoprotein induces cell division and prevents later stages of differentiation that require downregulation of the signaling cascade. The third sytem that controls differentiation is the genetic response activated by the first two systems. This response allows completion of the "execute genetic differentiation program—stop proliferation" steps, and numerous human oncogenes interfere with the ability of the cell to execute these terminal differentiation steps in re-

sponse to environmental morphogens and intrinsic selector gene expression. This article outlines key features of differentiation at the molecular level and strives to provide a context for understanding how human oncoproteins interfere with normal developmental programs.

II. HOX PROTEINS AND THEIR COFACTORS SELECT DEVELOPMENTAL PROGRAMS AND ARE HUMAN ONCOGENES

A. Hox Proteins and Their Cofactors in *Drosophila* Development

During embryogenesis, organisms must specify positional information in anterior/posterior, dorsal/ventral, and proximal/distal axes. Regardless of whether cells in a field are developing into body, leg, wing, or antenna, they must know where they lie so that they divide the correct number of times and express the correct pattern of genes required to perform their final function. This positional information is provided by morphogen gradients, which are concentration gradients of active factors that relay information concerning identity and position. Two types of morphogenetic gradients exist in *Drosophila*. The first is imparted to the egg by the mother and is composed of gradients of transcription factors that provide unique coordinates to each location within the egg. This information tells the nuclei how to respond to the second type of morphogenetic gradient, which is composed of extracellular signaling molecules, termed morphogens. Before nuclei become partitioned as cells, maternal transcription factor gradients are established in both anterior/posterior and dorsal/ventral axes of the egg and program each nucleus with permanent positional coordinants. Apical transcription factor morphogens orchestrate all facets of a differentiation response, and the gradient is essential to trigger different transcriptional responses at different distances from the source of the morphogen. In *Drosophila*, Bicoid is the apical anterior morphogen. Bicoid is a member of the homeodomain superfamily of transcription factors, each of which contains a DNA-binding domain of approximately 60 residues called the homeodomain (HD). *Bicoid* mRNA is anchored at the anterior of the egg, creating a gradient of Bicoid protein across the anterior/posterior axis that freely enters dividing nuclei within the egg prior to their cellularization. *Bicoid* loss of function mutants fail to develop anterior structures, and introduction of *bicoid* mRNA at the posterior induces development of anterior structures in the posterior; thus, Bicoid is necessary and sufficient for anteriorization. The importance of a gradient can be seen from gene dosage experiments, where increasing the concentration of anterior *bicoid* mRNA to levels twice or four times that of normal shifts the resulting zones of Hox gene expression posteriorly.

After cellularization, maternal transcription factor morphogens induce the expression of zygotic genes, which establish expression of eight Hox genes in overlapping zones across the anterior/posterior axis, including precursor cells of the imaginal discs, which develop into body appendages at metamorphosis. Hox genes represent a small, but very important subset of the hundreds of genes containing a homeobox, which encodes the HD. Hox genes reside at the apex of genetic programs, which, in response to environmental morphogens, specify the identity of body segments and body appendages across the anterior/posterior axis, as well as the number, size, and shape of cells within the developing structure. *Drosophila* Hox genes reside in the Antennapedia complex (ANT-C) and Bithorax complex (BX-C; Fig. 1). In mice and humans, four Hox loci (Hox A, B, C, and D) contain Hox genes similar to *Drosophila* BX-C and ANT-C genes in the amino acid sequence of their HDs. With the distinct exception of a highly conserved YPWMR or ANWL peptide motif (which binds Pbx cofactors,

see later), there is little sequence conservation among HD proteins outside their HD (Fig. 1).

While all Hox HDs bind sequences similar to TAAT, their transcriptional functions vary. By activating the expression of genes encoding extracellular morphogens (e.g., Hh, Dpp, Wg, Notch), as well as by functioning in concert with transcription factors activated by these morphogens, Hox proteins select the correct genetic programs that produce the correct structure. Mutations in Hox genes or ectopic expression of Hox genes has dramatic effects on development of both the *Drosophila* body and appendages. For example, the haltere is a tiny balancing organ positioned behind the wing. The Hox protein Ultrabithorax (Ubx) is expressed in the haltere and plays the essential role of suppressing a genetic program leading to wing development. In *Drosophila* containing loss of function *ubx* mutants, the haltere develops into a wing, producing spectacular four-winged flies. No Hox genes are normally expressed in developing wing, and ectopic expression of *ubx* transforms the wing into a haltere. These effects of abberant Hox gene expression are important in the context of cancer because the differentiation of hematopoietic progenitors (blood cell progenitors) can be arrested by ectopic Hox protein expression. In this light, it is important to note that while Hox proteins can induce differentiation programs in certain cell types, they are incapable of inducing them in other cell types; rather, they exhibit similar default functions that lack specificity (e.g., whereas *abdominal-A* and *abdominal-B* genes induce thoracic identities, they fail to induce any qualities of the thorax when expressed in wing; instead, like *ubx*, they repress wing development and produce a haltere-like appendage). Basic research in *Drosophila*, therefore, suggests that aberrant Hox gene expression in hematopoiesis may block differentiation by interference with genetic programs without necessarily specifying new ones.

During development, Hox proteins function in concert with two cofactors, Extradentical (Exd) and Homothorax (Hth), and human cognates of these genes are also involved in cancer. Exd and Hth are active in different regions of developing *Drosophila* embryos. They bind DNA as heterodimers with Hox proteins, change the DNA-binding specificity of Hox proteins, and therein shift the spectrum of genes activated or

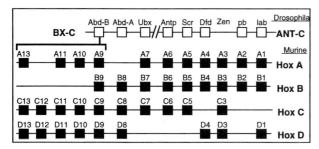

FIGURE 1 Comparison of *Drosophila* HOM-C and vertebrate Hox genes.

repressed by Hox proteins, thus changing the impact of Hox proteins in development. The regulation of biologically active Exd is controlled at the level of subcellular localization: in the absence of the Hth protein, Exd remains cytosolic and inactive, and in the presence of Hth, Exd is translocated to the nucleus. Exd is required for the development of most segments along the anterior/posterior axis of the embryo, functioning with Hox proteins in the selection, activation, or repression of specific genes (e.g., activation of teashirt in the visceral mesoderm, labial in the endoderm, and fork head in the ectoderm). In contrast, the presence or absence of nuclear Exd controls how appendages develop. A dramatic example of how Exd can reconfigure a genetic program is illustrated in antenna development. Antenna express *hth* and thus contain functional Exd. Removing nuclear exd from a developing antenna transforms it into a leg. This appears to be the molecular basis of the classic antennepedia mutation in which flies develop legs in the place of antenna. In this mutation, inappropriate expression of the Hox gene *antennepedia* in antennal progenitors eliminates nuclear Exd by repressing *hth* transcription. Without nuclear Exd, the antenna develops as a leg. Development of the distal portion of normal legs, as well as halters and wings, in contrast requires the absence of nuclear Exd, and enforced expression of *hth* in this zone, which induces nuclear translocation of Exd, results in leg truncations. Ectopic expression of *meis1*, a murine orthologue of *hth*, also triggers antennal development elsewhere in the fly. Ectopic expression of *hth* interferes with other developmental pathways as well, suppressing eye development and blocking the differentiation of wing cells along the anterior/posterior compartment boundary. These examples from fly development indicate that abnormal expression of human *pbx* and *meis* oncoproteins (human orthologues of *exd* and *hth*) could interfere with normal genetic programs in hematopoietic progenitors.

B. Vertebrate Hox Proteins and Cofactors are Structural and Functional Cognates of Their *Drosophila* Orthologues

The vertebrate genome contains 39 Hox genes; apparently, increased developmental complexity requires increased transcriptional selectivity. These genes are organized in clusters at four loci in an order colinear with that of *Drosophila* BX-C and ANT-C Hox genes in their degree of sequence homology. In mouse, Hox gene expression begins 8.0 days postconception in partially overlapping, spatially restricted domains along the A–P axis of the developing skeletal and central nervous system (CNS). Hox genes are also expressed during organogenesis (e.g., *hoxA5*, *hoxB5*, *hoxB6*, and *hoxB8* during lung development), during adipogenesis (*hoxA4*, *hoxA7*, and *hoxD4*), during skin differentiation (*hoxA4*, *hoxA5*, and *hoxA7*), and during limb regeneration and digit development (*hoxA9* and *hoxA13*). During development, Hox gene expression can drop (e.g., *hoxB7* in stomach and gut) or persist (e.g., *hoxA3*, *hoxA5*, *hoxA6*, *hoxB5*, *hoxB7*, *hoxB8*, and *hoxC8*, in the CNS). Vertebrate Hox genes are required for development, as their mutation alters the specification and development of structures along the anterior/posterior axis (e.g., disruption of *hoxA3*, *hoxA1*, or *hoxD3* produces defects in organ, neuronal, and skeletal development, including anterior transformations of the first and second vertebrae). Single Hox genes can be expressed in different tissues, and multiple Hox genes can be expressed simultaneously in single tissues. The combination of different Hox genes expressed within a single tissue may account for the specific developmental fate of cells.

Expression of Hox genes is also required during hematopoiesis, the process by which all blood cells differentiate from a common progenitor through "proliferate—execute genetic differentiation program—stop proliferation" cascades. Most *hoxA* and *hoxB* genes are expressed in the stem cell/CD34$^+$ population and downregulated when they leave the CD34$^+$ compartment. *hoxC4* and *hoxC8* are expressed during the maturation of B and T cells from CD34$^+$, CD38 low progenitors. *hoxA10* is expressed highly in CD34$^+$ progenitors, in normal myeloid progenitors, and in myeloid leukemias; is downregulated in CD34$^-$ marrow; and is absent in neutrophils, monocytes, and lymphocytes. Expression of some Hox genes is upregulated by activation programs that couple proliferation and differentiation (e.g., both *hoxD4* and *hoxC4* are induced by phytohemagglutinin (PHA) in peripheral blood lymphocytes). Some of the most striking data in this arena come from the analysis of *hoxB* gene expression in activated natural killer and peripheral T cells. When activated, these cells exhibit a 3′ to 5′ expression of B locus genes, beginning with activation of *hoxB1* and *hoxB2* by 10 min, continuing to activate *hoxB3, hoxB4,* and *hoxB5* transcription by 120 min, and later activating the transcription of *hoxB6, hoxB7,* and *hoxB9.* Genetic experiments also demonstrate the importance of hox genes in hematopoiesis. *hoxA9* knockout mice have suppressed counts of neutrophils, lymphocytes, and committed progenitors, suggesting that HoxA9 can regulate the balance of proliferation (self-renewal) and differentiation. While analysis of hox gene expression during normal hematopoiesis is still in an early stage, the lineage-specific expression of hox genes suggests that locus- and gene-specific expression contributes to both lineage definition and differentiation state.

C. Hox Genes and Cofactors Are Human Oncogenes

Persistent expression of normal or mutant Hox proteins, of normal or mutant Hox protein cofactors, or of mutant regulators of Hox gene expression are all oncogenic events in human leukemia. The impact of Hox oncogenes on hematopoietic "proliferate—execute genetic differentiation program—stop proliferation" programs was delineated using *in vitro* assays that sustain the proliferation and differentiation of committed progenitors cultured in the presence of a specific growth factor. For example, in marrow, myeloid progenitors differentiate into macrophages or neutrophils, cells that kill microorganisms. When removed from marrow and cultured in granulocyte–macrophage colony-stimulating factor (GM-CSF), a lymphokine whose receptor resides on the surface of maturing myeloid progenitors, such progenitors will execute a "proliferate—execute genetic differentiation program—stop proliferation" cascade, producing a colony after 14 days that contains hundreds of mature nonmitotic neutrophils and macrophages. Differentiation to either neutrophil or macrophage is accompanied by changes in nuclear morphology, cell size, and production factors involved in killing microorganisms (e.g., defensins, respiratory burst oxidase). In acute myeloid leukemia (AML), 80% or more of marrow cells are descendants of a single myeloid progenitor, and when removed from the marrow, these cells proliferate but fail to differentiate in GM-CSF, demonstrating that they contain a genetic

mutation(s) that blocks differentiation. The first example of an AML oncogene that arrested differentiation was *hoxB8,* whose transcriptional activation occurred concurrent with a transcriptional activation of the *interleukin-3 (IL-3)* gene. IL-3 induces proliferation and permits differentiation of a broad range of hematopoietic progenitors. Using retroviral vectors, persistent expression of *hoxB8* was proven to block differentiation to macrophages or neutrophils, permitting indefinite proliferation in GM-CSF or IL-3. Importantly, HoxB8 does not stimulate proliferation and does not sustain myeloid viability in the absence of GM-CSF or IL-3. Thus, HoxB8 specifically interdicts in the "execute genetic differentiation program" step of the differentiation cascade, preventing the cell from reaching "stop proliferation." How HoxB8 prevents differentiation is not yet understood. Ectopic expression of HoxB8 could compete with the normal function of an endogenous Hox protein or could target promoter motifs *de novo* with endogenous Pbx proteins. Understanding how HoxB8 prevents differentiation is an important question whose answer is likely to reveal how normal myeloid differentiation events are regulated.

Persistent activation of other Hox genes also arrests myeloid differentiation and, indeed, aberrant Hox gene expression may be a general mechanism underlying differentiation arrest in both human AML and human lymphoblastic leukemias (leukemias of B- and T-cell progenitors). The BXH strain of mice is prone to acquiring AML and, in most cases, *hoxA9* or *hoxA7* genes are activated in these AMLs. Retroviral-mediated expression of *hoxA9* and *hoxA7* (our unpublished results) precludes differentiation of myeloid progenitors but permits their indefinite growth in GM-CSF. Retroviral expression of *hoxA10* produces an expansion of multilineage progenitors and causes myeloid leukemia. In a small fraction of human AML, the t(7;11) chromosomal translocation fuses Nup98 sequences that function as a transcriptional activation domain to those encoding HoxA9, producing a Nup98–HoxA9 chimeric oncoprotein that blocks myeloid differentiation. Because *hoxA9* is expressed in immature CD34$^+$ progenitors and is transcriptionally downregulated during differentiation, and because HoxA9 is required for normal hematopoiesis, it is possible that HoxA9 both promotes early programming steps of immature progenitors and prevents their premature terminal differentiation. While mutations that activate the transcription of normal *hoxA9* have not been reported in human AML, virtually all human AMLs express *hoxA9*, suggesting that other oncogenes upstream of *hoxA9* may orchestrate its persistant expression. If these mutations prevent differentiation by maintaining *hoxA9* expression, inhibitors of HoxA9 could represent therapeutic agents for human AML. Also, understanding the mechanism by which *hoxA9* expression is maintained in such leukemias may lead to the identification of new "primary" oncogenes that function through *hoxA9* upregulation.

hox11 is an "orphan" gene of the Hox family not contained in the A-D loci that encodes an Antennapedia-type HD. *hox11* is essential for normal spleen development and is not expressed during hemato-poiesis. *hox11* transcription is activated by the t(10;14) translocation in 4–7% of pediatric T-cell leukemia and by other transcriptional mechanisms in one-third of cases, and its expression prevents the differentiation of IL-3-dependent myeloid progenitors.

Genes that regulate the expression of Hox genes are also oncogenes in human leukemia. During *Drosophila* development, the *polycomb* (*pc*) and *trithorax* (*ttx*) gene products maintain the silencing or activation of Hox gene transcription. Deletion of *pc* expands Hox gene expression zones, and deletion of *ttx* results constriction Hox gene expression zones. In approximately 20% of both AML and ALL, rearrangements occur in *mll*, a human *ttx* orthologue located on chromosome 11q23. These rearrangements fuse *mll* with over 40 other genetic loci, forming a family of fusion proteins that retain their ability to target DNA but have lost other regulatory functions. Mll-Enl prevents the differentiation of myeloid progenitors grown in IL-3 and activates expression of *hoxA7*, supporting the possibility that mutant Mll proteins may arrest differentiation through their aberrant activation of Hox genes. Future research should examine whether aberrant Hox gene expression is an important mediator of differentiation arrest by Mll oncoproteins.

pbx genes (*pbx1*, *pbx2*, and *pbx3*) are the human orthologues of *Drosophila exd*, and *meis* genes (*meis1*, *meis2*, and *meis3*) are the human orthologues of *Drosophila hth*. Pbx and Meis proteins bind DNA as heterodimers with each other as well as with Hox proteins, and both Pbx and Meis are oncoproteins. In 20% of pediatric pre-B ALL, the t(1;19) chromosomal translocation fuses the transcription activation domain of E2a to the majority of Pbx1, converting Pbx from a cofactor of Hox and Meis proteins into a persistent transcriptional activator that interacts only with Hox proteins. E2a-Pbx1 also blocks the differentiation of myeloid progenitors cultured in GM-CSF or IL-3. *meis* genes are coactivated with *hoxA9* and *hoxA7* in BXH mouse myeloid leukemia, and Meis proteins complement HoxA9 to produce overt leukemias in animal models.

How persistent expression of Hox genes prevents the "execute genetic differentiation program—stop proliferation" step in leukemia represents a completely open field for investigation. The mechanisms of transcriptional upregulation of terminal differentiation genes should be elucidated utilizing myeloid progenitor cell lines whose differentiation is arrested by conditional forms of Hox oncoproteins. It will then be possible to determine how Hox oncoproteins prevent these transcriptional events.

III. THE Hh, Wg, AND Dpp PATHWAYS IN DIFFERENTIATION AND CANCER

A. Role of Hh, Wg, and Dpp Morphogens in *Drosophila* Development

After the embryo has become cellularized, a second type of morphogenetic gradient—now in the form of extracellular factors—continues to relay positional information to cells in the developing body and appendages. The appendages develop from imaginal discs, groups of undifferentiated epithelial cells that proliferate and undergo patterning events that result in the formation of adult appendages at metamorphosis. Imaginal discs acquire disc-specific determination in the embryo as a result of specific homeotic selector gene function. Amazingly, both the trunk and appendages that develop from imaginal discs acquire positional information defining anterior/posterior, dorsal/ventral, and proximal/distal axes from the same group of morphogens—Hh, Wg, and Dpp—first identified for their requirement in establishing the correct polarity of segments in developing embryos (hence their assignment as "segment polarity" genes). Hh, Wg, and Dpp are extracellular signaling proteins that bind transmembrane receptors and transmit their signals through a cascade of intracellular proteins that activate the function of preexisting inactive transcription factors. Hh is a short-range morphogen that activates the transcription of *wg* and *dpp,* whose products function as long-range morphogens—the degree to which they activate their cascades is directly dependent on concentration gradients of their activities. The transcription factors newly activated by Hh, Dpp, and Wg work together with selector gene products (e.g., Hox proteins) to execute the correct "proliferate—execute genetic differentiation program—stop proliferation" program.

How do Hh, Wg, and Dpp control axis formation in the fly? The anterior/posterior axis of discs is established during embryogenesis so that when discs individualize, they are already composed of anterior and posterior compartments. The engrailed HD protein is the posterior-specifying factor, is produced in all discs only in posterior cells, and initiates organization of the dorsal/ventral axis by activating the transcription of Hh in the posterior compartment. In posterior cells, Engrailed also suppresses transcription of *cubitous interruptus,* which encodes the downstream transcription factor activated by Hh; thus, anterior cells, but not posterior cells, respond to Hh. Hh activates transcription of *dpp* in dorsal cells of the anterior compartment and *wg* in ventral cells of the anterior compartment. The expression of *wg* by ventral cells and *dpp* by dorsal cells is inherited from the embryonic ectoderm during development of the disc primordium, when *wg* is expressed in presumptive ventral cells. Because Dpp and Wg mutually antagonize each other's transcription, they maintain a sharp boundary between their expression zones.

Concentration gradients of Hh, Dpp, and Wg, as well as of factors that inhibit their function, diffuse across the developing limb, and the transcriptional response of a cell is dependent on the relative concentration of the *active* morphogen. The cell responds

to morphogenic gradients by activating expression of a profile of transcription factors and signaling genes that define what the cell will become and how its neighbors should develop. These transcription factors include members of the basic helix-loop-helix (bHLH), HD, and Zn finger families. Experiments in which Dpp and Wg signals are eliminated or ectopically expressed suggest that Dpp confers a dorsalizing activity and that Wg confers a ventralizing activity on surrounding tissues during appendage development. In *dpp* loss of function mutants in the leg, dorsal structures are replaced by symmetrically duplicated ventral structures. In larvae containing loss of function mutants for *wg* or for genes encoding signal transduction proteins in the Wg pathway, ventral structures are lost and are replaced by a symmetric duplication of dorsal structures. Ectopic expression of *wg* or activation of the Wg signal transduction pathway in cells on the dorsal side of the leg respecifies dorsal cells to ventral fate and causes dorsal/ventral axis duplication.

Hh, Dpp, and Wg signaling also initiates a cell division–cell quiescence program, a function that may be exploited by human oncoproteins that activate signaling components within these pathways (see later). In leg development, Dpp and Wg act jointly where their domains of expression meet, not only to specify structure formation, but also to induce distal growth along the proximodistal axis. Ordered activation of a "proliferate—execute genetic differentiation program—stop proliferation" cascade by Hh and Dpp is observed in a striking fashion during differentiation of the *Drosophila* retina. Differentiation starts at the posterior margin of the eye imaginal disc and progresses anteriorly over the course of 2 days. During this time, the disc increases in size eightfold while an indentation in the epithelium, designated the "morphogenetic furrow" (MF), demarcates the front of the differentiation wave. Undifferentiated cells lie anterior to the MF and differentiating photoreceptors lie posterior to the MF. Hh initiates all events of MF progression; when expressed ectopically, Hh initiates new MFs in the eye disc. Low concentrations of Hh and Dpp at further anterior points from the MF stimulate proliferation and expression of the bHLH repressor protein Hairy, which suppresses premature neuronal differentiation. As the MF approaches this mitotic zone, it has the short-range effects of inducing cell synchronization and quiescence, repression of *hairy*, and activation of another bHLH gene, *atonal (ato)*, which promotes neuronal development.

The target genes of Hh, Dpp, and Wg are often transcription factors that lie at the apex of developmental pathways. These factors are proposed to cooperate with Hox proteins to orchestrate development of the correct structure at appropriate positions within the segment or appendage. In the trunk, Wg in the ectoderm induces expression of the myogenic bHLH protein, *nautilus*, in somatic mesoderm progenitors, which subsequently develop into 30 somatic muscles of each abdominal segment. Wg, derived from either ectoderm or mesoderm, is also required to induce expression of the *S59* homeobox gene in muscle founder cells and of the *even-skipped* homeobox gene in heart and somatic muscle founders. Dpp in the dorsal ectoderm activates expression of the *tinman* and *bagpipe* homeobox genes in the underlying mesoderm, causing the mesoderm to separate into visceral mesoderm and dorsal mesoderm, which gives rise to cardiac mesoderm and the dorsal muscles of the body wall. In the wing, Hh induces expression of *collier*, which encodes a non-basic HLH transcription factor that controls formation of the central intervein of the wing by activating the transcription of *D-SRF*, which encodes the *Drosophila* orthologue of the human serum response factor. A current hypothesis is that developmental specificity in the appendages depends on a genetic program controlled by Hox proteins, Hox cofactors, and other selector gene products in conjunction with transcription factors activated by the Hh, Dpp, and Wg cascades.

B. Hh, Wg, and Dpp Feedback into Hox Selector Genes

Remarkably, the Hh, Dpp, and Wg signaling pathways, which define anterior/posterior and dorsal/ventral character, feed back into the Hox specificity system in a manner that defines the third axis (proximal/distal) by eliminating nuclear Exd in a large distal zone and by maintaining nuclear Exd in the proximal zone. Mosaic analysis using marked *exd* cells in different body regions has shown that Exd function

is not necessary in the distal regions of wings, halters, and legs, which is the same zone influenced most strongly by Hh, Dpp, and Wg signaling. Consistent with this observation, Exd resides in the inactive, cytoplasmic location in these distal zones. In fact, legs, wings, and halteres can only develop in the absence of Exd, and elimination of nuclear Exd is one of the first steps in generating an appendage. Exd must be functionally eliminated to allow the complete genetic response to the Hh, Dpp, and Wg signaling systems. Inactivation of Exd in the distal zone is accomplished by activating the Dpp and Wg pathways, which activate the expression of *distal-less (dll)*, which encodes a transcriptional repressor of *hth*. In the absence of Hth, Exd remains in the cytosol. The absence of Hth-Exd in distal zone nuclei permits Dpp and Wg to induce transcription of *dachshund (dac)* and *omb*, whereas nuclear Hth-Exd in the proximal zone prevents transcription of *dac* and *omb*, but does not alter transcription of Hh, Dpp, or Wg target genes. Therefore, the proximal/distal axis becomes subdivided according to *hth* expression and Hh-Dpp-Wg signaling. The proximal domain expresses *hth*, has nuclear Exd, and does not express a subset of target genes of Hh-Wg-Dpp signaling pathways. The distal domain does not express *hth*, has cytoplasmic Exd, and expresses the targets of Hh, Dpp, and Wg signaling. The profound developmental defects resulting from the enforced nuclear expression of Exd in the distal zone, therefore, result from reconfiguring the genetic targets of Hh, Dpp, and Wg signaling. Expression of E2a-Pbx in leukemia might also induce aberrant activation of morphogen target genes.

C. Vertebrate Orthologues of Hh, Wg, and Dpp Initiate and Organize Vertebrate Development

In vertebrates, Hh orthologues include Sonic hedgehog (Shh), Desert hedgehog (Dhh), and Indian hedgehog (Ihh); Dpp orthologues include transforming growth factor β (TGF-β), activin, and a large family of bone morphogenetic proteins (BMPs); Wg orthologues include over 18 members of the Wnt family. Like their *Drosophila* counterparts, activity gradients of these factors cooperate in patterning developing structures (e.g., the embryonic axis, the CNS, organs, and muscle) by activating the function of downstream transcription factors at different coordinates in the gradient fields. Early vertebrate development is unlike *Drosophila* development in an important respect. Early *Drosophila* development involves morphogenetic gradients of maternal transcription factors acting on 2000 nuclei in the egg prior to their cellularization, and, as a result, extracellular factors can not operate until after cellularization. In contrast, the vertebrate egg is a single cell at the outset, and the earliest organizational events, including the Hox gene and other selector gene expression, are specified by extracellular morphogens.

These concepts were first demonstrated in frogs in classic experiments by Hanna Speman and Hilde Mangold. During frog development, signals from the underlying vegetal hemisphere induce the formation of mesoderm at the equator between animal and vegetal hemisphere. A margin of approximately 60° of the mesoderm (the dorsal mesoderm) develops into notochord, and the remaining mesoderm is specified as ventral mesoderm. Interactions between the dorsal and the ventral mesoderm induce a process called "dorsalization," which involves the development of intermediate structures, such as somites (which differentiate into dermis, skeletal muscle, and cartilage), pronephros, and lateral plate. Speman and Mangold found that the dorsal mesoderm itself organizes all aspects of dorsalization. They grafted dorsal mesoderm from a lightly pigmented newt gastrula into the ventral side of a darkly pigmented gastrula of the same age and found that the resulting embryo developed a well-proportioned second dorsal axis in which a notochord formed from lightly pigmented cells, but intermediate structures developed from darkly pigmented cells. The ability of the donor dorsal mesoderm to specify the identity and to initiate differentiation of intermediate structures derived from cells of the recipient led Speman to designate this region as the organizer (hence the name Speman's organizer). It is now apparent that the organizer secretes a class of molecules that diffuse to form gradients and that these molecules bind and inhibit the function of BMP-4 and other TGF-β family factors. This process produces sharp gradients of active BMP-4 and TGF-β family factors, which directly pattern the embryo during gastrulation. Gradients of

Shh, Dhh, and Ihh also participate in this organizational process.

Hh orthologues regulate numerous developmental pathways in vertebrates, including patterning of the CNS and axial skeleton, generating anterior/posterior limb polarity, and normal development of the gastrointestinal tract, eye, lung, skin, and hair. At a high concentration, Shh, made by the notochord, induces development of the floor plate in the adjacent neural tube cells, whereas at a lower concentration, it specifies motor-neuron fate and induces sclerotome development in nonadjacent cells. A specific example of the interaction of Hh, Dpp, and Wg orthologues in development occurs during differentiation of a subset of somite cells into muscle. Wnt-1, produced in the dorsal neuronal tube, activates transcription of *myf5* in the dorsal/medial domain of the somite in regions that will differentiate to become muscles in the back. Wnt7a, produced in the dorsal ectoderm, "primes" somite cells in the dorsal/lateral domain for future expression of *myoD*; however, because these myogenic progenitors must migrate to the limb and body wall, where future differentiation will take place, the transcription of *myoD* is transiently repressed by bone morphogenetic protein 4 (BMP4), which is produced by lateral mesoderm. Removal of this signal after migration to the limb and body wall permits *myoD* expression and subsequent muscle differentiation. Shh, produced by the adjacent notochord and ventral neural tube, synergizes with both Wnt-1 and Wnt7a to augment activation of *myf5* and *myoD*. Understanding how the vertebrate orthologues of Hh, Dpp, and Wg proteins cooperate with selector genes in target gene activation continues to be an area of active research.

D. Human Oncogenes in Hh, Dpp, and Wg Signaling Pathways

1. Hh/Shh

The Hh signaling cascade is an example where *Drosophila* genetics assembled a pathway in the absence of biochemical data (Fig. 2, Table I). An important function of Hh in the *Drosophila* embryo is maintaining *wg* expression at 14 strips, where it specifies the character of the ectodermal cells that secrete the larval cuticle. Similar to *hh*, mutations in three

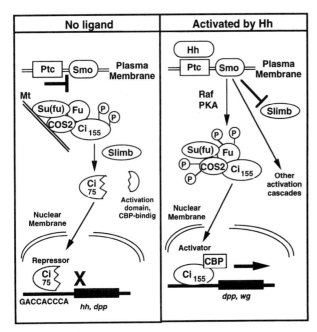

FIGURE 2 Hh/Shh signal transduction.

TABLE I

Drosophila–Human Orthologues in Morphogen Signal Transduction Pathways

Drosophila	Human
Hh/Shh	
Hh	Shh, Ihh, Dhh
Ptc	Ptc-1, Ptc-2
Smo	Smo
Fu	Fu
Su(fu)	Su(fu)
Cos2	Cos2
Ci	Gli, Gli2, Gli3
Slimb	Slimb
Wg/Wnt	
Wingless; Wg	Wnt
Frizzled; Frz	Frz
Dishevelled; Dsh	Dvl
Shaggy	GSK3
Armadillo	β-catenin
DAxin	Axin
DAPC	APC
Pangolin	TCF/LEF
Dpp/TGF-β/BMP	
Dpp	TGFβ, activin
	BMP
Mads	Smads

other segment polarity genes, *smoothened (smo)*, *fused (fu)*, and *cubitus interruptus (ci)*, eliminated wg transcription at parasegmental borders, whereas mutation of a fourth gene, *patched (ptc)*, permitted *wg* transcription in the absence of *hh*. These experiments were the first to suggest that Ptc is a persistent negative regulator of *wg* transcription and that inactivation of negative regulation required the functions of Hh, Smo, Fu, and Ci. Essentially, Hh regulates proteolytic processing that converts the zinc finger transcription factor, Ci, from a 150-kDa activator (Ci-150) to a 75-kDa repressor (Ci-75). In the absence of Hh, a domain of Ci-155 that intrinsically activates transcription and also binds the coactivator protein CBP is cleaved from the DNA-binding domain to form Ci-75, which functions as a transcriptional repressor of Hh responsive genes. Binding of Hh to Ptc suspends the inhibitory effect of Ptc on Smo. Active Smo prevents cleavage of Ci-155 through phosphorylation events regulated by protein kinase A (PKA), the serine/threonine kinase Fused (Fu), its regulator, Suppresser of Fused (Su[Fu]), and the kinesin-related protein Costal2 (Cos2). Ci-155 proceeds to activate Hh target genes *dpp* and *wg*.

Activation of signal transduction within the Hh pathway is a tumorigenic event. The Hh pathway is activated in humans through binding of Shh, Ihh, and Dhh to the Ptc-1 and Ptc-2 receptors (Ptc orthologues), and results in production of active forms of the Zn finger transcription factors, Gli, Gli-2, and Gli-3 (Ci orthologues). In humans, mutations producing truncated forms Gli-3 cause some forms of Pallister–Hall syndrome (postaxial polydactyly, cleft palate, and malformations in the larynx, heart, and genitourinary system), Greig cephalopolysyndactyly (axial skeletal deformities), and postaxial polydactyly type A. Inherited mutations in *ptc1* cause Gorlin or nevoid basal cell carcinoma syndrome (NBCCS/GS). NBCCS/GS is characterized by developmental defects and a disposition to a variety of tumors: basal cell carcinoma (BCC) in 97% of individuals; fibroma in 18%; menigioma in 5%; and meduloblastma, a very malignant tumor of the cerebellum, in 4%. Sporadic (noninherited) BCC is the most common type of human cancer, with over 750,000 cases per year in the

United States. Virtually all cases of BCC exhibit loss of function mutations in Ptc, activating mutations in Smo or Gli, or overexpression of *shh*. Amplification of *Gli* also occurs at a low frequency in rhabdomyosarcoma, osteosercoma, and malignant glioma, from which its name was derived. Thus far, the only proven target of Gli in vertebrates is HNF3beta, a member of the HNF family, another network of transcription factors that regulate early development. In addition to GLI proteins, which bind GACCAC-CCA, non-GLI transcription factors are also activated by Shh, such as COUP TFII. Therefore, important questions in the field of the effect of Shh signaling in development include identification of Gli target genes and an understanding of how Hox proteins modify this selection, as well as identifying non-Gli signaling mechanisms activated by Shh. From the context of oncogenesis, an important question is determining whether activation of the Shh cascade contributes to tumorigenesis principally because it stimulates cell proliferation (suggesting that other cooperating oncoproteins block differentiation) or whether chronic stimulation maintains cells in an early stage of the differentiation program that requires downregulation of the pathway for terminal differentiation and transition to the "stop proliferation" state. The latter mechanism may be operative because expression of *Gli* and *ptc-1* is only observed in proliferating cells adjacent to *shh*-expressing tissue during normal differentiation, suggesting that Gli-mediated transcription may need to be suppressed for cells to terminally differentiate.

2. Wg/Wnt

Wnt proteins share overall sequence identity and a conserved pattern of 23–24 cysteine residues. *Drosophila* contain at least 4 *wg* genes and mouse at least 18 *wnt* genes. The diversity of responses to Wnt ligands is likely due predominantly to the repertoire of Wnt receptors on the cell surface. Members of the *frizzled (Frz)* gene family encode Wnt receptors (Fig. 3; Table I). Wnt function is modulated extracellularly by a diverse group of inhibitors that bind Wnt proteins and inhibit their interaction with Frz (e.g., *Drosophila* Noggin). Activation of Frz receptors by Wnt proteins produces the same response: translocation of β-catenin to the nucleus where it converts

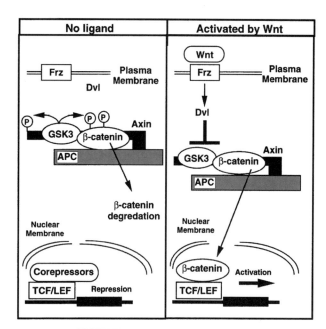

FIGURE 3 Wnt/Wg signal transduction.

the TCF/LEF DNA-binding factor from a transcriptional repressor into an activator. Therefore, the large repertoire or Wnt proteins and Frz receptors essential regulates a single parameter: the abundance of nuclear β-catenin. In the absence of Wnt proteins, Axin and adenomatous polyposis coli (APC) proteins serve as docking proteins that promote the phosphorylation of β-catenin by glycogen synthase kinase (GSK-3). Phosphorylation stabilizes Axin and targets β-catenin for ubiquitination and degradation through the proteosome pathway. Activation of Frz by Wnt prevents GSK-3 function through Dsh, resulting in the accumulation of nonphosphorylated β-catenin, which is not a target for ubiquitination. Dephosphorylation of Axin destabilizes the complex, releasing free β-catenin, which translocates to the nucleus and activates target gene transcription by binding TCF/LEF and other cofactors anchored to enhancer elements.

Three families of mutations that activate Wnt signaling are found in cancer: deletions in APC, stabilizing mutations in β-catenin, and activation of Wnt receptors. Each increases the concentration of nuclear β-catenin, solidifying the concept that oncoproteins within this pathway have the common impact of increasing nuclear levels of β-catenin. APC functions as a tumor suppresser protein because it acts as a negative regulator of nuclear β-catenin. Mutations that inactivate APC function are found in up to 80% of colon cancer. All mutations eliminate three or four 20 amino acid repeats that bind Axin. These mutations abrogate the ability of Axin to promote β-catenin phosphorylation and degradation, and promote nuclear accumulation of β-catenin. Mutations in β-catenin itself are found in colon carcinomas that lack mutations in APC. β-Catenin mutations occur at GSK-3 phosphorylation sites in the N-terminal "destruction box," whose phosphorylated form is recognized as a substrate for ubiquitin ligase and subsequent degradation by the proteosome pathway. The mutations abrogate β-catenin degradation, stabilizing the protein and promoting nuclear accumulation. Mutations at these phosphorylation sites and in this region of β-catenin occur in 5–20% of carcinomas of the colon, endometrium, liver, ovaries, prostate, and uterus. Activation of Wnt signaling by the ectopic expression of Wnt ligands, while demonstrated to induce mammary hyperplasia and mammary tumors in mouse models, has not yet been demonstrated in human cancer, despite numerous reports of sporadic aberrant expression of different *wnt* genes and *frz* receptors in small fractions of tumor cells. Many basic questions are yet unanswered concerning Wnt signaling. How does Frz transmit its signal? Are heterotrimeric G proteins coupled with Frz, as its seven transmembrane-spanning sequences would suggest? How are signals transduced from Frz to Dvl? How is β-catenin translocated to the nucleus?

3. Dpp/BMP/TGF-β

The TGF-β family of morphogens controls proliferation, differentiation, migration, and apoptosis of many different cell types. Receptors for the TGF-β family comprise type I (RI) and type II (RII) transmembrane proteins, both of which contain serine/threonine kinase activity (Fig. 4, Table I). There are at least six genes that encode RI receptors, denoted *alk1–alk6*. TGF-β and activin activate receptors Alk5 and Alk4, respectively, whereas BMPs activate Alk1, 2, 3, and 6. The ligand binds RII and catalyzes heterdimerization with a unique RI. Activated RI has a specific Smad substrate specificity. Smad1, 5, and 8 are substrates for the BMP receptors containing RI receptor kinases Alk2, 3, and 6, respectively. Smad2 and 3 are substrates for the TGF-β and activin complexes con-

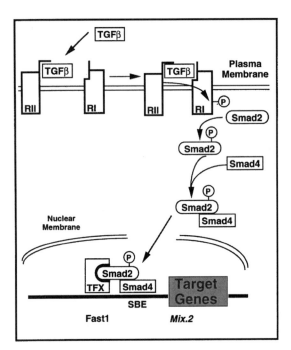

FIGURE 4   TGF-β/Dpp signal transduction.

taining RI receptors Alk5 and Alk4. After phosphorylation, Smad1, 2, 3, 5, and 8 heterodimerize with the common mediator Smad, Smad4. The complex between the unique Smad and Smad4 translocates to the nucleus and binds to promoters of specific target genes. DNA recognition is accomplished by a unique Smad4 domain that exhibits weak binding to Smad-binding DNA elements (SBE) whose consensus is GTCTAGNC. Interaction with other transcription factors (TFX in Fig. 4) is required for stable binding to target promoters, and the specific Smad component provides such interactions and therein provides a degree of selectivity in promoter targeting. Once bound, Smad proteins recruit coactivators or corepressors. Smad2 and Smad3 can recruit the coactivator CBP/p300, and Smad2 can also recruit the corepressor homeodomain protein TGIF. These cofactors, in turn, bind histone acetyltransferases that acetylate chromatin, loosen nucleosome packing, and promote transcriptional activation or histone deacetylases that deacetylate chromatin, tighten nucleosome packing, and repress transcription.

A classic example of transcriptional regulation by a Smad2–Smad4 complex is activation of the *mix.2* gene in *Xenopus*. Fast1 is a preexisting "winged helix" type transcription factor that binds the *mix.2* gene promoter but does not induce transcriptional activation. In response to either activin or TGF-β, the Smad2–Smad4 complex binds an SBE in the *mix.2* promoter and interacts with Fast1, inducing transcriptional activation. Antiproliferative responses to TGF-β are mediated by suppression of c-*myc* transcription and activation of transcription of the cell cycle suppresser gene *p21/Cip1* by Smad2–Smad4 complexes. Smad1 binds the HD of HoxC8, interferes with DNA binding by HoxC8, and therein counteracts repression of the osteopontin promoter by HoxC8. This is proposed to be the mechanism by which BMP2 upregulates *osteopontin* transcription during osteoblast differentiation and, importantly, establishes a mechanism by which Hox proteins as "selectors" interact with the transcription factors activated by TGF-β morphogens.

The involvement of TGF-β signaling in cancer was first discovered when a locus frequently deleted in pancreatic carcinoma (18q) was found to encode Smad4. Pancreatic cancers exhibited a high-frequency deletion of 17p, 9p, and 18q (90, 93, 50%). While eliminating the function of genes encoding the cell cycle regulators p53 (17p13) and *p16ink* (9p21) accounted for deletions at 17p and 9p, the presumptive tumor suppresser at 18q was unknown. The 18q gene was cloned by identifying the minimal common region eliminated in pancreatic tumors that harbored smaller chromosomal deletions. The gene was named *dpc4* ("deleted in pancreatic carcinoma locus 4) and, when sequenced, was found to encode a TGF-β responsive Smad protein. Further characterization of the Smad signaling system revealed this Smad to be the common Smad4 partner. Analysis of 35 pancreatic carcinomas that retained the *smad4* locus revealed that 9 contained mutations that abrogated the ability of Smad4 to heterodimerize with other Smad proteins, to translocate to the nucleus, to bind DNA, or to activate transcription. Cancers unresponsive to TGF-β, particularly those accompanying mutations in mismatch repair enzymes, also harbor inactivating mutations in the type II TGF-β receptor. Together, these mutations indicate that the transcriptional properties of Smad4 are essential for its tumor suppresser functions of promoting differentiation and suppressing proliferation.

Remarkably, oncogenic Ras mutations also target Smad4, causing its phosphorylation by MAP kinase at a site that prevents its nuclear import. Thus Ras, an oncoprotein classically associated with inducing proliferation, eliminates both cell cycle suppression and induction of cell differentiation by TGF-β family members. While perhaps counterintuitive, TGF-β overexpression is associated with a significant number of tumors of the pancreas, colon, stomach, lung, endometrium, prostate, breast, brain, and bone. In these cases, overexpression of TGF-β is preceded by mutations that make the cell unresponsive to growth suppression by TGF-β (e.g., Ras). Subsequent overexpression of TGF-β promotes tumor angiogenesis and has a potent immunosuppressive effect, including inhibition of natural and lymphocyte-activated T killer cells.

4. Human Oncogenes Target the Notch Morphogen Pathway

In *Drosophila*, Notch is a broadly expressed transmembrane receptor that binds two nondiffusible ligands, Serrate and Delta, which are anchored in the plasma membrane. Serrate and Delta are patterning morphogens. For example, differential signaling through Notch is required to establish the dorsal/ventral boundary of the wing margin. Coincident with ligand binding, the intracellular domain of Notch, denoted NIC, is released by proteolytic cleavage. NIC signals to multiple downstream effectors. In one pathway, NIC is translocated to the nucleus and binds the broadly expressed transcriptional repressor CBF-1, converting it to a transcriptional activator of genes whose promoters contain CBF-1-binding sites. NIC displaces corepressors (SMRT or N-CoR in vertebrates) that recruit histone deacetylase to CBF-1. Activation of Notch by Serrate and Delta is further regulated by Fringe, which can selectively bind and inactivate Delta.

Vertebrates broadly express four Notch receptors (Notch-1 through Notch-4), a family of Notch ligands ("Jagged" and "Delta-like"; orthologues of Serrate and Delta), and Lunatic Fringe, an orthologue of Fringe. Notch receptors and ligands are essential for embryonic development in mice; disruption of *notch-1* or *notch-2* genes or *jagged-1* or *jagged-2* ligand genes results in severe developmental defects and embryoic lethality. In many contexts, Notch activation inhibits or delays the differentiation of progenitors, therein allowing them to respond to stimuli that induce subsequent differentiation events. Activation of Notch suppresses muscle development by inducing transcription of HES-1, a bHLH protein that suppresses MyoD. Notch signaling by axons inhibits oligodendrocyte differentiation until specific neuronal signals trigger myelination. Notch-1 is expressed on CD34$^+$ cells, and ligand-induced activation of Notch-1 inhibits CD34$^+$ precursor maturation. When expressed in committed myeloid progenitors, NIC prevents terminal granulocytic differentiation, and expression of NIC in mouse bone marrow precursors permits development of immature T cells but completely prevents development of B cells.

Oncogenic *notch* genes encode truncated Notch proteins containing only NIC. In human immature T-ALL, the t(7;9) chromosomal translocation fuses a fragment of *notch-1* encoding NIC to the T-cell receptor β locus, which drives its constitutive expression. In cat T-cell leukemia, insertion of the feline leukemia provirus in genomic DNA induces persistent expression of the NIC of Notch-2. Mouse mammary tumor virus can initiate mammary carcinomas by integrating within *notch-4* and producing the Notch-4 NIC. Interestingly, expression of NIC in NIH3T3 fibroblasts also induces foci and growth in agar at levels comparable to activated Ras, demonstrating that Notch also regulates components of the cell cycle. Thus, tumorigenic properties of Notch include both repression of terminal differentiation and stimulation of cell division. This suggests that in at least certain normal developmental contexts, Notch couples stimulation of cell division with suppression of cell differentiation.

5. Human Oncogenes Prevent Differentiation Orchestrated by Selector Genes and Extracellular Morphogens

In addition to homologues of Hox selector proteins, their Ttx regulators, and the signaling components of the Hh, Dpp, Wg, and Notch pathways, mutant genes controlling differentiation downstream of these regulators are also oncogenes in human cancer. Dominant repressor versions of the retinoic acid receptor family of transcription factors (PML-RAR, PLZF-RAR) suppress differentiation in acute promyelocytic leukemia, and dominant-negative ver-

sions of the AML1 transcription factor (AML1-Eto, Tel-AML1) suppress normal differentiation in both human AML and ALL. The bHLH protein TAL1 interferes with differentiation in human stem cell and T-cell progenitor leukemias. Spi-1/Pu.1 prevents erythroid differentiation, leading to erythroleukemia. Indeed, it is almost certain that a large fraction of progenitor leukemias in which chromosomal translocations are not cytogenetically detectable (>50%) will contain oncogenes that arrest differentiation. Identifying such differentiation-arresting oncogenes and their biochemical mechanisms is an open field for future research.

6. Differentiation Therapy

The convergence of oncogene pathways on key regulatory factors suggests that inhibitors of these molecules may be potent cancer therapeutics. Inhibitors of GLI transcription factors, nuclear β-catenin, intracellular Notch domains, or Hox HD proteins could suppress proliferation and promote differentiation of a significant subset of carcinomas and leukemias. The rapid advances in methods to predict the structure of inhibitors (X-ray crystallography), to select inhibitors (chemical libraries and synthesis of predicted inhibitors), and to improve the potency of inhibitors (combinatorial chemistry) should make the identification of therapeutic drugs for many cancers a reality within this century.

See Also the Following Articles

Differentiation and the Role of Differentiation Inducers in Cancer Treatment • Tumor Suppressor Genes: Specific Classes

Bibliography

Barton, L. M., Gottgens, B., and Green, A. R. (1999). The stem cell leukaemia (SCL) gene: A critical regulator of haemopoietic and vascular development. *Intl. J. Biochem. Cell Biol.* **31,** 1193–1207.

Calonge, M. J., and Massague, J. (1999). Smad4/DPC4 silencing and hyperactive Ras jointly disrupt transforming growth factor-b antiproliferative responses in colon cancer cells. *J. Biol. Chem.* **274,** 33637–33643.

Casares, F., and Mann, R. S. (1998). Control of antennal versus leg development in *Drosophila*. *Nature* **392,** 723–726.

Collins, S. J. (1998). Acute promyelocytic leukemia: Relieving repression induces remission. *Blood* **91**, 2631–2633.

Cossu, G., and Borello, U. (1999). Wnt signaling and the activation of myogenesis in mammals. *EMBO J* **18**, 6867–6872.

Currie, P. D. (1998). Hedgehog's escape from Pandora's box. *J. Mol. Med.* **76**, 421–433.

Dale, L., and Wardle, F. C. (1999). A gradient of BMP activity specifies dorsal-ventral fates in early *Xenopus* embryos. *Cell Dev. Biol.* **10**, 319–326.

DiMartino, J. F., and Cleary, M. L. (1999). MLL rearrangements in haematological malignancies: Lessons from clinical and biological studies. *Br. J. Haematol.* **106**, 614–626.

Downing, J. R. (1999). The AML1-Eto chimaeric transcription factor in acute myeloid leukaemia: Biology and clinical significance. *Br. J. Haematol.* **106**, 296–308.

Gold, L. (1999). The role for transforming growth factor-β (TGF-β) in human cancer. *Crit. Rev. Oncogen.* **10**, 303–360.

Graba, Y., Aragnol, D., and Pradel, J. (1997). *Drosophila* Hox complex downstream targets and the function of homeotic genes. *BioEssays* **19**, 379–388.

Hahn, H., Wojnowski, L., Miller, G., and Zimmer, A. (1999). The patched signaling pathway in tumorigenesis and development: Lessons from animal models. *J. Mol. Med.* **77**, 459–468.

Hays, R., Buchanan, K., Neff, C., and Orenic, T. (1999). Patterning of *Drosophila* leg sensory organs through combinatorial signaling by Hedgehog, Decapentaplegic and Wingless. *Development* **126**, 2891–2899.

Kikuchi, A. (1999). Modulation of Wnt signaling by Axin and Axil. *Cytokine Growth Fac. Rev.* **10**, 255–265.

Mann, R. S., and Chan, S.-K. (1996). Extra specificity form extradenticle: The partnership between HOX and exd/Pbx homeodomain proteins. *Trends Genet.* **122**, 258–262.

Matise, M. P. and Joyner, A. L. (1999). Gli genes in development and cancer. *Oncogene* **18**, 7852–7859.

McGinnis, W., and Krumlauf, R. (1992). Homeobox genes and axial patterning. *Cell* **68**, 283–302.

Morata, G., and Sanchez-Herrero, E. (1999). Patterning mechanisms in the body trunk and the appendages of *Drosophila*. *Development* **126**, 2823–2828.

Polakis, P. (1999). The oncogenic activation of β-catenin. *Cur. Opin. Gen. Dev.* **9**, 15–21.

Shimamoto, T., Ohyashiki, K., Toyama, K., and Takeshita, K. (1998). *Int. J. Hematol.* **67**, 339–350.

Weinmaster, G. (1998). Notch signaling: Direct or what? *Curr. Opin. Genet. Dev.* **8**, 436–442.

Yang, X., Ji, X., Shi, X., and Cao, X. (2000). Smad1 domains interacting with Hoxc-8 induce osteoblast differentiation. *J. Biol. Chem.* **275**, 1065–1072.

Zakany, J., and Duboule, D. (1998). Hox genes in digit development and evolution. *Cell Tissue Res.* **296**, 19–25.

Zhou, S., Kinzler, K. W., and Vogelstein, B. (1999). Going Mad with Smads. *N. Engl. J. Med.* **341**, 1144–1145.

Differentiation and the Role of Differentiation Inducers in Cancer Treatment

Richard A. Rifkind
Victoria Richon
Paul A. Marks
Memorial Sloan-Kettering Cancer Center

Ronald Breslow
Columbia University

GLOSSARY

apoptosis Genetically programmed cell death triggered by cell-specific signals developmentally controlled, accompanied by, and recognized by a particular pattern of morphological changes and the digestion of chromatin into a discrete pattern of fragments.

carcinogenesis, oncogenesis The progressive acquisition, through the accumulation of mutations (in genes regulating genetic stability, cell proliferation and cell differentiation, cell-to-cell and cell-to-substrate adhesion, and perhaps other targets), of the capacity for unregulated proliferation and metastasis characteristic of cancers.

cell differentiation, cytodifferentiation, organogenesis The cellular and molecular process involving inter- and intracellular signaling mechanisms and the regulation of gene expression through controls that operate at the level of DNA (transcriptional controls) or at the level of mRNA or protein synthesis and stability (posttranscriptional controls), that transforms precursor cells, often with multilineage developmental potentialities, into phenotypically mature cells of the body's tissues and organs.

genotoxicity Damage to the genetic material, DNA.

growth factor Molecule, usually a polypeptide, that influences cellular proliferation (and often differentiation as well) through its binding to specific receptors.

kinase activity Enzymatic activity that transfers a phosphate group to the substrate of an enzyme, such as the protein substrate of a protein kinase, thereby altering the activity of the protein.

mutation Specific alterations to DNA, often as the result of genotoxic agents, but also due to errors during replication and to failures of the enzymatic machinery for error repair, which may be expressed as base substitutions, deletions, or transpositions in the genetic material.

oncogene Gene whose product potentiates the transformation of a normal cell to a cancer cell.

phase I, phase II clinical trials Trials designed to determine tolerable dose range and clinical toxicity (phase I) and to determine potential efficacy (phase II) of a therapeutic agent.

protooncogene Normal gene whose protein product often is an element in a signaling pathway regulating proliferation or differentiation, which, by alteration, can acquire the properties of an oncogene.

signaling pathway The molecular mechanism by which an extracellular condition, such as the attachment of a growth factor to its receptor, is translated through a cascade of molecular interations, often involving protein kinase activities and alterations in transcription factors, into a change in gene expression.

stochastic process A process whose kinetics is best described by a probability function.

transcriptional, posttranscriptional Describes the locus of control of gene expression at the level of synthesis of RNA from its DNA template (transcriptional control) or at subsequent levels, including the processing and stability of that RNA, the synthesis of protein from the RNA template, or the modification and/or stability of the protein product itself.

tumor suppressor gene A gene whose function diminishes the likelihood of a carcinogenic transformation of a normal to a cancer cell, often by coding for a product that blocks normal cell proliferation.

Cell differentiation plays an important role in the biology and genesis of cancer. Considerable evidence supports the concept that cancerous transformation of normal cells involves mechanisms that perturb the normal regulation of lineage-specific differentiation responsible for organogenesis. In addition, evidence also suggests that many, if not all, transformed cells, despite the carcinogenic lesions that they have sustained, still retain some capacity for normal differentiation, which can be triggered or revealed under appropriate conditions. This expression of normal differentiation can include as one manifestation both the suppression of proliferation and the triggering of apoptosis, which are the normal ultimate fates of

many fully differentiated tisssues. Many tumors retain, therefore, the capacity to suppress or lose the malignant properties that characterize the cancer. This fact has become the basis for current exploration of the potential of differentiation–induction by small chemical agents as a modality for the treatment, and possibly for the prevention, of cancer.

I. CANCER AS A DISORDER OF REGULATED DIFFERENTIATION

Almost all cancers contain a proportion of cells, sometimes large and more often small, which express some of the features characteristic of the tissue or organ of origin of the tumor. These are the features that the pathologist uses to identify the nature of a particular cancer, and staging a cancer according to the degree of expression of such differentiated features is standard clinical practice. The two principal biological implications of this observation are (1) that cancer involves a derangement of normal patterns and controls of differentiation and (2) that the derangement is not absolute; at least some, and perhaps all, cancer cells within a tumor population retain some capacity to express normal developmental features.

Additional evidence strengthening the conclusion that a blockade to normal differentiation underlies the phenomenon of neoplastic transformation comes from studies with temperature-sensitive oncogenic transforming viruses. Cells infected with such viruses display the normal development of differentiated features at one temperature but development is blocked and the cells display malignant properties at another temperature (the so-called "permissive" temperature). In this case, both malignancy and, conversely, differentiation are controlled by an environmental factor (in this case, heat) acting on the protein product of a transforming gene. It has also been shown that in some instances, neoplastic cells (teratocarcinomas, neuroblastomas, and leukemia cells have been tested) inserted into the normal embryonic environment of a mouse blastula, which is then reimplanted into a pregnant mouse, can differentiate normally, contributing progeny to the development of an apparently normal cancer-free mouse. Once again, evidence suggests that the blockade to normal differentiation associated with the neoplastic phenotype is not absolute but can be reversed under appropriate (in this case embryonal) environmental conditions. Further, as will be discussed at greater length here, several families of chemical agents also have the capacity to initiate normal differentiation and/or apoptosis in cancer cells, accompanied by the loss of their malignant characteristics or death of the cancer cells. For one such family of agents the intracellular molecular taret has been determined and such agents now form the basis for new chemotherapeutic strategies.

II. REGULATION OF DIFFERENTIATION AND CELL GROWTH

One of the principal linkages between cancer and differentiation resides in the relationship between cell differentiation and cell proliferation. Generally speaking, the more immature, less differentiated cells in a developmental lineage (the succession of cells that generate the mature functional cells of a particular organ or tissue) retain and exercise the capacity to undergo cell division and to replicate themselves, commonly under the influence of growth-regulating, hormone-like protein growth factors, which establish the rate of growth required to meet the needs of the organism and the organ or tissue for new cells. More mature, fully differentiated cells of a lineage, generally, have lost the capacity for continued cell division and no longer respond to lineage-specific growth factors. Many oncogenes and tumor suppressor genes whose activation or inactivation is implicated in malignant transformation control the production of growth factors (such as v-sis), the receptors for such growth factors (v-erbB, v-fms, v-kit), the intracellular signaling pathways responding to growth factor stimulation (v-src, v-ras, v-raf), and other critical proteins implicated in the regulation of cell proliferation and cell differentiation (pRB, p16, p53) or gene expression (transcription) factors, which represent the ultimate downstream activities in the signaling pathway. The result of altered expression of any or several of the genes for these regulatory elements is, frequently, a cell, arrested in its developmental pathway and which continues to replicate independent of the physiological signals controlling normal growth.

A second critical linkage between cancer and cell differentiation lies in the relationship, the profound significance of which has only recently become apparent, between cancer and the phenomenon of programmed cell death, known as apoptosis. Apoptosis can be viewed as a very particular form of cell differentiation which is triggered in response to the need to dispose, in an orderly fashion, of excess cells or cells that are at risk for or have sustained genotoxic damage. A growing number of both positive and negative genetic regulatory factors, which operate to control expression of the apoptotic pathway, have been identified. The c-myc protooncogene, whose protein product is a transcription-activating factor, is known to have growth-promoting functions accompanied by the capacity to initiate apoptosis. Suppression of the apoptosis program is the characteristic function of the product of the bcl-2 gene. Overexpression of the c-myc gene in combination with bcl-2 strikingly enhances tumor (lymphoma) formation in experimental animals, as a manifestation, presumably, of unregulated proliferation accompanied by the suppression of normal cell death. Another gene product, the p53 protein, loss of function of which, by mutation, is seen very frequently in a wide variety of cancers, is also implicated in the apoptosis pathway. The p53 protein acts, at least in part, as a cell cycle checkpoint regulator, designed to hold cells in G1 when they have sustained genotoxic damage (e.g., following τ-irradiation) and, presumably, require additional time for repair in order to avoid the accumulation of mutations. Evidence has accumulated suggesting that one outcome of this p53-mediated response to genotoxicity can be programmed cell death, the restriction of which, through defective p53 activity, may contribute to the accumulation of additional mutations leading to cancer.

III. DIFFERENTIATION-INDUCING CHEMICAL AGENTS

Taken together, current evidence suggests that cancer arises as the product of multiple mutational events involving the arrest of cells at an immature developmental stage, which retains the property of limitless proliferation, suppression of the normal developmental triggers for cell cycle withdrawal and apoptosis, which would protect the cells from accumulating additional carcinogenic mutations, and the effects of such additional mutations themselves. As already noted, it is evident that many, if not all, cancers, despite these developmental genetic lesions, still retain the capacity to express some developmentally normal characteristics and, under some circumstances, to suppress their malignant phenotype. Several classes of chemical agents, of which hybrid polar compounds (HPCs) [hexamethylene bisacetamide (HMBA), has become the prototype of this group) and retinoids (particularly, all-*trans* retinoic acid, ATRA) are the most studied examples, have the capacity to initiate such developmental programs in transformed cells. Other classes of agents with this property are known, including vitamin D3 analogs, certain tumor promoters of the phorbol ester class, cyclic AMP (cAMP) analogs, and a number of inhibitors of DNA and RNA synthesis (including some well-known cancer chemotherapeutic agents). Indeed, evidence shows that some of the effects of classical therapeutic agents, including irradiation as well as some chemotherapies, may not be mediated exclusively by direct cytotoxicity as is generally held, but also by triggering developmental programs, including differentiation, growth arrest, and/or apoptosis.

It may reasonably be assumed that differentiation-inducing agents, of the types noted, must act by influencing or modifying one or more of the several signaling pathways and the consequent pattern of gene expression responsible for cell differentiation and the linkages between and among differentiation, cell proliferation and apoptosis. With regard to these relationships and effects, studies on HMBA and related compounds, although not yet fully resolved with respect to their molecular mechanisms of activity, are the most complete at this time. HMBA was developed as a higher potency analog of dimethyl sulfoxide, which had been shown, by Charlotte Friend, to initiate apparently normal erythroid differentiation in a population of virus-transformed murine erythroleukemia cells (MELC) *in vitro*. Subsequently, even more potent HPCs have been synthesized (see later). This family of agents has been demonstrated to be active against a broad range of transformed cell targets, from man as well as mouse, and in cells de-

rived from many types of malignancies, including solid tumors as well as leukemias.

Although certainly not complete or proved, what is known of the mechanism of action of HMBA in inducing the differentiation of MELC may serve as a model for (1) projecting the molecular effects of other differentiation-inducing agents and (2) predicting some of the parameters that will be important when employing and studying these agents in the clinical setting. MELC are virus-transformed erythropoietic precursors, arrested at a developmental stage of the hematopoietic cell lineage approximating that of the colony-forming cell for erythropoiesis (CFUe), a precursor whose proliferation and further differentiation into red blood cells are normally controlled by a hormone, erythropoietin (Epo). Anemia or high altitude, e.g., lower oxygenation, induces the synthesis of Epo and stimulates the production of more red blood cells. Transformed MELC no longer respond to or require Epo for proliferation. Introduction of MELC into a susceptible mouse, either by virus infection (the Friend virus complex) or by transplantation, leads to a fatal leukemia of this cell type. MELC exposed *in vitro* to HMBA or related chemical compounds circumvent the blockade to normal differentiation and initiate a developmental sequence essentially identical to that seen in normal precursors. At the same time, these cells progressively lose the capacity to cause leukemia in a transplanted mouse, i.e., they lose their oncogenicity.

An important lesson is learned from observing the kinetics of HMBA-induced differentiation of MELC. It is a stochastic process; cells are progressively recruited, over time, to initiate the differentiation process. About 12 h of continuous exposure to HMBA is required before the first cells (about 10% of the population) are irreversibly committed to the developmental pathway. With further exposure, more and more cells are committed until almost all the cells have begun differentiation, by about 48 h. Experience has demonstrated that transformed cells of different lineages all require such continuous exposure to the differentiation inducer for protracted periods to achieve the maximum commitment of the cell population to differentiate and to lose oncogenicity; however, the *duration* of time required can vary greatly. MELC are about the fastest responding cells known.

At least for MELC, it appears, the cells must also be proliferating, i.e., in cell cycle, in order to respond to HMBA. MELC have a relatively short generation time (10–12 h) and virtually all the cells are in cell cycle, under test conditions. Both of these requirements, for prolonged administration to achieve full commitment to differentiate and for the tumor cells to be in cell cycle for the agent to be able to induce differentiation, if they hold true for human cancers *in vivo* as well, have profound implications for the clinical administration of differentiation inducers.

Although a discrete molecular target for HMBA has yet to be identified, a series of variants of HMBA, significantly more potent in their biological effects, have been synthesized, and a molecular target for their activities has been identified during the past decade. These compounds induce differentiation and inhibit the growth of cancer cells *in vitro* and in animal models of clinical cancer; several of these, all hydroxamic acid-based derivatives of the amide HMBA (Fig. 1), have been determined to function as potent inhibitors of a family of enzymes: the histone deacetylases (HDACs). For this reason, they are referred to as HDAC inhibitors. Histones are part of the core

Name	Structure	Opt. Conc.	% Diff.
SBHA	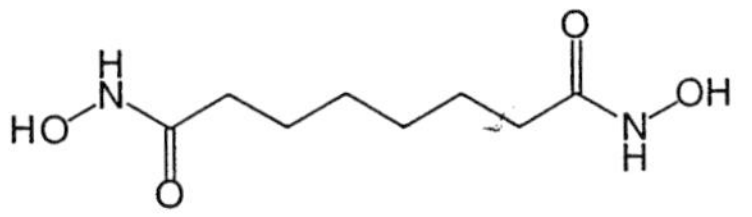	30 μM	90%
SAHA	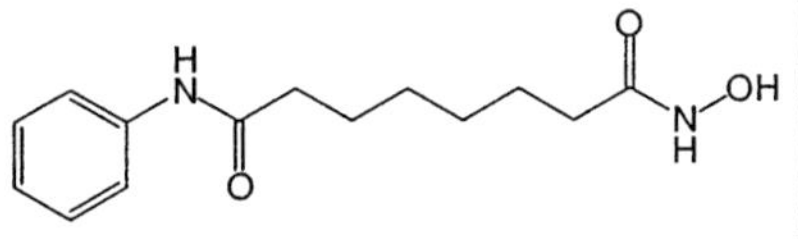	2.5 μM	68%
CBHA	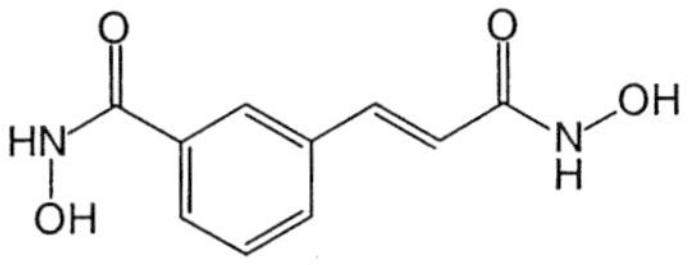	4.0 μM	73%
Pyroxamide	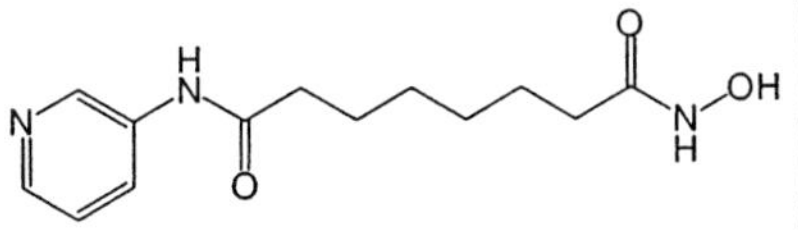	4.0 μM	51%

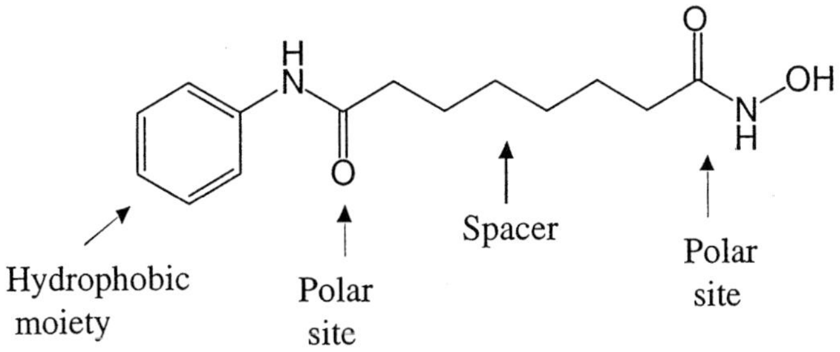

FIGURE 1 Hydroxamic acid-based hybrid polar compounds: SBHA, suberic bishydroxamic acid; SAHA, suberoyl anilide hydroxamic acid; CBHA, m-carboxy-cinnamic acid bishydroxamic acid.

proteins of nucleosome structures around which genomic DNA is wrapped to form chromatin. Acetylation and deacetylation of these nucleosomal proteins play a role in the regulation of gene expression by opening (acetylated form) and closing (deacetylated form) the chromatin, permitting and excluding penetration to the DNA of transcription factors needed for gene expression. Two classes of enzymes are involved in determining the state of acetylation of nucleosomal histones: histone acetyl transferases (HATs) and histone deacetylases. Several reports suggest that altered HAT or HDAC activity may be associated with cancers.

A. HDAC Inhibitors

A number of compounds have been shown to inhibit HDAC activity (Fig. 2). Butyrate and its analogs were

Name	Structure
Butyric Acid	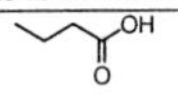
MS-27-275	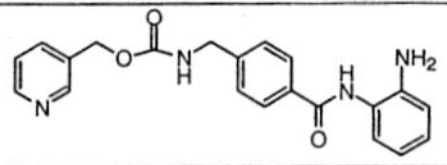
SAHA	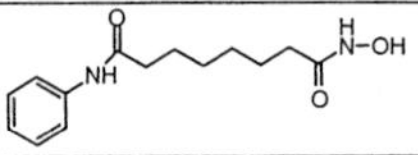
Trichostatin A	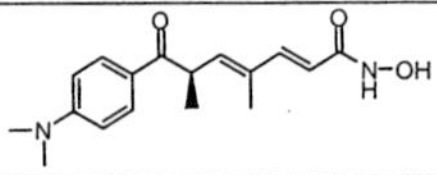
Oxamflatin	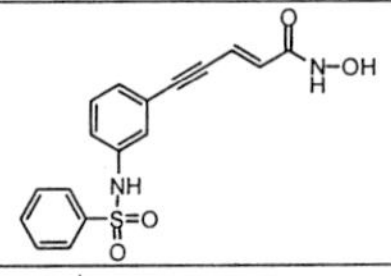
Apicidin	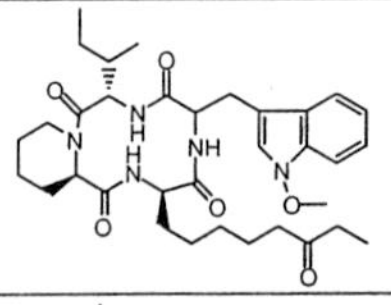
Depsipeptide	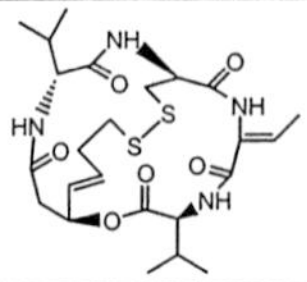
Depudecin	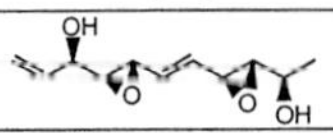
Trapoxin	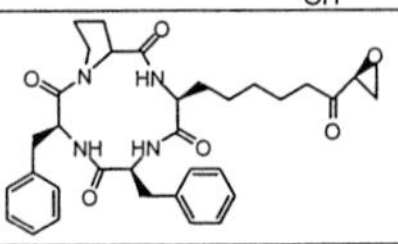

FIGURE 2 Histone deacetylase inhibitors. For SAHA, see Fig. 1.

among the earliest HDAC inhibitors identified. Butyrates are not very potent inhibitors and are active as HDAC inhibitors at millimolar concentrations, where they have been shown to have other cellular effects as well. Trichostatin A (TSA), originally developed as an antifungal agent, is a potent inhibitor of HDAC, active at nanomolar concentrations. HDACs are believed to be the critical molecular cellular target of TSA because cell lines selected for resistance to TSA have acquired an altered HDAC that is no longer inhibited by TSA. Apicidin is a fungal metabolite that exhibits potent, broad-spectrum, antiprotozoal activity and inhibits HDAC activity at nanomolar concentrations. Other HDAC inhibitors include depsipeptide (FR901228), a natural product isolated from chromobacterium violaceum; the benzamide MS-27-275; and oxamflatin. Trapoxin and depudecin form a class of natural product HDAC inhibitors, isolated from *Alternaria brassicicola*.

In our laboratories, a series of hydroxamide-based HPCs have been synthesized that inhibit HDACs, *in vitro* and *in vivo*, at micromolar concentrations and do so without substantial toxicity in animals (Fig. 1). Extensive structure–activity studies have been done with these hydroxamide-based HPCs. Essential characteristics of the compounds active as HDAC inhibitors are a polar site (the hydroxamide group), a six carbon hydrophobic spacer chain, a second polar site, and a terminal hydrophobic group. The prototype of this type of HDAC inhibitor is the compound suberoylanilide hydroxamic acid (SAHA), which bears some structural features in common with TSA but lacks the *in vivo* toxicities of TSA.

B. SAHA and TSA Bind to Histone Deacetylase

The structure of the histone deacetylase catalytic site in the HDAC core has been revealed by X-ray crystallography. HDACs share a roughly 390 amino acid region of homology, referred to as the deacetylase core. The residues that make up the active site are conserved across the HDAC family of proteins. The deacetylase core identifies a superfamily of genes, which includes an HDAC homologue in the hyperthermophilic bacterium A. acolicus. There is 35.2% base pair identity between the catalytic core of the

A. aecolicus HDAC-like protein and mammalian HDAC1. This bacterial HDAC homologue can deacetylate histones *in vitro*, with a specific activity equal to about 7.5% of that of partially purified mammalian HDACI. Its activity is inhibited by TSA and SAHA. Analysis of the deacetylase, and deacetylase complexed with TSA and with SAHA by X-ray crystallography, reveals that the active catalytic site in the HDAC homologue consists of a tubular pocket, at the base of which resides a zinc atom and two asparagine–histidine charge–relay systems. The hydroxamide ends of TSA and SAHA bind to the zinc molecule deep in the tubular pocket, while the carbon ring hydrophobic group projects out of the pocket and lies on the surface of the protein.

Hydroxamide-based HPCs, e.g., CBHA, SBHA, SAHA, and pyroxamide, inhibit partially purified HDAC1 and HDAC3 at concentrations that range between 0.01 and 1.0 μM. In support of the concept that HDAC inhibition is the principal molecular mechanism of action of these agents, a correlation has been demonstrated between the optimal concentration of the agent required for inducing MEL cell differentiation and that required for inhibition of the activity of partially purified HDAC1 or HDAC3 over a wide concentration range.

Employing MEL cells and T24 human bladder carcinoma cells in culture, the effects of SAHA and related hydroxamide-based HPCs on the acetylation of histones have been examined. It was found that SAHA, as well as pyroxamide, SBHA, and CBHA, causes an accumulation of acetylated histones. Using antibodies specific for each acetylated histone, SAHA leads to hyperacetylation of histones H2A, H2B, H3, and H4. These hyperacetylated histones can be detected as early as 1 h after the onset of exposure of MEL or T24 cells to SAHA or other hydroxamide-based HPCs. Acetylated histone accumulation reaches a maximum between 6 and 12 h and remains elevated for the duration of the culture with the inducer.

C. Activity of HDAC Inhibitors *in Vitro*

One of the most consistent molecular events in cells following exposure to these HDAC inhibitors is the induction of accumulation of the cyclin-dependent kinase inhibitor p21^{wafl}. The relation between HPC-mediated histone hyperacetylation and increased p21^{wafl} gene expression has been studied in SAHA-treated T24 cultured human bladder carcinoma cells. Evidence indicates that the induction of p21 by SAHA is governed, at least in part, by the acetylation of gene-associated histones (both promoter and structural sequences become associated with acetylated histones) and that this acetylation is gene specific in that genes not activated by SAHA do not display gene-associated histone acetylation. The increase in transcription of the p21 gene and the accumulation of p21 mRNA and p21 protein occur within 12 h of onset in culture with the HDAC inhibitor, and SAHA causes growth arrest of T24 cells in G1 within 12 to 24 h of onset of culture. It is likely that the induction of p21 plays an important, if not determinant, role in the cell growth arrest observed in these and other cell types.

Further evidence that the action of HDAC inhibitors is selective is the report of Verdin and colleagues: in cells cultured with TSA, only about 2% of genes show an increased or decreased expression compared to control cells. Our laboratory has obtained comparable results with transformed cells cultured with SAHA. The basis of this selectivity of SAHA or TSA is presently unknown.

D. *In Vivo* Studies with HDAC Inhibitors

The butyrate analog phenylbutyrate has been tested as an HDAC inhibitor in animals and in clinical acute promyelocytic leukemia, with mixed results. This agent is ineffective to moderately effective in inhibiting the growth of solid tumors or leukemias and relatively high doses are required. One report of a 13-year-old girl with relapsed acute promyelocytic leukemia unresponsive to retinoids (RA) alone reported that RA (45 mg/m^2) plus phenylbutyrate (150 mg/kg body weight) achieved a complete clinical remission, which persisted for 8 months before relapsing on treatment. The therapy did induce accumulation of acetylated histones in mononuclear blood cells during the period of clinical effectiveness.

TSA has been reported inactive against a human melanoma xenograft in nude mice, and azeloic bishydroxamate (ABHA, a variant of SAHA) caused significant inhibition of this tumor growth in the same animal model. Several other HDAC inhibitors have been shown to inhibit tumor growth in animal models. These include FR 901228, oxamflatin, MS-27-275, apicidin, and hydroxamide-based HPCs such as SAHA. Each of the HDAC inhibitors caused an accumulation of acetylated histones in the tumor tissue and/or normal tissues, e.g., spleen, bone marrow cells, and peripheral mononuclear cells.

Hydroxamic acid-based HPCs have been analyzed extensively in *in vivo* animal studies. For example, rats given N-methylnitrosourea (NMU) to induce mammary carcinoma were fed SAHA (900 ppm) continuously, beginning 7 days prior to administration of the carcinogen and thereafter. SAHA reduced the mammary tumor incidence by 40%, total tumors by 60%, and mean tumor volume by 78%, with no detectable side effects. A significant inhibition of tumor growth was also observed in animals fed SAHA beginning as late as day 18 or 28 after carcinogen. In another animal study, mice were treated with the tobacco-specific nitrosamine 4-(methylnitros-amino)-1-(3-pyridyl)-1-butanone (NNK) to induce lung tumors. Mice fed SAHA (900 ppm) continuously from 7 days prior to carcinogen administration showed significant inhibition of lung tumor formation again without toxic side effects. In a third rodent study, nude mice bearing transplanted CWR22 androgen-dependent human prostate tumors were administered SAHA (25, 50, or 100 mg/kg/day) by intraperitoneal injection daily for 3 weeks beginning with the first appearance of palpable tumors. SAHA suppressed tumor growth at all three doses, with 50 and 100 mg/kg/day causing a 97% reduction in the mean final tumor volume. Accumulation of acetylated histones H3 and H4 was found in CWR22 tumor cells within 6 h of SAHA administration. Similar effects on CWR22 tumor growth and histone hyperacetylation in this mouse model were observed using pyroxamide. There was no detectable toxicity with either agent as evaluated by weight gain and at necropsy of mice receiving the 50-mg/kg/day dose of these agents that had marked tumor growth inhibition. Taken together, these studies indicate that the hydroxamide-based HPCs, SAHA and pyroxamide, are promising agents to move forward into clinical trials. Based on these observations, SAHA and pyroxamide are now lead compounds from among the family of hydroxamide-based HPCs undergoing phase I clinical trials.

Bibliography

Ewen, M. E. (1994). The cell cycle and the retinoblastoma protein family. *Cancer Metast. Rev.* **13,** 45.

Hinds, P. W., and Weinberg, R. A. (1994). Tumor suppressor genes. *Curr. Opin. Genet. Dev.* **4,** 135.

La Thangue, N. B. (1994). DP and E2F proteins: Components of a heterodimeric transcription factor implicated in cell cycle control. *Curr. Opin. Cell Biol.* **6,** 443.

Marks, P. A, Richon V. M., and Rifkind, R. A. (2000). Histone deacetase inhibitors: Inducers of differentiation or apoptosis of transformed cells. *JNCI* **92,** 1210–1215.

Pierce, G. B., and Speers, W. C. (1988). Tumors as caricatures of the process of tissue renewal: Prospects for therapy by directing differentiation. *Cancer Res.* **48,** 1996.

Rifkind, R. A., and Marks, P. A. (1993). Induced differentiation: Molecular and Therapeutic Potential. In "The Pharmacology of Cell Differentiation" (R. A. Rifkind, ed.), p. 223. Elsevier Science Publishers B.V.

DNA-Based Cancer Vaccines

Jedd D. Wolchok
Alan N. Houghton

Memorial Sloan-Kettering Cancer Center and
Weill Medical College of Cornell University

GLOSSARY

cross-priming The process during which cells surrounding the site of DNA immunization become transfected and release preformed antigen through cell death or secretion. The antigen is then captured by antigen-presenting cells and is transported to draining lymph nodes for presentation to naïve T cells.

immunostimulatory sequences Unmethlyated cytosine–guanine sequences present normally in bacterial DNA, which result in the production of proinflammatory cytokines in mice and humans.

particle bombardment Process of introducing DNA vaccines during which plasmid conjugated to microscopic particles is delivered under high pressure to the skin.

plasmid DNA vaccine A circular piece of DNA purified from bacteria that contains elements required for the expression of genes for antigens of interest in eukaryotic cells.

xenogeneic immunization Vaccination with a homologous gene or protein derived from an organism of a different species.

Plasmid DNA vaccines represent a relatively new approach to immunization against antigens present on cancer cells. DNA vaccines are relatively simple to prepare and administer and present multiple epitopes within the complete coding sequence of an antigen. Immunostimulatory sequences naturally occurring in bacterial DNA may add to the ability of DNA vaccines to induce both antibody and T-cell responses. The results of experiments using mouse melanoma models have suggested that DNA immunization is a promising new approach to cancer vaccine therapy.

I. BACKGROUND

A. Cancer Vaccines: Introduction

A marked evolution has taken place in the field of cancer vaccines since the 1970s. A brief history of the field reveals that the earliest attempts to vaccinate against cancer were based on seminal observations of tumor rejection in inbred strains of mice by Prehn, Main, and others. These early models demonstrated that mice bearing a particular type of chemically induced tumor, which was subsequently surgically excised, could reject the same type of tumor when injected at a later time. However, injection of a different type of tumor was not observed, suggesting a tumor-specific immune response. It is then quite understandable that interest developed in the possibility of creating cancer vaccines for human clinical use, especially given the remarkable safety and efficacy of vaccination for infectious diseases.

B. Melanoma as a Model for Cancer Vaccine Investigation

The majority of clinical trials for cancer vaccines have involved melanoma, based on several lines of circumstantial evidence implicating the immune system in the biology of the disease. The natural history of melanoma in individual patients can be unpredictable, with some patients surviving many years with relatively stable metastatic disease. Melanoma is one of the few cancers in which rare, but well-documented, instances of spontaneous regression occur. Serum and T cells from individual melanoma patients have been intensively studied and found to contain antibodies and CD4$^+$ and CD8$^+$ T lymphocytes that recognize melanoma cells, and numerous antigens capable of immune recognition have been identified on melanoma cells (summarized in Table I). Also, the most active current therapies for metastatic melanoma utilize the immunologic agents interferon-α and interleukin-2. Although vaccines are also being investigated for many other malignancies, including breast, prostate, colorectal, and lung cancers, this article focuses on melanoma, as most of preclinical as well as clinical trial data are derived from studies of this disease.

TABLE I
Types of Antigens

Cateogry	Examples
Mutated proteins	CDK4, β-catenin
Differentiation antigens	Tyrosinase family, MART-1, gp100, gangliosides
Cancer-testis antigens	MAGE, BAGE, NY-ESO-1

C. Cellular Vaccines

Initial clinical trials have involved whole cell, cell lysate, or shed antigen vaccines from either autologous or allogeneic melanomas. Many preliminary trials have been completed with such vaccinees, and current phase III trials are underway for the allogeneic CancerVax and Melacine, as well as the NYU polyvalent shed antigen vaccine. These vaccines have the advantage of containing many potential antigenic targets. Disadvantages include an inability to specifically quantify response, as the exact molecular components of such vaccines are unknown. In addition, immunity to irrelevant allogeneic antigens may be induced.

D. Ganglioside Vaccines

The identification of potential antigenic targets was facilitated initially by the intensive study of sera from melanoma patients. Commonly identified antigens from this serologic screening program included the gangliosides. One of the earliest trials of a monoclonal antibody for cancer utilized R24, a mouse monoclonal antibody (mAb), which recognizes GD3 ganglioside. Clinical trials using R24 and other mAbs demonstrated a reproducible response rate of 10% in patients with advanced metastatic melanoma, confirming the importance of gangliosides in immunotherapy of melanoma and the ability of mAbs to shrink bulky tumors. The logical next step was to develop vaccines for active immunization against gangliosides. One such vaccine is a conjugate of the GM2 ganglioside with keyhole limpet hemocyanin as a carrier (GMK vaccine), which has been studied in a phase III trial as an adjuvant therapy for patients at high risk for recurrence of a surgically resected melanoma.

E. Peptide Vaccines

Advances in molecular biology since the 1980s have allowed for an unprecedented increase in understanding the events involved in the generation of an immune response. By application of such techniques to individual patient samples, several groups have identified peptides derived from antigens recognized by T cells from patients with cancer. Several different categories of antigens have been recognized, which are presented in Table I. In the area of melanoma, tyrosinase and tyrosinase-related protein-2 (TRP-2), components of normal and transformed melanocytic cells, have been demonstrated to be targets for CD8$^+$ T cells. These antigens, along with Melan-A/MART-1 and gp100, represent examples of melanocytic differentiation antigens. Antigens such as the MAGE family constitute the so-called cancer-testis antigens, as their expression is found only on normal spermatogonia and malignant cells. Other antigenic targets found include mutated self proteins such as CDK4 and β-catenin. Peptides that bind to specific HLA class I molecules can be readily synthesized; however, peptide vaccination is limited by the need for potent immunologic adjuvants.

II. DNA VACCINES

A. Introduction

All of the vaccination strategies just described have relative advantages and disadvantages. Cell-derived vaccines have a composition that is difficult to precisely define and with that comes risk of transmission of unknown pathogens. However, these vaccines contain numerous potential antigenic targets, which provide an advantage over the carbohydrate vaccines. Peptide vaccines are simple to produce but require adjuvants and are only effective in certain HLA types.

Several years ago, researchers interested in vaccines for infectious disease began to experiment with the possibility of injecting DNA coding for antigens of interest directly into animals. Advances in molecular biology had made available DNA plasmids containing constitutively active promoters, and such plasmid DNA is simple and inexpensive to produce. Intramuscular injection of plasmid DNA had already been shown to result in uptake of the DNA and expression of the encoded gene of interest by myocytes. The work of Ulmer and colleagues demonstrated the first successful immunization of mice with DNA encoding influenza A nucleoprotein, resulting in the production of antigen-specific antibodies, cytotoxic T lymphocytes (CTLs), and protection from subsequent viral challenge. The use of plasmid DNA for vaccination was therefore practical and effective.

DNA immunization has several advantages over more conventional means of vaccination (summarized in Table II). In contrast to peptide vaccines, which are MHC restricted and only present a single epitope, full-length DNA vaccines contain numerous epitopes, both known and unknown. Because the antigen is being transcribed and translated by host cells, it is more likely to be presented in the proper context of MHC and costimulatory molecules. Most methods for delivery of DNA vaccines (described later) involve the transfection of bone marrow-derived antigen-presenting cells, which contributes to the ability of DNA vaccines to generate potent immune responses. The precise mechanism of immunization following introduction of DNA remains to be elucidated, but it is known that at least a small percentage of antigen-presenting cells are directly transfected. Other surrounding cells may release antigen through cell death or secretion, facilitating a process known as cross-priming during which preformed antigen is captured by antigen-presenting cells and transported to draining lymph nodes for presentation to naïve T cells.

Another property unique to DNA vaccines is the presence of immunostimulatory sequences (ISS) within bacterial DNA. It has long been known that unmethylated CpG motifs in prokaryotic DNA are highly inflammatory and lead to the activation of B cells and the release of cytokines, including IL-6, IL-12, and both type I and II interferons. This inherent immunogenicity of DNA vaccines allows for their delivery without the need for immunologic adjuvants.

Based on the exciting initial studies of DNA vaccines for infectious diseases, several groups began to investigate the possibility of using DNA vaccines to

TABLE II
Relative Advantages of DNA-Based Vaccines

Capable of eliciting both antibody and T-cell responses

Simple to prepare

Long shelf life

Relatively inexpensive

Multiple potential epitopes: HLA restriction not required

Adjuvant effect of immunostimulatory sequences (CpG motifs)

generate antitumor immunity. The first studies performed with DNA vaccination in the authors' laboratory used a model mouse tumor antigen system in which P13.1 tumor cells express β-galactosidase. Mice were immunized with a plasmid encoding β-galactosidase by a gene gun system in which DNA conjugated to gold particles is propelled into depilated epidermis using helium gas. The results of these experiments confirmed the ability of DNA immunization to generate potent CTL responses and also demonstrated that mice could be protected from challenge with tumor expressing a model antigen. In addition, established tumors (3 or 7 days after subcutaneous injection) could be rejected after as few as one immunization with the β-galactosidase gene.

B. Plasmid DNA Vaccines: Preclinical Mouse Melanoma Studies

Data just presented clearly demonstrate the ability of DNA immunization to generate antitumor immunity using a model antigen system. In an attempt to apply this technique to more biologically relevant situations, attention was turned to a mouse melanoma system. The components of melanocytic cells that constitute the melanin synthetic machinery (tyrosinase and tyrosinase-related proteins −1 and -2 (gp75^{TRP-1} and TRP-2), gp100) have been identified a targets for both antibodies and T cells in patients with melanoma. Immunization of mice with xenogeneic human gp75 results in the production of Th2 antibodies, which recognize both human gp75 and mouse gp75, as well as protection from tumor challenge with a syngeneic B16 mouse melanoma. Tumor immunity was accompanied by an autoimmune depigmentation of coat, which had been previously observed in studies using injection of an anti-gp75 monoclonal antibody. Tumor protection was shown to require natural killer cells, CD4 cells, and intact Fcγ receptors. No CTL response to gp75 has been detected, and CD8 cells are not required. An immune response could only be generated with the use of xenogeneic human gp75. Injection of syngeneic mouse gp75 DNA did not elicit an antibody response and did not result in tumor protection or depigmentation.

TRP-2 is another melanosomal membrane glycoprotein that shares approximately 50% homology with gp75. Immunization of mice with human TRP-2 results in rapid depigmentation and tumor protection from syngeneic B16 challenge. In contrast to gp75, TRP-2 elicits a potent CTL response, which requires CD4 cells, CD8 cells, and perforin to achieve tumor protection. Although Th2 antibodies are generated by immunization with both human gp75 and TRP-2, only gp75 requires antibodies to mediate tumor protection. Thus, experiments with TRP-2 show that DNA immunization can result in a Th1 CTL response, as well as a Th2 antibody response. This ability to mobilize multiple arms of the immune system represents an additional advantage of DNA vaccines. These mouse melanoma studies also document the ability of DNA vaccines to mediate potent immune responses to otherwise poorly immunogenic "self" molecules.

C. DNA Vaccines: Other Tumor Systems

In addition to the melanoma model described earlier, DNA vaccines have been investigated using antigens from other types of cancer. Carcinoembryonic antigen (CEA) is a 200-kDa glycoprotein produced in large quantities by the first and second trimester fetus. In the adult, elevated levels of CEA can be detected in patients with adenocarcinomas as well as chronic obstructive pulmonary disease and cirrhosis. Immunization of mice with human CEA DNA results in the production of both antibodies and T cells, which recognize human CEA. The gene encoding MUC-1, an epithelial mucin expressed on a variety of adenocarcinomas, has also been used in DNA vaccination studies and was shown to induce protection from tumor challenge with a syngeneic MUC-1 expressing tumor.

B-cell lymphomas express distinct immunoglobulin molecules on their surface (idiotypes), which can serve as true tumor-specific antigens. Idiotypes from individual lymphomas can be cloned and inserted into expression vectors for use as DNA vaccines. Various constructs containing heavy chain, light chain, or single chain Fv (scFv) can be used, and some groups have even produced fusion proteins composed of idiotype and granulocyte-macrophage colony stimulating factor (GM-CSF). Immunization of mice with idiotype DNA vaccines results in an idiotype-specific antibody response, which can provide protection from challenge with the original lymphoma.

D. DNA Vaccines: Delivery Systems

The first studies of DNA vaccines were done simply by injecting plasmid intramuscularly (im) in mice. Subsequently, other routes for needle/syringe injection have been explored, including intradermal, intravenous, intraperitoneal, and subcutaneous injection. There is inconsistency in the literature as to which route is optimal for antibody versus CTL responses; however, most investigators have focused on intradermal and intramuscular injections. Administration of DNA using jet injection devices has also been investigated in both preclinical and clinical trials. Such devices may lead to more potent immune responses and have the important safety advantage of needle-free design. Application of DNA to oral, vaginal, and rectal mucosal surfaces for the purpose of inducing mucosal immunity has also been explored.

The development of the gene gun has popularized the technique of particle bombardment for the delivery of DNA vaccines. DNA conjugated to micron-sized gold particles can be delivered to the epidermis by high-pressure helium gas. Relatively small quantities of DNA are needed for gene gun immunization (1 μg vs 100 μg for im). This method of immunization has the added advantage of accessing epidermal dendritic (Langerhans) cells, which are among the most potent antigen-presenting cells.

A recently described method of DNA immunization uses a live attenuated strain of *Salmonella typhimurium* to deliver plasmid orally. The bacteria is used as a carrier for DNA transfer and has the advantage of acting as an adjuvant through the release of numerous cytokines. Both antibody and T-cell responses have been documented with this system, and tumor protection using a model tumor antigen system was also demonstrated.

E. DNA Vaccines: Clinical Trials

As of the writing of this volume, several clinical trials for DNA vaccines have been completed in the area of infectious disease (malaria and HIV). These trials have documented the safety and immunogenicity of DNA vaccines. Study of the malaria circumsporozoite vaccine clearly demonstrated the advantages of DNA vaccines, especially the ability to generate CTL responses to multiple MHC-restricted epitopes. In the area of DNA-based vaccines for human cancer, the only completed studies are those involving Allovectin-7, a liposomally encapsulated plasmid containing the HLA-B7 gene. The goal of the Allovectin-7 trials was to stimulate an immune response to injected tumors based on recognition of the allogeneic HLA-B7 molecule. These trials documented the safety of intratumoral plasmid DNA injection, as well as suggesting efficacy of the local antitumor effect. Ongoing clinical trials of DNA vaccines for cancer include idiotype DNA vaccines at Stanford University and a gp100 DNA vaccine study at the National Cancer Institute. Further trials are expected to begin shortly for other melanosomal antigens, as well as for CEA.

See Also the Following Articles

ANTIBODIES IN THE GENE THERAPY OF CANCER • ANTI-IDIOTYPIC ANTIBODY VACCINES • CANCER VACCINES: GENE THERAPY AND DENDRITIC CELL-BASED VACCINES • CANCER VACCINES: PEPTIDE- AND PROTEIN-BASED VACCINES • CARBOHYDRATE-BASED VACCINES • MELANOMA: CELLULAR AND MOLECULAR ABNORMALITIES • RESISTANCE TO ANTIBODY THERAPY • TUMOR ANTIGENS

Bibliography

Bowne, W. B., Srinivasan, R., Wolchok, J. D., Hawkins, W. G., Blachere, N. E., Dyall, R., Lewis, J. J., and Houghton, A. N. (1999). Coupling and uncoupling of tumor immunity and autoimmunity. *J. Exp. Med.* **190**, 1717–1722.

Donnelly, J. J., Ulmer, J. B., Shiver, J. W., and Liu, M. A. (1997). DNA vaccines. *Annu. Rev. Immunol.* **15**, 617–648.

Huygen, K., Content, J., Denis, O., Montgomery, D. L., Yawman, A. M., Deck, R. R., DeWitt, C. M., Orme, I. M., Baldwin, S., D'Souza, C., Drowart, A., Lozes, E., Vandenbussche, P., Van Vooren, J. P., Liu, M. A., & Ulmer, J. B. (1996). Immunogenicity and protective efficacy of a tuberculosis DNA vaccine. *Nature Med.* **2**, 893–898.

Ugen, K. E., Nyland, S. B., Boyer, J. D., Vidal, C., Lera, L., Rasheid, S., Chattergoon, M., Bagarazzi, M. L., Ciccarelli, R., Higgins, T., Baine, Y., Ginsberg, R., Macgregor, R. R., and Weiner, D. B. (1998). DNA vaccination with HIV-1 expressing constructs elicits immune responses in humans. *Vaccine* **16**, 1818–1821.

Ulmer, J. B., Donnelly, J. J., Parker, S. E., Rhodes, G. H., Felgner, P. L., Dwarki, V. J., Gromkowski, S. H., Deck, R. R.,

DeWitt, C. M., Friedman, A., *et al.* (1993). Heterologous protection against influenza by injection of DNA encoding a viral protein. *Science* **259,** 1745–1749.

Wang, R., Doolan, D. L., Le, T. P., Hedstrom, R. C., Coonan, K. M., Charoenvit, Y., Jones, T. R., Hobart, P., Margalith, M., Ng, J., Weiss, W. R., Sedegah, M., de Taisne, C., Norman, J. A., and Hoffman, S. L. (1998). Induction of antigen-specific cytotoxic T lymphocytes in humans by a malaria DNA vaccine. *Science* **282,** 476–480.

Weber, L. W., Bowne, W. B., Wolchok, J. D., Srinivasan, R., Qin, J., Moroi, Y., Clynes, R., Song, P., Lewis, J. J., and Houghton, A. N. (1998). Tumor immunity and autoimmunity induced by immunization with homologous DNA. *J. Clin. Invest.* **102,** 1258–1264.

DNA Damage, DNA Repair, and Mutagenesis

Miriam C. Poirier

National Cancer Institute

Ainsley Weston

National Institute for Occupational Safety and Health

I. Introduction
II. DNA Damage
III. DNA Repair
IV. Mutagenesis

GLOSSARY

carcinogen–DNA adducts Addition products that typically form as a result of covalent binding between a chemical carcinogen and a DNA base.

DNA damage Consists of (a) formation of carcinogen–DNA adducts and other chemical modifications of DNA bases and (b) alterations in DNA ultrastructure (DNA strand cross-links/DNA strand breaks/chromatid exchanges/chromosomal loss).

DNA mismatch mutations Unconventional base pairings, which can be *transitions* (purine to purine or pyrimidine to pyrimidine change resulting in two possible mispairings: G-T and A-C) or *transversions* (purine to pyrimidine or pyrimidine to purine resulting in six possible mispairings: A-A, C-C, G-G, T-T, A-G, or C-T).

DNA repair Consists of multiple different mechanisms for re-

moving DNA damage from the genome and is a critical component in the maintenance of genomic integrity.

mutagenesis A permanent alteration in DNA structure that produces miscopying of information during DNA replication and yields abnormal gene products (proteins).

DNA damage consists of (a) formation of carcinogen–DNA adducts and other chemical modifications of DNA bases and (b) alterations in DNA ultrastructure (DNA strand cross-links/DNA strand breaks/chromatid exchanges/chromosomal loss). DNA damage can be induced by endogenous processes and by exogenous chemical and physical agents. A potential consequence of DNA damage is *mutagenesis*, i.e., a permanent alteration in DNA structure that produces miscopying of information during DNA replication and yields abnormal gene products (proteins). The process of carcinogenesis is considered to require mutations in multiple critical genes, and the risk of cancer is reduced when potentially mutagenic DNA damage is removed by DNA repair.

I. INTRODUCTION

DNA damage and the consequential mutagenic events are considered to bring about changes in gene expression that produce a loss of growth control, a clonal growth of cells, and ultimately a tumor. A substantial period of time is required for a tumor to become evident, and DNA damage is considered to be necessary but not sufficient for tumorigenesis, as other events, such as mutagenesis and cell proliferation, must also take place. DNA adduct levels, measured at any point in time, reflect tissue-specific rates of damage processing, which include carcinogen activation, DNA repair, adduct instability, tissue turnover, and other events. In experimental models, dose–response associations have been observed for DNA damage, mutagenesis, and tumorigenesis. Reductions in tumor incidences have been observed when DNA damage has been lowered, either by DNA repair processes or by administering compounds that inhibit DNA adduct formation (chemoprevention).

II. DNA DAMAGE

A. DNA-Damaging Agents

Agents that damage DNA can be either endogenous or exogenous, and they can be either direct acting or require metabolic activation. Arguably the most frequent endogenous mechanisms by which the integrity of DNA is compromised include deamination (cytosine or methylcytosine to form uracil or thymine) and depurination. The endogenous formation of reactive oxygen species and other free radicals, and exogenous exposure to irradiation (ultraviolet light, radon, X rays), can act to damage DNA directly producing cross-links, strand breaks, chromosomal aberrations, and other structural changes. Normal endogenous metabolic processes, e.g., lipid peroxidation, redox cycling, and endogenous nitrosation, can produce oxygen-free radicals, oxidative DNA adducts, etheno adducts, and nitrosamine adducts. Pathways that lead to the formation of oxygen radicals include degradation of organic peroxides (catechol, hydroquinone, and 4-nitroquinoline-N-oxide), hydrogen peroxide, lipid peroxidation, and the catalytic cycling of some enzymes. The role of endogenous nitric oxide is un-

clear because while there is the potential for oxyradical formation, nitric oxide is an effective scavenger of superoxide, resulting in nitrogen dioxide formation. Exposure to tumor promoters indirectly increases oxyradical formation; examples include the action of phorbol esters, mediated by protein kinase C, and inflammation mediated by nitric oxide. Oxygen free radicals produce multiple DNA adducts, including 8-hydroxy-deoxyguanosine, thymine glycol, 5-hydroxy-uracil, 5-hydroxymethyl-uracil, and 6-hydroxy-5,6-dihydro-cytidine.

Exogenous (xenobiotic) DNA-damaging agents that are highly reactive and direct acting include radon, ultraviolet light, the nitrosoureas, some nitrosamines, ethylene oxide, and ozone. However, most exogenous chemical carcinogens are inert, such as the polycyclic aromatic hydrocarbons (PAHs), and require metabolic activation in order to become adducted to DNA. Inert exogenous agents are altered metabolically by families of enzymes that convert a small fraction of the initial dose to highly reactive intermediate metabolites that react directly with specific bases in nucleic acids. Examples of exogenous carcinogens are some plant and fungal products (aflatoxins, ochratoxins, hydrazines), pyrolysis products from cooking (heterocyclic amines, PAHs), industrial combustion products (aromatic amines, PAHs, nitro-PAHs, benzene, vinyl chloride, nitrosamines, ethylene oxide), urban pollution contaminants (PAHs, nitro-PAHs, aromatic amines), and contents of tobacco smoke (PAHs, nitosamines, aromatic amines). In addition, oxyradical formation may result from futile redox cycling that occurs through the metabolic activation of otherwise inert chemical carcinogens.

B. DNA Adduct Structures

There are a wide variety of DNA adduct structures, and some examples are shown in Fig. 1. Alkylation occurs when a portion of a chemical carcinogen, such as a methyl or ethyl moiety, becomes covalently bound to DNA. Alkyl radicals form during the metabolic activation of certain N-nitrosamines or spontaneously in the case of N-alkylureas (N-methyl-N-nitrosourea) and N-nitrosoguanidines. Protonated alkyl functional groups, which become available to modify DNA, attack nucleophilic centers on DNA bases. There are 10 of these: N1, N3, and N7 of adenine; N3 of cyto-

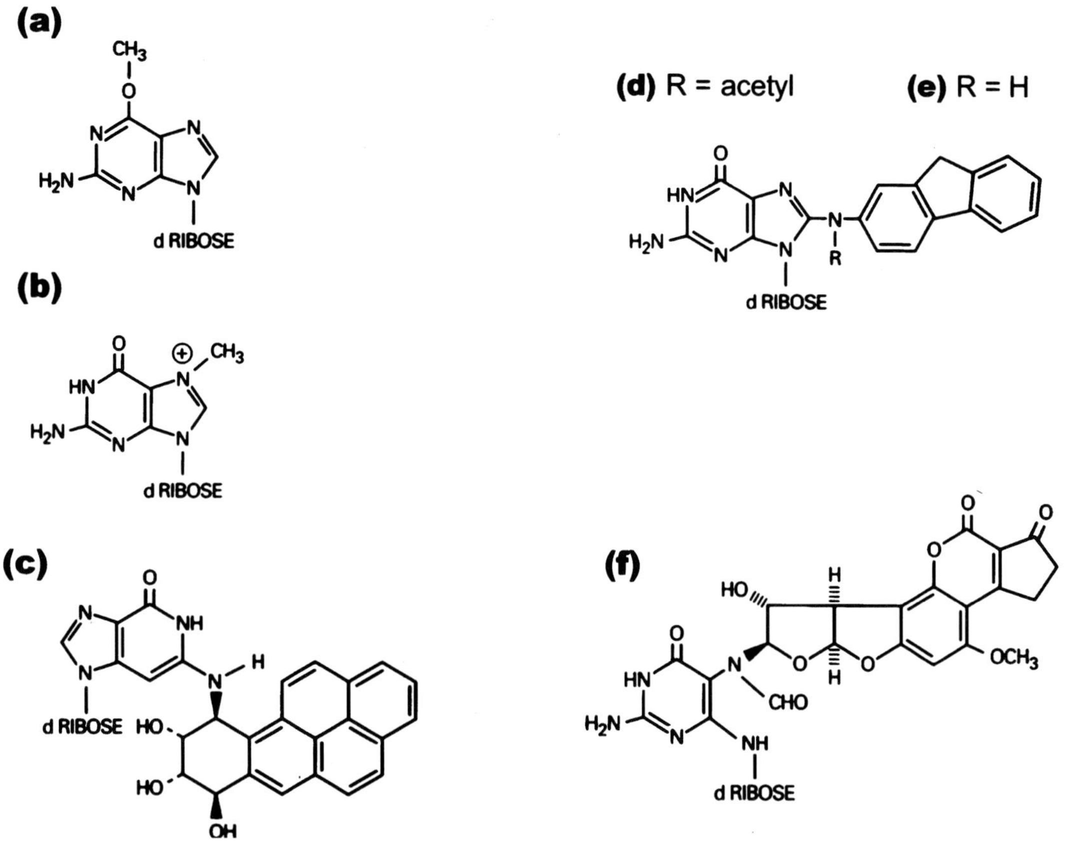

FIGURE 1 DNA adduct structures: (a) O^6-methyldeoxyguanosine; (b) N^7-methyldeoxyguanosine; (c) (7R)-N^2-(10[7β,8α,9α-trihydroxy-7,8,9,10-tetrahydro-benzo[α]pyrene]yl)-deoxyguanosine; (d) N-(deoxyguanosin-8-yl)-2-(acetylamino)fluorene; (e) N-(deoxyguanosin-8-yl)-2-(amino)fluorene; and (f) 8,9-dihydro-8-(N^5-formyl- 2′, 5′, 6′-triamino-4′-oxo-N^5-pyrimidyl)-9-hydroxy-aflatoxin B_1.

sine; N2, O6, and N7 of guanosine; and O2, N3, and O4 of thymidine. Repair of some of these lesions is correlated with mutagenicity; e.g., O6-methyldeoxyguanosine (Fig. 1a) can be repaired and is a promutagenic lesion, whereas N7-methyldeoxyguanosine (Fig. 1b) is neither repaired nor mutagenic.

Larger, aromatic-type ("bulky") DNA adducts are formed by covalent binding between the whole carcinogen molecule and DNA. The resulting three-dimensional structures reside either in the minor or in the major groove of the DNA helix and may cause distortion. Activated benzo[a]pyrene binds preferentially to the exocyclic (N2) amino group of deoxyguanosine (Fig. 1c). Guanine is a preferred site for modification by most PAHs, but covalent binding to deoxyadenosine and deoxycytosine is also possible. The major aromatic amine DNA adducts form at the C8 position of deoxyguanosine (Fig. 1d), but adducts

are possible at the C8, N2, and O6 positions of deoxyguanosine and deoxyadenosine. Activation of aflatoxin B_1 produces adduction primarily at the N7 position of deoxyguanosine (Fig. 1e). As with smaller molecular weight adducts, the correlation among DNA adduct formation, mutagenicity, and DNA repair is not always predictable, and certain adducts appear to be more closely associated with mutagenicity than others.

C. Methods for DNA Adduct Determination

Methods currently used alone for carcinogen–DNA adduct detection include radiolabeling, immunoassays, immunohistochemistry, ^{32}P-postlabeling, fluorescence and phosphorescence spectroscopy, mass spectrometry, atomic absorbance spectrometry, electrochemical conductance, and accelerator mass spectrometry. These methods work well for animal models where only one agent is under study, but in human tissues they are often unable to distinguish individual adducts, as multiple human exposures typically produce multiple DNA adducts. Success in the characterization of individual human DNA adducts has been obtained by combining preparative methods (immunoaffinity chromatography, high-performance liquid chromatography or gas chromatography) with immunoassays, ^{32}P-postlabeling, synchronous fluorescence spectrometry, or mass spectrometry. Most DNA adduct assays are able to detect as little as 1 adduct in 10^9 nucleotides using ~5–100 μg of DNA. Novel and sophisticated mass spectrometry-based methods have sensitivities similar to those found with more conventional assays, and accelerator mass spectrometry can detect 1 adduct in 10^{12} nucleotides but requires administration of exceedingly low levels of radioactively labeled compounds.

III. DNA REPAIR

The capacity for DNA repair, or removal of DNA damage, is a critical component in the maintenance of genomic integrity and stability. A diminished capacity for DNA repair is associated with carcinogenesis, birth defects, premature aging, and a foreshortened life span. There are six known basic DNA repair mechanisms: direct DNA repair, base excision repair, nucleotide excision repair, mismatch repair, homologous recombination, and nonhomologous end joining. In order to accomplish this range of DNA repair mechanisms cells employ complex protein–protein and protein–nucleic acid interactions. Hitherto, at least 125 genes have been implicated, either directly or indirectly in DNA repair. A list of human DNA repair genes, together with structural and functional information and potentially associated diseases, has been published.

A common thematic scenario, in the presence of genetic damage, is the implementation of cell cycle delay for the purpose of allowing DNA repair to take place. In this scenario, a damage recognition sensor triggers a signal transduction cascade and downstream effectors direct G_1 or G_2 arrest in concert with the

proteins operationally responsible for the repair process. Although each repair mechanism is different, the DNA repair process is typically composed of some or all of several generic steps, which include damage recognition, damage removal or excision, resynthesis or patch synthesis, and ligation. These processes proceed efficiently because of the existence of multiprotein complexes comprising all of the machinery necessary to complete all of the DNA repair steps.

A. Direct DNA Repair

Alkyltransferases are suicide enzymes that commute alkyl groups from alkylated bases (O^6-methyldeoxyguanosine, Fig. 1a) to a cysteine residue. This process occurs in the active site in the enzyme in the absence of strand scission (Fig. 2a). One molecule of alkyltransferase is consumed during repair of one alkyl lesion in DNA; hence the term suicide enzyme.

B. Base and Nucleotide Excision Repair

Base and nucleotide excision repair processes are similar in that they both require strand scission, removal of a DNA segment containing the damaged base, reconstruction of the lost bases (repair patch), and ligation. A major difference is the size of the repair patch, which is about 3 bases in base excision repair and approximately 30–50 bases in nucleotide excision repair. The cell appears to choose one or the other based on the molecular size of the damage, as base excision repair is typically used to remove alkylation, whereas nucleotide excision repair is employed with large molecular weight ("bulky") carcinogens.

In base excision repair (Fig. 2bi), a glycosylase discards a damaged base, typically containing an adducted methyl, ethyl, or hydroxyl group. An apurinic endonuclease complexed with a 3′ repair diesterase displaces the glycosylase, degrading one to three bases on the damaged strand. The repair patch is typically synthesized by DNA polymerase β. Ligation is accomplished by one of a number of possible ligases that include LIG1, LIG3α, or LIG3β. An additional ligase variant, LIG 2, is formed through the proteolytic modification of LIG3.

Nucleotide excision repair (Fig. 2bii) proceeds by preincision lesion recognition, usually in response to

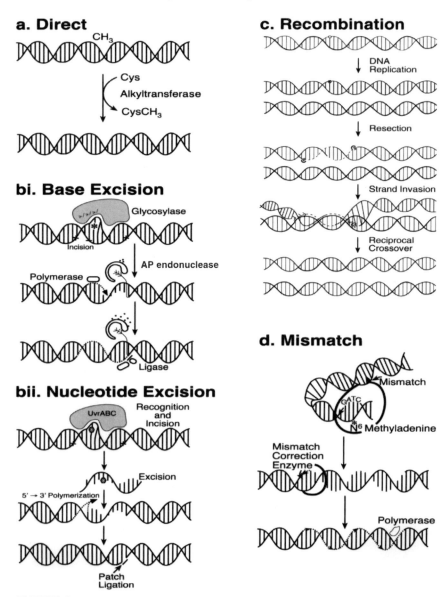

FIGURE 2 Mechanisms of DNA repair: (a) direct repair catalyzed by alkyltransferase; (bi) base excision repair, catalyzed by a glycosylase and an apurinic endonuclease; (bii) nucleotide excision repair, catalyzed by an endonuclease complex (e.g., UvrABC); (c) homologous recombination, catalyzed by a helicase complex; and (d) mismatch repair, catalyzed by a proofreading complex containing a correctional enzyme (e.g., hMLH1).

the formation of a bulky DNA adduct or ultraviolet damage (see Section II.B). Excinuclease complexes (e.g., UvrABC) are able to recognize such damage and excise a portion (30–50 bases) of the affected strand. For example, the XPC.RAD23 recognition complex recruits XPA.TFIIH to the repair location. An endonuclease, such as XPF, XPG, or FEN, clips out the damage. A 5′ - 3′ polymerase [e.g., polII ac-

tivated through phosphorylation by CDK activating kinase (CAK), a member of the TFIIH complex] fills in the gap using the undamaged strand as a template. Ligation completes the closure at the 3′ junction. This type of DNA repair is generally strand specific, and the transcribed strand is preferentially repaired over the nontranscribed or non-DNA coding strand. In addition, transcribing regions of the DNA are often repaired preferentially (transcription-coupled repair), compared to the whole genome (global genomic repair). Nucleotide excision repair is critical in humans. Loss of function of this pathway causes sensitivity to ultraviolet light, as evidenced in the clinic by the disease xeroderma pigmentosum. The clinical syndrome can involve loss of function of various proteins necessary for the nucleotide excision repair pathway, but all affected individuals experience early onset of skin cancer as a result of sun exposure.

C. Homologous Recombination and Postreplication Repair

Homologous recombination (Fig. 2c) occurs in response to DNA double strand breaks or the DNA damage tolerance mechanism known as postreplication repair. In postreplication repair, the replication polymerase either stops at the replication fork when DNA damage is detected or proceeds past the damaged base, leaving a gap. The gap can be filled with an adenine residue, potentially creating a mismatch (see Section III.D) or homologous recombination may occur. Thus, this mechanism is likely to introduce DNA sequence errors. Ionizing radiation, oxidative or mechanical stress, and some toxic chemicals can cause DNA double strand breaks, which also stimulate homologous recombination.

Homologous recombination is mediated by a helical nucleoprotein, such as the mammalian *RAD51*, which is homologous to *RecA* of *Escherichia coli*. The first step involves simultaneous 5′ - 3′ resection of both strands catalyzed by a nuclease (e.g., nibrin complexed with RAD50/MREII). The 5′ tails of the disrupted DNA species invade the homologous duplex DNA and polymerization occurs using the appropriate, undamaged duplex strands as templates. Ligation and Holliday junction resolution occur on completion of polymerization through the action of an endonuclease. This can either result in a reciprocal crossover event or can be accomplished without crossover.

D. Mismatch Repair

DNA mismatches are unconventional base pairings, which can be transitions (purine to purine or pyrim-

idine to pyrimidine change resulting in two possible mispairings: G-T and A-C) or transversions (purine to pyrimidine or pyrimidine to purine resulting in six possible mispairings: A-A, C-C, G-G, T-T, A-G, or C-T). These can occur through mistakes in normal DNA repair processes or as a result of replication on a damaged template. For example, in postreplication repair (see Section III.C), the single nucleotide gaps that may be left are always filled by DNA polymerases with an adenine residue. This type of damage can also result from deamination of cytosine or 5-methylcytosine, which leaves a thymidine residue. Transversion mispairs are repaired more efficiently than transition mispairs, as a probable consequence of differential recognition.

Both nucleotide excision repair and mismatch repair have the common features that a large piece of the damaged strand is degraded and resynthesis occurs on the intact strand followed by ligation. However, a major difference is the mechanism of recognition (Fig. 2d). In mismatch repair the recognition protein complex (e.g., MLH1-MSH2-MSH6-PMS1 or MLH1-MSH2-MSH6-PMS2) binds simultaneously to the mismatch and the nearest unmethylated adenine in the recognition sequence GATC. The whole intervening strand sequence is excised, and the proliferating cell nuclear antigen can be recruited as a sliding clamp, providing a support for the action of DNA polymerases δ or ε. Ligation may be brought about by a ligase complexed to the polymerase (e.g., LIG1 complexes with polδ). This mechanism of DNA repair is critical in humans, and mutations in *hPMS1*, *hPMS2*, *hMLH1*, *hMLH2*, and *hMLH3* can predispose to cancers of the bowel and brain. Such mutations are relatively common, and 1 in ~200 persons are carriers.

E. Nonhomologous End Joining

Nonhomologous end joining is responsible for the repair of double strand breaks. This is a distinct but complementary mechanism to homologous recombination. The mechanism is homology independent because repair occurs without copying an undamaged template. Unless ligation of two complementary or blunt ends can restore the original sequence, a deletion mutation will result. Consequently, this mechanism is sometimes referred to as "illegitimate." The process of nonhomologous end joining is mediated by XRCC4 and the DNA-dependent protein kinase holoenzyme. The site of a double strand break may be blunt or asymmetric. In the event of asymmetry, resection occurs with the purpose of creating a pair of blunt ends, which are then joined by LIG4 (XRCC4 is an essential cofactor for LIG4). Because nonhomologous end joining may require limited nucleotide degradation before ligation can occur, it is therefore error prone, leading to small deletions.

IV. MUTAGENESIS

A. Definition, Cause, and Evolutionary Importance

A mutation is a change in the sequence of DNA that results in alterations in the transcribed RNA and the translated protein (Fig. 3). Mutagenic DNA damage can be caused by endogenous and exogenous chemical and physical agents (see Section II.A) and typically consists of small molecular changes involving a few nucleotides (substitutions/insertions/deletions) or changes involving the gain or loss of large groups of nucleotides (large insertions/deletions/strand breaks/chromatid exchanges). Mutations can also occur as a result of cellular efforts to repair DNA (see Sections III.C, III.D, and III.E). During mutagenesis, structural changes in the DNA will result in the translation of proteins that have a loss of function, a gain of function, or no functional change. Mutagenesis is a major mechanism of evolution; typically mutations that lead to beneficial function will be selected for and others that lead to deleterious traits will be selected against.

B. Nature of Mutations and Mechanisms of Mutagenesis

Mutations involving small molecular changes consist of single base substitutions, as well as small insertions and deletions. Single base substitutions, missense mutations, are designated transitions if the original base and the new base are both either purines or pyrimidines (e.g., a G → A transition). However, a change from a purine to a pyrimidine or vice versa (e.g., G → T) is designated a transversion. Single base substitu-

tions may have a rate of reversion similar to the original mutation rate. Insertions and deletions occur due to slippage and misrecognition by the polymerase, and such changes in the DNA structure may cause alterations in the DNA "reading frame," i.e., the sequence of nucleotides coding for a functional protein. For example, a normal reading frame contains signals for starting and stopping transcription that may be lost, and loss or gain of a critical amino acid in the coded protein may result in a change of catalytic activity. Mutations that change the reading frame of a protein are termed frameshift mutations.

Large DNA sequence rearrangements by recombination, chromatid exchange, or other copying errors can produce the accumulation of multiple mutations and genomic instability, as well as acceleration of the carcinogenic process. For example, large insertions and deletions can lead to chromosomal aberrations, and as the damaged cells attempt to divide, chromosomal DNA fragments can become translocated to unaccustomed positions and expressed inappropriately. Progressive genetic instability is a prominent feature of the carcinogenic process, resulting in the frequent occurrence of aneuploidy, gene amplification, microsatellite instability, chromosomal aberrations, and chromosomal loss in malignant tumors. The process of tumor progression appears to select for cells that are mutated in genes that function to ensure the stability of the genome, thus giving rise to the suggestion that most human cancers progress because they acquire a "mutator phenotype."

Mutagenesis has been dissected on a molecular level by site-specific studies in which an oligonucleotide carrying a specific damaged base or DNA adduct has been repaired by mammalian cultured cells and, after fixation, the resulting DNA mutations have been revealed by polymerase chain reaction and sequencing of the oligonucleotide target. Hemminki and colleagues have summarized mutagenic DNA adducts of various carcinogens elucidated by site-specific investigations. This type of study has demonstrated that the ability of an adduct to induce mutagenesis depends upon the DNA sequence context, the specific site that is modified on the base, the size and three-dimensional conformation of the modified base, conformational attributes of the adduct (tautomerization, ionization, rotation), and the polymerase involved.

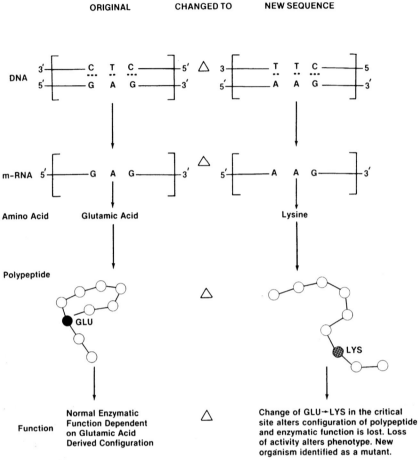

FIGURE 3 Schematic representation of a change in DNA sequence (CTC becomes TTC), which results in a miscoding of mRNA and a change in amino acid sequence (primary protein structure), whereby a glutamine residue is replaced by a lysine residue. This change in protein primary structure could lead to an alteration in protein folding and/or catalytic capacity.

Mutation "hot spots," or highly mutable sequences, have been observed in both site-specific mutagenesis and conventional mutagenesis assays and may occur for some of the reasons mentioned earlier. Frequently, a single carcinogen will produce multiple types of DNA adducts and mutations; however, it is occasionally possible to deduce the identity of a mutagenic DNA damaging agent by the mutations observed.

C. Measurement of Mutations

Mutations are typically measured in a specific target gene in cultured cells by growing mutagen-exposed cells in a selective medium that supports the growth of mutant but not normal cells, and growing normal cells in an optimal medium. Mutant frequencies are expressed as the number of mutated cell clones per 10^6 normal growing cell clones. Mutagen-induced reversion in the mutated histidine gene of *Salmonella typhimurium* comprises the basis of the Ames assay, which has been widely used to screen chemicals for potential genotoxicity.

In mammalian cells, a frequently investigated mutational target is the hypoxanthine–guanine phosphoribosyl–pyrophosphate (HPRT) gene, which produces a protein involved in the incorporation of nucleotides into nucleic acids. Normal cells are selectively inhibited by the aberrant base analog 6-thioguanine, but cells that have a mutated HPRT enzyme grow well because the drug is not incorporated into nucleic acids. In addition to experimental models, *HPRT* mutagenesis in human peripheral T-cell lymphocytes is frequently used as a human biomarker, and studies in the general population show that the individual burden of *HPRT* mutations increases with age.

An additional human mutational biomarker is glycophorin A, a glycoprotein on the surface of red blood cells. Approximately 50% of the population are heterozygous, expressing both M and N alleles. The mutations scored are typically deletions of the M allele, which can be found by flow cytometry using specific antibodies. As the mutant clones persist, an age-related increase in glycophorin A mutant burden has been observed in the general population.

In addition to the classical methods for detecting mutagenesis, newer methods include sequencing-based molecular biology approaches and transgenic mice carrying the *Lac* locus. Mutations can be evaluated in any organ of a mouse carrying *Lac* as a target gene, as the locus can be packaged into a phage vector. After exposure of the whole mouse to a mutagen, DNA is extracted and cloned into the phage and mutations are determined by the clonal growth of colored colonies.

D. Mutations and Cancer

Mutations in the genes responsible for growth control allow uncontrolled clones of cells to become tumors. Hereditary cancers in children can be caused by mutations occurring in germline cells; however, somatic mutations occurring as a result of chemical or physical exposures will also destroy the normal cellular control of growth and cause cancer later in life. Typically, the critical target genes mutated in the process of tumorigenesis are protooncogenes and tumor suppressor genes. These genes have normal growth controlling functions; however, the mutated forms are activated oncogenes that have growth-enhancing properties and lost or inactivated tumor supressor genes that no longer have the capacity to control growth. Certain tumor supressor genes not only lose growth repression function, but can, in addition, gain oncogenic function; some *TP53* mutants are prone to this dual mechanism because their normal function involves transcriptional activation.

See Also the Following Articles

CARCINOGEN–DNA ADDUCTS • CELLULAR RESPONSES TO DNA DAMAGE • CHEMICAL MUTAGENESIS AND CARCINOGENESIS • DNA METHYLATION AND CANCER • HEREDITARY COLON CANCER AND DNA MISMATCH REPAIR • MISMATCH REPAIR: BIOCHEMISTRY AND GENETICS • RESISTANCE TO DNA-DAMAGING AGENTS

Bibliography

Brusick, D. J. (1999). Genetic Toxicology. *In* "Toxicology," p. 127. Academic Press, San Diego.

Cotton, R. G. H. (1997). "Mutation Detection." Oxford Univ. Press, Oxford.

Friedberg, E. C., Walker, G. C., and Seide, W. (eds.) (1995). Introduction to mutagenesis. *In* "DNA Repair and Mutagenesis," p. 59. American Society for Microbiology Press, Washington, DC.

Hemminki, K., Koskinen, M., Rajaniemi, H., and Zhao, C. (2000). DNA adducts, mutations and cancer 2000. *Regu. Toxicol. Pharmacol.* **32,** 264–275.

Khanna, K. K., and Jackson, S. P. (2001). DNA double-strand breaks: Signaling, repair and the cancer connection. *Nature Genet.* **27,** 247–254.

Loeb, K. R., and Loeb, L. A. (2000). Significance of multiple mutations in cancer. *Carcinogenesis* **21,** 379–385.

Pfeiffer, P., Goedecke, W., and Obe, G. (2000). Mechanism of DNA double-strand break repair and their potential to include chromosomal aberrations. *Mutagenesis* **15,** 289–302.

Poirier, M. C., Santella, R. M., and Weston, A. (2000). Carcinogen macromolecular adducts and their measurement. *Carcinogenesis* **21,** 353–359.

Provost, G. S., Kretz, P. L., Hamner, R. T., Mathews, C. D., Rogers, B. J., Lundberg, K. S., Dycaico, M. J., and Short, J. M. (1993). Transgenic systems for in vivo mutation analysis. *Mutat. Res.* **288,** 133–149.

Ronen, A., and Glickman, B. W. (2001). Human DNA repair genes. *Environ. Mol. Mutagen.* **37,** 241–283.

Singer, B., and Kuśmierek, J. T. (1982). Chemical Mutagenesis. *Annu. Rev. Biochem.* **52,** 655–693.

Watson, J. D., Hopkins, N. H., Roberts, J. W., Steitz, J. A., and Weiner, A. M. (eds.) (1987). The mutability and repair of DNA. *In* "Molecular Biology of the Gene," p. 339. Benjamin/Cummings, Menlo Park, CA.

DNA Methylation and Cancer

Peter A. Jones
University of Southern California

GLOSSARY

CpG island A region of vertebrate DNA about 0.5–2 kb in length that does not show the 80% suppression in the frequency of occurrence of this dinucleotide observed in bulk DNA. CpG islands are often associated with genes and are not methylated in the germline.

de novo methylation New methylation of previously unmethylated CpG sites. It occurs during development, particularly on genes located on the inactive X chromosome in female mammals on imprinted genes and commonly occurs in cancer cells.

DNA methyltransferases Enzymes that transfer the methyl group from S-adenosyl-L-methionine to the 5 position of cytosine show a marked preference for CpG palindromes in double-stranded DNA in which one cytosine is already methylated. Three active mammalian enzymes have been identified so far: DNMT-1, 3a, and 3b.

hypermethylation A process of increased methylation of a region of DNA or an individual CpG site.

hypomethylation A process of decreased methylation of a region of DNA or an individual CpG site.

5-Methylcytosine The only modified base in vertebrate DNA; found almost exclusively at CpG sites and is formed by the enzymatic transfer of a methyl group from S-adenosyl-L-methionine to the 5 position of the cytosine ring in newly synthesized DNA. About 4% of cytosines are modified in this way, and 5-methylcytosine makes up 1% of the bases in human DNA.

5-Methylcytosine, which is the only modified base found in human DNA, occurs predominantly at the sequence CpG. DNA methylation has been shown to be essential for vertebrate development where its major role seems to be as a mediator of gene suppression. Pervasive changes in DNA methylation patterns take place during the process of oncogenic transformation. These changes, involving focal hypermethylation at the same time as the overall level of methylation is decreased, may be responsible for causing the permanent inactivation of tumor suppressor genes and in altering chromosome stability. 5-Methylcytosine also participates in the generation of a high percentage of point mutations that inactivate tumor-suppressor genes in the germline and somatic cells, thus contributing very significantly to oncogenic transformation and progression.

I. INTRODUCTION

5-Methylcytosine is formed by the postsynthetic modification of cytosine residues at the CpG dinucleotide sequence in double-stranded DNA in a reaction catalyzed by DNA methyltransferase enzymes. The three known enzymes (DNMT-1, DNMT-3a, and DNMT-3b) apply a methyl group from S-adenosylmethionine to the 5 position of the cytosine ring, and this modification is the only naturally occurring covalent base change seen in vertebrate DNA. Interest in the field of DNA methylation has been stimulated by observations that DNA methylation contributes to the silencing of genes on the inactive X chromosome, imprinted genes, and intragenomic parasites. DNA methylation is essential for vertebrate development, as mice lacking functional DNA methyltransferase genes do not survive gestation.

In addition to its role in suppressing the expression of genes by interfering with the function of promoters, DNA methylation plays a role in the stability of repetitive DNA sequences and may also be involved in processes resulting in allelic loss. Changes in gene expression and losses of chromosomes are fundamental to the development of neoplasia and thus DNA methylation is likely to play an important part in generating the oncogenic phenotype.

5-Methylcytosine is inherently mutagenic in both prokaryotes and eukaryotes and contributes to more than one-third of all of the point mutations that cause human genetic diseases. Thus the modified base, which constitutes only 1% of human DNA, is the site of more than 30% of all point mutations. An important discovery has been the observation that a significant number of inactivating point mutations in tumor suppressor genes, which are responsible for tumor

initiation and progression, also occur at DNA methylation sites in somatic cells. DNA methylation therefore influences several key molecular events known to contribute to carcinogenesis.

II. CpG ISLANDS

Almost all of the 5-methylcytosine present in vertebrate DNA is found at the simple palindromic sequence CpG. This site is the preferred substrate for the DNA methyltransferases, one of which (DNMT-1) shows a marked preference for hemimethylated CpG palindromes created after DNA replication. The DNMT-1 enzyme is considered to function as a "maintenance enzyme" and is thought to copy preexisting patterns of methylation after DNA replication. The majority of CpG sites that contain 5-methylcytosine in vertebrate cells are methylated at both cytosine residues, and half (or hemi) methylation has been infrequently observed. Two methylation states are therefore seen in cells; full methylation of both cytosines or complete unmethylation. The patterns and distribution of methylation vary during development and two enzymes (DNMT-3a and DNMT-3b) have been discovered that may function as "*de novo*" methyltransferases and be responsible for the establishment of DNA methylation patterns during development. However, because all three known enzymes have both "*de novo*" and "maintenance" activities, the precise roles of the enzymes in setting up and copying the patterns are not yet known.

The CpG site is the only dinucleotide sequence underrepresented in vertebrate DNAs and occurs at approximately one-fifth the frequency expected on a random statistical basis. Interestingly, the distribution of CpG sites is not random. Most DNA shows a substantial CpG suppression, whereas the remaining 1% of DNA shows no such suppression; these regions are called CpG islands. CpG islands are approximately 0.5–2.0 kb in length and show the expected frequency of occurrence of CpG relative to GpC and are often associated with genes.

The suppression of CpG is thought to be due to the fact that 5-methylcytosine has an increased potential to deaminate spontaneously to thymine, which, being a normal DNA constituent, is more difficult for the cell to repair than uracil formed by the deamination of cytosine. CpG islands are thought to exist because they have never been methylated in the germline and thus have not been subjected to the same evolutionary mutagenic pressure that would have led to their eventual disappearance from DNA. The frequent association of CpG islands with genes has proven to be useful in the isolation and identification of genes where they are often, but not exclusively, associated with promoter regions. Two kinds of promoters therefore have to be considered in any discussion of DNA methylation, those that are CpG poor and those that are CpG islands.

III. TRANSDUCTION OF THE METHYLATION SIGNAL

Two general pathways by which methylation of promoter elements could block transcription have been proposed. First, modification of a cytosine residue at the recognition site for a specific transcription factor might interfere directly with factor binding, thus resulting in transcriptional inactivity. In this regard, it has been shown that the binding of some transcription factors, such as c-*myc*, are inhibited by the presence of 5-methylcytosine at the cognate sequence, whereas SP1 binds equally well to both methylated and unmethylated DNA. Methylation of promoter elements might therefore actively inhibit transcription, but the responses of individual factors to methylation vary.

The second mechanism by which DNA methylation acts to inhibit the transcriptional activity of promoters is by a mechanism in which the binding of "methylated CpG-binding proteins" is encouraged by DNA methylation, thus blocking access by transcription factors. The laboratory of Adrian Bird showed that the methylation of CpG islands leads to an altered chromatin structure with ensuing promoter inactivity. Exciting new work has shown that binding of one such protein (MeCP2) to methylated CpG islands results in the recruitment of histone deacetylase and other transcriptional inactivators to the promoter, resulting in a condensed, transcriptionally inactive promoter. This mechanism is likely to be of particular importance in ensuring the heritable quiescence of promoters such as those associated with the inactivated X chromosome.

Most of the documented examples of methylation of CpG islands in normal cells are on genes located on the inactive X chromosome and on imprinted genes. It remains controversial as to whether this methylation follows or precedes the inactivation of the X chromosome at an early stage of embryonic development. However, it has been conclusively shown in appropriate gene transfer experiments that once methylation has occurred, it can strongly suppress the activity of the promoter. The facts that methylation of CpG islands suppresses gene activity and that these islands become extensively methylated during development, when the X chromosome is inactivated, strongly suggest that methylation reinforces gene silencing and has developmental significance.

In contrast to the situation on inactive X chromosomes, there is little evidence that CpG islands become methylated on autosomal genes in normal tissues. It therefore seems unlikely that the activities of these genes are subject to methylation "control" as part of normal development. Exceptions to this generality are the methylation of CpG-rich regions in some genes subject to genomic imprinting.

IV. METHYLATION CHANGES IN TUMOR TISSUES

Early studies on methylation changes in human tumors demonstrated a hypomethylation associated with the malignant state, and a generalized decrease in the amount of 5-methylcytosine per genome occurs in cancer cells. However, more detailed studies have shown that although hypomethylation of the genome occurs, the change in distribution of methyl groups within transformed cells is not random. Some areas of DNA, such as CpG islands, show hypermethylation, even though the total amount of 5-methylcytosine per cell decreases. Often, multiple CpG islands become concurrently methylated in a given tumor, leading to the suggestion that they harbor a "hypermethylation phenotype." The mechanisms underlying these changes remain unknown; however, these data suggest that early changes in the DNA methylation machinery accompany and may directly participate in the process of transformation.

The fact that changes in the methylation of CpG islands located in the promoters of growth regulatory genes can result in their permanent inactivation has led to the idea that abnormal hypermethylation should be considered one of the pathways resulting in tumor-suppressor gene inactivation as outlined by Alfred Knudson. Knudson proposed that two hits were required for the full inactivation of a tumor suppressor gene and this has been shown to be correct in almost all cancers that have been examined for mutations and losses of heterozygosity. Most of the focus in cancer research until now has been on the roles of intragenic mutations and loss of chromosomal material (LOH). However, as indicated in Table I, it has been found that the abnormal methylation of wild-type alleles of tumor suppressor genes occurs in both familial and sporadic cancers harboring mutations in the other allele. Hypermethylation should therefore be considered one of the pathways to cancer development, and this abnormal methylation is increasingly being recognized as an important molecular pathway to satisfy Knudson's hypothesis (Fig. 1).

Mechanisms responsible for the abnormal methylation of tumor suppressor genes in human cancer are not understood. However, methylation changes can be present in the apparently normal epithelium of certain tissues in a process associated with aging. Jean-Pierre Issa and colleagues have found widespread *de novo* methylation of normally unmethylated CpG islands in the colonic epithelium of older patients. Conceivably, these methylation changes could be responsible for setting up a field defect, resulting in the predisposition of large areas of epithelia to subsequent transformation. While it is not clear what causes CpG islands to become *de novo* methylated, it is probable that the DNA methyltransferase enzymes described earlier play an important role in this process. However, it remains to be seen whether the changes are due to abnormalities in the regulation of these enzymes or are due to changes in chromatin structure that predispose CpG islands to become abnormally methylated during the process of cell transformation.

While the mechanisms for abnormal promoter methylation remain to be unraveled, the process of biological selection probably plays an important role in the final pattern of methylation observed in a given cancer tissue. Thus, the gradual silencing of growth regulatory genes by ever-increasing methylation may result in the selection of cells with enhanced growth potential within the tumor. The actual pattern of growth regulators silenced in this way will most likely be a reflection of their relative importance in the control of growth in a particular differentiated cell type. Evidence for this has come from studies comparing leukemia cells to solid tumors where the pattern of genes inactivated by promoter hypermethylation varies, suggesting that the scenario just described may be correct.

V. METHYLATION AND GENOMIC INSTABILITY

The focus of work in the DNA methylation field has concentrated on the potential for methylation to control gene activity; however, evidence suggests that methylation may also play a role in ensuring chromosomal stability. Methylation changes may play a role in the instability of microsatellites in human DNA in diseases such as the fragile X syndrome and mutations in the DNMT-3b enzyme led to the development of chromosomal abnormalities in the ICF syndrome. Changes in methylation seen in human tumors may also result in a generalized destabilization of the genome, allowing for further downstream chromosomal alterations. Regional DNA hypermethylation on chromosome 17 precedes structural changes in the progression of renal tumors, suggesting that these changes may constitute a molecular change associ-

TABLE I

Examples of Cancer-Related Genes
Whose CpG Island Promoters Become
Abnormally Methylated in Cancer

Gene	Tumor type
Retinoblastoma gene	Retinoblastoma
Von Hippel Lindau gene	Kidney tumors
p15	Leukemias
p16	Lung and colon tumors
p14	Colorectal tumors
hMLH1	Colorectal tumors
E-cadherin	Gastric cancers
APC	Colorectal tumors

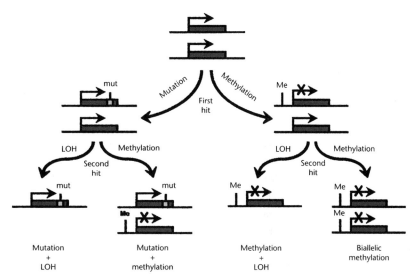

FIGURE 1 Knudson's two-hit hypothesis revised. Two active alleles of a tumor-suppressor gene are indicated by the two boxes shown at the top. The first step of gene inactivation is shown as a localized mutation on the left or by transcriptional repression by DNA methylation on the right. The second hit is shown by either LOH or transcriptional silencing. From Jones, P. A., and Laird, P. W. (1999). *Nature Genet.* **22,** p. 165, with permission.

ated with genetic instability. Similar results have been found with neural tumors, suggesting that methylation changes could play an important part in generating allelic loss in addition to being involved in the stability of other chromosomal elements such as the microsatellites. However, the mechanisms by which DNA methylation changes could contribute to genomic instability are entirely unknown.

VI. THE ROLE OF 5-METHYLCYTOSINE AS A MUTAGEN

Methylation sites contribute to the generation of an extraordinarily high percentage of point mutations in prokaryotes and eukaryotes. Methylation sites were first recognized as hot spots for mutation in *Escherichia coli* where it was proposed that their enhanced mutability was due to the fact that thymine, the deamination product of 5-methylcytosine, is inherently more difficult for the cell to recognize and excise than uracil, the corresponding deamination product of unmethylated cytosine.

Methylation of a cytosine residue is thought to increase the potential for a $C \rightarrow T$ or corresponding $G \rightarrow A$ transition mutation by 12- to 30-fold, which is consistent with the fact that more than 30% of all human germline point mutations occur at CpGs. This enhanced mutability is thought to have been responsible for the substantial suppression of CpGs in organisms that methylate their DNAs and for the frequent occurrence of restriction fragment length polymorphisms at CpGs. Thus, 5-methylcytosine, which constitutes 1% of the base composition of human DNA, contributes to more than 30% of germline point mutations, despite the existence of an efficient repair system with the capacity of restoring T:G mispairs specifically back to C:G pairs.

The isolation and characterization of the oncogenes and tumor-suppressor genes frequently mutated in human cancers have been a major achievement. Analysis of the mutational spectra in these genes should allow for an analysis of what caused the mutations and hence acted as a carcinogen in particular tumor types. The spectrum of point mutations in tumor-suppressor genes such as *p53*, which is frequently inactivated in human tumors, has shown that CpG is a major hot spot for mutation in human somatic cells. Analysis of the point mutations sustained in the *p53* gene in human colon cancer, for example, shows that more than half of all mutations are sustained at CpG sites. The frequency at which mutations are sustained at CpG sites is less in other kinds of cancer (e.g., lung cancer). However, approximately one-third of all inactivating point mutations in the *p53* gene occur at methylation sites if all human tumors are considered together.

Codons 175 and 273, which represent strong hot spots for mutation in colon cancer, have been shown to be methylated in human DNA by direct genomic sequencing. This led us to hypothesize that 5-methylcytosine should be considered an endogenous mutagen, as it is likely that these mutations do not require the direct interaction of a carcinogenic substance with DNA for their generation. The role of cytosine methylation in inducing mutations in tumor suppressor genes is not confined to the *p53* gene, as genes such as APC and retinoblastoma frequently contain mutations at CpG sites in the human germline and in sporadic tumors.

Work by Pfeiffer and colleagues has led to the realization that the methylation of CpG sites increases the binding of chemical carcinogens to guanine residues as well as increasing the susceptibilities of the cytosine residues to the formation of pyrimidine dimers by UV light. This methylation can increase the frequencies of both endogenous and exogenous mutagenesis.

VII. REVERSING METHYLATION CHANGES

The hypermethylation of CpG islands in the promoters of tumor-suppressor genes results in their inactivation and is potentially reversible by the appropriate drug treatment. This represents an exciting new therapeutic option, which is likely to be exploited in the future as a new way to treat human cancer. It has been known since the early 1980s that the drug 5-aza-2'-deoxycytidine is incorporated effectively into DNA of replicating cells where it acts as a powerful inhibitor of DNA methyltransferase enzymes. The fact that the incorporated drug forms a strong complex with DNA methyltransferases results in a substantial hypermethylation of DNA synthesized in the absence of further drug treatment following removal of the drug. Because the methylation patterns are copied, hypomethylation induced by drug treatment can be inherited and genes can be rapidly activated from

their hypermethylated states following drug treatment. Thus, genes such as MyoD1, growth control genes such as p16, p14, and p15, and DNA repair genes such as hMLH1 have been shown to be activated by drug treatment. Importantly, it has also been shown that this treatment results in the restoration of gene activity to the cells, e.g., in cells with hMLH1 silenced by promoter methylation. Thus, new protocols are likely to be developed with DNA methyltransferase inhibitors that restore the activities of silenced genes.

VIII. CONCLUSIONS AND PERSPECTIVES

Pervasive changes in DNA methylation accompany the process of oncogenic transformation. These alterations are likely to have significant roles in the generation of the tumorigenic state and are summarized in Table I. The ability of 5-methylcytosine to silence the activities of promoters, particularly promoters containing CpG islands, could cause the permanent inactivation of growth-regulating genes. DNA methylation changes can be detected in bodily fluids using sensitive techniques, giving rise to new approaches for the detection of cancer. Changes in DNA methylation may generate genomic instability, facilitating the allelic loss that is common in tumorigenesis. The fact that one-third of all the point mutations occurring in the p53 tumor suppressor gene in human cancers are sustained at methylated CpG sites suggests that this base adds a substantial mutagenic load on these genes.

Despite the importance of methylation in the initiation and progression of cancer, many fundamental questions regarding the biochemistry of this process remain unknown. For example, virtually nothing is known of the mechanisms governing the establishment and changing of methylation patterns during development, and our knowledge of mutagenic mechanisms at methylation sites remains obscure. The mechanisms by which methylation may be involved in genomic stability are also completely unknown. The fact that DNA methylation changes are almost universal in tumors and often can be observed at a very early stage in the transformation process suggests a causal relationship between this epigenetic process and neoplastic development.

See Also the Following Articles

TP53 Tumor Suppressor Gene: Structure and Function • Tumor Cell Motility and Invasion • Tumor Suppressor Genes: Specific Classes

Bibliography

Antequera, F., Boyes, J., and Bird, A. P. (1990). High levels of *de novo* methylation and altered chromatin structure at CpG islands in cell lines. *Cell* **63,** 503–514.

Baylin, S. B., Herman, J. G., Graff, J. R., Vertino, P. M., and Issa, J. P. (1998). Alterations in DNA methylation: a fundamental aspect of neoplasia. *Adv. Cancer Res.* **72,** 141–196.

Bird, A. P. (1987). CpG islands as gene markers in the vertebrate nucleus. *Trends Genet.* **3,** 342–347.

Bird, A. P. (1992). The essentials of DNA methylation. *Cell* **70,** 5–8.

Feinberg, A. P., and Vogelstein, B. (1983). Hypomethylation distinguishes genes of some human cancers from their normal counterparts. *Nature* **301,** 89–91.

Harrington, M. A., Jones, P. A., Imagawa, M., and Karin, M. (1988). Cytosine methylation does not affect binding of transcription factor Sp1. *Proc. Natl. Acad. Sci. USA* **85,** 2066–2070.

Issa, J. P., Ottaviano, Y. L., Celano, P., Hamilton, S. R., Davidson, N. E., and Baylin, S. B. (1994). Methylation of the oestrogen receptor CpG island links ageing and neoplasia in human colon. *Nature Genet.* **7,** 536–540.

Jones, P. A., and Laird, P. W. (1999). Cancer epigenetics comes of age. *Nature Genet.* **21,** 163–167.

Jones, P. A., Rideout, W. M., Shen, J.-C., Spruck, C. H., and Tsai, Y. C. (1992). Methylation, mutation and cancer. *BioEssays* **14,** 33–36.

Jones, P. A., and Taylor, S. M. (1980). Cellular differentiation, cytidine analogs and DNA methylation. *Cell* **20,** 85–93.

Jones, P. L., Veenstra, G. J., Wade, P. A., Vermaak, D., Kass, S. U., Landsberger, N., Strouboulis, J., and Wolffe, A. P. (1998). Methylated DNA and MeCP2 recruit histone deacetylase to repress transcription. *Nature Genet.* **19,** 187–191.

Li, H., Bestor, T. H., and Jaenisch, R. (1992). Targeted mutation of the DNA methyltransferase gene results in embryonic lethality. *Cell* **69,** 915–926.

Makos, M., Nelkin, B. D., Chazin, V. R., Cavenee, W. K., Brodeur, G. M., and Baylin, S. B. (1993). DNA hypermethylation is associated with 17p allelic loss in neural tumors. *Cancer Res.* **53,** 2715–2718.

Nan, X., Ng, H. H., Johnson, C. A., Laherty, C. D., Turner, B. M., Eisenman, R. N., and Bird, A. (1998). Transcriptional repression by the methyl-CpG-binding protein MeCP2 involves a histone deacetylase complex. *Nature* **393,** 386–389.

Okano, M., Xie, S., and Li, E. (1998). Cloning and characterization of a family of novel mammalian DNA (cytosine-5) methyltransferases. *Nature Genet.* **19,** 219–220.

Pfeifer, G. P., Tang, M.-S., and Denissenko, M. F. (2000). Mutation hotspots and DNA methylation. *In* "DNA Methylation and Cancer" (P. A. Jones and P. K. Vogt, eds.), p. 1. Springer-Verlag, Berlin.

Rideout, W. M., Coetzee, G. A., Olumi, A. F., and Jones, P. A. (1990). 5-Methylcytosine as an endogenous mutagen in the human LDL receptor and p53 genes. *Science* **249,** 1288–1290.

Yu, S., Mulley, J., Loesch, D., Turner, G., Donnelly, A., Gedeon, A., Hillen, D., Kremer, E., Lynch, M., Pritchard, M., Sutherland, G. R., and Richards, R. I. (1992). Fragile X syndrome: Unique genetics of the heritable unstable element. *Am. J. Hum. Genet.* **50,** 968–980.

DNA Tumor Viruses: Adenovirus

Hwei-Gene Heidi Wang
Bristol Myers Squibb, Wallingford, Connecticut

Brad Zerler
Locus Discovery Inc., Blue Bell, Pennsylvania

Elizabeth Moran
Temple University School of Medicine, Philadelphia, Pennsylvania

GLOSSARY

apoptosis or programmed cell death A genetically controlled response to induce cell death as a normal part of development or as a defense against the growth of tumorigenic or virus-infected cells.

cyclin A protein that periodically rises and falls in concentration in step with the eukaryotic cell cycle. Cyclins activate crucial protein kinases (called cyclin-dependent protein kinases) and thereby help control progression from one stage of the cell cycle to the next.

cyclin dependent kinases (Cdks) Protein kinases that have to be complexed with a cyclin protein in order to perform their function in protein phosphorylation. Different Cdk–cyclin complexes are thought to trigger different steps in the cell division cycle by phosphorylating specific target proteins. They are inactive when their cyclin partners are not present or when one of a class of small proteins known as "cyclin-dependent kinase inhibitors" joins the complex.

S phase The period of the cell cycle during which actively proliferating cells synthesize new DNA.

tumor suppressor gene, or tumor susceptibility gene Gene whose functional product reduces the likelihood of transformation of normal cells to tumor cells.

H uman adenovirus is a small DNA virus, classified as a tumor virus because it can induce tumors in rodents and immortalize primary cells *in vitro*. Small DNA tumor viruses have provided the basis for much of our current understanding of the molecular mechanisms of cancer. Adenovirus in particular, because of its ease of culture and relatively small genome size, has served as a convenient and sensitive probe for cellular mechanisms that control gene expression during carcinogenesis and the interactions of tumorigenic cells within the host organism. Adenovirus is not associated with cancer in humans, but the basic molecular strategies used by adenovirus to induce terminally differentiated cells to resume proliferation are common to a number of DNA tumor viruses, including ones clearly associated with human tumorigenesis, such as human papillomavirus. Moreover, adenovirus gene products interact so intimately with the molecular mechanisms of the host cell that their study offers important basic insights into cell growth control and tumorigenesis. The importance of these insights extends far beyond the significance of the virus itself as an agent of human carcinogenesis. The ease of genetic manipulation and the ability to infect many different types of cells that make adenovirus useful for studying the mechanisms of carcinogenesis also make adenovirus a promising vector for use in gene therapy against a number of diseases, including cancer. This article (1) focuses on the insights adenovirus has provided into the host cell mechanisms that regulate gene expression in cancer cells and the host response to carcinogenesis and (2) reviews the role of adenovirus as a gene therapy vector.

I. INTRODUCTION: THE ADENOVIRUS GENOME

Adenoviruses are a family of small DNA viruses with a genome size of about 36 kb, known to infect a range of mammalian species and birds. Exposure to the virus is widespread, and the majority of the human population is positive for adenovirus antibodies. Approximately 40 different serotypes of adenovirus have been isolated from humans, including intestinal forms as well as the more common respiratory forms. Of these, human adenoviruses types 2 and 5 are by far the best studied. They have been used in numerous laboratory studies, are entirely sequenced, and have been sub-

jected to intensive mutagenesis and recombinant studies. Essentially all of the information reviewed here is derived from studies with types 2 and 5. These two serotypes are almost identical in their sequence and are not distinguished here.

The adenovirus genome encodes several primary transcription units that are expressed in a regulated order during the virus replication cycle. Transcription of the virus genome is entirely dependent on host cell factors, although a few virus-encoded factors act to moderate the host response. Much of the adenovirus genome is devoted to encoding the structural proteins required to form the capsids of new virus particles. These products are produced from the major late promoter (MLP). The remainder of the viral genome consists of early transcription units, which encode a variety of small proteins that dramatically modify host cell mechanisms to serve the needs of the virus.

The adenovirus genome is not sufficient to encode the many factors required for DNA replication. Like other small DNA viruses, adenovirus relies almost entirely on host cell DNA synthesis factors to replicate the viral genome. However, adenovirus is not limited to infecting proliferating cells because adenovirus early proteins are capable of activating cell cycle-specific transcription in a wide variety of quiescent host cells. It is this activity of the viral early genes that has made adenovirus such a valuable probe for the mechanisms regulating cell cycle-specific gene expression.

Each of the virus early region genes encodes multiple proteins as a consequence of differential splicing. Depending on the effects of the splicing pattern and the frame in which translation is initiated, proteins from each transcription unit can show a close relationship or be entirely unrelated. In either case, proteins from each region usually have related functions.

Early region 1A (E1A), the first transcription unit expressed, encodes proteins that subvert host cell transcription controls and activate cell cycle-specific gene expression. E1A products also activate host cell transcription factors required for expression of the remainder of the viral genome. The products of early region 1B (E1B) suppress the apoptotic response that is often induced when DNA synthesis is activated against prevailing molecular signals in mammalian cells.

Early region 2 (E2) encodes the few products that adenovirus contributes to its own replication. The major product is a 72K DNA-binding protein, produced in very large amounts. This protein binds single-stranded DNA and helps open the DNA duplex so replication can proceed. The E2 gene also encodes a DNA polymerase and a third product, designated terminal protein, that binds to the adenovirus linear ends to help initiate replication. The major importance of the E2 transcription unit to carcinogenesis studies derives not from its encoded products but from its promoter. The promoter is activated by E1A in concert with host genes required for DNA synthesis. Because activation of the E2 transcription unit is closely tied to the activation of host cell S phase genes, the study of this promoter has played a central role in developing our understanding of cell cycle-specific transcription in the host. The host factor responsible for its activation was named for the viral transcription unit, hence the designation E2F. E2F activation is a function of E1A and is considered in more detail in the section on E1A.

Early region 3 (E3) encodes several small proteins with the general function of countering host cell immune responses designed to act against infected or inappropriately proliferating host cells. Early region 4 (E4) encodes a variety of small proteins that help fine-tune the interaction between host and virus factors. The remaining transcription unit in adenovirus does not encode a protein, but instead produces two small RNA species (the VA RNA molecules) that oppose the host interferon response. A simplified transcription map of the adenovirus genome is shown in Fig. 1.

From the perspective of the biological effects of the virus early genes, it is clear why their study has contributed so much to our understanding of the molecular mechanisms involved in carcinogenesis. In the following sections, viral products important to the tumorigenic effects of the virus are considered in turn.

II. VIRUS INTERACTIONS WITH HOST IMMUNE RESPONSES

Adenovirus can persist for years in its human host. The continued presence of the virus requires the ability to evade host immune defenses. Adenovirus encodes products capable of protecting infected cells from lysis mediated by tumor necrosis factor (TNF), Fas ligand, and TRAIL (tumor necrosis factor-related apoptosis-inducing ligand treatment) and from cytotoxic T lymphocytes (CTLs). The virus also encodes products that oppose the antiviral effects of interferons. The host mechanisms that attack cells infected with a foreign agent such as a virus are similar to mechanisms that guard against the emergence of cells with tumorigenic potential. Thus, virus studies offer insight into the means by which tumor cells can evade host responses, as well as the mechanisms by which potentially tumorigenic viral agents can persist. In addition, attempts to use adenovirus as a vector for gene therapy against diseases, including malignancies, must consider the immune responses active at the tumor site and aspects of the host response that may affect the ability of the virus to deliver exogenous gene products to their target sites.

Much of the ability of adenovirus to guard against the TNF- and CTL-mediated response resides in the products encoded by the E3 region. Awareness of the role of the E3 region has had a curious history in adenovirus studies. Because E3 function is largely related to the host response at the organism level, it is dispensable to the virus life cycle in tissue culture. dl309, a commonly used laboratory strain of adenovirus and one that is often regarded as a "wild type," does not actually contain the E3 region. dl309 was generated by selection against all but a single *XbaI* restriction endonuclease site at the left end of the wild-type virus genome. It was developed to facilitate recombinant strategies involving the E1 region and, because of its usefulness in this regard, has become a widely used vector in laboratory studies. The selection resulted in the loss of the E3 region. Because it did not affect the ability of the virus to grow in tissue culture, the deletion was not considered to be of major importance initially. Many gene therapy strategies employing adenovirus vectors have used dl309 in order to take advantage of the useful single *XbaI* site as the site of insertion for the exogenous gene or because the missing adenovirus sequences provide more room for insertion of larger fragments of heterologous DNA, which could not otherwise be accommodated within the encapsidation limits of the virus. However, as knowledge

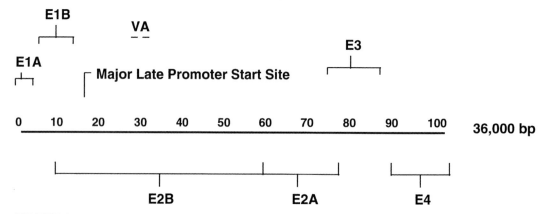

FIGURE 1 The linear, 36,000-bp adenovirus genome is represented (in percentages of length) showing the positions of the early viral genes and the start site of the major late transcription unit. (Adapted from A. J. Levine *Viruses*. Scientific American Library. W. H. Freeman and Co., New York, NY.)

about the activity of the E3 region has expanded, the decision to include the E3 region or not has become an important consideration in designing adenovirus vectors for therapeutic uses.

One mechanism by which the E3 region may protect infected cells from lysis by CTLs is by reducing the surface expression of major histocompatibility complex (MHC) class I antigens. Recognition of infected cells by CTLs requires that viral peptide antigens be displayed on the cell surface in a complex with an MHC class I antigen. The E3-encoded 19-kDa glycoprotein (E3 19K), the most abundant of the E3-encoded products, binds to the peptide-binding domain of MHC class I antigens and localizes to the membrane of the endoplasmic reticulum, preventing the transport of MHC antigens to the cell surface. Reduced expression of class I antigens on the cell surface is expected to inhibit the ability of CTLs to recognize infected cells. Experiments to test this mechanism in the commonly studied human viruses have mostly relied on infection of rodents. It is not yet clear how significant reduced surface expression of MHC class I antigens is to viral persistence in the natural host. Adenovirus does not reduce surface expression of MHC class I antigens in all laboratory cell lines tested, and mouse adenovirus, which establishes a persistent infection in its natural host, does not appear to reduce surface levels of MHC antigens.

Adenovirus can also counteract the cytolytic effects of TNF-α. This activity appears to be mediated by E3 and E1B gene products. Several E3 proteins (14.7K, 10.4K, and 14.5K) are involved in this pathway. The 14.7K protein, or a heterodimeric complex between the 14.5K protein and the 10.4K protein, can protect infected cells against TNF-α-mediated cytolysis. Although the mechanism of action needs to be fully determined, the anticytolytic effects of the E3 proteins may be a consequence of their ability to inhibit the release of arachidonic acid following the stimulation of phospholipase A_2 by TNF-α. Inhibition of arachidonic acid release correlates with reduced cytokine production and inhibition of the TNF-α-induced inflammatory response as well as reduced cytolysis. TNF-α kills some cells by necrosis and others by apoptosis. As discussed later, products encoded by the adenovirus E1B region can inhibit apoptosis, and the E1B 19K protein can protect human cells in culture from TNF-α-induced cytolysis. Thus, adenovirus has at least three protein mechanisms able to counteract the effects of TNF-α. The three functions do not all prevent TNF-α-mediated cytolysis in all cell types examined, which perhaps explains the need for partially redundant mechanisms.

The E3 transcription unit encodes at least three additional protein products: 11.6K, 6.7K, and 12.5K. The 11.6K product accumulates to high levels at very late stages of infection and promotes cell lysis, allowing mature virus to be released from infected cells. The 11.6K product has been named the adenovirus death protein (ADP). The roles of E3 6.7K and 12.5K proteins are not yet known. Their significance may become more apparent with increasing use of adenovirus vectors in vaccine and gene therapy.

Yet another adenovirus defense against the host immune response is encoded by the virus-associated (VA) RNA transcription unit, which antagonizes the host interferon response. VA RNAs are not translated products. They comprise two extremely abundant short RNA species: VA RNAI and VA RNAII. Interferons induce a protein kinase that is activated by double-stranded RNA (which often is formed during virus infections due to transcription off both strands of the viral genome). The kinase shuts down protein synthesis in the infected cell by phosphorylating an elongation factor, eIF-2, leading to inhibition of a recycling factor required for protein synthesis. Activation of the kinase depends on its binding to double-stranded RNA as a dimer and undergoing auto-phosphorylation. VA RNAs are short molecules that form double-stranded hairpin structures that bind the kinase but prevent autophosphorylation. In this situation, the kinase is not activated and protein synthesis continues in the infected cell.

III. VIRAL MECHANISMS THAT OPPOSE THE HOST APOPTOSIS RESPONSE: E1B GENE PRODUCTS

Two major products, a 55-kDa protein (55K) and a 19-kDa protein (19K), are produced from the E1B transcription unit by alternate splicing. (The 19K product of E1B is entirely distinct from the E3 19K product.) E1B splice products initiate translation in different reading frames so that they have no overlapping sequence. Each is unique with respect to the other through its entire protein sequence. Although they are not structurally related, these proteins have complementary functions. They serve to oppose the host cell apoptosis response. Apoptosis, or programmed cell death, is a genetically controlled response whereby cells die either as a normal part of development or as a defense against the proliferation of tumorigenic or infected cells. Apoptosis is particularly characterized by fragmentation of the host DNA. E1B

products have provided genetic tools that have played an important role in dissecting the molecular basis of apoptosis and in revealing the relationship between suppression of apoptosis and tumorigenesis.

A. E1B 19K and the Bcl-2 Pathway

The Bcl-2 gene was first identified as part of the most common translocation in human B-cell follicular lymphoma. The translocation results in higher than normal cellular levels of Bcl-2, which had the unusual biological property of extending cell survival rather than stimulating cell proliferation. Bcl-2 was soon found to inhibit apoptosis induced by a variety of stimuli in a wide range of cell types, indicating that this product acts at a controlling point in the pathway to programmed cell death. In general, an inappropriate gain of Bcl-2 function is associated with the genesis of cancer, whereas a loss of Bcl-2 function impairs normal development. The observation that mice lacking the Bcl-2 gene survive with only relatively minor developmental anomalies suggested that other molecules can supply Bcl-2-like functions, and indeed a family of Bcl-2-like proteins is now recognized, with both positive- and negative-acting members. Multiple sequence alignment of Bcl-2 family members and mutagenesis have identified three conserved regions, Bcl-2 homology regions 1, 2, and 3 (BH1, BH2, and BH3), that are required for the regulation of apoptosis. Studies indicate that Bcl-2 family signals converge on a series of proteases, designated caspases, that degrade cellular proteins and activate a DNase.

The developing understanding of Bcl-2-related products in cells was enhanced with the realization that the E1B 19K protein is a member of the Bcl-2 family. The biological phenotype of adenoviruses unable to express normal E1B 19K protein first suggested that 19K is an inhibitor of cell death. In the absence of the 19K product, adenovirus can initiate proliferation in quiescent primary cells, but the cell population does not increase readily due to extensive apoptosis. Failure to suppress apoptosis in productively infected cells compromises virus production because of the premature death of the infected host cell. Further studies showed that E1B 19K and increased

Bcl-2 expression are functionally interchangeable in adenovirus infection and transformation. Regions of 19K identified as important for structure and function are homologous to functional regions in Bcl-2. Studies with 19K have helped to identify other Bcl-2 family members and interacting proteins.

B. E1B 55K and the p53 Pathway

p53 is a protein whose wild-type form has DNA binding activity and both positive and negative effects on transcription, as well as the ability to suppress aspects of the transformed cell phenotype. Functional domains identified within p53 include a sequence-specific DNA-binding domain, an amino-terminal transcriptional activation domain, and a carboxy-terminal oligomerization domain. The extremely widespread occurrence of p53 mutations in naturally occurring tumors implies strongly that alteration of a cellular pathway involving p53 is essential for the formation of most tumors. Almost all p53 mutations sequenced from human tumors map within the DNA-binding domain of p53, indicating that this domain is essential for the tumor-suppressing activity of p53. Mutant forms of p53 act as dominant suppressors of wild-type p53 tumor suppression and transcription activities, presumably because of the oligomerization activity. Overexpression of p53 in some situations results in growth arrest, but in other situations it induces not just cessation of growth but apoptosis, suggesting that p53 plays a regulatory role in this process. p53-mediated apoptosis is most often associated with specific damage to the cell or its genome, such as occurs during ionizing radiation. Developmentally regulated pathways of apoptosis, those mediated by Bcl-2-like proteins, can operate independently of p53-mediated apoptosis, although p53 may be able to influence the expression level of these proteins. p53 was among the first cloned cellular products to be recognized as a tumor suppressor gene product.

The transcription activating function of p53 appears to be central to its ability to arrest cell growth. One gene that is activated by increased p53 expression is p21/WAF-1/cip-1, a cyclin-dependent kinase inhibitor, which is thought to be largely responsible for the inhibition of cell cycle progression mediated by p53. The transcription-regulating function of p53 also appears to be important in apoptosis, possibly by altering the ratio of expression of Bcl-2-related proteins. Whether apoptosis or growth arrest is the eventual outcome of increased p53 expression may depend on whether the apoptosis signals are strong enough to prevail. Growth arrest would be the result if apoptosis does not occur.

Interest in p53 originated when this product was observed as a cellular protein bound to the transforming gene product (T antigen) of SV40, a DNA tumor virus of the class papovaviridae. Subsequently, other DNA tumor viruses, including human papillomavirus (HPV) and adenovirus, were also found to encode products that targeted p53. The consistent targeting of p53 by the DNA tumor viruses engendered study of this protein even when its cellular role was completely unknown. DNA tumor viruses use a variety of mechanisms to interfere with p53 function. In HPV infection, a ubiquitin-mediated pathway is used to cause p53 degradation. In adenovirus infection, the E1B 55K protein targets p53 by binding to the p53 acidic activation domain. This domain, like the DNA binding domain, is required for the transcription-regulating activity of p53. Mutations in 55K that render adenovirus transformation defective are consistently deficient in blocking the transcription stimulating activity of p53, even in a case where the mutant 55K retains the ability to bind p53. The Ad12 homologue of Ad2 E1B 55K does not bind p53 at all. Nevertheless, it is able to block p53-stimulated transcription activity by a mechanism not yet known. These results indicate that blocking p53-mediated transcription effects is an integral part of the mechanisms by which the E1B 55K product contributes to transformation.

This mechanism of virus–host interaction suggested that an E1B 55K-defective adenovirus might be able to replicate successfully in p53-deficient cells, while it is unable to replicate in normal cells. Given that most tumor cells are defective in p53-mediated responses, this could be used as a selective means to kill tumor cells. This strategy is discussed further in Section VI.

p53 is now known to have two genetic paralogues, p63 and p73. The adenovirus E1B 55K protein is helping to distinguish related and distinct functions in these p53 family members.

IV. E1A PRODUCTS AS MODULATORS OF GENE EXPRESSION IN NORMAL VERSUS TRANSFORMED CELLS

A. Activation of Cell Cycle-Specific Gene Expression

E1A products initiate the dramatic changes in host cell gene expression that are the basis for the transformed phenotype. E1A proteins act by binding directly to cellular proteins involved in transcription complexes, thus altering their activity. A leading contribution of adenovirus studies to the broader understanding of the molecular basis of tumorigenesis was identification of the mammalian transcription factor, E2F, as a major activator of cell cycle-specific gene expression, and the concomitant identification of the product of the retinoblastoma tumor susceptibility gene (pRb) as a negative modulator of E2F function, which itself is regulated by cyclin-dependent kinases. The role of E1A in activating E2F complexes is discussed in more detail later.

Four or five proteins are expressed through differential splicing from the E1A transcript. Early in infection, two E1A proteins predominate, a 13S and a 12S product (named for the sedimentation coefficients of their respective mRNAs). The 13S and 12S products are sufficient for virtually all known E1A activities. The role of the additional proteins is not yet clear. The 12S product is translated in the same frame as the 13S and is distinguished by an internal deletion of 46 amino acids. Each of these small proteins has multiple functional domains, revealed by site-specific mutagenesis. E1A products have been particularly amenable to genetic analysis because their functional sites consist of discrete amino acid segments that are functionally stable even in a context of major deletions.

Most E1A studies have focused on the 12S and 13S products from Ad2 and Ad5. However, the E1A sequence has been determined in several adenovirus serotypes, revealing the presence of three highly conserved amino acid regions, designated conserved regions (CR)1, CR2, and CR3. All of these regions occur in the first exon of the 12S and 13S products; the second exon does not show such a high level of sequence conservation.

E1A products are expressed constitutively in a variety of cells, but activation of the remainder of the virus genome requires the 13S product. The 12S product is inefficient in activating most of the virus transcription units, but is similar to the 13S product in stimulating the transcription of all host cell genes required for cell cycle progression and proliferation in quiescent rodent cells. In contrast to this widely studied effect in rodent cells, the 12S product shows relatively little cell cycle-promoting activity in the absence of the 13S product when the host cell is of human origin.

Site-specific mutagenesis of E1A products combined with adenovirus promoter analysis has linked individual E1A functional domains with the modulation of specific host transcription complexes. Most of the adenovirus promoters contain a sequence element recognized by host transcription factors of the ATF/CREB family. The sequence had previously been described as an element that could confer cAMP inducibility on a number of cellular genes. Although at least 20 cellular members of the ATF/CREB family are known that can bind this site, the major one responsive to 13S activation is ATF-2. The requirement for the 13S product in activating virus genes suggested that the 13S unique region was largely responsible for activation through the viral ATF sites. The 13S unique region, which is essentially colinear with CR3, has the structure of a "zinc finger," a DNA- and protein-binding motif that forms a loop or "finger" when a molecule of zinc is bound between specific amino acid residues on the sequence. A number of studies combine to suggest that the zinc finger of the 13S product binds the basal transcription factor, TBP, whereas sequences immediately downstream of the zinc finger bind ATF-2. In this manner, the 13S product bridges a physical interaction between these proteins on a promoter, presumably facilitating the signals by which ATF-2 recruits the basal transcription machinery to initiate active transcription. The 13S unique region has also been shown to bind additional upstream transcription factors, distinct from the ATF/CREB family, in combination with TBP. Although it is not clear how such limited E1A sequences can bind a number of unrelated proteins, their binding is consistent with observations that the 13S product can activate transcription through a number of distinct promoter elements.

Sequences common to the 12S and 13S products are more closely linked with the activation of cell cycle-specific transcription complexes. The E2 transcription unit is unusual among adenovirus genes in that it is efficiently activated by E1A 12S, probably because it encodes the adenovirus replication proteins, and has therefore been linked by the virus with the expression of host cell S-phase genes. The host cell transcription factor that binds to the activation element in the E2 promoter is termed E2F. Sequences in the 12S product required to induce proliferation in quiescent rodent cells align very closely with conserved regions 1 and 2 and also include the relatively less conserved amino terminus. The same regions are required for binding to certain host cell proteins observed in immune complexes with E1A. Identification of one of these products as pRb, the product of the retinoblastoma tumor susceptibility gene, provided the first evidence of the molecular basis of pRb function. When genetic mapping revealed that the pRb-binding motif in E1A proteins is specifically required for E2 activation, pRb was implicated as a negative regulator of E2F. E2F-binding elements have since been recognized in a number of genes expressed in a cell cycle-specific manner. A general model for pRb function in E2F regulation is that pRb binds E2F complexes on the promoter in an inactive form. Dissociation of pRb, either by E1A binding or by normal cellular mechanisms designed to trigger the cell cycle, allows E2F to signal activation of the basal transcription machinery.

Other cellular products bound by E1A through the pRb-binding motif have been identified as pRb-related proteins or as cyclin-dependent kinase complexes bound to E1A indirectly through association with products of the pRb family. Largely as a result of these studies, cyclin-dependent kinases have been recognized as normal cellular regulators of the pRb family. Additionally, the recognition of multiple pRb family members prompted the subsequent recognition of multiple E2F family members. Current models of cell cycle regulation postulate that individual members of the E2F family act sequentially to affect the ordered expression of cell cycle-specific genes. Different pRb family members modulate the activity of specific E2F members and are in turn regulated by a series of cyclin-dependent kinases. The ability of another tumor suppressor, p53, to affect this pathway was indicated earlier. p53 can increase expression of the p21 inhibitor of cyclin-dependent kinases, thus arresting cell growth.

E2F proteins are by no means the only cellular proteins regulated by pRb, but detailed knowledge of the E2F/pRb/cyclin-dependent kinase interactions fostered by E1A studies has provided a number of new cellular targets for tumor diagnosis and potential therapies. The fine-tuned mapping of the pRb-binding motif in E1A has also prompted the recognition that this motif is common to the transforming proteins of other DNA tumor viruses, including the E7 product of human papillomavirus (HPV). The carcinogenic potential of the various types of HPV linked with human cervical cancer correlates closely with the affinity of the respective E7 products for pRb.

A second functional domain in 12S products is also linked with cell cycle activation. This site binds a large nuclear phosphoprotein, termed p300, that occurs *in vivo* in cellular complexes with the basal transcription factor, TBP, in the presence or absence of E1A. p300 is highly homologous to a product that binds to activated forms of the cyclic AMP response element binding protein (CREB) and which was therefore named CREB-binding protein (CBP). E1A binds both p300 and CBP. A major link between transcriptional control at promoter sites and the modification of chromatin during regulated gene expression was forged with the discovery that p300 contains intrinsic histone acetyltransferase activity. p300-mediated acetylation also appears to regulate key transcription factors, including p53.

In primary rodent cells, either the pRb-binding activity or the p300-binding activity is sufficient to drive the cells into S phase, but with only one or the other site operable, the cell cycle is abortive and few cells go on to divide successfully. Efficient E1A-mediated induction of proliferation requires not just that E1A binds both pRb and p300, but that the E1A products be capable of binding both proteins on the same E1A molecule, implying that there is some interaction between pRb and p300 in the normal course of the cell cycle. Recent studies indicate that pRb activity is modified by acetylation and that E1A stimulates acetylation of pRb by recruiting p300 and pRb into a multimeric protein complex.

The second exon sequences of E1A proteins also influence gene expression in the host cell. These C-terminal sequences are not highly conserved and are dispensable for the ability of E1A to stimulate initial rounds of proliferation in primary rodent cells. However, the C-terminal region plays a powerful role in downregulating certain host cell properties associated with the transformed phenotype. Deletion of the second exon does not reduce the ability of E1A to cooperate in the transformation of rat cells, but its absence correlates with the greatly increased oncogenicity of these cells. In cell culture, this phenotype correlates with an increased invasive potential and a defect in the downregulation of stromelysin I. The biological properties of exon 2 have been linked genetically and biochemically with binding to a cellular phosphoprotein of ~48 kDa. Characterization of this C-terminal binding protein (CtBP) has led to the recognition of a new family of transcriptional corepressors. The CtBP family binds transcription factors via a Pro-X-Asp-Leu-Ser motif, first defined in E1A. The mechanisms by which the CtBP family influences transcription are not yet clear, but they have significant homology to certain dehydrogenases, suggesting that they might recruit enzymatic activities distinct from phosphorylation and acetylation to transcription sites.

B. Suppression of Tissue-Specific Gene Expression

E1A mechanisms that activate the cell cycle are also capable of interfering with cellular differentiation in a process that mimics the general loss of differentiation markers seen in tumorigenesis. For this reason, E1A mutants are being used with increasing frequency to help decipher the molecular pathways controlling terminal differentiation. In simplest terms, proliferation and terminal differentiation are mutually exclusive. E1A-mediated inhibition of differentiation generally results from a combination of suppressing tissue-specific gene expression while activating cell cycle-specific gene expression. The ability of E1A to affect either process is closely linked with binding to the p300 and/or pRb protein families. This implies that these products are likely to be the main control points in the transcription pathways that coordinate

suppression of cell cycle activity with activation of tissue-specific gene expression during terminal differentiation. Expression of E1A mutants allows investigators to view the effect of disrupting these controls, and possibly to determine which changes in gene expression are linked with one pathway versus the other.

The normal targets of adenovirus type 2/5 infection are epithelial cells of the respiratory tract. However, adenovirus can infect a wide range of tissue types. In addition, the ability to express E1A stably or transiently through plasmid transfection has permitted the use of E1A as a probe in virtually any type of tissue that can be handled in the laboratory. In almost all cases, E1A expression inhibits major aspects of tissue-specific gene expression, implying that the roles of p300 and pRb are almost universal in contrast with the tissue-specific expression of certain transcription factors. Individual transcription factors may be severely limited in expression among tissue types, but whether they are active may be the result of signals controlled by p300 and pRb. The specific effects of E1A are not exactly the same in each system studied, presumably because the effects of pRb and p300 vary to some extent according to the combination of tissue-specific factors present in any cell type.

Several investigators have shown that E1A can inhibit the differentiation of myoblasts and mediate the repression of skeletal muscle-specific gene expression by inhibiting the activity of myogenic transcription factors containing basic helix–loop–helix regions (bHLH). Subsequent studies with E1A mutants indicate that the ability of E1A to suppress the expression of specific differentiation markers correlates with binding to p300 and not to pRb. In a ventricular myocyte system, E1A mutations affecting association with either p300 or pRb were able to suppress transcription of the cardiac and skeletal actin gene to levels observed with wild-type E1A. E1A transfection assays have shown that p300 binding without pRb binding can repress the melanocyte tissue-specific TRP-1 gene almost as well as wild-type E1A, whereas pRb binding has only a partial repression effect. In pancreatic cells, E1A suppresses insulin gene expression in a manner dependent on the p300-binding site. In osteoblasts, E1A blocks differentiation to the mineralization phenotype and suppresses expression of specific markers, including the early osteoblast differentiation marker alkaline phosphatase. E1A mutants have also been used to assess the roles of pRb and p300 in growth control and tissue-specific gene expression in mouse keratinocytes treated with TGF-β1, in PC12 cells induced to differentiate by exposure to nerve growth factor (NGF), and in P19 cells induced to differentiate into neuroectoderm or mesoderm by respective exposure to retinoic acid or dimethyl sulfoxide. A search for pRb-interacting factors revealed an E1A-like inhibitor of differentiation (EID-1) capable of binding both pRb and p300 and of inhibiting transactivation by myoD. Thus, E1A studies continue to illuminate cellular mechanisms.

C. Use of Adenovirus to Establish Cell Lines from Primary Tissue

Understanding the molecular basis of tissue pathogenesis and subsequent drug development is often hindered by the lack of appropriate cell lines that maintain the phenotype of the primary tissue. To circumvent this shortcoming, investigators have taken advantage of the ability of E1A to establish an extended cycle of cell proliferation in terminally differentiated nonmitotic cells to develop tissue-specific cell lines that retain many of the properties exhibited by the parental primary tissue.

This may at first seem contradictory to the effects of E1A in blocking differentiation when expressed in progenitor cells, but it has been found generally that the effect of E1A expression is less severe in cells that are already terminally differentiated. Certain markers may be lost, but others may remain intact. Also, other parameters, such as the level of E1A expression, may limit the effect on tissue-specific gene expression such that individual lines can be selected that retain the ability to express at least a subset of tissue-specific markers on induction. E1A has been used to generate hepatocyte cell lines that retain the ability to express several liver-specific genes, including albumin, transferrin, hemopexin, and the third component of complement. A number of other examples illustrate the range of this application. Glial progenitor cell lines have been developed from primary embryonic rat brain cells that are capable of expressing tissue-specific markers and genes. Rat intestinal epithelial cell lines have been developed that retain characteristics of parental intestinal mucosa cells, including cytoplasmic villin, cytokeratins, enkephalinase, and sensitivity to vasoactive intestinal peptide (VIP). A pulmonary alveolar type II cell line has also been isolated from primary tissue, and rat endometrial cell lines have been developed that will be used to analyze endometrium-specific gene expression and as model systems for endometrial carcinoma.

V. E4 OPEN READING FRAMES

The E4 transcription unit of Ad2/5 encodes six partially overlapping open reading frames (ORFs) generating a series of small proteins ranging in size from 10 to about 35 kDa. These proteins contribute to the viral replicative cycle in various ways. Recent results suggest that they contribute significant tumorigenic functions as well. While the well-studied Ad2/5 type ade-noviruses are not tumorigenic *in vivo*, Ad9 selectively induces mammary tumors in injected rats. This activity does not require the Ad9 E1 region, but instead requires E4-ORF1. The tumorigenic activity of the Ad9 E4-ORF1 protein is such that an E1-deficient Ad5 vector engineered to express the Ad9 E4-ORF1 protein becomes tumorigenic in rats and, like Ad9, promotes solely mammary tumors.

Ad2/5 E4-ORFs may have tumorigenic functions as well. The products of E4-ORF6 and E4-ORF3 can cooperate with E1A proteins to transform primary rat cells in a manner analogous to E1B cooperation with E1A. For ORF6 at least, the underlying mechanism may be related to the effect of E1B-55K, as ORF6 can also interact directly with p53 and promote p53 degradation. E4-ORF6 and E1B-55K may be designed to act in tandem, as E4-ORF6 forms a complex with E1B-55K. While the physiological functions of the E4 open reading frames are not yet fully understood, their continued study can be expected to shed new light on cellular growth regulatory processes.

VI. ADENOVIRUS AS A GENE THERAPY VECTOR

The ease with which the adenovirus genome can be manipulated using recombinant DNA techniques, along with its tissue promiscuity and ability to infect postmitotic, nondividing cells, has led to the use of adenoviruses as vectors for expression of heterologous genes, and as delivery systems for gene therapeutics and recombinant vaccines. Adenovirus is not associated with serious illness in immunocompetent individuals. For more than two decades unattentuated adeno-viruses have been used successfully as oral vaccines, offering strong evidence of the safety of such vectors as potential gene therapy tools. Since the initial construction and *in vitro* expression of recombinant adenovirus vectors containing the SV40 T-antigen and herpes simplex virus thymidine kinase genes and, in 1990, the groundbreaking use of adenoviruses to deliver the gene for ornithine transcarbamylase (OTC) in mice harboring a genetic OTC defect, adenovirus has been used to deliver numerous genes in *in vivo* preclinical models.

Replication-defective adenoviruses have been used for the delivery of genes encoding immune-modulating cytokines and growth factors to tumor sites to increase tumor susceptibility to host defenses. Because adenovirus infects terminally differentiated postmitotic cells, it represents an attractive vector system for delivery of these cytokines into normal cells juxtaposed to the tumor, ensuring constant cytokine production to stimulate the host cellular defense system. In addition, adenoviruses have been used as vectors to deliver therapeutic cell cycle-regulating genes intratumorally to attempt to restore proliferative control as well as to deliver genes encoding factors that augment and sensitize tumors to various chemotherapeutic regimens.

Another approach to the treatment of tumors is the use of replication-competent adenoviruses. An adenovirus E1B-55-kDa gene deletion mutant (dl1520) was the first genetically constructed adenovirus to be administered to humans. As discussed in Section III,B, the E1B-55-kDa product is required to inactivate the p53 cellular tumor suppressor and to enable subsequent adenoviral replication in host cells. It follows that an adenovirus harboring a mutation in the EIB-55-kDa gene is unable to replicate in normal host cells that contain a functional p53 gene product, but can replicate very efficiently in host tumor cells that have defective p53. Thus, such a virus has the potential to lyse tumor cells without killing normal cells.

Initial clinical studies with replication-selective adenoviruses have shown that this type of therapy is relatively safe and holds promise as a feasible approach in cancer treatment. It even appears that a combination treatment regimen involving replication-sensitive adenoviruses, along with standard chemotherapy, is synergistic over either treatment alone. The optimal use of these types of adenoviruses in the clinic will undoubtedly require several different strains tailored to the specific therapeutic application. Adenoviruses will be engineered to contain transgenes that augment antitumor response and suppress the antiviral response. In addition, replication-selective adenoviruses can also contain genes encoding factors that sensitize tumors to chemotherapeutic agents, thereby providing the additive effect of a multidrug regimen consisting of viral-mediated cell lysis and standard cytotoxic drug-mediated cell killing. The amount of genetic material that can be packaged into a mature adenovirus particle is limited to about 105% of the genome. Therefore, there are limitations to the size and number of transgenes that can be introduced into the genome. However, as more detail becomes known about the necessary adenoviral genes required for effective therapy, more efficient viruses will be generated and several adenoviruses harboring different complementary genetic compositions can be coadministered.

See Also the Following Articles

ADENO-ASSOCIATED VIRUS: A VECTOR FOR HIGH-EFFICIENCY GENE TRANSDUCTION • BCL-2 FAMILY PROTEINS AND THE DYSREGULATION OF PROGRAMMED CELL DEATH • PAPILLOMAVIRUSES • RETROVIRUSES • TP53 TUMOR SUPPRESSOR GENE: STRUCTURE AND FUNCTION • VIRAL AGENTS

Bibliography

Bayley, S. T., and Mymryk, J. S. (1994). Adenovirus E1A proteins and transformation (Review). *Int. J. Oncol.* **5,** 425–444.

Beck, G. R., Jr., Zerler, B., and Moran, E. (1998). Introduction to DNA tumor viruses: Adenovirus, simian virus 40, and polyomavirus. *In* "Human Tumor Viruses" (D. J. McCance, ed.), pp. 51–86. ASM Press.

Chan, H. M., Krstic-Demonacos, M., Smith, L., Demonacos, C., and La Thangue, N. B. (2001). Acetylation control of the retinoblastoma tumour-suppressor protein. *Nature Cell Biol.* **3,** 667–674.

Graham, F. L., and Prevec, L. (1995). Methods for construction of adenovirus vectors. *Mol. Biotech.* **3**, 207–220.

Graña, X., and Reddy, E. P. (1995). Cell cycle control in mammalian cells: Role of cyclins, cyclin-dependent kinases (CDKs), growth suppressor genes and cyclin dependent kinase inhibitors (CKIs). *Oncogene* **11**, 211–219.

Hermiston, T. (2000). Gene delivery from replication-selective viruses: Arming guided missiles in the war against cancer. *J. Clin. Invest.* **105**, 1169–1172.

Horwitz, M. S. (2001). Adenovirus immunoregulatory genes and their cellular targets. *Virology* **279**, 1–8.

Irwin, M. S., and Kaelin, W. G. (2001). p53 family update: p73 and p63 develop their own identities. *Cell Growth Differ.* **12**, 337–349.

Katakura, Y., Alam, S., and Shirahata, S. (1998). Immortalization by gene transfection. *Methods Cell Biol.* **57**, 69–91.

Levine, A. J. "Viruses." Freeman, New York.

MacLellan, W. R., Xiao, G., Abdellatif, M., and Schneider, M. D. (2000). A novel Rb- and p300-binding protein inhibits transactivation by MyoD. *Mol. Cell Biol.* **20**, 8903–8915.

Mathews, M. B. (1995). Structure, function, and evolution of adenovirus virus-associated RNAs. *In* "Current Topics in Microbiology and Immunology" (W. Doerfler and P. Böhm, eds.), Vol. 199, pp. 173–187. Springer, Berlin.

Moran, E. (1994). Mammalian cell growth controls reflected through protein interactions with the adenovirus E1A gene products. *Semin. Virol.* **5**, 327–340.

Querido, E., Morisson, M. R., Chu-Pham-Dang, H., Thirlwell, S. W., Boivin, D., and Branton, P. E. (2001). Identification of three functions of the adenovirus e4orf6 protein that mediate p53 degradation by the E4orf6-E1B55K complex. *J. Virol.* **75**, 699–709.

Shenk, T. (2001). Adenoviridae: The viruses and their replication. *In* "Fundamental Virology" (B. N. Fields, D. M. Knipe, and P. M. Howley *et al.*, eds.), 4th Ed. Lippincott-Raven, Philadelphia.

Smith, K., and Spindler, K.R. (1997). Pathogenesis and persistence of mouse adenovirus infections. In "Persistent Viral Infections" (R. Ahmed and I. Chen, eds.), pp. 477–484. John Wiley & Sons.

Sparer, T. E., and Gooding, L. R. (1998). Suppression of MHC class I antigen presentation by human adenoviruses. *Curr. Top. Microbiol. Immunol.* **232**, 135–147.

Steele, T. A. (2000). Recent developments in the virus therapy of cancer. *Proc. Soc. Exp. Biol. Med.* **223**, 118–127.

Swanton, C., and Jones, N. (2001). Strategies in subversion: De-regulation of the mammalian cell cycle by viral gene products. *Int. J. Exp. Pathol.* **82**, 3–13.

Thomas, D. L., Schaack, J., Vogel, H., and Javier, R. (2001). Several E4 region functions influence mammary tumorigenesis by human adenovirus type 9. *J. Virol.* **75**, 557–568.

Turner, J., and Crossley, M. (2001). The CtBP family: Enigmatic and enzymatic transcriptional co-repressors. *Bioessays* **23**, 683–690.

White, E. (1996). Life, death, and the pursuit of apoptosis. *Genes Dev.* **10**, 1–15.

Wold, W. S., Doronin, K., Toth, K., Kuppuswamy, M., Lichtenstein, D. L., and Tollefson, A. E. (1999). Immune responses to adenoviruses: Viral evasion mechanisms and their implications for the clinic. *Curr. Opin. Immunol.* **11**, 380–386.

Dosimetry and Treatment Planning for Three-Dimensional Radiation Therapy

Howard Amols

Memorial Sloan-Kettering Cancer Center

GLOSSARY

beams eye view Computer rendition of tumor and patient anatomy from the direction of a proposed radiation treatment portal.

digitally reconstructed radiograph (DRR) Computer reconstruction (from CT data) of a 2D X-ray projection image.

dose Amount of energy absorbed by the patient from the radiation per unit mass. Measured in units of gray (Gy), defined as 1 Joule of energy per kilogram of tissue. One Gy = 100 centigray (cGy), or 100 rad.

dose-volume histogram (DVH) Two-dimensional table quantifying the variation in dose for a particular structure. DVH gives the number of Gy received by different volume fractions of the organ.

dynamic multileaf collimator (DMLC) Device on linear accelerator, which permits computer control of X-ray beam shape and dose intensity.

electronic portal imaging device Similar to a digital X-ray imaging plate used to obtain 2D transmission X rays of the treatment beam on a linear accelerator.

energy Measured in units of MeV, is a function of the voltage and frequency of the X-ray production, and relates to the penetrability of the X-ray beam.

forward planning Radiation therapy treatment planning wherein the planner manually adjusts beam parameters to obtain an optimum plan.

intensity modulated radiation therapy (IMRT) Radiation therapy delivered with beams having continuously varying radiation intensity. See also DMLC.

inverse planning Radiation therapy treatment planning wherein the computer iteratively adjusts beam intensities from the DMLC to obtain an optimum plan.

linear accelerator Device used to produce high-energy X-ray beams.

normal tissue complication probability Estimation of the probability of normal tissue damage from a particular dose of radiation.

objective function Mathematical expression used in inverse treatment planning that quantifies the degree to which a plan matches the prescription criteria.

sliding window Type of IMRT beam delivery where the DMLC leaves are in continuous motion.

step and shoot Type of IMRT beam delivery where the MLC leaves move in discrete steps, with a fraction of the irradiation occurring at each step.

teletherapy Radiation therapy delivered with external beams of X rays aimed at the tumor.

three-dimensional computerized radiation therapy treatment planning Highly conformal radiation therapy achieved via the use of 3D image sets to precisely define the shape of the radiation beam to best avoid normal tissue irradiation.

tumor control probability Estimation of the probability of tumor control from a particular dose of radiation.

tumor volume The tumor, as visualized from various diagnostic studies. Differentiated into gross tumor volume (GTV, defined as gross tumor visible on CT); clinical tumor volume (CTV, equal to GTV plus margins for regions at risk); and planning target volume (PTV, equal to CTV plus margins for setup uncertainties).

virtual simulation Designing treatment beams from 3D CT data only, without use of conventional X-ray films.

X rays or γ rays Also referred to as photons. High-energy electromagnetic radiation produced by linear accelerators or by decay of radioisotopes.

The goal of radiation therapy is to deliver maximal doses to tumors while avoiding, as much as possible, overdosing intervening and surrounding normal tissues. For many treatment sites the success of radiation therapy is limited by the side effects of radiation on normal tissues. Recent advancements in high-energy X-ray equipment and computer technology now permit radiation therapy to be delivered with highly conformal megavoltage X-ray beams. New technologies such as three-dimensional (3D) tumor imaging, 3D conformal radiation therapy, intensity modulated radiation therapy, and inverse treatment planning enable customized beams and treatment plans for each patient to provide exquisite avoidance of normal tissue irradiation with ensuing reductions in treatment complications. This in turn permits escalation of prescribed tumor doses, which leads to improved local control for many tumor sites. This article reviews the development and applica-

tions of these new treatment modalities in radiation therapy.

I. INTRODUCTION

Radiation therapy began at the end of the 19th century immediately after the discoveries of X rays by Wilhelm Roentgen in 1895 and radium by Marie and Pierre Curie in 1897. Since then, advancements in radiation therapy have paralleled advancements in radiation physics, high voltage engineering, computer science, and diagnostic radiology. Computers, in particular, have enabled the development of three-dimensional computerized radiation therapy (3DCRT) treatment planning and intensity modulated radiation therapy (IMRT). The heart of these processes is computer-generated patient images, computer-controlled linear accelerators, and dynamic multileaf collimators (DMLC). Prior to 3DCRT and IMRT, the success of radiation therapy has been limited by the side effects of radiation on normal tissues. Higher energy X rays, improved imaging, and computer technology now permit avoidance of normal tissue irradiation to levels not previously achievable, opening new horizons in radiation therapy. A recent clinical trial in cancer of the prostate, for example, has tested escalation of prescription dose to as high 86.4 Gy via a combination of 3DCRT and IMRT compared to 65–75 Gy using conventional treatment planning and beam delivery techniques.

The technological development of radiation therapy is summarized in Table I.

II. RADIATION DOSIMETRY

A. X Rays, γ Rays, and Dose

Therapeutic ionizing radiation is most commonly in the form of X rays or γ rays (also referred to as photons) delivered via the use of external beams of X rays aimed at the tumor, so-called "teletherapy." Alternatively therapy may be via the implantation of radioactive isotopes directly into tumor tissue, called "brachytherapy." This article discusses only teletherapy.

X and γ rays are forms of high-energy electromagnetic radiation, similar in physical nature to mi-

TABLE I
Evolution of Radiation Therapy and Treatment Planning

Year	Tools	Techniques
1895	Low-energy X-ray tubes	"Clinical" beam setup, beams of poor penetrability, elementary dosimetry
1960	Cobalt-60, simulators, early computers	Simulation X-ray films used to design beams, better treatment planning with 2D dose calculations, more precise dosimetry
1975	High-energy linear accelerators, CT scanners, faster computers	Beam design from CT-generated beams eye view (BEV) computer renditions, faster 2.5D dose calculations and dose volume histograms
1995	MR+PET scanners, MLC, faster computers, improved graphics, IMRT	BEV + "virtual simulation" from CT, MRI, and PET, dose volume constraints and computer-optimized inverse treatment planning, 3D dose calculations, DMLC intensity modulated dose delivery

crowaves, visible light, ultraviolet, etc. The distinction between X and γ rays lies only in the source of origin: X rays originate from atoms and γ rays emanate from nuclear decay. The high-energy linear accelerators used in modern radiotherapy produce X rays.

Two different quantities are used to describe radiation. The amount of radiation prescribed is quantified by dose, which is equal to the energy absorbed by the patient from the radiation rather than the actual physical quantity of radiation used. The unit of dose in the international system of measurements (all units based on meters-kilograms-seconds) is the gray (Gy), defined as 1 Joule of energy absorbed per kilogram of tissue. One gray equals 100 centigray (cGy), or 100 Rad. Rad is an older unit being phased out of use. The absorbed radiation dose in a patient is a complicated function of the type and energy of the radiation, the geometry of the radiation source, its distance from the patient, and the shape and chemical composition of the patient. Different body tissues such as muscle, fat, and bone absorb different doses when exposed to the same radiation conditions. The energy of a photon is determined by the voltage (or sometimes frequency) of the production source, measured in volts, or, more commonly, million electron volts (MeV, or MV). In general, higher MV or energy means deeper tissue penetration. Thus, higher energy photons are required to treat deeper seated tumors. Modern teletherapy is usually administered with X rays from a linear accelerator having energies between 1 and 20 MV.

B. Dose Measurements

Radiation dosimetry is the science of determining the dose and dose distribution absorbed by a patient from ionizing radiation. *In vivo* measurements of dose are usually time-consuming and/or impractical. Also, the variations of radiation dose within a patient can be significant. *In vivo* dosimetry is therefore usually confined to occasional single point measurements for confirmation of calculated doses. Clinical radiation dosimetry is mostly confined to dose measurements in simple geometric phantoms, such as aquarium-like water tanks or tissue equivalent (TE) plastic. Calculational models of radiation transport are used to extrapolate phantom measurements to patient doses. Various devices have been developed for measuring radiation dose as well as complex computational algorithms. Phantom dose measurements serve two purposes: (1) to verify the accuracy of the computational algorithms and (2) as a routine quality assurance (QA) system to assess the functionality of all radiation delivery systems, including linear accelerators, CT machines, and so on.

The most common type of radiation detector is the ionization chamber, which consists of a small (typically <1 cm³) gas cavity (typically air) surrounded by a thin wall (typically 1–10 mm thick) of tissue-equivalent electrically conductive material. For dosimetry purposes, tissue equivalent means similar in atomic number and composition to muscle or water. A typical ionization chamber is shown schematically in Fig. 1. Operation of the ion chamber is based on the phenomenon that as X rays penetrate tissue, they scatter with molecular electrons producing ionizations, which produce free radicals and other chemical reactions, which results in biological damage to the irradiated tissue. Ions produced in the gas cavity of the ionization chamber by the X rays are "collected" by a voltage potential applied across the gas cavity,

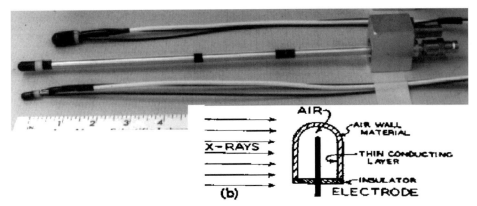

FIGURE 1 Examples of thimble-type ionization chambers (top), and schematic of X-ray beam irradiation of chamber to produce ionizations (lower right). (Reproduced courtesy of Charles C. Thomas, Springfield, IL.)

thus producing a measurable electrical current proportional to the radiation dose. Many other types of dosimeters are used in radiation therapy for special purposes, including thermolumenescent dosimeters (TLD), diodes, and radiographic film. Details can be found in the literature.

The shape of the dose distribution in a patient is a complicated function of radiation type, energy, and tissue composition. A typical dose distribution for a 22-MV X-ray beam is shown in Fig. 2. Note that the dose first rapidly increases with depth and then gradually decreases with depth because the X rays are attenuated by the tissue. There is also a sharp penumbra on the lateral edges of the beam produced by adjustable lead collimators in the accelerator, which precisely define the shape of the beam.

III. THREE-DIMENSIONAL COMPUTERIZED RADIATION THERAPY AND INTENSITY MODULATED RADIATION THERAPY

A. Treatment Planning Concepts

Conventional radiation therapy entails irradiation of the patient from multiple beam directions (the accelerator rotates about the patient), using beams similar to that shown in Fig. 2. All beams are "aimed" at the tumor, which is denoted as the "isocenter." Even though the intervening superficial tissues receive higher radiation doses for each single beam than the tumor, the summation of all beams results in a higher dose to the tumor. 3DCRT entails more sophisticated

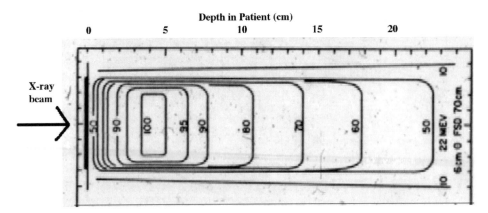

FIGURE 2 Typical 2D isodose distribution in a water phantom for 22-MV X-ray beam, entering phantom from the left. Note initial dose buildup to a maximum of 100% at a depth of approximately 5 cm and gradually decreasing dose at greater depths. (Reproduced courtesy of Charles C. Thomas, Springfield, IL.)

shaping of the dose distribution than conventional radiation therapy because the collimation, or shaping, of the beam and the selection of beam directions are designed with the advantage of 3D imaging data to best avoid normal tissue irradiation. IMRT goes one step beyond 3DCRT by, in addition, enabling variations of the *dose intensity* within each beam via use of the DMLC. A typical IMRT irradiation geometry and dose distribution for treatment of the prostate is shown in Figure 3 (discussed in more detail later). Briefly, this process of 3DCRT and IMRT can be summarized as follows.

1. Patient setup and immobilization.
2. CT imaging and "virtual" simulation, sometimes augmented by MRI and/or PET.
3. Delineation of treatment volume and normal tissue structures from various imaging modalities.
4. Design of treatment portals using computerized BEV, specification of desired doses to tumor and normal tissues.
5. Iterative optimization of treatment beams to obtain the "best" possible plan.

6. Treatment plan evaluation via analysis of dose distributions and DVH.
7. For IMRT (but not 3DCRT) calculation of DMLC "leaf sequence files."
8. Patient treatment using beams designed from the treatment-planning process.
9. Dosimetric and QA tasks for verification that all equipment is functioning properly and that the specifics of the dose prescription and treatment plan are accurately delivered to the patient on a daily basis.

These steps are discussed in more detail.

B. Simulation and Virtual Simulation

A course of radiation therapy may entail in excess of 40 daily treatments over a 6- to 10-week period. Each treatment must duplicate as precisely as possible the setup geometry of the original CT simulation planning session. Minimizing setup uncertainty is even more important in 3DCRT and IMRT than in conventional radiotherapy due to the improved

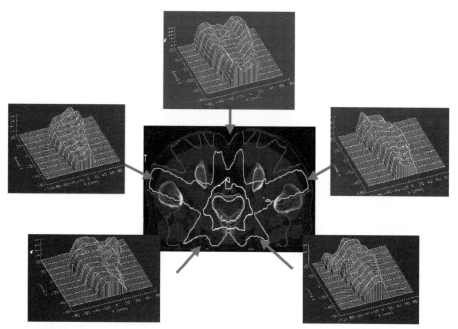

FIGURE 3 Isodose distribution in the transverse plane for IMRT prostate treatment to 81 Gy with five beams. Also shown are the intensity modulated beam profiles for each field. Patient is in the prone position. Increasing dose levels are represented by concentric contours.

conformality of the dose distribution. Thus, immobilization devices such as molds and body casts, plus precise positioning procedures, are used throughout the process of image acquisition, simulation, and treatment.

A complete 3D CT image set is obtained with the patient in the treatment position. CT slice thickness is typically 3–5 mm or less, with smaller slice thicknesses being desirable for better contour definition, and also higher resolution digitally reconstructed radiographs (DRR). DRRs are computer-rendered 2D projection images similar to conventional X-ray films, which enable the planner to "view" the patient from any beam direction. For some sites, MRI and PET are complementary to CT and are especially useful when used with image correlation software, which permits fusing data from multiple imaging studies.

DRRs allow us to use the CT imaging session as a replacement for the conventional simulation process, in effect combining the two processes into one so-called "virtual simulation" (VS), which is carried out on a computer workstation. For any set of treatment parameters or desired beam directions, the CT data set becomes the virtual patient and is used to reconstruct DRRs and BEV images in order to visualize the patient anatomy and simulate the treatment. Structures are defined by contouring each tissue of interest on a series of 2D axial CT images. Tumor volumes are defined according to the ICRU Report 50 nomenclature:

a. Gross tumor volume (GTV) is defined as gross tumor visible on CT (or other imaging modality).
b. Clinical tumor volume (CTV) is the visualized GTV plus regions at risk (microscopic disease, etc.).
c. Planning target volume (PTV) is CTV plus setup and other uncertainties, typically 5–15 mm.

In addition to the PTV, contours are needed for the skin, bone, lungs, and air cavities, plus any tissues that may be dose limiting vis a vis therapy such as spinal cord, kidneys, and rectum. These objects are often displayed in BEV as color-coded wire frames or solid structures. The manual delineation of these structures is time-consuming, although computerized tools such as edge detection algorithms and autosegmentation can automate the process for outer skin and air cavities. Improvements in these algorithms will likely make this process easier in future, although human intervention will probably always remain a necessary component. The treatment planner must define the number, energy, and orientation of all radiation beams in the treatment. Selection of beams is based on a combination of experience, (sometimes) standard protocols, and patient-specific anatomy.

C. Dose Calculations and Optimization

After the beams are specified (as described earlier), the 3DCRT and IMRT planning processes diverge. 3DCRT, like more conventional treatment planning, entails so-called forward planning wherein the user defines the intensity of or dose to be delivered from each beam. The computer then calculates the dose distribution resulting from these beams, including doses to the PTV and all normal tissues defined by contours. Based on these calculated doses, the user adjusts the intensity or shape of any or all treatment beams in order to "improve" the dose distribution to best meet prescription criteria. The computer recalculates the dose each time the user changes a beam, and the process is repeated until an "optimal" dose distribution is obtained. This approach is sensitive to the experience of the planner and can be very time-consuming.

For IMRT planning, the user does not attempt to optimize or readjust beam intensities. Instead, after defining the orientation and energy of all beams (but *not* their intensities), the planner specifies the doses *desired* for the PTV and all tissues of interest. The *computer* then iteratively calculates the optimum beam intensities to achieve this distribution. This process is called inverse treatment planning. The most distinguishing feature in IMRT planning, however, is not inverse planning, but rather the use of *intensity modulation* to improve the dose distribution. In this approach, the computer algorithm divides each beam into individual rays or beamlets and iteratively alters the ray weights until the composite dose distribution best meets the specified objectives. Unlike 3DCRT, which is limited to beams of uniform intensity, IMRT beams have significant intensity variation throughout.

A typical radiation therapy treatment plan may entail anywhere from two to eight treatment fields. In conventional forward planning, the total dose from each field is the major "adjustable" parameter available to the planner. For inverse planning and IMRT, however, the computer divides each treatment field into several hundred individual beamlets, each with a different intensity, thus providing an order of magnitude more control over the resulting dose distribution. Obviously the success of inverse IMRT treatment planning hinges on the practicality of being able to deliver an intensity modulated beam. This is accomplished with the use of computer-controlled linear accelerators and DMLC (as described later).

Also central to the success of computer optimization is some quantitative measure of the "goodness" of a treatment plan. For inverse planning, "goodness" is specified as a mathematical objective function (OF) that the computer attempts to minimize (or maximize, depending on definitions). At present, most OFs are based on dose or DVH to the PTV and normal tissues of interest. The use of biologically weighted objective functions is in principle more relevant, but is currently limited by the lack of validated biophysical models on tumor control and organ toxicity.

The "heart" of inverse treatment planning is minimization of the OF. The OF can have many mathematical definitions, but is typically of the form:

$$OF = \sum_i w_i * P(D_{prescribed} - D_{delivered})_i$$

where $D_{prescribed}$ is prescription dose to the ith CT voxel in the patient. $D_{delivered}$ is calculated dose to the ith voxel from the current beam and beamlet parameters. This dose is a complicated function of the radiation beam parameters (energy, orientation, etc.), the voxel coordinates in space relative to the beamlet, and the voxels position within the patient. $P(\delta D)$ is penalty function, which quantifies the "undesirability" of having a difference between the prescribed dose and the delivered dose of δD. The penalty function can take many mathematical forms, as described more fully later and in Fig. 4. w_i is weight, or relative importance of the ith voxel. The weight assigned, for example, to the spinal cord may be greater than the weight to the bowel, or vice versa.

In practice, doses to any tissue structure are rarely uniform, and specifying the OF simply as a summation of $P(D_{prescribed} - D_{delivered})_i$ is overly simplistic

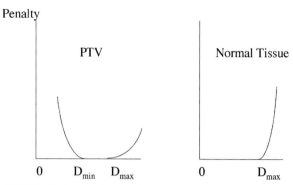

FIGURE 4 Sample objective functions. For PTV there is no penalty if dose is within an allowable window, but larger penalties are assessed for underdose than overdose. For normal tissue penalty is applied only for overdose.

because biological response is *not* linearly proportional to dose. Therefore, it is often more meaningful to specify desired doses in terms of dose-volume constraints such as no more than x% of an organ may receive a dose greater than d_{max} or no less than x% of the PTV may receive a dose less than d_{min}.

Figure 4 graphs two typical objective functions. For the PTV, Fig. 4 illustrates the concept of "allowable inhomogeneity." That is, if the dose is between an acceptable lower and upper limit there is no penalty, and a larger penalty can be assigned to an underdose than to an overdose. For an organ at risk there is no penalty for an underdose, but a rapidly increasing penalty for overdose.

After computer optimization, the planner must evaluate the plan. The tools used for treatment plan evaluation are similar for 3DCRT and IMRT. They consist of:

a. Two-dimensional dose distributions superimposed onto CT images (as shown in Fig. 3 for treatment of prostate).
b. Three-dimensional volumetric rendering of dose distribution, PTV, and critical organs (as shown in Fig. 5 for treatment of nasopharynx).
c. DVH for PTV and critical organs, as shown in Fig. 6 for treatment of prostate.
d. Predicted values of normal tissue complication and tumor control probabilities (NTCP and TCP).

With these tools the planner evaluates the treatment design and, if necessary, via either forward

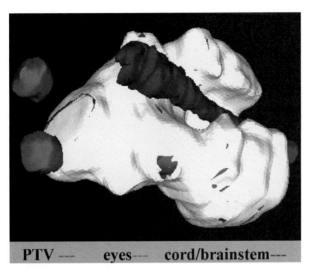

FIGURE 5 Display of 65-Gy isodose contour (white) for na-sopharynx irradiation showing target volume, brain stem/spinal cord, and eyes.

(3DCRT) or inverse (IMRT) planning, tries to make improvements. Improving an unacceptable IMRT plan can often be difficult because one may not know a priori whether the calculated plan is "bad" because of inappropriately chosen beams, dose volume constraints, penalties, and so on or because the dose parameters "requested" are physically impossible to achieve. Our past experience in conventional 3DCRT treatment planning is only of marginal help in assessing IMRT plans. We are still on the learning curve!

D. IMRT Treatment Delivery and Verification

At present there are three primary methods of IMRT beam delivery: (a) IMRT fields at fixed gantry angles delivered with DMLC using the "sliding window" technique, (b) IMRT fields at fixed gantry angles delivered with MLC using the "step and shoot" technique, and (c) tomotherapy using beams from 360° and modulated by a slit multileaf collimator.

Most of our discussion focuses on the first approach. The "sliding window" technique permits continuous variation in the intensity distribution within each field by customized motion of the individual leaf pairs of the MLC. The desired 2D intensity distribution for each field (see, e.g., the intensity profiles in Figure 3) is divided into 1D intensity profiles, with each profile delivered by one leaf pair of the DMLC. Figure 7 shows a cutout view of a DMLC mounted in the head of a linear accelerator with the individual leaf pairs and control motors. With the sliding window method, the leaves are in continuous motion during radiation delivery such that at any instant in time the "open" portion of the field is an irregularly shaped slit (Fig. 8). The dose received by any point in the patient is proportional to how long that point spends under the open portion of the slit. By controlling the movement of the leaves and therefore the "exposure" or duration, one can deliver virtually any desired dose to any point in the patient. In practice, a separate computer program (different from the inverse planning algo-

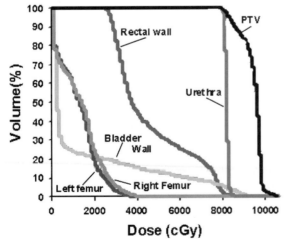

FIGURE 6 DVHs for the 81-Gy IMRT plan illustrated in Fig. 3. DVH is plotted for PTV, rectum, urethra, bladder, and femurs.

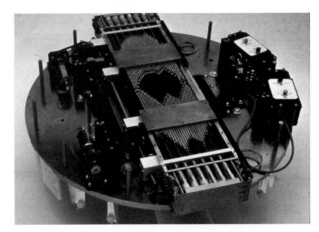

FIGURE 7 DMLC located in "head" of linear accelerator. Note multiple leaf pairs and individual control motors for each leaf. (Reproduced by courtesy of Varian Medical Systems, Palo Alto, CA.)

Delivery of IMRT with
continuous leaf motion

• Each leaf pair forms a window which slides across the field.

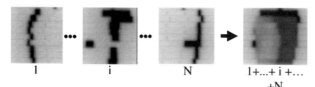

• The final dose distribution is the summation from all "segments"

FIGURE 8 At any instant in time the IMRT field is an irregular slit (panels 1–3 on the left). The total dose from this beam is the summation of all segments, as indicated in gray scale (white, low dose; black, high dose) in panel 4 on the right.

rithm), sometimes called the "leaf-sequencer," is used to translate the intensity profiles of the IM beam into the so-called DMLC file, which contains data for the leaf positions as a function of treatment time.

The MLC can also be used to deliver IMRT via the delivery of multiple static fields of different shapes; the so-called step-and-shoot mode. In this mode, the MLC travels in a stepwise manner to discrete positions, with the beam turned off during the stepwise movement.

For both 3DCRT and IMRT, data on beam shapes, directions, and dose are transferred from the treatment planning system to the computer that controls the linear accelerator. For IMRT the leaf motion files for the DMLC must also be transferred. This is done via floppy disk or network transfer. A separate "record and verify" computer monitors all treatments and data transfer to ensure accuracy.

In addition to the computer-oriented treatment planning process, IMRT entails extensive dosimetry and QA. Treatments are more complex than 3DCRT, and a great reliance is placed on sophisticated computer technology, particularly the integrity of the large volumes of data transferred between the treatment planning system and the linear accelerator computers. In addition, for IMRT it is virtually impossible to check computer dose calculations "by hand" or with any simple algorithm. Thus unlike conventional forward planning, IMRT treatments are often impossible to verify by conventional dosimetric or calculational techniques.

Verification of IMRT doses therefore relies largely on measurements, which may include the use of radiographic film, ion chamber dosimetry, and electronic portal imaging devices (EPID). A typical geometry for performing film and/or ion chamber dosimetry tests is shown in Fig. 9. Installing and commissioning

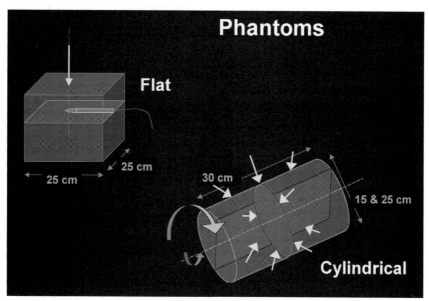

FIGURE 9 Schematic of rectangular and cylindrical plastic phantoms for ion chamber or film dosimetry.

a DMLC system also require extensive mechanical and dosimetric measurements, including mechanical calibration of leaf positions and dosimetric characterization of the MLC. The latter is done using a combination of ion chambers and radiographic film.

IV. SUMMARY

Engineering advancements and computer technology now permit radiation therapy to be delivered with highly conformal radiation beams to provide exquisite avoidance of normal tissue irradiation and ensuing complications. New technologies such as 3DCRT, IMRT, and inverse treatment planning enable customized beams and treatment plans for each patient. This in turn permits escalation of prescribed tumor doses, which it is hoped will lead to improved local control for many tumor sites.

See Also the Following Articles

LATE EFFECTS OF RADIATION THERAPY • MOLECULAR ASPECTS OF RADIATION BIOLOGY • PHOTODYNAMIC THERAPY: CLINICAL APPLICATIONS • PROTON BEAM RADIATION THERAPY • RADIATION RESISTANCE • STEREOTACTIC RADIOSURGERY

Bibliography

Brahme, A. (1988). Optimization of stationary and moving beam radiation therapy techniques. *Radiother. Oncol.* **12**, 129–140.

Chui, C. S., LoSasso, T., and Spirou, S. (1994). Dose calculations for photon beams with intensity modulation generated by dynamic jaw or multi-leaf collimations. *Med. Phys.* **21**, 1237–1243.

Gagliardi, R., and Almond, P. (eds.) (1996). "A History of the Radiological Sciences: Radiation Physics." Radiology Centennial, Reston, VA.

Gagliardi, R., and Wilson, J. F. (eds.) (1996). "A History of the Radiological Sciences: Radiation Oncology." Radiology Centennial, Reston, VA.

Goitein, M., Abrams, M., Rowell, D., *et al.* (1983). Multidimensional treatment planning. II. Beam's eye view, back projection and projection through CT sections. *Int. J. Radiat. Oncol. Biol. Phys.* **9**, 789–797.

ICRU Report 50 (1993). "Prescribing, Recording, and Reporting Photon Beam Therapy." International Commission on Radiation Units and Measurements, Bethesda, MD.

Johns, H., and Cunningham, J. (1983). "The Physics of Radiology," 4th Ed. Charles C. Thomas, Springfield, IL.

Leibel, S. A., Zelefsky, M. J., Kutcher, G. J., et al. (1994). The biological basis and clinical application of three-dimensional conformal external beam radiation therapy in carcinoma of the prostate. *Semin. Oncol.* **21**, 580–597.

Ling, C. C., Chui, C., LoSasso, T., et al. (2000). Intensity-modulated radiation therapy (IMRT). *In* "Cancer: Principles and Practice of Oncology" (V. DeVita, S. Hellman, and S. Rosenberg, eds.), 6th Ed. Lippincott, Philadelphia.

LoSasso, T., Chui, C. S., Kutcher, G. J., *et al.* (1993). The use of a multileaf collimator for conformal radiotherapy of carcinoma of the prostate and nasopharynx. *Int. J. Radiat. Oncol. Biol. Phys.* **25**, 161–170.

LoSasso, T., Chui, C. S., and Ling, C. C. (1998). Physical and dosimetric aspects of a multileaf collimation system used in the dynamic mode for implementing intensity modulated radiotherapy. *Med. Phys.* **25**, 1919–1927.

Lyman, J. T. (1985). Complication probability as assessed from dose volume histograms. *Radiat. Res.* **8**, 113.

McShan, D. L., Fraass, B. A., and Lichter, A. S. (1990). Full integration of the beam's eye view concept into computerized treatment planning. *Int. J. Radiat. Oncol. Biol. Phys.* **18**, 1485–1494.

Niemierko, A., Urie, M., and Goitein, M. (1992). Optimization of 3D radiation therapy with both physical and biological end points and constraints. *Int. J. Radiat. Oncol. Biol. Phys.* **23**, 99–108.

Spirou, S. V., and Chui, C. S. (1998). A gradient inverse planning algorithm with dose-volume constraints. *Med. Phys.* **25**, 321–333.

Zelefsky, M. J., Leibel, S. A., Gaudin, P. B., *et al.* (1998). Dose escalation with three-dimensional conformal radiation therapy affects the outcome in prostate cancer. *Int. J. Radiat. Oncol. Biol. Phys.* **41**, 491–500.

Drug Resistance: DNA Sequence Amplification

Joyce L. Hamlin

University of Virginia School of Medicine, Charlottesville

GLOSSARY

abnormally banding region (ABR) An expanded chromosomal region displaying a banding pattern different from that of the normal chromosome when subjected to the Giemsa-staining protocol, usually as the result of gene amplification. When these ABRs contain large numbers of amplicons, they stain homogenously and are known as homogenously staining regions *(HSRs)*.

amplicon The unit-repeating sequence that is amplified.

anti-oncogene or tumor suppressor gene A gene whose loss is involved in the acquisition of cancer.

DNA amplification A process in which the copy number of a subchromosomal length of DNA is selectively increased relative to flanking DNA sequences.

double minute chromosome A small chromosome-like body that lacks a centromere and consists of multiple tandem amplicons.

genetic variant A cell line that has suffered a mutation or DNA sequence rearrangement which results in a heritable, altered phenotypic property.

genome The entire nuclear DNA content of a cell.

nondisjunction A process in which a replicated chromosome, or a part thereof, fails to separate at mitosis so that both copies are distributed to one daughter cell.

oncogene A gene encoding a positive growth factor or growth factor receptor which, when activated or amplified, can contribute to tumorigenesis.

DNA sequence amplification is a process whereby the copy number of a large but subchromosomal length of DNA is selectively increased—sometimes by more than a thousandfold. With only a few exceptions, the phenomenon is unique to tumor cells. Amplification was discovered in cultured mammalian cell lines selected for resistance to anti-cancer agents, and these variants were subsequently shown to have amplified the gene encoding the corresponding target protein. Each unit of amplification (amplicon) can range in length from a few hundred kilobase pairs to tens of megabases. Amplicons are organized into tandem arrays, either in the body of chromosomes as abnormally banding or homogenously staining regions or as autonomous episomal elements known as double minute chromosomes. The most popular models for initiating and propagating amplification to a high copy number have invoked overreplication. However, recent studies employing high resolution fluorescence *in situ* hybridization (FISH) argue strongly that amplification may usually be initiated by classic bridge–breakage–fusion cycles. Thus, amplification can now be understood as yet another example of the untoward consequences accruing in cancer from the loss of DNA damage-sensing pathways that prevent replication prior to the repair of chromosome breaks.

I. INTRODUCTION

As discussed elsewhere in this volume, drug resistance is a serious clinical problem that has plagued oncologists since the advent of cancer chemotherapy. The design of more rational drug therapies in the future will require a thorough understanding of the molecular mechanisms responsible for drug resistance. Beginning in the early fifties, investigators employed cultured mammalian cell lines as simplified model systems in which to recreate and study the phenomenon. Since most cultured cells are tumorigenic and since amplification is virtually unique to tumor cells, these model systems have provided a basis for understanding drug resistance in all it forms at the molecular level. However, as discussed in this article, tumor context in the body may modulate the degree of amplification or the choice of mechanism. Hence, results obtained in these model systems will ultimately have to be interpreted in light of the *in vivo* milieu.

In addition, initial experimental approaches were directed toward understanding the development of resistance to selective agents in cultured cells. It is therefore interesting that well-documented clinical examples of drug resistance acquired by the amplification mechanisms uncovered in this approach are extremely rare. Rather, the most frequently amplified sequences in human tumors turn out to be cellular oncogenes, the products of which contribute to the

transformed state. Thus, investigations that were initiated in the drug resistance arena may explain critical first steps in oncogenesis.

II. DEFINING THE PROBLEM

Since the acquisition of drug resistance in cultured cells and tumors is heritable, it was assumed from the outset to be a genetic change. One can imagine at least four different ways in which a cell could acquire resistance to a drug: (1) by mutating a membrane carrier so that the drug is not transported into the cell; (2) by mutating or increasing the amount of an efflux protein so that the drug is more rapidly pumped out of the cell; (3) by modifying the target enzyme or protein so that it no longer binds or is inhibited by the drug; and/or (4) by increasing the concentration of the target protein and overtitrating the ambient drug concentration.

A common form of resistance to chemotherapeutic agents in human tumors is the multidrug-resistance phenotype, which is acquired by increasing the level of the broad spectrum drug efflux transporter, P-glycoprotein (but not by amplifying its gene). Each of the other possible modes of drug resistance has been detected in experimental circumstances, and the development of resistance to the antifolate drug, methotrexate (MTX), which is apparently not recognized by the P-glycoprotein carrier, can serve as an example.

In a typical selection protocol, a cultured mammalian tumor cell line is exposed to stepwise increases in MTX concentration over the period of many months. A series of increasingly more resistant variants is selected in which the most resistant can survive MTX concentrations thousands of times higher than the starting cells. One curious feature is that even at the first selection step, the number of resistant variants recovered is of the order of 10^{-4}–10^{-5} per cell generation—a frequency much higher than expected if resistance is acquired by point mutation of a single gene. This suggested that mutations in any one of several genes could result in drug resistance. However, very early on it was discovered that only a minority of resistant variants sustain mutations in genes encoding either drug carriers or the target proteins themselves. Rather, the majority of independently isolated variants displayed increased levels of dihydrofolate reductase (DHFR) enzyme activity, which was subsequently shown to correspond to increased levels of wild-type DHFR protein.

Understanding the nature of the genetic changes responsible for the overproduction of DHFR protein in the majority of variants was attendant on two important developments in the seventies: recombinant DNA technology and high resolution chromosome-banding methods. Robert Schimke's group at Stanford pioneered the molecular biological approach by first purifying the messenger RNA (mRNA) from a MTX-resistant murine cell line and using solution hybridization and *in vitro* translation approaches to show that the mRNA encoding DHFR is also overproduced. In simpler genetic systems such as bacteria, the only precedents for mRNA overproduction were mutations that increase the efficiency of transcription of the gene in question.

However, at about the same time, June Biedler and Barbara Spengler at Sloan-Kettering Memorial Institute made a seminal observation which argued that a totally different kind of genetic anomaly might be re-sponsible for drug resistance in most cases. In G-banded mitotic chromosome preparations of a series of MTX-resistant Chinese hamster cell lines, they noticed a strong correlation between drug resistance and the presence of expanded, abnormally banding regions (ABRs) on one or more chromosomes. In highly resistant cell lines, these ABRs either stained uniformly or displayed a regular series of fine dark bands superimposed on a uniform background (unlike the irregularly alternating light and dark bands that characterize normal chromosomes in these preparations). Hence, they were called homogenously staining regions (HSRs). An example of an HSR is shown in Fig. 1A. Biedler and Spengler made the additional observation that ABRs/HSRs often resided on chromosome 2, the chromosome that was subsequently shown to carry the normal DHFR gene. They suggested that these structures might correspond to arrays of amplified copies of the DHFR gene.

Proof for this contention followed rapidly. A complementary DNA (cDNA) copy of the murine DHFR mRNA was cloned by Schimke's group, which provided a specific radioactive probe for *in situ* hybridization studies on the mitotic chromosomes of a

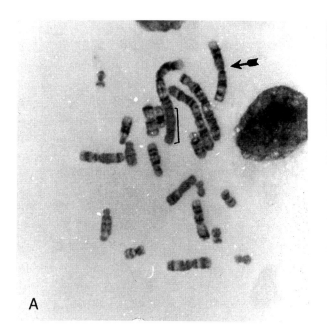
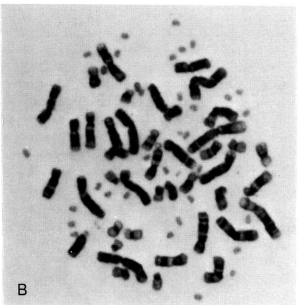

FIGURE 1 Giemsa-banding patterns of ABR- and DM-containing rodent cells. (A) The Giemsa-staining pattern of a mitotic chromosome spread of a MTX-resistant Chinese hamster lung fibroblast (courtesy of J. Biedler, Memorial Sloan-Kettering Institute). The bracket indicates the ABR containing amplified DHFR genes. (B) A Giemsa-stained chromosomal spread showing numerous small DMs that stain to an intermediate degree.

MTX-resistant Chinese hamster cell line. In all cases, large numbers of silver grains were localized to each ABR or HSR, indicating that each contained multiple copies of the DHFR gene. In MTX-resistant murine cell lines, the multiple extrachromosomal double minutes (DMs) were separated by size on a sucrose gradient and were shown to contain amplified copies of the murine DHFR gene. With these experiments, the field of DNA sequence amplification was essentially launched.

III. EXAMPLES OF DNA SEQUENCE AMPLIFICATION

Right from the beginning, investigators looked for models from nature that could provide insight into the mechanisms of amplification. In fact, there are more than a few natural situations in which organisms selectively amplify a section of the genome in order to increase the rate of protein synthesis. In several species, ribosomal RNA genes (rDNA) are amplified during early cleavage stages in the embryo in order to cope with the tremendous demand for proteins. Interestingly, in the oxytrich *Tetrahymena*, the genome is fragmented into thousands of gene-sized pieces at an early stage of development; the rDNA fragments are then selectively amplified by overreplication. In contrast, frogs increase the number of rDNA genes in early cleavage stages by synthesizing extra copies of the rDNA genes and releasing them as episomes that continue to be replicated by a rolling-circle mechanism. Yet another variation occurs in the egg shell chambers of *Drosophila*, in which the chorion genes are selectively amplified prior to egg laying by an onionskin mode of rereplication in which the extra copies of the chorion genes lay side by side in the genome. Onionskin replication also occurs in the salivary glands of sciarid flies, amplifying genes encoding cocoon proteins. Thus, Mother Nature has developed several different mechanisms for amplifying specific stretches of genomic DNA under well-controlled circumstances.

There are many archaeological relics of probable aberrant amplification events in mammalian genomes. Presumably, all multigene families (including, e.g., histones, globins, and immunoglobulins) were originally generated by the same mechanisms that are re-sponsible for the acute amplification of drug-resistance genes under selective pressure in cultured cells. Evolution would then have a chance to work on each copy independently to diversify gene function without losing the original function.

It appears that almost any DNA sequence can be amplified under experimental circumstances, as long as there is some method for identifying (i.e., selecting) cells that have undergone amplification at that locus. Table I provides an incomplete list of genes that have been amplified in various mammalian cell lines isolated by selection on increasing concentrations of the indicated agents. In each case, the selective agent is a good competitive inhibitor of the protein or enzyme encoded by that gene. With the exception of the MDR gene, none of these resistant variants (amplicants) are cross-resistant to any other drug. However, variants selected with one of a number of alkaloids and antibiotics of plant and fungal origin can acquire resistance to other structurally unrelated members of this group, due to the amplification of the MDR gene. The MDR gene encodes a broad-spectrum drug efflux transporter.

TABLE I

Examples of DNA Sequence Amplification
in Drug Resistance

Drug	Gene
Methotrexate	Dihydrofolate reductase
PALA	Multienzyme CAD complex
FUdR	Thymidylate synthetase
Albiizin	Asparagine synthetase
Coformycin/adenine	Adenylate deaminase
Deoxycoformycin	Adenosine deaminase
Hydroxyurea	Ribonucleotide reductase
Compactin	HMG-CoA reductase
Heavy metals	Metallothionein
Ouabain	Na,K-ATPase
Colchicine	Microtubular proteins
Nitrogen mustards	Glutathione-S-transferase
Pyrazofurine	UMP synthetase
Methyl sulfoximine	Glutamine synthetase
α-CH₃-ornithine	Ornithine decarboxylase
Mycophenolic acid	IMP-5′-dehydrogenase
Tunicamycin	N-Acetylglucosaminyl transferase
Borrelidin	Threonyl-tRNA synthetase
Alanosine	Adenylosuccinate synthetase

All of the resistant cell lines in Table I have undergone neoplastic transformation prior to amplification, either in the animal as a tumor prior to *in vitro* culture or while in culture after the crisis and genetic rearrangement that normal mammalian cell types must undergo before they can be successfully adapted to long-term culture. In fact, it took a while to realize that nontransformed cells do not amplify DNA (or, if they do, they do not stably maintain the extra DNA in the genome). There have been several carefully designed studies comparing the frequency with which transformed and nontransformed cultured cells amplify the CAD gene in response to selection with phosphonacetyl-L-aspartic acid (PALA). This drug was chosen because amplification of the CAD gene is the only known mode of developing resistance to PALA. The frequencies of resistant colony formation (and, ergo, CAD gene amplification) for tumorigenic cell lines ranged from 10^{-3} to 10^{-4}, while the corresponding numbers for minimally transformed cell lines were less than 10^{-9}.

Interestingly, to date, there is only one documented account of gene amplification occurring in apparently normal cells in humans. In certain areas in Israel (and presumably other geographic locations as well) in which the insecticide parathion is used on agricultural crops, the gene encoding butyryl cholinesterase was shown to be amplified approximately 100-fold in a family residing near and working in the fields. As the potential for gene amplification in response to chemicals in the environment is appreciated, this isolated instance will surely be accompanied by other examples in the future.

Although the topic of this article is DNA sequence amplification in drug resistance, it is impossible to overlook another class of genes that is amplified routinely in human tumors. Indeed, the first examples of gene amplification were detected in the fifties in cytological preparations from tumor cells as expanded chromosomes and double minutes. Although at the time there was no way to know that these abnormal entities contained amplified DNA, they were added to the catalogue of chromosome rearrangements (along with translocations, deletions, and inversions) that could be discerned in a large percentage of tumor samples.

By partially purifying double minute chromosomes from the human HL60 tumors, Donna George and colleagues were able to clone some of the corresponding DNA sequences and show that they contain the cellular proto-oncogene, c-myc. This important contribution led the way to the discovery that the majority of human tumors have amplified some proto-oncogene. The partial list in Table II shows that the variety of tumor types and oncogenes is almost endless. As more and more oncogenes are identified and cloned, providing probes for detecting increased copy numbers in tumor DNA, it is likely that the majority of tumors will be shown to have amplified at least one oncogene.

As discussed earlier, amplification of a given marker under selective conditions only occurs at a frequency of 10^{-4}–10^{-5} per cell generation, but drug selection allows enrichment of amplicants by killing off those cells with diploid copy numbers. Why do tumor cells amplify DNA and, in the case of a neoplastic cell, what selection pressures operate to allow the infrequent cell with an amplified oncogene(s) to survive? These are fascinating and important questions that

TABLE II
Oncogene Amplification in Human Tumors

c-myc	Breast carcinoma
	Osteosarcoma
	Lung carcinoma
	Non-Hodgkin's lymphoma
	Adenocarcinoma
	Myeloid leukemia
N-myc	Neuroblastoma
	Small cell lung carcinoma
c-myb	Small cell lung carcinoma
Ki-ras/n-ras	Ovarian carcinoma
	Lung carcinoma
	Adrenocortical tumor
	Embryonal carcinoma
Ha-ras	Carcinogen-induced tumors
ets-1	Myelomonocytic leukemia
erbB-2 (neu/Her2)	Gastric carcinoma
	Breast carcinoma
	Lung carcinoma
	Adenocarcinoma
erbB-1	Squamous cell carcinoma
	Breast carcinoma
	Lung carcinoma
	Glioma
Hist-1/Int-2	Stomach carcinoma
	Esophageal carcinoma
c-abl	Myelogenous leukemia

probe the heart of the cancer problem. However, it is reasonable to assume that the genetic instability that characterize tumor cells renders them capable of amplifying DNA, including oncogenes. Once a cell has more than the usual two copies of these positive growth factor genes, it may have a slight growth advantage and, given enough time, will eventually win out in the competition for scarce blood supply, etc.

Thus, it is ironic that studies on DNA amplification began by examining resistance to single drugs in cultured cells since this kind of resistance has turned out not to be very important clinically; rather, amplification of oncogenes is a far more frequent occurrence in human tumors. As we will see, however, concentrating on the single drug approach has helped to understand the molecular mechanisms responsible for initiating amplification, and these mechanisms are likely to apply to any DNA sequence.

IV. THE NATURE OF AMPLIFIED DNA

When it was fully appreciated that most experimentally developed drug-resistant cell variants had amplified the gene encoding the target protein, it became important to define the properties of the amplified DNA. The obvious place to begin this analysis was the HSRs and DMs that bear the amplicons in highly resistant cell lines.

The first question is why there are two different chromosomal forms. The answer is presently not known. Chinese and Syrian hamster cells virtually always carry amplified DNA sequences in chromosomal ABRs or HSRs, but the physical properties of these entities vary. At low levels of drug resistance, ABRs appear as elongated chromosomal regions with altered Giemsa-staining bands and are identified by their patchy hybridization patterns with radioactive gene-specific probes. Highly resistant variants usually display at least one and usually more marker chromosomes with extended HSRs (i.e., regions that stain homogeneously to an intermediate degree). A curious observation is that HSRs in highly MTX-resistant Chinese hamster cells also stain by the C-banding technique, which is normally thought to preferen-

tially illuminate condensed, inactive heterochromatin. Other than the rather different staining patterns, the HSRs in metaphase chromosomes of highly resistant variants appear to be condensed to the same degree as the rest of the chromosome complement. In cell lines bearing hundreds of copies of the amplicon in question, the amplified DNA can approach 10% of the total genomic DNA content of the cell. HSRs are usually stable for months or even years in the absence of the selective agent, but eventually they are partially or completely lost.

Drug-resistant murine, rat, and human lines in culture can exhibit either ABRs/HSRs or DMs, even when amplifying the same gene. There have been reports in which MTX-resistant murine cell lines that originally carried the DHFR amplicons in DMs eventually gave rise to a stable chromosomal HSR after a lengthy interval in culture. However, the presence of ABRs/HSRs and DMs in the same cell has rarely been reported.

The term *double minute (DM) chromosomes* is used to refer to relatively small, extrachromosomal, acentromeric chromosome fragments. Those that are visible in the light microscope after staining probably have to be >5 MB in length. The number of DMs per cell can range from only one or two to many thousands (see Fig. 1B). In general, the larger the number, the smaller the DM. There is some semantic confusion between what constitutes a very large DM and a small, acentromeric chromosome fragment since they are essentially featureless blobs of chromatin that usually stain to an intermediate degree with Giemsa, just as do HSRs. It may turn out that they are one and the same. Most DMs appear in the light microscope as if they were a cross section between the two chromatids of a chromosome, although many single minutes can usually be observed in the same cell. The single form most likely represents the condensed chromosome structure of a single chromatid.

DMs have been shown to replicate once per cell cycle and to be carried as clusters into daughter cells by attachment to normal chromosomes, usually near the telomeres. As a consequence, they are not distributed uniformly to daughter cells. Furthermore, it has been demonstrated that cells bearing DMs grow considerably more slowly than matched cell lines that contain no DMs. Therefore, it is not surprising that

DMs are quickly diluted out in an expanding cell population in the absence of drug. Indeed, all detectable DMs can be lost within a matter of 20 or 30 cell generations.

Electron microscope investigations have suggested that DMs are actually circular, consisting of many tandemly arranged amplicons per DM. Much smaller circular, autonomously replicating episomes in the range of 600–800 kb have also been observed in several human and rodent cell lines displaying only moderate degrees of drug resistance. These episomes have been suggested to increase in size with time and ultimately to become DMs, but other studies suggest the opposite, i.e., that episomes actually arise from larger initial amplicons. Neither the significance nor the generality of these interesting entities is yet known.

An important point made by Geoffrey Wahl and colleagues is that biopsied human tumors display DMs more often than ABRs/HSRs; thus, it is suggested that efforts should be concentrated on understanding the genesis of amplified DNA via DMs. However, Levan and co-workers have shown that a drug-resistant murine tumor cell line displays either ABRs/HSRs or double minutes depending on whether it is propagated in plastic dishes or as an ascites tumor, respectively. Since the cell presumably did not cast off the ABRs/HSRs and restart the amplification process from scratch when reintroduced into the animal, the two forms are likely to be interconvertible. This, in turn, suggests that the differences between ABRs/HSRs and DMs may be a question of maintenance in stable arrays as opposed to two different mechanisms of generation. This suggestion is supported by the observation that introduction of a Chinese hamster chromosome bearing an HSR into a murine cell line causes the HSR to disproportionate into DMs. Nevertheless, these interesting observations point out that the milieu of the cell plays a major role in the nature of the amplification process and/or the maintenance of amplified DNA.

With regard to the genesis and stability of amplified DNA, Schimke and colleagues performed an interesting series of experiments with a fluorescent-activated cell sorter (FACS) in which they monitored changes in DHFR gene copy number in individual CHO cells. They first showed that when cells are incubated with an extremely low (nonselective)

concentration of fluorescein isothiocyanate-labeled methotrexate, the level of fluorescent DHFR protein is usually proportional to the DHFR gene copy number. A naive population of CHO cells that had never been treated with MTX was then exposed to the fluorescent compound and sorted according to DHFR gene copy number. Surprisingly, the population contained cells with vastly different numbers of DHFR genes, ranging from the usual 2 to more than 20. In fact, it was estimated that the frequency of spontaneous amplification of the DHFR gene in CHO cells was on the order of 10^{-3} per cell generation, an unusually high incidence of genetic variation.

When cells with high copy numbers were isolated with the FACS and cultured in the presence of selective concentrations of MTX, the frequency of MTX-resistant amplicants was greatly increased, showing that this population is capable of giving rise to the amplicants isolated in the usual way. More importantly, when cells with elevated DHFR gene copy numbers were cultured in the absence of MTX, they were seen to both lose and gain DHFR genes at a rapid rate.

This apparent instability in copy number mimicked the behavior of DMs in highly resistant murine cells in the absence of drug selection and suggested that even in CHO cells, which maintain amplified genes as "stable" ABRs, early amplification events might release extrachromosomal copies of the DHFR gene. Presumably, these would eventually reintegrate into a chromosome to become the familiar ABRs that signal amplification in this cell line. This proposal will be revisited in a later section on mechanisms.

It is reasonable to assume that sequence arrangements of the amplicons themselves might give a clue to the mechanism(s) responsible for generating these arrangements. Thus, considerable effort has been expended characterizing amplified DNA in selected drug-resistant variants by molecular cloning and mapping strategies. By estimating the DHFR gene copy number in solution hybridization studies and by knowing the length of the chromosomal HSRs in one MTX-resistant Chinese hamster cell line, it was possible to show that each amplicon is approximately 500 kb in length. In another MTX-resistant cell line containing 1000 copies of the DHFR amplicon, the restriction pattern of the amplified unit could actually be discerned in restriction digests separated on agarose gels and stained with ethidium bromide; based on the lengths and numbers of these restriction fragments, the amplicon in this cell line appeared to be at least 150 kb in length. Therefore, at the time these studies were initiated, cloning such large amounts of DNA represented a rather formidable task. Moreover, since the murine and Chinese hamster DHFR genes are only 32 and 26 kb in length, it was clear that large amounts of flanking DNA are coamplified with the gene selected by the drug treatment regimen.

In initial attempts by the Schimke laboratory to clone the amplified DNA from MTX-resistant murine cells, double minute chromosome fractions were partially purified on sucrose gradients based on their small size relative to the other chromosomes, and recombinant DNA libraries were constructed. By using the murine DHFR cDNA to isolate clones containing the DHFR gene and by extending the map outward by chromosomal walking, it was possible to isolate approximately 200 kb of DNA from the murine DHFR locus. However, several branch points were encountered during this cloning process, suggesting that the amplicons in a single murine cell line were not identical in size; thus it was not possible to isolate a single amplicon type by this approach. When the resulting clones were utilized to probe restriction digests of DNA from several independent, MTX-resistant murine cell lines, amplicon heterogeneity was detected not only in other murine cell lines that carry amplified sequences on double minute chromosomes, but also in lines containing HSRs: all of the amplicons necessarily contained the DHFR gene, but the amount of DNA flanking the gene on either side varied considerably, with amplicons ranging from 40 kb to more than 200 kb in length. Interestingly, however, one or a few amplicon arrangements predominated, and the minor types were themselves amplified to some degree (i.e., the junction fragments between them were amplified). Thus, it could be concluded that the endpoints of amplicons are probably not dictated by the amplification mechanism itself; in fact, it appeared that there might be an almost infinitely complex array of amplicons in any given cell line. There was even some evidence from mapping studies that DNA from unrelated sites could become joined to sequences from the DHFR locus to fabricate new amplified units.

Almost 200 kb of amplified DNA sequence from the CAD locus has also been cloned from PALA-resistant Syrian hamster cell lines by George Stark and colleagues. The amplicons here are maintained in stable ABRs/HSRs. Again, several novel junction fragments were isolated, indicating amplicon heterogeneity, and no single amplicon type has yet been cloned in its entirety from these highly resistant derivatives.

However, an important insight was gained from efforts to clone amplified sequences from much less resistant variants isolated earlier in the PALA treatment program: the very small number of junction fragments encountered relative to unrearranged fragments that derive from internal positions suggested that the initial units of amplification could be as large as 10,000 kb! If this number were to be accurate, it would imply that amplicons start out being very large, but are somehow trimmed to smaller sizes as the copy number increases to account for the much more frequent occurrence of interamplicon junction fragments in clones from highly-resistant variants.

Another thought-provoking observation was made by Ford and Fried, who used a snap-back hybridization procedure to show that the CAD amplicons in some PALA-resistant variants, as well as the amplicons containing c-myc in several human tumor cell lines, are arranged as inverted repeats in the genome. Although it was not possible to determine from this approach the size of the average amplicon, nor what percentage of the amplicons is actually arranged in this way, this important observation would have to be explained by any proposed mechanism for gene amplification.

The Hamlin laboratory was ultimately able to clone the equivalent of several different DHFR amplicon types in their entirety from highly resistant Chinese hamster cell lines. The first amplicon type was cloned from the CHOC 400 cell line, is 240 kb in length, and represents approximately 75% of the amplified units in CHOC 400 cells. Interestingly, these units are organized into alternating head-to-head and tail-to-tail arrays in the chromosome. A second amplicon type representing about 5% of the amplified units was cloned from the same cell line. This amplicon is 273 kb in length and is organized in head-to-tail arrays. Its arrangement clearly shows that it gave rise to the

240-kb amplicon by an internal deletion and subsequent rearrangement. The remaining amplicons in this cell line represent a heterogenous collection, most of which are larger.

It was subsequently possible to isolate overlapping recombinant cosmid clones representing a complete copy of a 450-kb DHFR amplicon from the independently isolated MTX-resistant Chinese hamster lung fibroblast, DC3F/A3. This 450-kb version constitutes 20% of the total in this cell line. More than 500 kb of a contiguous DNA sequence from the remaining amplicons has been cloned without reaching the endpoints of additional amplicons; thus the majority are extremely large and very homogenous within this 500-kb core sequence, i.e., they represent exactly the same arrangement as the parental, unamplified DHFR locus.

The ability to isolate these amplicon types by cloning depended on their relatively small size, their prevalence in the particular cell of origin, and the remarkable homogeneity. The 240-kb DHFR amplicons from the CHOC 400 cell line, which constitute 75% of the total, appear to be virtually identical to one another, including the junction fragments that join the units together. Thus, the mechanism of amplification to high copy number somehow must involve the perfect reproduction of a subset or subsets of existing amplicons (by whatever means).

V. PROPOSED MECHANISMS

The diagrams in Fig. 2 illustrate the four most popular models that have been suggested by various

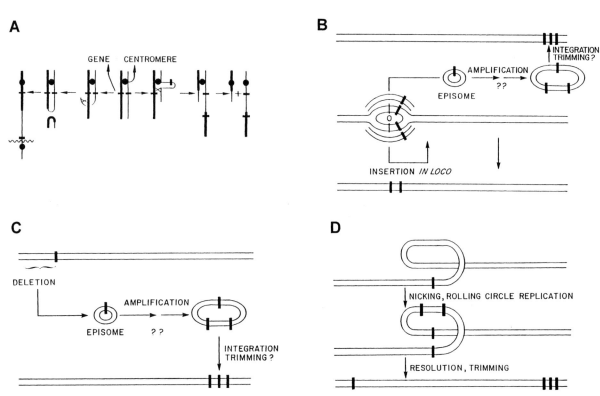

FIGURE 2 Models for initial amplification events in CHO cells. (A) Two different unequal sister chromatid exchange events that would lead to an initial duplication of the DHFR gene. (B) An overreplication model that would lead to amplification either *in loco* if the extra duplexes were integrated close to the original locus or at a distant position if the extra duplexes had a finite extrachromosomal existence. The length of the amplicons may be shortened during the process. (C) A deletion model in which the deleted locus forms an episome that increases in size and gene copy number, possibly by rolling circle replication; the episome then either remains extrachromosomal or reintegrates into the same or another chromosome, possibly after having been trimmed. (D) A conservative transposition model in which extra copies of the locus in question are generated by a roll-in replication mechanism analogous to transposition of bacteriophages, but the original locus remains intact.

investigators to explain the initiation of DNA sequence amplification in mammalian cells. These models actually fall into two groups: (1) those in which copy numbers are increased by an overreplication mechanism, and (2) those in which copy numbers are increased in only one daughter cell by a nondisjunction event.

Probably the most popular model has been the onionskin overreplication model (Fig. 2B) in which multiple initiations occur at a local origin of replication in a single cell cycle. This model obviously originates from the natural example of chorion gene amplification in Drosophila. The extra daughter duplexes would then somehow have to be integrated in tandem arrays in the body of the chromosome to become an ABR, either near to or far from the original locus. Alternatively, each extra copy of the original amplicon could peel away from the chromosome, circularize, and spend its lifetime as an episome, increasing the number of amplicons per episome by some means and eventually becoming a microscopically visible DM.

A second overreplication model suggests that amplification could be initiated by a modification of rolling-circle replication analogous to some forms of transposition in bacteria. In this relatively complicated mechanism (Fig. 2D), an internal loop is formed in a chromosome; at the crossover position, the 3' and 5' ends of two single-stranded nicks become ligated to one another to form a single-stranded circle. The remaining free 3' end then serves as the primer for continuous replication of the circular template by a strand displacement mechanism. In bacteriophage μ, after one traverse of the template, a specific endonuclease usually ends the cycle, thereby generating an integrated, unit-sized, double-stranded phage. In the absence of such a nuclease, the cycle could presumably continue around the circular template many times to give long tandem arrays.

The first example of a nondisjunction model for amplification is pictured in Fig. 2A. Here it is suggested that an unequal sister chromatid exchange occurs after replication but prior to separation of the centromeres at mitosis. In the direct exchange pictured on the right, an incorrect alignment of chromatids allows a crossover to occur in such a way as to transfer both copies of the selectable marker to one chromatid. The daughter cell that loses the marker (along with flanking DNA) would therefore die under selective conditions, while the

daughter receiving two copies would survive. No inherent genetic instability should accrue to the survivor after such an exchange. Presumably, once this large, direct repeat is formed, subsequent unequal sister chromatid exchanges mediated by slippage in homologous pairing should become easier and easier, just as there are many ways to incorrectly align a shirt with many buttons and buttonholes.

In the hairpin exchange pictured on the left, one chromatid actually reverses direction and recombines with the other at positions distal to the markers, again transferring both markers to one chromosome. In this arrangement, the acentromeric chromosome fragments distal to the crossovers will be lost from the daughter cells. In addition, however, a giant inverted duplication in the form of a dicentric chromosome is produced. Unlike the direct unequal exchange, this situation is highly unstable since the dicentric must break somewhere during mitosis as the two centromeres attempt to go to the opposite poles. If the break occurs between the marker and the centromere on one chromosome, both copies of the marker will end up in one cell on a chromosome with an atelomeric, double-stranded, frayed end. This highly recombinogenic end can be healed after replication by fusion with the other chromatid or with another frayed end elsewhere in the genome.

An alternative nondisjunction model is pictured in Fig. 2C and suggests that the original locus in question is deleted from the chromosome and then has an independent existence as an autonomously replicating episome. This acentromeric episome is then partitioned randomly to the two daughter cells during mitosis, but continuing drug selection pressure ensures that only those receiving a large number of copies survive. The model further suggests that the episomes can recombine with one another to increase in internal amplicon copy number, eventually becoming microscopically visible DMs; alternatively, they may integrate into the body of a chromosome to become an ABR or HSR.

VI. TESTING THE MODELS

The Schimke and Varshavsky laboratories devoted considerable effort to testing various predictions of the onionskin overreplication (replicon misfiring) model. For example, they proposed that any treatment that stalls or slows replication forks should increase the frequency of amplification by allowing more time for reinitiation to occur. Indeed, it was found that pretreatment of rodent cells with hydroxyurea, methotrexate, or ultraviolet light dramatically increased the frequency of DHFR gene amplification when they were subsequently selected on methotrexate. These agents inhibit DNA replication by interfering with deoxynucleotide metabolism or by introducing adducts into the DNA template. However, pretreatment with a variety of other agents, including phorbol esters, some hormones, and hypoxia, also increased the frequency of DHFR gene amplification, and it is not obvious why this should be so. Furthermore, treatment with many of these agents could have multiple effects on DNA, including the introduction of single-strand breaks. Thus, it is not possible to prove the operation of an overreplication mechanism by this approach.

Other observations are difficult to reconcile with a straightforward onionskin overreplication mechanism. Stark's estimates for the size of initial amplified units in PALA-resistant hamster cells are on the order of 10,000 kb, about 100-fold larger than the average replicon in mammalian cells. Furthermore, the Hamlin laboratory has shown directly that some amplicons have more than one origin of replication. To accommodate these data in an overreplication model, many adjacent origins would have to misfire simultaneously. Alternatively, one origin could misfire and the adjacent replicons would then have to be replicated passively by forks emanating from that origin; with a replication fork rate of 3 kb/min and an S period lasting 8–10 hr in mammalian cells, this would limit the size of initial amplicons to about 3600 kb.

To address the possibility that repeated unequal sister chromatid exchange might mediate the amplification process, Chasin and colleagues compared the frequency of sister chromatid exchange in HSRs to those occurring in other parts of the genome. In the MTX-resistant Chinese hamster cell lines that they examined, the number of exchanges per metaphase was actually lower in HSRs than in other chromosomal locations. Thus, the unequal sister chromatid exchange model lost its appeal as a viable model.

It is hard to imagine how one might design experiments to test directly whether either roll-in replication or deletion and episome formation are involved in the amplification process. In fact, it is difficult to devise conclusive tests for any of the four general models for the simple reason that the event of interest is so rare (on the order of one per 10^3 cells per generation). Furthermore, as long as one examines a population of cells (as opposed to a single cell), the heterogeneity and instability of amplified sequences would render it impossible to paint a clear picture of the chromosome rearrangements that occur in the first steps of the amplification process.

What was needed was a high-resolution technique for examining the chromosomes in single cells at the time of, or shortly after, the event that initiates the first duplication. In fact, a method has been developed that has done a great deal to rejuvenate the DNA sequence amplification field. This FISH method is a modification of the *in situ* hybridization technique that has been around for years. However, instead of using radioactive hybridization probes for the gene of interest to detect chromosomal rearrangements, the probes are labeled with biotinylated dUTP and are detected with fluorescein-labeled avidin or with avidin and fluorescent anti-avidin.

The difference in the information content of images attained with either radioactive or fluorescent DHFR-specific probes is illustrated in Figs. 3A and 3B, respectively, in which mitotic chromosome spreads from the same MTX-resistant CHO cell line were hybridized under similar conditions. Not only is the resolution vastly improved with the fluorescent detection method, allowing the precise location and relative gene copy number to be assessed, but the sensitivity is high enough to allow detection of single copy loci.

By applying the FISH technique to nine independent MTX-resistant CHO cell lines selected very early in the amplification process, Trask and Hamlin were able to detect several similarities in rearrangements involving the DHFR gene: (1) in agreement with earlier studies, the majority of resistant cell lines become so by amplifying the DHFR gene; (2) the DHFR amplicons in these resistant amplicants are most often on the same chromosome arm as the original single copy DHFR locus, but usually very far away from it at

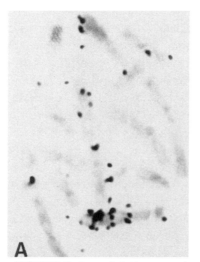 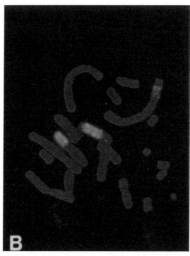

FIGURE 3 *In situ* hybridization with radioactive and fluorescent probes. The MTX-resistant CHO cell line CHOC 400 was hybridized with a DHFR-specific recombinant cosmid that was labeled by nick-translation either with [³H]dCTP (A) or with biotin-dUTP (B). The radioactive probe was detected by autoradiography and the biotin-labeled probe was detected with an avidin and fluorescein-labeled anti-avidin.

the terminus, and sometimes further out than the original end of the chromosome; (3) the single copy DHFR locus on the involved chromosome usually remains intact and single copy; (4) even at the lowest selective drug concentration, the DHFR gene copy number can vary from five to as many as a hundred or more, suggesting that once started, the mechanism of amplification may be self-propagating; (5) the DHFR amplicons are arrayed either as clusters of a few copies spaced at 5 to 10-MB intervals along the chromosome or as homogenous regions with large numbers of closely spaced amplicons; (6) a large degree of heterogeneity was detected in amplicon arrangements, even among the products of a single clone, suggesting that amplicons continue to rearrange with time even at a single drug level; and (7) many examples of translocations of amplicons to other chromosomes were detected, and, remarkably, almost 20% of all mitotic figures examined in the nine independently isolated resistant cell lines displayed dicentric chromosomes or chromosomes with fused termini.

Utilizing FISH techniques to follow early CAD gene amplification events in Syrian hamster cells, Stark and colleagues detected very similar rearrangements, with initial amplicons residing on elongated chromosomes near the terminus and retention of the single copy locus.

Taken at face value, these data appeared to rule out the deletion and episome formation model as a potential mechanism for initiating events in hamster cells since the single copy locus appeared to be retained in almost all cases. In addition, it was difficult to reconcile the onionskin overreplication model with the large amounts of extra, nonamplicon DNA that appeared to intervene between the single copy locus and the amplified arrays.

It therefore seemed more likely that amplification is initiated either by unequal sister chromatid exchange or, conceivably, by some form of roll-in replication mechanism that would subsequently engender further rearrangements. Of the two modes of unequal sister chromatid exchange pictured in Fig. 2A, only the reverse exchange could lead to the instability displayed by amplicons early in the amplification process.

In Fig. 2D, it can be seen that the roll-in replication mechanism would likely yield head-to-tail amplicon arrays that would essentially be direct repeats of the single copy locus in question. However, a reverse sister chromatid exchange would form a giant inverted duplication centered at the exchange points on the two chromatids. To examine these possibilities in more detail, the DHFR amplicants that were analyzed by single color FISH were reinvestigated utilizing a series of additional recombinant clones situated at intervals along the involved arm of chromosome 2. Each of these probes (marked with red fluorescence) was paired with the DHFR-specific probe (marked with green fluorescence), and the mixture was hybridized to mitotic chromosome spreads.

The resulting fluorescent images show clearly that the initial event in the generation of extra copies of the DHFR gene in CHO cells is the formation of a giant inverted duplication. As shown in the diagram in Fig. 4, in all but one case, the duplication appears to be symmetrical. The center of the duplication can be positioned either near to or far from the DHFR gene in independent amplificants.

Remarkably similar images were obtained when a two-color FISH approach was utilized by DeBatisse, Buttin, and their co-workers to examine early events in the amplification of the adenylate deaminase 2 gene in CHO cells. In addition, some chromosomes displayed several small tandemly arranged inverted duplications, again localized near the end of the chromosome.

These patterns strongly suggest a mechanism in which an initiating break occurs somewhere below the gene, leaving a truncated chromosome that is missing its telomere (Fig. 5). The chromosome is then replicated during the S period and the atelomeric ends become fused to one another by repair processes to form a dicentric chromosome. Alternatively, an already replicated chromosome could break at approximately the same position on both chromatids and these frayed ends could fuse. The dicentric chromosome thus formed then breaks during the next mitosis, and if the break occurs between the marker and the nearest centromere, both copies of the gene will be transferred to one chromosome, thus constituting the first amplification event. The frayed, atelomeric end of this chromosome is then likely to fuse again to repeat the classic bridge–breakage–fusion cycles that were originally described by McClintock to explain certain examples of genetic instability in maize.

This model is attractive because it accommodates almost all of the FISH data obtained in several different laboratories, but also much of the other data that has been obtained over the years. For example, the obligate loss of the telomere in the initial amplification step would generate the subsequent instability that has been observed in virtually all systems, even those in which the amplicons are borne on

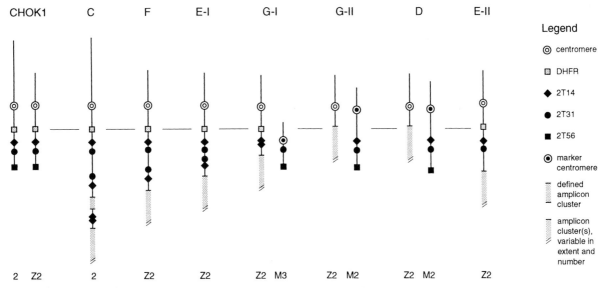

FIGURE 4 Model chromosomes from several independently isolated DHFR amplificants. The average distances between chromosome features (centromere, probes, amplicon cluster boundaries, and termini) were compiled to produce model chromosomes for each class. Although the three 2T probes were not hybridized simultaneously to cells, the distances obtained with each probe individually (Fig. 5) were consistent with the combined patterns shown here. Both chromosomes are shown for normal CHO-K1 cells. The marker chromosome (M1), whose short arm hybridized with 2T56 in CHO-K1 and all of the variants, as well as the unaffected chromosome in the amplificants (Z2 in class C and 2 in all the other classes), is omitted for simplicity.

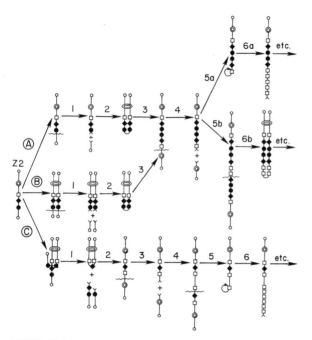

FIGURE 5 Proposed mechanisms for initiating amplification of the DHFR locus in CHO cells. In this diagram, a single line is equivalent to a double helix, telomeres are denoted by the small open circles, and frayed ends are indicated with a Y. The other symbols correspond to individual hybridization probes from different parts of the long arm of chromosome 2. (Mechanism A) The unreplicated chromosome (Z2 in this case) suffers a break distal to the 2T31 marker (step 1), followed by terminal fusion, either by repair or during the subsequent S period (step 2). The resulting dicentric then breaks between one centromere and a DHFR gene (step 4), resulting in the transfer of both copies of the DHFR gene to one chromatid, which now has a frayed end. The near-terminal DHFR gene can now be amplified by a roll-in replication mechanism (step 5a). Alternatively, the frayed ends can fuse again to form a dicentric (step 5b), which then breaks asymmetrically again to transfer all four copies of the DHFR gene to one chromatid (step 6b), etc. (Mechanism B) The replicated Z2 chromosome breaks at the same place on both chromatids (step 1), the ends fuse (step 2), and the bridge–breakage–fusion cycle continues as in Mechanism A (step 3). (Mechanism C) An asymmetrical reverse sister chromatid exchange takes place below the 2T14 marker on one chromatid but above 2T14 on the other (step 1), resulting in the formation of a dicentric chromosome with an asymmetric-inverted duplication (step 2). This dicentric chromosome then breaks between one DHFR gene and a centromere (step 3), transferring both copies of the DHFR gene to one chromosome. Terminal fusion of the frayed ends then occurs (step 4), leading to subsequent bridge–breakage–fusion cycles, possibly interspersed with roll-in replication cycles (step 6).

"stable" chromosomal ABRs or HSRs. It also explains why the amplicons are most often found on the same chromosome arm as the parental locus and why initial amplicons are extremely large (the initial duplication can involve more than half of a chromosome

arm, depending on the position of the initiating break); subsequent breaks can also occur at relatively long distances from the original duplicated marker gene to yield amplicons that are in the megabase range (see Fig. 5). Finally, the chromosome breakage model may partly explain why the frequency of amplification of any particular marker is so high: the initiating break can occur at any one of a number of positions along the chromosome arm bearing the gene as long as it is distal to the gene; once this break occurs, the instability engendered by the frayed, atelomeric end could account for frequent additional amplifications.

However, some aspects of the FISH data are not easily explained by the chromosome breakage model. For example, it is easy to see how amplicons would tend to become smaller (at least those in cells that survive drug selection) since chromosome breaks presumably can occur at random positions, but the smaller the amplicons produced at each new step, the more the cell can accommodate in a single chromosome.

However, it is not so easy to explain how the high copy number amplicons that are detected in highly resistant variants become so uniform in structure. One possibility is that additional mechanisms take over at some point early in the process. An attractive possibility is roll-in replication since one of the required initiating breaks (see Fig. 2D) would be provided by the broken, atelomeric chromosome end. Presumably, the frayed end could invade the chromosome above an amplicon or two and initiated several cycles of rolling circle replication, which could amplify perfect copies of a single unit or inverted dyad. Only time and clever experimental protocols will determine whether this or another mechanism is involved in rapidly generating high copy numbers of uniformly sized amplicons.

Another unknown is whether murine and human cell lines that normally carry amplified sequences on DMs utilize the same initiating mechanism to produce the first copies of the selected gene. It should be relatively easy to answer this question with the same FISH techniques that provided so much information when applied to ABR/HSR-containing cell lines. It is conceivable, for example, that a chromosome break initiates the first few intrachromosomal duplication events, in the process truncating the length of individual amplicons; for unknown reasons, however, the extra copies are not as easily accommodated in the body of murine and human chromosomes as they are in hamster chromosomes. Once released from the chromosome, these initial amplicons would be free to circularize and recombine with one another to increase their internal copy number (becoming heterogenous and scrambled in the process); ultimately, they would form the larger DMs that characterize most human and murine cell lines.

There is one other observation that particularly deserves comment. The FISH studies on CHO cells showed that when the breakpoint occurs relatively far away from the single copy DHFR gene, the acentromeric chromosome fragment lying distal to the breakpoint is lost from the cell. However, when the breakpoint is close to the DHFR gene, the distal atelomeric fragment is recovered as a translocation to another chromosome. This observation suggests that there is a gene lying close to DHFR that is required in two copies for cell survival.

This emphasizes the important point that many factors in any drug selection regimen (or during amplification of an oncogene) play a role in determining whether the gene is amplified and, if so, how many times. For example, if a particular gene is far out on the end of a chromosome, a break distal to the marker is unlikely to happen very often; by the same token, being close to the centromere on a long chromosome arm would appear to favor initiating events. However, these factors would be tempered by the nature of the genes lying distal to the marker that would be lost (or have to be retained by transposition to another chromosome).

These considerations could explain a seeming dichotomy that exists between the FISH data cited earlier and a study performed by Geoffrey Wahl and coworkers. They selected MTX-resistant variants from a hemizygous CHO cell line that had lost one copy of the DHFR gene and large amounts of flanking DNA by deletion. This cell line was chosen because it would eliminate any complications arising from the presence of the second allele. Using the FISH technique with a DHFR-specific probe to examine early amplificants, they detected small, DHFR-containing chromosome fragments resembling DMs. Moreover,

the single copy DHFR locus was deleted from the chromosome.

How is it possible to reconcile these data with those obtained with MTX- and coformycin-resistant CHO cells and PALA-resistant Syrian hamster cells in which the single copy loci were clearly retained in their usual positions? The answer may be that the hemizygote has already lost many of the markers surrounding the DHFR gene on one chromosome, thus it cannot survive the loss of the second copy of these markers by the common chromosome breakage route that characterizes diploid CHO cells. Perhaps the only cells to survive MTX selection are those that experience a double break encompassing the DHFR gene, which releases the DHFR amplicon as a transient episome or DM, but leaves the flanking (required) genes intact.

VII. IMPLICATIONS AND FUTURE DIRECTIONS

It is clear that we are only beginning to understand some of the machinations involved in generating high copy numbers of a gene under selective conditions. Several different mechanisms may be operative, depending on the starting cell line, the position of the gene on the chromosome, and the stage of amplification. However, the most plausible mechanisms for explaining all of the extant data initially involve chromosome breaks, which was suggested by Schimke and by Wahl even before FISH data were available.

The reason the chromosome breakage model makes so much sense in that it fits perfectly into another recent discovery that may explain why only tumor cells commonly amplify DNA and, indeed, why tumor cells are so unstable genetically. Vogelstein and colleagues, as well as others, have accumulated overwhelming evidence that a majority of human tumors have suffered the loss of wild-type p53 activity. As discussed elsewhere in this volume, p53 is classified as a tumor suppressor gene, and Kastan and co-workers have obtained evidence that it is involved in a DNA damage-sensing pathway that arrests cells in the G1 part of the cell cycle in response to ionizing radiation and other insults. In addition, the laboratories of Thea Tlsty and Geoffrey Wahl have each shown that, by in large, only cells lacking wild-type p53 activity can amplify genes.

Thus, an attractive model emerges in which a normal cell sustains single-strand DNA breaks, probably from natural processes, such as DNA replication, recombination, or repair, and the cell suppresses replication in the face of such damage until it can be repaired. When the p53 pathway is nonfunctional (as in a cancerous or precancerous cell), replication proceeds unimpeded through these lesions, converting them to double-stranded chromosome breaks. These breaks then lead to a variety of chromosomal aberrations, including translocations, deletions, inversions, and amplification. In the latter instance, chromosomal breakage could lead to amplification of an oncogene since (1) there are so many of them, (2) the very large initial amplicons would often include an oncogene, and (3) increasing the copy number of an oncogene could provide a selective growth advantage.

A model of this kind leads to specific predictions, many of which are now testable with FISH techniques utilizing the large variety of recombinant clones available from the human genome project. Other fresh approaches from a new generation of investigators will undoubtedly yield even more surprises. It seems clear, however, that the study of DNA sequence amplification will continue to contribute to, and benefit from, studies in the general field of tumor biology.

See Also the Following Articles

C-MYC PROTO-ONCOGENE • RESISTANCE TO TOPOISOMERASE-TARGETING AGENTS

Bibliography

Hamlin, J. L., Vaughn, J. P., Leu, T.-H., Ma, C., and Dijkwel, P. A. (1991). The use of cell lines carrying amplified DNA sequences for studying chromosome structure and function. *Prog. Nucleic Acids Res.* **41,** 203.

Kellems, R. E. (ed.) (1993). "Gene Amplification in Mammalian Cells." Dekker, New York.

Stark, G. R., DeBatisse, M., Guilotto, E., and Wahl, G. M. (1989). Recent progress in understanding mechanisms of mammalian DNA amplification. *Cell* **57,** 901.

Schimke, R. T. (1988). Gene amplification in cultured cells. *J. Biol. Chem.* **263,** 5989.

Wahl, G. M. (1989). The importance of circular DNA in mammalian DNA amplification. *Cancer Res.* **49,** 1333.

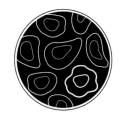

Endocrine Tumors

James E. Gervasoni, Jr.
*Robert Wood Johnson Medical School/
University of Medicine and Dentistry of New Jersey*

Blake Cady
*Brown University School of Medicine and
Women & Infants Hospital, Providence*

GLOSSARY

ACTH Adrenal corticotrophin hormone.
APUD Amine precursor uptake and decarboxylation.
FNAB Fine-needle aspiration biopsy.
MEN Multiple endocrine neoplasia.
TSH Serum thyrotropin.
ZES Zollinger-Ellison syndrome.

$\mathbf{T}$umors of the endocrine system are rare and account for approximately 1.2% of the estimated 1.25 million cases of cancer, excluding skin cancers diagnosed per year in the United States. In addition, these tumors are only responsible for about 0.3% of the estimated 550,000 cancer deaths in the United States per year. However, these cancers present interesting challenges in genetics, pathophysiology, diagnosis, and treatment. They often present initially with hypersecretion of hormones that pose a more immediate threat to the patient than the cancer itself, as with islet cell carcinoma and parathyroid carcinoma. As is the case with many cancers, a multidisciplinary approach is essential for adequate care of the patient with an endocrine gland tumor, with treatment and close follow-up from the surgeon, medical oncologist, and the endocrinologist. This article reviews several endocrine gland cancers, including those arising from the thyroid and parathyroid, the adrenal cortex and medulla (pheochromocytoma) pancreatic islet cells and also carcinoid tumors, and the multiple endocrine neoplasias.

I. THYROID CANCERS

Thyroid cancer is by far the most common type of endocrine malignancy and accounts for most deaths caused by all of the endocrine tumors combined. The thyroid is composed histologically of two main parenchymal cell types. The follicular cells line the colloid follicles concentrate iodine and are predominantly involved in production of the thyroid hormone. These cells give rise to the differentiated and anaplastic thyroid cancers. The second is the parafollicular or C cell responsible for production of calcitonin and medullary thyroid cancer. There are estimated to be approximately 19,500 new thyroid cancers diagnosed in 2001, 90% of which are well-differentiated thyroid cancers. About 5% are medullary and 1 to 3% are anaplastic cancers. One to 3% are lymphomas and sarcomas.

Well-differentiated thyroid cancers are subdivided histologically into three basic categories: papillary, follicular, and Hurthle cell. Papillary cancers account for the majority (up to 80%) of thyroid cancers and 90% of radiation-associated thyroid cancers. These cancers are generally slow growing and are multicentric in about 15% of cases; the predominant mode of spread is via the lymphatics. The prognosis for papillary cancer is excellent, with an overall mortality rate of approximately 6% at 30 years. Papillary thyroid cancer occurs in all age groups, but with a peak incidence in the third and fourth decades of life. The male to female ratio is about 1:5, but the 30-year cancer mortality is greater in men. Ten percent of thyroid papillary cancers occur in children or adolescents less than 20 years of age. Cervical lymph node metastases occur frequently, approaching 90% in children compared to 50 to 70% in adults up to 40 to 50 years of age. Risk factors associated with an increased proportion of papillary cancer are therapeutic radiation exposure, which is no longer a problem in the United States where that practiced ceased in the 1950s, and adequate iodine intake.

II. PAPILLARY THYROID CANCER

Papillary cancers usually present as an asymptomatic hypofunctioning nodule that does not respond to thyroid suppression. Diagnosis is usually made by fine-needle aspiration biopsy (FNAB) of solitary thyroid nodules. There are four FNAB results reported: malignant, indeterminate, benign or unsatisfactory. Surgery should be recommended for malignant and indeterminate aspirates, whereas repeat biopsy should be recommended for an unsatisfactory specimen. An adequate FNAB reported as benign is over 99% accurate if experienced cytologists interpret the sample.

The prognosis of papillary cancer depends on several factors, which have been combined into a number of scoring systems: AGES and MACIS (Mayo Clinic), AMES (Lahey Clinic), TNM staging, and the EORTC system. The most important factors in these scoring systems are age and the extent and size of the tumor. The AGES (age, grade, extent, size) score includes tumor grade as a factor, whereas the AMES (age, metastases, extent, size) score ignores grade and particularly notes distant metastases. Both systems identify low- and high-risk groups; the low-risk group makes up the vast majority of patients, 80 to 90% with only a 1 or 2% death rate.

The primary treatment for papillary thyroid cancer is surgical excision, but there is considerable controversy concerning the most appropriate operation. "Occult" papillary thyroid cancers 1.0 to 1.5 cm in maximum diameter can be treated with a lobectomy and isthmusectomy. High-risk papillary cancers should be preferably treated by a total or near total thyroidectomy. Modified lymph node dissection of the central and cervical lymph node basins should be performed for clinically palpable metastases by modified resection of lymphatic tissue with sparing of other structures. Postoperatively following total thyroidectomy, patients must receive thyroid replacement or suppression. If patients undergo radioactive iodine ablation therapy, serum thyrotropin (TSH) levels should be greater than 35 μU/ml by stopping thyroid hormone or giving TSH injections before the ^{131}I diagnostic and therapeutic total body scan is carried out.

III. FOLLICULAR THYROID CANCER

The treatment of follicular and Hurthle cell cancers is by subtotal or total thyroidectomy, depending on the risk group. The cervical lymph nodes should not be routinely resected unless there are clinically positive nodes. Many follicular cancers suspected on FNAB are found to be follicular variants of papillary cancer.

Postoperatively, follicular cancers are frequently treated with ^{131}I radioablation.

Follicular carcinomas constitute approximately 10 to 20% of differentiated thyroid cancers diagnosed in the United States; Hurthle cell carcinomas are a form of follicular cancers. While follicular cancers are generally thought of as being more aggressive than the papillary type, the risk group assignment is still completely appropriate. Follicular cancers are unifocal and have a male to female ratio of 3:1. These tumors usually spread hematologically and are occasionally found to be metastatic to the lung and bone at initial presentation; lymph node metastases are uncommon.

Follicular lesions remain a common cause of thyroid nodules in the United States. No diagnostic modality, including FNAB, is sufficiently reliable to distinguish between follicular hyperplastic nodules in goiter, follicular adenomas, and follicular cancers. Therefore, FNAB with a microfollicular pattern of cells are called suspicious and should be removed. The diagnosis of cancer is established by invasion of the tumor pseudo-capsule or blood vessel invasion. Follicular cancers diagnosed with minimal pseudo-capsular involvement or minor blood vessel involvement seldom, if ever, cause death.

IV. MEDULLARY THYROID CANCER

Medullary thyroid cancer arises from parafollicular C cells, neural crest derivation (ultimobranchial body), and are considered part of the amine precursor uptake and decarboxylation (APUD) system of neuroendocrine cells. Medullary thyroid cancers secrete various substances, including calcitonin, carcinoembryonic antigen (CEA), histaminase, serotonin, somatostatin, and thyroglobulin. These tumors develop as unifocal (sporadic) or multifocal (heredity) cancers that spread to lymph nodes of the perithyroidal, paratracheal, jugular, and mediastinal chains frequently. Medullary cancer may remain confined to the neck clinically for long periods of time, but metastases are found in lungs, liver, or bone.

Medullary cancers occur in sporadic (90%) and hereditary forms (10%). The sporadic cases are unifocal, usually presenting as a thyroid or lymph node mass at a median of 45 years of age, and carry a guarded prognosis. In the hereditary form, patients present with multifocal disease at a median of 35 years of age or are detected in a preclinical stage by calcitonin detection and carries a better prognosis. Hereditary medullary cancers of the thyroid are associated with multiple endocrine neoplasia (MEN) types 2A and 2B. In the MEN 2A syndrome, medullary cancers may accompany pheochromocytoma and parathyroid hyperplasia. MEN 2B patients also may develop pheochromocytoma, but multiple mucosal neuromas and intestinal ganglioneuromas occur as a hallmark.

The primary treatment of all medullary thyroid cancers is total thyroidectomy with central node dissection, as any case presenting clinically may be an index case for a family. Patients that have clinically palpable cervical lymph nodes require a modified radical neck dissection.

Radioactive iodine is not useful in the treatment of medullary cancers because parafollicular cells do not take up iodine. Postoperatively, patients are followed clinically but also with calcitonin and CEA levels for recurrence detection. Patients who present with increased CEA or calcitonin may have localization studies to include ultrasonography, computed tomography (CT) scanning, and nuclear imaging studies for anatomic localization of disease. However, if adequate surgery of the thyroid and cervical lymph nodes has been performed initially, a rising CEA or calcitonin indicates distant metastatic disease, which rarely can be subjected to curative surgery.

Data indicate that genetic screening is helpful in detecting carriers of a defect in the RET protooncogene almost universally found in patients with MEN 2A, MEN 2B, and familial non-MEN medullary thyroid cancer.

V. ANAPLASTIC THYROID CANCER

Anaplastic thyroid cancer is one of the most aggressive and difficult malignancies to treat and has a median survival of 4 to 5 months from diagnosis, with uncommon long-term survivors. In the United States they represent between 1 and 3% of thyroid cancers. Anaplastic thyroid cancer occurs more commonly in iodine-deficient areas with endemic goiter and often occurred on a background of persistent or recurrent differentiated papillary thyroid cancer, but this seldom occurs now.

The clinical presentation of anaplastic thyroid cancer reflects its aggressive nature with a rapidly growing mass with invasive characteristics. Core needle or FNAB of the mass usually establishes the diagnosis. In the past, the majority of patients died of local and regional spread, primarily with upper airway respiratory obstruction. Synchronous pulmonary metastases are common at diagnosis. Aggressive combined modality treatment by external-beam radiation and doxorubicin-based chemotherapy is the most appropriate current treatment for patients and usually prevents death from airway obstruction. Surgery plays a minor role, as these lesions seldom can be resected.

VI. PARATHYROID CANCER

Parathyroid carcinoma is a rare endocrine malignancy and usually presents as severe primary hyperparathyroidism. Hyperparathyroidism results from four general disease presentations: single parathyroid adenoma (85% of cases), double adenomas (5%), multiglandular hyperplasia (10%), and parathyroid cancer (<1%). Parathyroid cancer clinically presents with signs and symptoms related to hyperparathyroidism. Most patients with parathyroid cancer present with renal disease associated with hypercalcuria and hypercalcemia such as renal stones, renal insufficiency, renal colic, and nephrocalcinosis. In long-standing disease, patients with parathyroid cancer may present with bone disease related to calcium absorption with osteoporosis and bone pain. Patients with both renal and bone disease are unusual in adenomas currently, but are found in up to 50% of patients with parathyroid cancer, an indication of the more severe hyperparathyroidism usually accompanied by very elevated levels of calcium (>14 mg/dl) and a gland larger than 3 cm.

The surgeon usually makes the diagnosis of parathyroid cancer because of large size and adherence and involvement of surrounding fat, muscles, or structures.

The treatment of parathyroid cancer is complete surgical resection if possible to include the adherence to surrounding tissue. Routine lymphadenectomy is not performed unless there is clinical evidence of regional nodal spread. Long-term survival in patients with parathyroid cancer ranges between 18 and 78% with 5- and 10-year survival rates in one report of 57 and 39%, respectively. Recurrent disease is treated with attempted aggressive reresection. Metastatic disease is treated medically for the signs and symptoms of hypercalcemia. Implantation of benign parathyroid adenoma tissue presenting as recurrent hyperparathyroidism has been reported and must be distinguished from cancer.

VII. ADRENAL CORTICAL CANCER

Adrenal cortical carcinomas are rare and constitutes 0.05 to 0.2% of all cancers. Functional tumors are more common in women and are found most frequently in two age groups: under 5 or in the 4th and 5th decades of life. Adrenal cortical cancers are highly malignant, with 5-year survival rates between 20 and 30%. Approximately 50% of patients have metastatic disease at the time of diagnosis. Adrenal cortical hyperplasia and adenomas can produce excess hormone, such as hypercortisolism (Cushing's syndrome) and primary aldosteronism (Conn's syndrome) and must be differentiated from cancer.

VIII. CUSHING SYNDROME; CUSHING'S DISEASE

Cushing's syndrome results from adrenal corticotrophin hormone (ACTH) secretion by a pituitary tumor, by cortisol release from an adrenal neoplasm, or by ectopic secretion of ACTH. To determine the actual cause of the hypercortisolism often requires multiple tests. The most common cause of hypercortisolism is a pituitary tumor that produces excessive ACTH, termed Cushing's disease.

The most common symptom of patients with hypercortisolism is progressive weight gain and facial rounding. The weight gain is truncal, and patients usually have disproportionally slender extremities due to muscular wasting. Other signs and symptoms include hypertension, hirsutism, virilization, glucose intolerance, menstrual irregularity, mental status changes, hypokalemia, and decreased immune responsiveness.

The diagnosis of hypercortisolism is established with a 24-h urinary-free cortisol measurement. An inappropriate response to an overnight dexamethasone suppression test is the most useful study in establishing hypercortisolism. Urinary 17-hydroxysteroid-free cortisol is usually reduced when normal patients receive a low dose (2 mg) of dexamethasone. In Cushing's syndrome, this suppression of urinary-free cortisol does not occur. High-dose dexamethasone (8 mg) will suppress free cortisol to less than 50% of baseline levels with pituitary-dependent hypercortisolism (Cushing's disease). This high-dose dexamethasone will not suppress patients with primary adrenal disease or ectopic ACTH syndrome.

Radiographic localization studies of adrenal neoplasms consist of a CT scan, magnetic resonance (MR), radioisotope imaging with labeled iodocholesterol, and venous sampling.

Treatment is surgical *en bloc* resection of the adrenal cancer and adjacent structures. However, metastatic disease is found in many patients at diagnosis of adrenal cortical cancers. Chemotherapeutic agents used for recurrent or metastatic adrenal cortical carcinoma are mitotane and doxorubicin-based chemotherapy. Adjuvant therapy has not proven to be successful.

IX. HYPERALDOSTERONISM

Overproduction of aldosterone is the etiology of hypertension in patients with primary aldosteronism or Conn's syndrome. Aldosterone-producing adenoma is the most common cause of primary aldosteronism, with idiopathic hyperplasia second and carcinoma third.

The diagnosis of hyperaldosteronism requires hypertension, hypokalemia, increased levels of aldosterone, and decreased plasma rennin levels. The plasma aldosterone/rennin ratio is usually greater than 30. Additional evidence for the diagnosis of primary hyperaldosteronism is the inability of the ACE inhibitor captopril to lower plasma aldosterone levels

and raise plasma rennin activity. The clinical signs are mostly due to the hypokalemia and include muscle cramps and weakness, polyuria, and polydipsia.

Following the diagnosis of primary hyperaldosteronism, the differentiated diagnosis between idiopathic adrenal cortical hyperplasia (IAH) or a tumor producing aldosterone must be made, as IAH is treated medically and a tumor is surgically resected. A mass can be identified by CT scan 75 to 95% of the time if there is an aldosteronoma. An imaging study utilizing ^{131}I-β-iodomethyl-19-nocholesterol (iodocholesterol) gives functional information about the adrenal gland. Patients with IAH demonstrate bilateral symmetrical uptake, whereas adenomas display uptake unilaterally and carcinomas demonstrate no uptake. The single most sensitive study in equivocal situations is differentiated adrenal vein aldosterone levels.

IAH responds medically to spirononlactone or amiloride in conjunction with other antihypertensive drugs. A laparoscopic surgical approach is preferable in patients with small benign adenomas, but a formal *en bloc* resection of the adrenal gland is the best approach to adrenal carcinomas.

X. ADRENAL MASSES DISCOVERED INCIDENTALLY

Incidental adrenal masses found on abdominal CT scans (incidentaloma) may need to be evaluated further for function or cancer depending on size and symptoms. The initial steps in the evaluation of an incidentaloma include a careful history and physical examination. The maximum diameter of the mass is based on the CT scan. Laboratory studies should include 24-h urine collection for free cortisol, vanylmendelic acid (VMA), metanephrines, and catecholamines. Any lesion greater than 5 to 6 cm should be resected, as the incidence of cancer in a solid adrenal mass greater than or equal to 6 cm is high. Lesions less than 5 cm on a CT scan are usually benign adenomas, but may be functional. If the tumor is functional, adrenalectomy is indicated. If the tumor is less than 5 cm and nonfunctional, repeat CT scans at 6 and 12 months are indicated; surgical resection is indicated if the lesion increases in size.

XI. ADRENAL MEDULLA LESIONS

Pheochromocytomas are rare tumors that originate from chromaffin cells of the adrenal medulla. These tumors may be found in other locations also, wherever chromaffin cells reside, such as the organ of Zuckerkandl (found near the origin of the inferior mesenteric artery to the left of the aortic bifurcation). Pheochromocytomas cause intermittent, episodic, or sustained hypertension due to the release of catecholamines. Of the patients diagnosed with hypertension, only a few are found to have elevated urinary catecholamines from a pheochromocytoma. Pheochromocytomas are malignant in a substantial proportion. It is important to diagnose, localize, and treat these tumors early to lessen the probability of sudden death from uncontrolled hypertension. Malignant pheochromocytomas are more common among extraadrenal tumors. Pheochromocytomas are a component of some inherited disorders, such as MEN 2a and 2b, familial pheochromocytoma, Von Hippel–Lindau's disease, neurofibromatosis, and von Recklnghausen's disease.

Typical clinical presentation of patients with pheochromocytomas consists of mild to severe hypertension, bouts of paroxysmal headaches, pallor, palpitations, weight loss, and diaphoresis. Patients may also present with signs of hypovolemia and orthostatic hypotension or lactic acidosis secondary to excess catecholamines stimulation and vasoconstriction, and sudden death may occur.

The diagnosis of pheochromocytoma is made by measuring 24-h urine for catecholamines, metanephrines, and VMA. In addition, the clonidine suppression test can be used on patients that demonstrate a borderline plasma or urine level of catecholamines. Patients with pheochromocytoma will not suppress their levels of catecholamines following administration of clonidine, whereas normal patients will.

Localization studies are essential for pheochromocytomas utilizing a CT scan and MRI, which are quite sensitive and usually able to detect lesions 1 cm or greater in diameter. MRI has greater specificity because of the increased signal intensity on the T2-weighted imaging. Nuclear scanning using labeled metaiodobenzylguanidine (MIBG) is an excellent means of localizing adrenal and extraadrenal pheochromocytomas not otherwise visualized or in abnormal locations.

The preoperative management of pheochromocytoma consists of α-adrenergic blockade for several weeks prior to surgery. If tachycardia develops, β-adrenergic blocking agents are added before surgery. Propranolol (β-adrenergic blocker) should never be started before an α-adrenergic blocker because unopposed vasoconstriction may cause a hypertensive crisis. Intraoperatively, tumor manipulation may cause a release of catecholamines that increase the blood pressure and should be controlled with agents that relax arterial and venous smooth muscle cells, such as nitroprusside.

Surgical resection should be carried out for pheochromocytomas via a transabdominal incision, either bilateral subcostal or midline. A small pheochromocytoma can be resected using laparoscopic techniques. No surgical procedure should be carried out until the patient is adequately prepared by blocking its endocrine function.

XII. PANCREAS

Pancreatic endocrine tumors are all similar in that the cell of origin is an APUD neuroendocrine cell. In 60% of the cases these tumors are malignant, except for insulinomas (10%), and they demonstrate similar radiographic appearances with a high degree of vascularity and a similar metastatic pattern (regional lymph nodes and liver). These tumors may be either clinically functional or nonfunctional depending on the quantitative secretion of ectopic hormone production and symptom generation.

A. Gastrinomas

Gastrinomas are rare tumors and derive their name from the overproduction of the hormone gastrin. Zollinger and Ellison first described this tumor in 1955 in two patients with severe peptic ulcer disease treated by total gastrectomy. The Zollinger–Ellison syndrome (ZES) is estimated to occur in 0.5 to 3 cases per 100,000 population per year in the United States.

The clinical signs of patients with ZES are due to the elevated gastrin levels causing the hypersecretion of gastric acid. The basic treatment of ZES is to reduce the amount of gastric acid secreted, which abrogates the clinical manifestations, such as peptic ulcer disease or diarrhea. There is a slight male predominance with a mean age at diagnosis of 45 to 50 years. Approximately 20% of the patients with ZES also have MEN 1. Most patients present with abdominal pain similar to peptic ulcer pain, but may present with diarrhea and esophageal reflux symptoms. A diagnosis of ZES should be suspected if a patient presents with both abdominal pain and diarrhea, particularly with recurrent or persistent peptic ulcer disease, or a peptic ulcer in an unusual location, and in patients with a family history.

A diagnosis of ZES is made by demonstrating a fasting gastrin level of greater than 1000 pg/ml and a basal acid output (BAO) of at least 15 mEq/h in patients without and at least 5 mEq/hr in patients with previous acid reduction surgery. If a fasting gastrin level is greater than 200 pg/ml, but less than 500 pg/ml, a provocative test including a secretin test, a calcium test, or a meal test is required. The provocative test will differentiate between ZES and antral G-cell hyperplasia, which can mimic ZES clinically with elevated BAO and fasting plasma gastrin levels. Antral C-cell hyperplasia will have a positive meal test and a negative secretin test (no increase in gastrin levels following secretin injection).

Tumor localization studies are very important in the evaluation of patients with gastrinomas. Approximately 80 to 85% of gastrinomas localize within the gastrinoma triangle, the area defined by the common bile duct, the first, second, and third portions of the duodenum, and the head of the pancreas. The first localization study is usually a CT or MRI scan, but these studies fail to locate the tumor approximately 75% of the time, as gastrinomas may be very small. A newer method is the use of radiolabeled octreotide, a somatostatin analog, to scan the patient.

Surgical resection represents the only chance of cure and is the standard of care, unless there is evidence of extensive disease to the liver. Preoperatively, patients should be prepared with antacid therapy with H_2 blockers or omeprazole. Patients with active ulcers should receive 6 weeks of medical management to allow ulcers to heal. The procedure of choice is a local resection or enucleation if small and duodenal. If the tumors are large, a formal pancreatic resection should be performed, including a pancreaticoduodenectomy if necessary. Nodal resection should be performed. If liver metastases are few, hepatic resection or oblation can be considered.

B. Insulinoma

Insulinomas are the second most common pancreatic islet cell tumor. The clinical symptoms are related to hypoglycemia and include sweating, palpitations, nervousness, blurred vision, and mental status changes. The classic (Whipple's) triad consists of mental status changes during a fasting serum glucose level less than 50 mg/dl, with relief of symptoms after glucose ingestion.

Insulinomas usually occur in patients between the ages of 20 and 57 years of age. The incidence is 0.8 cases per 1,000,000 population in the United States each year. Insulinomas are usually less than 1.5 cm, usually benign, solitary intrapancreatic lesions. Insulinomas are found throughout the pancreas. Only 5% of patients with an insulinoma also have the MEN 1 syndrome.

A diagnosis of insulinoma is confirmed by a fasting insulin–glucose ratio of greater than 0.3 μU/ml/mg% glucose with an elevated level of C peptide.

Localization of insulinomas can be difficult because they are often too small to be found by a CT scan. Arteriography and portovenous sampling can be very helpful. Recent data support the primary use of intraoperative ultrasound (IOUS) with careful palpation after complete mobilization of the pancreas at surgery. More than 90% of tumors can be located in this fashion.

As with gastrinomas, insulinomas are cured with surgical excision. These tumors can be enucleated from the pancreas because they are benign, but care must be taken not to injure the pancreatic duct. Larger tumors are treated with formal resection.

C. Glucagonomas

Glucagonomas occur in older individuals. Less than 20% of patients are less than 40 years of age. Most of these tumors are large and found in the tail of the pancreas, although they do occur in the proximal duodenum. The most common site of metastasis is the liver. Symptoms are related to increased levels of glucagon; clinically, patients present with dermatitis, diabetes mellitus, glucose intolerance, diarrhea, abdominal pain, weight loss, thromboembolic disease, and mental status changes. Cutaneous lesions often precede the diagnosis of glucagonoma for several years. Once the diagnosis is suspected, glucagon levels over 200 pg/ml are confirmatory. Following the diagnosis, these tumors are localized using similar imaging studies as the other pancreatic islet cell tumors, including CT scan, MRI, angiogram, octreotide scans, and IOUS.

As with the other pancreatic islet cell tumors, this disease is treated by surgical resection, with octreotide therapy reserved for metastatic disease.

D. Somatostatinoma

Somatostatinomas occur in the pancreas and the proximal small bowel. They are usually solitary and are metastatic at diagnosis in the majority of cases. Metastases are usually hepatic and regional lymph nodes; less commonly bone metastases occur. Somatostatin inhibits both exocrine and endocrine processes. Patients with somatostatinomas usually present with diabetes mellitus, abdominal pain, gallbladder disease, diarrhea, weight loss, steatorrhea, and hypochlorhydria, all symptoms of altered hormonal activity.

The diagnosis of somatostatinomas is often made at the time of surgery for gallbladder disease or following imaging studies of the gastrointestinal tract. An elevated serum somatostatin level is essential for diagnosis. Unlike somatostatinomas in the pancreas, duodenal and small bowel tumors do not always demonstrate elevated plasma somatostatin levels.

As with the other pancreatic islet cell tumors, the mainstay of treatment is surgical resection. Survival data of patients with these tumors demonstrate that approximately 60% of these patients are alive at least 5 months to 6 years after diagnosis.

E. VIPomas

VIPomas, first described by Verner and Morrison, are very rare tumors and have a clinical presentation of watery diarrhea, hypokalemia, and achlorhyria, giving the acronym for this disease as WDHA. These patients usually demonstrate elevated plasma levels of vasoactive intestinal peptide (VIP). In adults the mean age of diagnosis is approximately 50 years of age, with a range of 30 to 80 and a female predominance. In children the mean age is 4 years, with a range of 10 months to 9 years.

Demonstrating elevated serum levels of VIP and the presence of a large volume of secretory diarrhea make the diagnosis of VIPomas.

Treatment of patients with VIPomas consists of fluid resuscitation and electrolyte correction due to severe hypokalemia, dehydration, and acidosis. Following medical treatment, imaging studies including a CT scan to localize the tumor are performed following surgical excision for cure in all patients that do not have metastatic disease. As with the other pancreatic islet cell tumors, metastatic disease is treated by chemotherapy, including agents such as streptozotocin, dacarbazine, doxorubicin, 5-fluorouracil, interferon-α, and somatostatin analogs. In addition, hepatic artery embolization, liver resection, and transplant have all been used with moderate results.

XIII. MULTIPLE ENDOCRINE NEOPLASIAS

MEN syndromes are composed of three types: MEN 1, 2A, and 2B. The MEN 1 syndrome is inherited as an autosomal-dominant trait. The MEN 1 syndrome consists of parathyroid hyperplasia (88 to 97% of patients with MEN 1), pancreatic endocrine tumors (80 to 100% of patients with MEN 1), and pituitary tumors (54 to 80% of patients with MEN 1). In addition, adrenal abnormalities and thyroid adenomas may occur in 27 to 36% and 5 to 30% of patients with MEN 1, respectively. The peak incidence of symptoms in women is during their 3rd decade of life and in men it is in their 4th decade of life. Clinical signs and symptoms include hypercalcemia, kidney stones, peptic ulcer disease, hypoglycemia, hypopituitarism, headache, acromegaly, Cushing's syndrome, and galactorrhea–amenorrhea. There is a decreased life expectancy in patients with MEN 1, with a 50% mortality by the age of 50 years of age. Most of these patients die from a malignance.

The other two MEN syndromes are MEN 2A and MEN 2B. MEN 2A consists of hyperparathyroidism due to parathyroid hyperplasia, medullary carcinoma of the thyroid, and pheochromocytomas. MEN 2B consists of parathyroid hyperplasia, medullary carcinoma of the thyroid, and multiple mucosal neuromas. Patients that have either MEN 2A or 2B syndromes can present with any of the neoplasms described, but a hallmark feature is that medullary carcinoma of the thyroid presents in 100% of affected individuals. Some characteristics of patients with MEN 2B are that medullary carcinoma of the thyroid presents at an earlier age and appears to be more aggressive. Patients usually present initially with complaints of dizziness, headache, or symptoms of nervousness and irritability. Patients with the MEN 2A syndrome usually present initially with symptoms related to parathyroid disease.

See Also the Following Articles

CORTICOSTEROIDS • GERM CELL TUMORS • PANCREAS AND PERIAMPULLARY TUMORS • STEROID HORMONES AND HORMONE RECEPTORS • THYROID CANCER

Bibliography

Fraker, D. L. (1997). Parathyroid tumors. *In* "Cancer: Principles and Practice of Oncology" (V. T. DeVita, S. Hellman, and S. A. Rosenberg, eds.), 5th Ed., pp. 1652–1659. Lippincott-Raven, Philadelphia.

Fraker, D. L., and Jensen, R. T. (1997). Pancreatic endocrine tumors. *In* "Cancer: Principles and Practice of Oncology" (V. T. DeVita, S. Hellman, and S. A. Rosenberg, eds.), 5th Ed., pp. 1678–1704. Lippincott-Raven, Philadelphia.

Fraker, D. L., Skarulis, M., and Livolsi, V. (1997). Thyroid tumors. *In* "Cancer: Principles and Practice of Oncology" (V. T. DeVita, S. Hellman, and S. A. Rosenberg, eds.), 5th Ed., pp.1629–1652. Lippincott-Raven, Philadelphia.

Haller, D. G. (1993). Endocrine neoplasms: Neoplasms of the endocrine and reproductive systems. *In* "Medical Oncology: Basic Principles and Clinical Management of Cancer" (P. Calabresi and P. S. Schein, eds.), 2nd Ed., p. 795. McGraw-Hill, New York.

Kulke, M. H., and Mayer, R. J. (1999). Carcinoid tumors. *N. Engl. J. Med.* **340**(11), 858–868.

Norton, J. A. (1997). Adrenal tumors. *In* "Cancer: Principles and Practice of Oncology" (V. T. DeVita, S. Hellman, and S. A. Rosenberg, eds.), 5th Ed., pp. 1659–1677. Lippincott-Raven, Philadelphia.

Norton, J. A., and Jensen, R. T. (1997). Multiple endocrine neoplasias. *In* "Cancer: Principles and Practice of Oncology" (V. T. DeVita, S. Hellman, and S. A. Rosenberg, eds.), 5th Ed., pp. 1723–1729. Lippincott-Raven, Philadelphia.

Endometrial Cancer

Richard R. Barakat

Memorial Sloan-Kettering Cancer Center

GLOSSARY

adenocarcinoma A malignant neoplasm of epithelial cells in glandular or gland-like pattern.

androstenedione An androgenic steroid of weaker biologic potency than testosterone, secreted by the testis, ovary, and adrenal cortex.

anovulation Suspension or cessation of ovulation.

bilateral salpingo-oopherectomy Removal of ovaries and fallopian tubes.

brachytherapy Radiotherapy in which the source of irradiation is placed close to the surface of the body or within a body cavity.

dilation and curretage Dilation of the cervix and curettement of the endometrium.

endogenous Originating or produced within the organism or one of its parts.

estrone A metabolite of 17β-estradiol, commonly found in urine, ovaries, and placenta; with considerably less biological activity than the parent hormone.

hysterectomy Removal of the uterus.

intraperitoneal Within the peritoneal cavity.

laparoscopy Examination of contents of the peritoneum with a laparoscope (a type of endoscope) passed through the abdominal wall.

laparotomy Incision into the loin.

lymphadenectomy Removal of the lymph nodes.

metastatic disease Shifting of a disease or its local manifestations from one part of the body to another.

myometrium The muscular wall of the uterus.

pelvic exenteration Removal of all of the organs and adjacent structures of the pelvis.

peritoneum The serous sac, consisting of mesothelium and a think layer of irregular connective tissue that lines the abdominal cavity and covers most of the viscera contained therein; it forms two sacs: the peritoneal sac and the omental bursa connected by the epiploic foramen.

progestin Generic term for any substance, natural or synthetic, that affects some or all of the biological changes produced by progesterone.

retroperitoneal nodal metastasis Disease growth occurring posterior to the peritoneum.

tamoxifen An antiestrogen agent used in the treatment of breast cancer.

Cancer of the epithelial lining (endometrium) of the uterine corpus is the fourth most common malignancy in women and ranks seventh among causes of female cancer deaths. Since 1972, it has been the most common female pelvic malignancy with the American Cancer Society, which estimates that in 2000 there will be 36,100 newly diagnosed cases along with 6500 deaths in the United States. The majority of cases occur in postmenopausal women who usually present with abnormal vaginal bleeding and are, therefore, detected at an early stage when they are highly curable. Nonetheless, approximately 6000 patients will die annually from this disease. Over the past decade the management of endometrial cancer has evolved from the inaccurate method of clinically staging patients to a newly developed surgical staging system. Contemporary surgical issues include the increasing use of minimal access surgery, including laparoscopically assisted vaginal hysterectomy and lymph node sampling. Another area that continues to evolve is the role of postoperative adjuvant therapy, including radiation and chemotherapy. The optimal management of patients with metastatic/recurrent disease also continues to be defined. Hormones continue to play a prominent role in endometrial cancer. A great deal of attention has been paid to the possible induction of endometrial cancer by the antiestrogen tamoxifen and has led to the development of new selective estrogen receptor modulators (SERMs). Controversy still exists regarding estrogen replacement therapy in the management of women with a history of endometrial cancer, and it is hoped that a large cooperative group trial currently underway will clarify this issue as we enter the next century.

I. EPIDEMIOLOGY

Endometrial cancer is primarily a disease of postmenopausal women, although 25% occur in premenopausal patients, with 5% occurring in patients younger than 40 years. It is widely held that there are two types of endometrial cancers with differing prognoses. Type I cancers are due to unopposed endogenous or exogenous estrogen and are clinically associated with obesity, nulliparity, diabetes, and hypertension. Increased endogenous estrogen exposure can be associated with chronic anovulation as occurs with Stein–Leventhal syndrome or estrogen-producing tumors such as granulosa cell tumors of the ovary. Peripheral conversion of androstenedione to estrone by extraglandular aromatization in adipose tissue accounts for the higher rate of endometrial cancer in obese women.

Unopposed estrogen administration is associated with a four- to eightfold increased risk of developing endometrial carcinoma, usually consisting of early stage, low-grade lesions that have a favorable prognosis. This risk can be almost completely prevented by the addition of progesterone to combat the carcinogenic effect of unopposed estrogen.

II. TAMOXIFEN AND ENDOMETRIAL CANCER

Following the initial report by Killackey and colleagues on endometrial cancer occurring in three breast cancer patients receiving antiestrogens, numerous studies have appeared implicating tamoxifen as a causal agent in the development of endometrial cancer. Perhaps the strongest data initially implicating tamoxifen use and the subsequent development of endometrial cancer were published in 1989 by Fornander and co-workers. The authors reviewed the frequency of new primary cancers as recorded in the Swedish Cancer Registry for a group of 1846 postmenopausal women with early breast cancer who were included in a randomized trial of adjuvant tamoxifen. They noted a 6.4-fold increase in the relative risk of endometrial cancer in 931 tamoxifen-treated patients compared to 915 patients in the control group. The dose of tamoxifen in this study was 40 mg/day, and the greatest cumulative risk of developing endometrial cancer was after 5 years of tamoxifen use.

Fisher and colleagues published the most compelling data to date regarding the association between tamoxifen use and the development of endometrial cancer when they reported the findings of the National Surgical Adjuvant Breast and Bowel Project (NSABP) B-14 trial. Data regarding the rates of endometrial and other cancers were analyzed on 2843 patients with node-negative, estrogen receptor-positive, invasive breast cancer randomly assigned to placebo or tamoxifen (20 mg/day) and on 1220 tamoxifen-treated patients registered in NSABP B-14 subsequent to randomization.

The average annual hazard rate for endometrial cancer in the placebo group was 0.2/1000 and 1.6/1000 for the randomized tamoxifen-treated group. The relative risk of endometrial cancer occurring in the randomized, tamoxifen-treated group was 7.5. Similar results were seen in the 1220 registered patients who received tamoxifen. Any conclusions regarding the risks of tamoxifen treatment inducing endometrial cancer must weigh the benefits of tamoxifen in reducing breast cancer recurrence and new contralateral breast cancers. In the B-14 trial, the cumulative rate/1000 of breast cancer relapse was reduced from 227.8 in the placebo group to 123.5 in the randomized tamoxifen-treated group. In addition, the cumulative rate of contralateral breast cancer was reduced from 40.5 to 23.5, respectively, in the two groups. Taking into account the increased cumulative rate of endometrial cancer, there was a 38% reduction in the 5-year cumulative hazard rate in the tamoxifen-treated group. These results led the authors to conclude that the benefit of tamoxifen therapy for breast cancer outweighs the potential increase in endometrial cancer being reported.

There is no proven benefit to screening women for endometrial cancer currently undergoing tamoxifen treatment for breast cancer. The ultimate goal of any cancer screening program is to detect disease at an earlier stage when it is more curable. Because tamoxifen-associated endometrial cancers appear to have a similar stage, grade, and histology as endometrial cancers occurring in the general population, their prognosis is generally good and early detection will probably not improve outcome significantly. Because the annual risk of endometrial cancer is 2/1000 in this population, and approximately 15% of these cancers will result in the patient's death, annual screening could potentially decrease mortality in only $0.002 \times 0.15 = 0.0003$, or 0.03% of all tamoxifen-treated patients.

Because approximately 80,000 women begin tamoxifen treatment annually in the United States, the cost to undertake screening for endometrial cancer in this population may be prohibitively high. All women with breast cancer, regardless of whether they are receiving tamoxifen, should be encouraged to undergo an annual gynecologic evaluation. Endometrial sampling should be reserved for patients with any sign of abnormal vaginal bleeding, including spotting or brownish vaginal discharge.

A. Staging

The primary surgical approach for endometrial cancer led the International Federation of Gynecology and Obstetrics (FIGO) to switch from an inaccurate clinical staging system developed in 1978 (Table I) to a primary operative staging system in 1988 (Table II). This new system incorporated many of the prognostic factors based in part on two large prospective staging trials reported by the Gynecology Oncology Group in 1984 and 1987. These studies helped define the prognostic factors of endometrial carcinoma and the current treatment approach for patients with this

TABLE I
Corpus Cancer Clinical Staging (FIGO, 1971)

Stage	Histologic subtype of adenocarcinoma	Characteristic
I		The carcinoma is confined to the corpus
IA		The length of the uterine cavity is 8 cm or less
IB		The length of the uterine cavity is more than 8 cm
	G1	Highly differentiated adenomatous carcinoma
	G2	Differentiated adenomatous carcinoma with partly solid areas
	G3	Predominantly solid or entirely undifferentiated carcinoma
II		The carcinoma involves the corpus and cervix
III		The carcinoma extends outside the uterus but not outside the true pelvis
IV		The carcinoma extends outside the true pelvis or involves the bladder or rectum

disease. In addition to evaluating the factors of age, race, and endocrine status, these studies confirmed that patient prognosis is directly related to the presence or absence of easily determinable uterine and extrauterine risk factors. Uterine factors were histologic cell type, tumor grade, depth of myometrial invasion, occult extension to the cervix, and vascular space invasion. Extrauterine prognostic factors are adnexal metastases, other extrauterine intraperitoneal spread, positive peritoneal cytology, pelvic lymph node metastases, and aortic lymph node involvement. Uterine size was previously believed to be a risk factor; however, recent information indicates that uterine size is not an independent risk factor, but rather relates to cell type, grade, and myometrial invasion.

Cell type and grade are factors that can be determined before hysterectomy, although grade as determined by dilatation and curettage in some series has

an overall 31% inaccuracy rate compared with grade in the hysterectomy specimen, and grade 3 tumors have a 50% inaccuracy rate. Recognition of all the other factors require an exploratory laparotomy, peritoneal fluid sampling, and hysterectomy with careful pathologic interpretation of all removed tissue.

B. Surgical Staging

To appropriately stage by FIGO criteria, the surgical procedure includes abdominal exploration, sampling of peritoneal fluid for cytologic evaluation (intraperitoneal cell washings), and abdominal and pelvic exploration with biopsy or excision of any extrauterine lesions suspicious for tumor. Total abdominal hysterectomy and bilateral salpingo-oophorectomy are the standard operative procedures for carcinoma of the endometrium, although ovarian preservation is

TABLE II
Corpus Cancer Surgical Staging (FIGO, 1988)[a,b]

Stage	Characteristic
IA G123	Tumor limited to endometrium
IB G123	Invasion to <1/2 myometrium
IC G123	Invasion to >1/2 myometrium
IIA G123	Endocervical glandular involvement only
IIB G123	Cervical stromal invasion
IIIA G123	Tumor invades serosa or adenexae or positive peritoneal cytology
IIIB G123	Vaginal metastases
IIIC G123	Metastases to pelvic or paraaortic lymph nodes
IVA G123	Tumor-invaded bladder and/or bowel mucosa
IVB	Distant metastases including intraabdominal and/or inguinal lymph node
Histopathology: Degree of differentiation	
Cases should be grouped by the degree of differentiation of the adenocarcinoma:	
G1	5% or less of a nonsquamous or nonmorular solid growth pattern
G2	6–50% of a nonsquamous or nonmorular solid growth pattern
G3	More than 50% of a nonsquamous or nonmorular solid growth pattern

[a]Notes on pathologic grading: Notable nuclear atypia, inappropriate for the architectural grade, raises the grade of a grade 1 or grade 2 tumor by 1. In serous adenocarcinomas, clear cell adenocarcinomas, and squamous cell carcinomas, nuclear grading takes precedence. Adenocarcinomas with squamous differentiation are graded according to the nuclear grade of the glandular component.

[b]Rules related to staging: Because corpus cancer is now surgically staged, procedures used previously for the determination for stages are no longer applicable, such as the finding of fractional D&C to differentiate between stages I and II. It is appreciated that there may be a small number of patients with corpus cancer who will be treated primarily with radiation therapy. If that is the case, the clinical staging adopted by FIGO in 1971 would still apply, but designation of that staging system would be noted. Ideally, width of the myometrium should be measured, along with the width of tumor invasion.

occasionally performed in premenopausal patients with early stage disease. In some cases, pelvic lymph node sampling is indicated. In a lymph node sampling procedure, it is important to try to achieve an adequate sample of nodes from the common iliac, external iliac, and obturator regions, but no attempt is made to perform a complete lymphadenectomy. Because lymph node sampling is not routinely performed by the general gynecologist, it is important to identify the subset of patients that will benefit from selective lymphadenectomy, which may require further surgical expertise from a gynecologic oncologist. If there is no gross intraperitoneal tumor noted at the time of laparotomy, pelvic and paraaortic lymph nodes should be sampled for the following indications: (1) myometrial invasion greater than one-half (outer half of myometrium); (2) tumor presence (regardless of tumor grade) in isthmus-cervix, adnexal, or other extrauterine metastases; (3) presence of serous, clear cell, undifferentiated or squamous types, and lymph nodes that are visibly or palpably enlarged.

For patients in whom paraaortic node sampling is indicated, sampling can be performed through a midline peritoneal incision over the common iliac arteries and aorta. Node sampling can also be performed on the right by mobilizing the right colon medially and on the left by mobilizing the left colon medially. In each case, a sample of lymphatics and lymph nodes is resected along the upper common iliac vessels on either side and from the lower portion of the aorta and vena cava. After these procedures, the patient is surgically staged according to 1988 FIGO criteria. The overall surgical complication rate after this type of staging is approximately 20%. The serious complication rate is 6%.

In the Gynecologic Oncology Group study, 46% of positive paraaortic lymph nodes were enlarged, and 98% of the cases with aortic node metastases came from patients with positive pelvic nodes, adnexal or intraabdominal metastases, or outer one-third myometrial invasion. These risk factors affected only 25% of the patients, yet they yielded most of the positive paraaortic node patients. Overall, 5 to 6% of patients with clinical stage I and II (occult) endometrial carcinoma have tumor spread to these lymph nodes. The key to the surgical management of patients with endometrial cancer is identifying patients at risk for

retroperitoneal nodal metastasis, as both patients with pelvic and aortic disease can be salvaged with adjuvant radiotherapy. Postoperative irradiation to the pelvis and aortic area appears to be effective. In the Gynecologic Oncology Group study, 37 of 48 patients with positive paraaortic nodes received postoperative irradiation and 36% remain tumor free at 5 years. Potish and others reported a 5-year survival rate of 47% in a smaller group of patients who were also treated with postoperative irradiation. Although this accounts for only 5 to 6% of patients with early stage endometrial cancer, it is important that patients with metastatic spread to the paraaortic nodes be identified, as approximately 40% will be salvaged with extended field radiotherapy.

Regardless of grade, lymph nodes need not be sampled for tumor limited to the endometrium because less than 1% of these patients have disease spread to pelvic or paraaortic lymph nodes. An area of frequent indecision regarding lymph node sampling is represented by patients whose only risk factor is inner one-half myometrial invasion, particularly if the grade is 2 or 3. This group has 5% or less chance of node positivity. Lymph node sampling should be performed in these instances if there seems to be any question about the degree of myometrial invasion. This includes invasion that approaches one-half of the myometrial thickness in patients who are medically fit to undergo the sampling procedures.

The depth of myometrial invasion can be assessed easily at the time of surgery. The excised uterus is opened, preferably away from the operating table, and the depth of myometrial penetration and the presence or absence of endocervix involvement are determined by clinical observation or by a microscopic frozen section. Doering and others reported a 91% accuracy rate for 148 patients for determining the depth of myometrial invasion by gross visual examination of the cut uterine surface.

Nine percent of patients with endometrial carcinoma have positive pelvic lymph nodes (stage IIIC). The incidence is increased to 51, 32, and 25%, respectively, in patients with extrauterine metastases, adnexal involvement, and deep myometrial invasion. Patients with this as their only high-risk factor should be treated with postoperative whole pelvic irradiation. In the Gynecologic Oncology Group study, 13

(72%) of 18 patients were disease free 5 years after treatment. Potish and others reported a 5-year survival rate of 67% in a smaller series of similarly treated patients.

III. LAPAROSCOPIC SURGERY

An alternative method of surgically staging patients with clinical stage I endometrial cancer is gaining in popularity. This approach combines laparoscopically assisted vaginal hysterectomy with laparoscopic lymphadenectomy. Childers and colleagues described their experience with this procedure in 59 patients with clinical stage I endometrial carcinoma. The laparoscopic procedure included a thorough inspection of the peritoneal cavity, obtaining intraperitoneal washings, and performing a laparoscopically assisted vaginal hysterectomy. Laparoscopic pelvic and aortic lymph node sampling were performed in all patients with grade 2 or 3 lesions as well as those patients with grade 1 lesions who were found to have greater than 50% myometrial invasion on frozen section. In two patients, laparoscopic lymphadenectomy was precluded by obesity.

Six patients who were noted to have intraperitoneal disease at laparoscopy underwent exploratory laparotomy. Two additional patients required laparotomy for complications including a transected ureter and a cystotomy. The mean hospital stay was 2.9 days.

Laparoscopically assisted surgical staging is feasible in select groups of patients. However, it is not known whether it is applicable to all patients with clinical stage I disease. In particular, two groups of patients may not be ideal candidates because of their weight or the presence of intraabdominal adhesions. Paraaortic lymphadenectomy is technically more difficult through the laparoscope. To obtain adequate exposure, it is necessary to elevate the mesentery of the small bowel into the upper abdomen, which becomes increasingly difficult as the patient's weight increases, especially for patients whose weight exceeds 180 lbs.

For those patients that are eligible, advantages of the laparoscopic approach include a reduction in the length of hospitalization and fewer complications. Boike and colleagues compared 23 patients who underwent laparoscopic management of endometrial cancer with 21 who underwent laparotomy during the same time period. The laparoscopy group weighed significantly less than the laparotomy group. There was no significant difference in the number of lymph nodes obtained from the pelvic or paraaortic regions between the two groups. The mean length of stay was 2.7 days for the laparoscopy group vs 5.9 days for the laparotomy group.

Although laparoscopically assisted vaginal hysterectomy with surgical staging may provide an alternative approach to the management of endometrial cancer, its equivalency in terms of cancer outcome to the standard laparotomy approach remains unproven and the abdominal approach is still considered to be standard therapy. The Gynecology Oncology Group is conducting a randomized trial of these two approaches to help answer this question.

IV. ROLE OF POSTOPERATIVE THERAPY

The postoperative treatment approach in patients with endometrial cancer is tailored to various prognostic factors. Patients with grade 1 or 2 lesions whose disease is confined to the endometrial cavity (stage IA) are considered low risk and do not appear to benefit from postoperative radiation. In the GOG experience, there were no recurrences in 72 of these patients who received no radiation compared with 19 who received either pelvic or vaginal radiation. One of 5 patients with a stage IA, grade 3 lesion who was not irradiated recurred, but the number of these patients was too small to draw any firm conclusions.

Patients with less than 50% myometrial invasion (stage IB) or greater than 50% (stage IC), along with those who have endocervical glandular (IIA) or stromal (IIB) involvement, are considered to be of intermediate risk. The value of adjuvant pelvic radiation in this group of patients is of questionable benefit. A randomized trial from the Norwegian Radium Hospital revealed no difference in survival between 277 patients with clinical stage I endometrial cancer treated with vaginal radium only and 263 patients who received 4000 rads of whole pelvis radiation as well. Although the patients who received pelvic irradiation had a lower incidence of pelvic recurrences, this was offset by a higher frequency of distant failures. The GOG recently completed protocol 99, a randomized trial of no additional treatment versus 5040 rads of pelvic radiotherapy in patients with intermediate risk endometrial cancer. The estimated 2-year progression-free interval was 88% in the no-treatment group versus 96% in the radiation arm. The majority of the 17 recurrences in the no-treatment arm were pelvic or vaginal. Because most of these were salvaged with radiation therapy, the study did not show any survival benefit to adjuvant radiation, with 96% of patients who received adjuvant radiation being alive at 3 years compared to 89% of patients who did not receive radiation up front. Because toxicity was greater in the pelvic radiation group, perhaps the greatest therapeutic benefit to be achieved would be with vaginal brachytherapy. Further studies in this intermediate risk group of patients will need to be designed to answer this question.

The significance of positive peritoneal cytology in the absence of extrauterine disease is unclear. The benefit of adjuvant therapy, including intraperitoneal chromic phosphate or other therapeutic modalities, such as whole abdominal radiation, is unproven. Many clinicians will opt to treat such patients with oral progestins.

Patients with extrauterine disease, including intraperitoneal spread or spread to retroperitoneal lymph nodes, are considered high risk and will benefit from adjuvant treatment. Patients with positive pelvic lymph nodes are treated with postoperative whole pelvis radiation. In the GOG study, only 5 of 18 patients treated in this manner recurred. Aortic nodal metastasis is a very important prognostic factor. In the GOG experience, patients with grossly positive pelvic lymph nodes, gross adnexal metastasis, or outer one-third myometrial invasion had a 55, 43, and 18% incidence of aortic node metastasis, respectively. The importance of aortic nodal sampling in this group relates to the ability to salvage approximately 40% of this group of patients with adjuvant therapy. Of 48 patients in the GOG study with documented aortic nodal metastases, 37 received extended field radiation therapy to include the paraaortic region and 36% remained tumor free at 5 years.

The ideal treatment for patients who present with intraabdominal disease remains to be determined.

Those patients with residual disease following surgery may benefit from whole abdominal radiation or cytotoxic chemotherapy. It is hoped that results of a GOG trial comparing whole abdominal radiation versus combination chemotherapy with cisplatin and doxorubicin in patients with stage III or IV disease and less than 2 cm residual disease following surgery will shed some light on this topic in the near future.

V. RECURRENT DISEASE

Various treatment strategies exist for patients with recurrent endometrial cancer. Aalders and co-workers reported on 379 patients with recurrent disease treated at the Norwegian Radium Hospital. Local recurrence was noted in 50% of patients, whereas 28% experienced distant recurrence and 21% had both local and distant failure. The median time to recurrence was 14 months for patients with local recurrence and 19 months for those with distant metastases.

Patients with isolated vaginal recurrences are salvageable with radiation therapy in approximately 40% of cases. Kuten and others noted a 40% progression-free 5-year survival in patients with an isolated vaginal recurrence treated with pelvic radiotherapy. If the disease extended into the pelvis, however, this rate fell to 20%.

Hormonal therapy, including progestins and the antiestrogen tamoxifen, has proven useful in patients with recurrent endometrial cancer. About one-third of patients with recurrent disease will respond to progestins, with the highest responses being observed in patients with well-differentiated lesions that tend to be estrogen and progesterone receptor positive. In a review of 17 trials consisting of 1068 patients, Kaupila noted a 34% response rate to progestins with a 16- to 28-month duration of response and average survival of 18–33 months. Because of their low toxicity, many oncologists favor the use of progestins initially in patients with recurrent disease with cytotoxic chemotherapy being reserved for treatment failures or symptomatic patients. A long disease-free interval (exceeding 2 or 3 years), well-differentiated histologic type, and positive estrogen or progesterone receptor status have all been associated with increased frequency of response to progestins. Response rates of approximately 22% have been noted with tamoxifen, with the majority of responses occurring in women with well-differentiated tumors or those who have previously responded to progestins.

Cytotoxic chemotherapy is most often used for patients with advanced or recurrent disease who have failed hormonal therapy. A large variety of chemotherapeutic agents have been tested in patients with endometrial cancer with variable results. Doxorubicin is generally considered the most active agent in endometrial cancer, with an overall response rate of approximately 26%. Thigpen and colleagues reported the GOG experience comparing doxorubicin with doxorubicin and cisplatin in patients with advanced or recurrent endometrial cancer. The combination had a higher overall response rate (45% vs 27%) and complete response rate (22% vs 8%) than doxorubicin alone. At this point, the most active chemotherapeutic regimen for advanced endometrial cancer would appear to be the combination of cisplatin and doxorubicin.

Paclitaxel (Taxol) appears to be a promising agent for the treatment of endometrial cancer. In a phase II trial conducted by the Gynecologic Oncology Group, Ball and colleagues reported on 28 patients with recurrent or advanced endometrial cancer treated with 24-h paclitaxel at a dose of 250 mg/m^2 every 21 days. Patients who had received prior pelvic radiation were treated at an initial dose of 200 mg/m^2. Complete responses were noted in 4 patients (14%) and partial responses in 6 (21%) for an overall response rate of 36%. Results of a GOG trial evaluating paclitaxel in combination with doxorubicin compared to doxorubicin plus cisplatin will be important in determining the most active regimen for patients with advanced disease.

VI. SURGERY FOR RECURRENT DISEASE

One of the modifications many institutions have made is to reserve pelvic exenteration for the treatment of centrally recurrent cervical carcinoma. The rationale to excluding patients with endometrial cancer is that the procedure is unlikely to be curative in these patients, as those who recur tend to have extrapelvic and/or disseminated disease. However, reports have demonstrated that in highly selected patients with centrally recurrent endometrial cancer, adequate long-term survival can be achieved.

Morris and associates reported on 20 patients who underwent pelvic exenteration for recurrent endometrial cancer at four major institutions. The 5-year disease-free survival rate was 45% with a complication rate of 60%.

In the largest series of pelvic exenterations for recurrent endometrial cancer, Barakat and colleagues reported a 20% 5-year survival rate in 44 patients. With a major complication rate of 80%, the authors emphasized that highly specific selection criteria are needed in the selection of candidates for pelvic exenteration for recurrent endometrial cancer. They recommend a full evaluation to rule out metastatic disease, including diagnostic imaging with computed tomography of the chest, abdomen, and pelvis. Because patients who have pelvic sidewall involvement are not considered candidates for exenteration, magnetic resonance imaging of the pelvis can be used to detect pelvic sidewall disease and can thereby reduce the number of patients undergoing unnecessary exploration. At the time of exploration, if the patient has tumor fixed to the pelvic sidewall, intraabdominal metastases, or positive lymph nodes, the exenteration is generally aborted.

VII. ESTROGEN REPLACEMENT THERAPY IN WOMEN WITH A HISTORY OF ENDOMETRIAL CANCER

In the 1970s, reports in the medical literature began to link the use of exogenous estrogen to an increased incidence of endometrial cancer. However, these patients were found to have superficial, well-differentiated endometrial cancers that were highly curable. Furthermore, it was subsequently demonstrated that the addition of progestational agents abrogated this increased risk. Estrogen replacement offers important health benefits to women, including alleviation of hot flashes, prevention of osteoporosis, and protection from cardiovascular disease. The risk of major coronary disease for women who currently take estrogen has been demonstrated to be 0.56 of the risk for nonusers. Despite the known benefits of estrogen-replacement therapy, women with a history of endometrial carcinoma are usually denied this therapy because adenocarcinoma of the endometrium is considered an estrogen-dependent neoplasm. However, no scientific data exist to support the contention that estrogen replacement is dangerous for this group of patients.

Several retrospective studies have looked at the issue of estrogen replacement after surgical treatment of early stage endometrial adenocarcinoma. In 1986, Creasman and colleagues reported on 221 patients with stage I endometrial cancer, of whom 47 (21%) received postoperative estrogen replacement for a median of 26 months. Estrogen was applied vaginally for 34 of these patients. A multivariate analysis revealed no differences in tumor grade, myometrial invasion, nodal metastasis, or peritoneal cytology between the 47 patients who received estrogen-replacement therapy and the 174 who did not. In fact, the rate of recurrence was higher in the nontreated group (15%) than in the treated group (2%), and 26 deaths occurred in the nontreated group versus only 1 death in the group that received estrogen. The median time between surgery and initiation of estrogen-replacement therapy was 15 months. In 1989, Lee and associates reported on 44 patients with a history of stage I endometrial carcinoma who were selected to undergo estrogen replacement for a median of 64 months. No recurrent endometrial cancers or intercurrent deaths occurred in the treated group. In this study, 43% of patients waited 1 year before starting estrogen and 34% waited at least 2 years. Because the majority of recurrences of endometrial cancers occur within the first 2 years following surgery, a selection bias exists in these two studies, as many patients who would have recurred were not included in the study. Most recently, Chapman and colleagues compared 62 women with stage I and II endometrial cancer who received estrogen replacement following surgery with 61 who did not. The median interval to initiation of estrogen in this study was 8 months, and there was no increase in recurrences or deaths due to endometrial cancer in the estrogen-treated group. These patients did have a greater incidence of early stage disease with less myometrial invasion.

While not proving the safety of estrogen replacement in this population, these studies do, however, indicate that the safety of estrogen replacement therapy in women with a history of endometrial cancer should be determined in a prospective randomized trial. For this reason, the Gynecologic Oncology Group is undertaking a prospective, randomized, double-blinded study of estrogen replacement therapy versus placebo for patients with surgical stage IA, IB, IIA, or IIB endometrial carcinoma. The study will look to accrue 2206 patients who will receive treatment for 3 years and be followed for an additional 2 years. Patients considered ineligible include those with known or suspected carcinoma of the breast, patients with acute liver disease, those receiving any other form of hormonal therapy, and those with a history of thromboembolic disease.

This study should have the statistical power to prove the safety of estrogen replacement in this population and lead to similar trials being conducted in women with breast cancer. As we enter the next century, quality-of-life issues will play an increasing role in the management of patients with cancer. For the patient with early stage endometrial cancer, prospective trials will help define the need, or lack of need, of adjuvant therapy. Increasing knowledge of biomarkers of disease recurrence should help refine this area.

See Also the Following Articles

CISPLATIN AND RELATED DRUGS • ESTROGENS AND ANTI-ESTROGENS • HORMONAL CARCINOGENESIS • OVARIAN CANCER: EPIDEMIOLOGY

Bibliography

Aalders, J., Abeler, V., and Kolstad, P. (1984). Recurrent adenocarcinoma of the endometrium: A clinical and histopathological study of 379 patients. *Gynecol. Oncol.* **17,** 85.

Aalders, J., Abeler, V., Kolstad, P., *et al.* (1980). Postoperative external irradiation and prognostic parameters in stage I endometrial carcinoma. *Obstet. Gynecol.* **56,** 419–426.

Ball, H., Blessing, J. A., Lentz, S., and Mutch, D. (1995). A Phase II trial of Taxol in advanced and recurrent adenocarcinoma of the endometrium: A Gynecologic Oncology Group study. *In* "Proceedings of the Society of Gynecologic Oncologists Annual Meeting," 102. [Abstract #69]

Barakat, R. R., Goldman, N. A., Patel, D. A., *et al.* (1999). Pelvic exenteration for recurrent endometrial cancer. *Gynecol. Oncol.* **75,** 99.

Boike, G., Lurain, J., and Burke, J. (1994). A comparison of laparoscopic management of endometrial cancer with a traditional laparotomy. *Gynecol. Oncol.* **52,** 105.

Chapman, J. A., DiSaia, P. J., Osann, K., *et al.* (1996). Estrogen replacement in surgical stage I and II endometrial cancer survivors. *Am. J. Obstet. Gynecol.* **175,** 1195–2000.

Childers, J. M., Brzechffa, P. R., Hatch, K. D., *et al.* (1993). Laparoscopically assisted surgical staging (LASS) of endometrial cancer. *Gynecol. Oncol.* **51,** 33–38.

Childers, J. M., Hatch, K. D., Tran, A., *et al.* (1993). Laparoscopic para-aortic lymphadenectomy in gynecologic malignancies. *Obstet. Gynecol.* **82**(5), 741–747.

Creasman, W. T., Henderson, D., Hinshaw, W., *et al.* (1986). Estrogen replacement therapy in the patient treated for endometrial cancer. *Obstet. Gynecol.* **67,** 326–330.

Creasman, W. T., Morrow, C. P., Bundy, B. N., *et al.* (1987). Surgical pathologic spread patterns of endometrial cancer (a Gynecologic Oncology Group study). *Cancer* **60,** 2035.

Doering, D. L., Barnhill, D. R., Weiser, E. B., *et al.* (1989). Intraoperative evaluation of depth of myometrial invasion in stage I endometrial adenocarcinoma. *Obstet. Gynecol.* **74,** 930.

Elwood, J. M., and Boyes, D.A. (1980). Clinical and pathological features and survival of endometrial cancer patients in relation to prior use of estrogens. *Gynecol. Oncol.* **10,** 173–187.

FIGO (1971). Classification and staging of malignant tumors in the female pelvis. *Int. J. Gynaecol. Obstet.* **9,** 172.

FIGO (1989). Corpus cancer staging. *Int. J. Gynecol. Obstet.* **28,** 190.

Fisher, B., Costantino, J. P., Redmond, C. K., *et al.* (1994). Endometrial cancer in tamoxifen-treated breast cancer patients: Findings from the National Surgical Adjuvant Breast and Bowel Project (NSABP) B-14. *J. Natl. Cancer Inst.* **86,** 527–537.

Fornander, T., Rutqvist, L. E., Cedermark, B., *et al.* (1989). Adjuvant tamoxifen in early breast cancer occurrence of new primary cancers. *Lancet* **21,** 117–120.

Gallup, D. G., and Stock, R. J. (1984). Adenocarcinoma of the endometrium in women 40 years of age or younger. *Obstet. Gynecol.* **64,** 417.

Greenlee, R. T., Murray, T., Bolden, S., *et al.* (2000). Cancer statistics, 2000. *CA Cancer J. Clin.* **50,** 7.

Kauppila, A., Janne, O., Kujansuu, E., *et al.* (1980). Treatment of advanced endometrial adenocarcinoma with a combined cytotoxic therapy. *Cancer* **46,** 2162–2167.

Killackey, M. A., Hakes, T. B., and Pierce, V. K. (1985). Endometrial adenocarcinoma in breast cancer patients receiving antiestrogens. *Cancer Treat. Rep.* **69,** 237–238.

Kuten, A., Grigsby, P. W., Perez, C. A., *et al.* (1989). Results of radiotherapy in recurrent endometrial carcinoma, a retrospective analysis. *Int. J. Radiat. Oncol. Biol. Phys.* **17,** 29.

Lee, R. B., Burke, T. W., and Park, R. C. (1990). Estrogen replacement therapy following treatment for stage I endometrial carcinoma. *Gynecol. Oncol.* **36,** 189–191.

Malviya, V. K., Deppe, G., Malone, J. M., Jr., *et al.* (1989). Reliability of frozen section examination in identifying poor prognostic indicators in stage I endometrial adenocarcinoma. *Gynecol. Oncol.* **34,** 299.

Morrow, C. P., Bundy, B. N., Kumar, R. J., *et al.* (1991). Relationship between surgical-pathological risk factors and outcome in clinical stages I and II carcinoma of the endometrium: A Gynecologic Oncology Group study. *Gynecol. Oncol.* **40,** 55.

Morris, M., Alvarez, R. D., Kinney, W. K., *et al.* (1996). Treatment of recurrent adenocarcinoma of the endometrium with pelvic exenteration. *Gynecol. Oncol.* **60,** 288.

Potish, R. A., Twiggs, L. B., Adcock, L. L., *et al.* (1985). Para-aortic lymph node radiotherapy in cancer of the uterine corpus. *Obstet. Gynecol.* **654,** 251.

Roberts, J. A., Brunetto, V. L., Keys, H. M., *et al.* (1998). A phase III randomized study of surgery vs. surgery plus adjunctive radiation therapy in intermediate risk endometrial carcinoma (GOG 99). *In* "Proc SGO Fourth Annual Meeting," 70. [Abstract #35].

Saint Cassia, L. J., Weppelmann, B., Shingleton, H., *et al.* (1989). Management of early endometrial carcinoma. *Gynecol. Oncol.* **35,** 362.

Thigpen, T., Blessing, J., Homesley, H., *et al.* (1993). Phase III trial of doxorubicin +/− cisplatin in advanced or recurrent endometrial carcinoma: A Gynecologic Oncology Group (GOG) study. *Proc ASCO* **12,** 261.

Whitaker, G. K., Lee, R. B., and Benson, W.L. (1986). Carcinoma of the endometrium in young women. *Milit. Med.* **151,** 25.

Epstein–Barr Virus and Associated Malignancies

Eric Johannsen
Fred Wang

*Brigham and Women's Hospital and
Harvard Medical School*

GLOSSARY

episome A circular viral genome that replicates autonomously and is characteristic of the latent phase of Epstein-Barr virus infection.

Epstein–Barr virus A γ herpesvirus with genetic information in the form of DNA, whose primary host is humans. It is associated with infectious mononucleosis, lymphomas, nasopharyngeal carcinoma, and various other neoplasms.

latent viral genes Viral genes that are expressed when a virus is in a latent state, i.e., not producing virus particles.

lytic infection The expression of viral genes involved with DNA replication and the production of structural proteins, with resultant assembly of virus particles. The initiation of this viral program results in cell death.

E pstein–Barr virus (EBV; human herpesvirus 4; HHV-4) is a human herpesvirus that infects most humans by adulthood and is associated with a number of different cancers. Like other herpesviruses, EBV has a large (~180 kb), double-stranded DNA genome that encodes approximately 100 different gene products. Most of these viral genes are expressed during lytic viral replication and are common to other herpesviruses, e.g., proteins that are important for transcriptional regulation, nucleic acid metabolism and synthesis, and virus structure. Herpesviruses are differentiated based on genetic and biologic properties. EBV is classified with the Kaposi's sarcoma herpesvirus (KSHV; HHV-8) in the γ herpesvirus subfamily based on genetic similarities and common biologic predisposition for latent infection and lymphocyte cell tropism. EBV is unique among herpesviruses in its ability to infect and immortalize B cells. A repertoire of latent infection viral genes unique to EBV is expressed in immortalized B cells, and these genes are likely to be important for transformed cell growth and EBV-induced malignancies.

I. PRIMARY AND PERSISTENT EPSTEIN–BARR VIRUS (EBV) INFECTION

Primary EBV infection is most often acquired by oral transmission and is the most common cause of the infectious mononucleosis (IM) syndrome. The IM syndrome, characterized by fever, malaise, splenomegaly, lymphadenopathy, and atypical lymphocytosis, is due in large part to the vigorous T-cell response to the sudden appearance of EBV-infected B cells in the peripheral blood of a naive host. As many as 1 in 100 B cells are EBV infected during IM, but the atypical lymphocytosis, splenomegaly, and lymphadenopathy result from the vigorous T-cell activation. Over time, EBV-specific T-cell responses develop and help resolve acute EBV infection. Despite the development of EBV-specific humoral and cellular responses, the immune system is unable to purge the host of EBV. Thus in most adults, EBV infection persists as a latent infection in a small number of B cells (1 in 10^6 B cells) and as a lytic infection in the oropharynx, resulting in viral shedding in oral secretions. A benign virus:host relationship is maintained in most humans by a balance between the EBV-specific immune response and viral strategies to evade the immune response.

II. EBV-ASSOCIATED MALIGNANCIES IN IMMUNOSUPPRESSED HOSTS

EBV-associated malignancies can occur in hosts with immune defects where this homeostasis is disturbed and EBV-infected B cells are allowed to proliferate. EBV-infected B-cell lymphomas occur in patients with congenital immunodeficiencies, e.g., severe combined immunodeficiency, Wiskott–Aldrich syndrome, ataxia-telangiectasia, X-linked lymphoproliferative disease, and in patients with acquired immunodeficiencies (e.g., HIV infection or posttransplant drug-

induced immunosuppression). Less aggressive, polyclonal B-cell proliferation may respond to a reduction of the immunosuppression if possible, e.g., lowering the dose of immunosuppressive drugs. More aggressive, monoclonal cell proliferations may be difficult to treat even with chemotherapeutic agents. The importance of the immune system is highlighted by the increased risk of EBV-induced lymphoproliferative disease in posttransplant patients with more intense immunosuppression and the decreased incidence of EBV-induced lymphomas in AIDS patients treated with highly active antiretroviral therapy. The adoptive transfer of EBV-specific T cells expanded *in vitro* has been used as an effective treatment in some patients with EBV-induced lymphoproliferative disease.

A. X-Linked Lymphoproliferative Disease

An unusual congenital immunodeficiency occurs in boys who appear otherwise healthy, but have a unique susceptibility to EBV infection. Patients with this X-linked lymphoproliferative (XLP) syndrome are able to control other viral and bacterial infections normally, but when they acquire EBV infection, approximately one-third succumb to a fatal IM syndrome, one-third develop EBV-induced B-cell lymphomas, and one third develop bone marrow aplasias. This spectrum of clinical presentations is unusual because in some instances it suggests an overactive immune response, e.g., bone marrow suppression, whereas in others it suggests an inadequate immune response, e.g., B-cell lymphomas. A genetic defect responsible for many cases of XLP has been described, and the affected gene (known as SAP, SH2D1A, or DSHP) is believed to be important for regulating the intensity of the immune response. Why this gene is so critical for the control of EBV infection remains to be determined.

III. EBV-ASSOCIATED MALIGNANCIES IN IMMUNOCOMPETENT HOSTS

A. Burkitt's Lymphoma

A variety of EBV-associated malignancies occur in patients with no overt immunosuppression. EBV was originally discovered by Dr. Anthony Epstein as a herpesvirus infecting Burkitt's lymphoma tumor cells, the most common pediatric malignancy in Africa. Dr. Epstein, in association with colleagues Yvonne Barr and Dr. Bert Achong, was able to propagate tumor cell lines from Burkitt tumor biopsies and identify infecting herpesvirus particles by electron microscopy. In collaboration with Drs. Gertrude and Werner Henle, they were able to identify the virus as a new human herpesvirus. Subsequently, it was shown that EBV infects every tumor cell and that the cells are infected with a clonal population of virus. This suggested that virus infection precedes the malignant conversion as a potential causal factor in the tumorigenesis and does not occur as a secondary infection after malignant transformation. A two-step model for tumorigenesis was proposed. African children are infected early in life with EBV. Frequent infections, such as malaria, stimulate the proliferation of EBV-infected B cells, increasing the risk for a second event. The frequent finding of chromosomal translocations between the c-myc gene and immunoglobulin loci in Burkitt tumor cells suggests that the combination of EBV infection and deregulated c-myc expression are important steps for tumorigenesis.

B. Nasopharyngeal Carcinoma

EBV infection is also associated with the development of nasopharyngeal carcinomas (NPC). Like Burkitt's lymphoma, EBV infection is also found in all tumor cells, is monoclonal, and precedes malignant conversion. Similarly, the occurrence of EBV-infected tumors many years after initial EBV infection of the host suggests that EBV acts in conjunction with other factors to increase the risk of tumorigenesis. No specific chromosomal translocations have been identified in nasopharyngeal carcinomas, but the high frequency of EBV-infected NPC in southeast China, northern Africa, and Inuit populations has suggested the possibility of dietary or genetic (HLA) cofactors.

C. Hodgkin's Disease and Gastric Carcinomas

EBV infection has also been linked to other malignancies of B-cell and epithelial cell origin, including Hodgkin's disease and gastric carcinomas. EBV infection is associated with 40–60% of Hodgkin's disease cases and most often with the mixed cellularity subtype. Monoclonal EBV DNA can be detected in Reed–Sternberg cells. Reed–Sternberg cells are believed to represent the malignant cell population in Hodgkin's disease and are probably of B-cell origin. The mixed cell population of other reactive cells in these tumors is notable because EBV-infected tumors are typically associated with a reactive lymphocytic infiltrate, e.g., the lymphoepithelioma-like phenotype for NPC. EBV infection in a subset of gastric carcinomas was first observed in the Far East, but it is now recognized that EBV infection is present in approximately 10% of gastric carcinomas around the world. Similarly, a lymphoepithelioma-like phenotype is characteristic. The association of EBV infection with different B-cell and epithelial cell malignancies may represent the risk of persistent infection in these cell types.

D. Other Tumors

EBV infection is also associated with other unusual malignancies such as leiomyosarcomas in immunosuppressed AIDS and transplant patients, natural killer lymphomas, and T-cell lymphomas. The role of EBV infection in the development of these tumors is interesting because these cell types are not thought to represent natural reservoirs of persistent infection. EBV infection has also been implicated in the development of other malignancies, e.g., breast cancer. However, because EBV infection is present in most adults, establishing a potential causal association between EBV infection and a certain type of malignancy requires careful investigation.

IV. MOLECULAR BIOLOGY

Much of our insight into EBV-associated oncogenesis stems from the observation that the EBV infection of primary B lymphocytes results in their immortalization into lymphoblastoid cell lines (LCLs). During B lymphocyte infection, most EBV gene expression is turned off and the genome is maintained in the nucleus by cellular machinery as a circular piece of DNA termed an episome. Because viral particles are not being produced, this state is termed "latent infection." Investigation into the LCL phenomenon has revealed that EBV latent infection is anything but passive. In fact, the observed growth transformation is a direct result of the limited number of EBV that are expressed during latency. These include two latent membrane proteins (LMP1 and LMP2), six nuclear proteins (EBNA-1, 2, 3A, 3B, 3C, and EBNA-LP), and two abundant, noncoding RNAs called EBERs. Reverse genetic analysis has established that LMP2A, EBNA-3B, and the EBERs are not required for LCL transformation, although they may play an important role in EBV biology *in vivo*. The role of the remaining genes in transformation/oncogenesis has been the study of intensive investigation.

A. Latent Infection Membrane Protein 1 (LMP-1)

The membrane protein LMP-1 plays a central role in EBV-mediated growth transformation. It can act as a classical oncogene in standard assays, and its expression in transgenic mice results in B-cell lymphomas. The C-terminal cytoplasmic tail of LMP-1 is able to interact with proteins responsible for transducing signals from the tumor necrosis factor (TNF) family of receptors, such as CD40. LMP-1 has no extracellular domain for ligand binding, but instead appears to be capable of sending a constitutive growth-promoting signal via this pathway. Thus B cells can proliferate in the absence of exogenous growth signals such as the CD40 ligand found on helper T cells.

B. Epstein-Barr Virus Nuclear Antigen 2 (EBNA-2)

EBNA-2 is the lynch pin of the EBV transformation program. Along with EBNA-LP, it is the first EBV protein expressed during latent B-cell infection. It has been shown to be an acidic transactivator of transcription and is critical for the expression of all the EBV latent genes and may upregulate the expression of important growth-promoting cellular genes. Surprisingly, EBNA-2 lacks sequence-specific DNA-binding capacity and is instead targeted to DNA by efficiently binding to the cell DNA-binding protein

RBP-Jκ (also called CBF-1 by some investigators). EBNA-LP appears to act cooperatively with EBNA-2 to promote transcription from specific promoters.

C. EBNA-1

EBNA-1 functions to ensure that the viral episome is maintained by the cellular machinary. It has specific DNA-binding protein activity and recognizes a sequence found within the EBV genome. EBNA-1 binding near the origin of replication is thought to be important for relaxing of the DNA and the recruitment of cellular DNA replication machinery. Binding of EBNA-1 to chromosomes or chromosome-associated proteins appears to form a bridge between the viral episome and host cell chromosome, thus ensuring that episomes are properly segregated into the nuclei of each daughter cell.

D. EBNA-3A, -3B, and -3C

The role of the family of related proteins EBNA-3A, EBNA-3B, and EBNA-3C in transformation is not clear. All three can bind to the same cellular DNA-binding protein, RBP-Jκ, which targets EBNA-2 to DNA. In the context of most promoters, this appears to lead to a reduction in the ability of EBNA-2 to stimulate transcription. However, in at least one context, the LMP-1 promoter EBNA-3C displays synergistic activity with EBNA-2. This had led to speculation that EBNA-3 may serve to modulate or fine-tune the effects of EBNA-2 at specific promoters. It should be mentioned that despite their apparent similarity in structure and function, EBNA-3 proteins do not appear to be extensively redundant. Deletion of EBNA-3A or EBNA-3C from the virus results in a complete loss of transforming ability, whereas removal of EBNA-3B had no apparent effect.

Other EBV genes expressed in latency also appear to be dispensable for B lymphocyte transformation. These included the high abundance, noncoding EBER RNAs and the LMP2 membrane protein. Although these proteins are not required for LCL transformation, they may be important for the biology of EBV *in vivo*. For example, LMP2 has been shown to interact with signaling proteins downstream of the B-cell receptor to prevent B-cell activation. Because this signal frequently induces lytic replication, the purpose of LMP2 may be to preserve EBV in a latent state of infection.

V. PATHOGENESIS

The study of EBV-associated tumors has consistently shown that EBV is present in a latent state of infection. Terminal repeat analysis has been used to demonstrate that the EBV infection of these tumor lines is clonal and therefore was present at or before the time of neoplastic conversion. Moreover, continued expression of particular latent genes is seen in any given tumor type. What is remarkable is that between tumor types there are considerable differences in latent gene expression. The patterns of expression fall into a few broad groups and have been termed type I, type II, and type III latency (Table I). Expression of the full repertoire of latent genes or type III latency typical of the *in vitro* LCL system is observed during lymphoproliferative disease in immunosuppressed patients. Type III latency is also transiently observed in the peripheral blood of normal hosts during IM and has been reported in the tonsilar B cells of healthy carriers.

More limited gene expression is seen in NPC, HD, and peripheral T-cell lymphomas. In these tumors, LMP1 likely continues to play its central role in oncogenesis, although the control of its expression is clearly different as many of the EBNAs are not expressed.

This is likely the result of immune pressure against expression of these antigens.

Ironically, the role of EBV in Burkitt's lymphoma, the tumor in which the virus was discovered, is least well understood. Only the most limited EBV gene expression is seen—EBNA-1 and the EBERs, called type I latency. Neither of these genes has a clearly established role in growth transformation. The consistent finding of c-*myc* translocation suggests that EBV plays a secondary role in growth transformation.

VI. SUMMARY

EBV is a common herpesvirus that normally maintains a benign, but persistent infection in nearly all adults. However, EBV infection is also associated with a wide variety of malignancies. In immunosuppressed hosts, tumorigenesis is probably due to the direct B-cell growth-transforming properties of the virus that can be reproduced by virus-immortalized B cells in tissue culture. This *in vitro* system has provided much information about the cellular pathways usurped by specific EBV genes to alter normal cell growth. In patients with EBV-associated malignancies and no overt immunosuppression, the role of virus infection is more complicated, with differing patterns of viral gene expression, long periods between initial virus infection and tumorigenesis, and possible requirement of other cofactors, such as chromosomal translocations, for malignant transformation.

TABLE I
Latent Gene Expression[a]

Latency pattern	LMP-1	LMP-2	EBNA-1	EBNA-2 EBNA-LP	EBNA-3	EBER	Occurrence
Type I	−	−	+	−	−	+	Burkitts lymphoma
Type II	+	+	+	−	−	+	NPC Hodgkins disease Peripheral T-cell lymphoma
Type III	+	+	+	+	+	+	IM, LCLs AIDS-associated DLCL XLPD, PTLD
	−	−	+	−	−	+	+ Healthy carrier

[a]LMP, latent membrane protein; EBNA, EBV nuclear antigen; EBER, EBV-encoded RNA; NPC, nasopharyngeal carcinoma; IM, infectious mononucleosis; LCL, lymphoblastoid cell line; DLCL, diffuse large cell lymphoma; XLPD, X-linked lymphoproliferative disease; PTLD, posttransplant lymphoproliferative disease.

See Also the Following Articles

GASTRIC CANCER • HEPATITIS B VIRUSES • HEPATITIS C VIRUS • HIV • HUMAN T-CELL LEUKEMIA/LYMPHOTROPIC VIRUS • LYMPHOMA, HODGKIN'S DISEASE • PAPILLOMA-VIRUSES • RETROVIRUSES

Bibliography

Coffey, A. J., Brooksbank, R. A., Brandau, O., Oohashi, T., Howell, G. R., Bye, J. M., Cahn, A. P., Durham, J., Heath, P., Wray, P., Pavitt, R., Wilkinson, J., Leversha, M., Huckle, E., Shaw-Smith, C. J., Dunham, A., Rhodes, S., Schuster, V., Porta, G., Yin, L., Serafini, P., Sylla, B., Zollo, M., Franco, B., Bentley, D. R., *et al.* (1998). Host response to EBV infection in X-linked lymphoproliferative disease results from mutations in an SH2-domain encoding gene. *Nature Genet.* **20,** 129–135.

Epstein, A. (1999). On the discovery of Epstein-Barr Virus: A memoir. *Epstein-Barr Virus Report* **7,** 58–63.

Grossman, S. R., Johannsen, E., Tong, X., Yalamanchili, R., and Kieff, E. (1994). The Epstein-Barr virus nuclear antigen 2 transactivator is directed to response elements by the J kappa recombination signal binding protein. *Proc. Natl. Acad. Sci. USA* **91,** 7568–7572.

Henkel, T., Ling, P. D., Hayward, S. D., and Peterson, M. G. (1994). Mediation of Epstein-Barr virus EBNA2 transactivation by recombination signal-binding protein J kappa. *Science* **265,** 92–95.

Izumi, K. M., and Kieff, E. D. (1997). The Epstein-Barr virus oncogene product latent membrane protein 1 engages the tumor necrosis factor receptor-associated death domain protein to mediate B lymphocyte growth transformation and activate NF-kappaB. *Proc. Natl. Acad. Sci. USA* **94,** 12592–12597.

Kieff, E., and Richinson, A. B. (2001). Epstein-Barr virus and its replication. *In* "Fields Virology" (D. M. Knipe, P. M. Howley, D. E. Griffin, R. A. Lamb, M. A. Martin, B. Roizman, and S. E. Strauss, eds.), pp. 2511-2574. Lippincott, Williams, & Wilkins, Philadelphia.

Kulwichit, W., Edwards, R. H., Davenport, E. M., Baskar, J. F.,

Godfrey, V., and Raab-Traub, N. (1998). Expression of the Epstein-Barr virus latent membrane protein 1 induces B cell lymphoma in transgenic mice. *Proc. Natl. Acad. Sci. USA* **95,** 11963–11968.

Mosialos, G., Birkenbach, M., Yalamanchili, R., VanArsdale, T., Ware, C., and Kieff, E. (1995). The Epstein-Barr virus transforming protein LMP1 engages signaling proteins for the tumor necrosis factor receptor family. *Cell* **80,** 389–399.

Nichols, K. E., Harkin, D. P., Levitz, S., Krainer, M., Kolquist, K. A., Genovese, C., Bernard, A., Ferguson, M., Zuo, L., Snyder, E., Buckler, A. J., Wise, C., Ashley, J., Lovett, M., Valentine, M. B., Look, A. T., Gerald, W., Housman, D. E., and Haber, D. A. (1998). Inactivating mutations in an SH2 domain-encoding gene in X-linked lymphoproliferative syndrome. *Proc. Natl. Acad. Sci. USA* **95,** 13765–13770.

Papadopoulos, E. B., Ladanyi, M., Emanuel, D., Mackinnon, S., Boulad, F., Carabasi, M. H., Castro-Malaspina, H., Childs, B. H., Gillio, A. P., Small, T. N., *et al.* (1994). Infusions of donor leukocytes to treat Epstein-Barr virus-associated lymphoproliferative disorders after allogeneic bone marrow transplantation. *N. Engl. J. Med.* **330,** 1185–1191.

Purtilo, D. T., DeFlorio, D., Hutt, L. M., Bhawan, J., Yang, J. P., Otto, R., and Edwards, W. (1977). Variable phenotypic expression of an X-linked recessive lymphoproliferative syndrome. *N. Engl. J. Med.* **297,** 1077–1080.

Rooney, C. M., Smith, C. A., Ng, C. Y. Loftin, S., Li, C., Krance, R. A., Brenner, M. K., and Heslop, H. E. (1995). Use of gene-modified virus-specific T lymphocytes to control Epstein-Barr-virus-related lymphoproliferation. *Lancet* **345,** 9–13.

Sayos, J., Wu, C., Morra, M., Wang, N., Zhang, X., Allen, D., van Schaik, S., Notarangelo, L., Geha, R., Roncarolo, M. G., Oettgen, H., De Vries, J. E., Aversa, G., and Terhorst, C. (1998). The X-linked lymphoproliferative-disease gene product SAP regulates signals induced through the co-receptor SLAM. *Nature* **395,** 462–469.

Yates, J., Warren, N., Reisman, D., and Sugden, B. (1984). A cis-acting element from the Epstein-Barr viral genome that permits stable replication of recombinant plasmids in latently infected cells. *Proc. Natl. Acad. Sci. USA* **81,** 3806–3810.

Esophageal Cancer: Risk Factors and Somatic Genetics

Michael T. Barrett

Fred Hutchinson Cancer Research Center
Seattle, Washington

GLOSSARY

p16^{cdKn2a} Cyclin-dependent kinase inhibitor that regulates the transition of cells through the G_1 phase of the cell cycle by inhibiting the association of cyclin D and CDK4. This tumor suppressor gene is located on 9p21, which is disrupted in multiple types of human cancers.

p53 Key regulatory gene that controls pathways regulating several cellular functions, including cell cycle progression, apoptosis, and response to DNA damage. It is the most frequently mutated tumor suppressor gene in human cancer located on 17p13.1.

CpG island Small regions of genomic DNA containing high G+C content typically associated with promoter regions of genes. Methylation of these regions is associated with the inactivation of gene expression.

aneuploidy DNA content less than or greater than normal 2N content in human diploid cells.

loss of heterozygosity Loss of genetic information at a given chromosomal locus typically detected by a polymorphic marker(s).

The pattern and the prevalence of esophageal cancer in western countries, including the United States, have undergone dramatic changes since the 1970s. Once considered a relatively rare diagnosis, esophageal adenocarcinomas (EA) now comprise more than three of every five new esophageal cancers. The highest rate occurs among white males, whose incidence increased more than 350% in the United States between 1974 and 1994. Similar increases have been observed for white females (300%), although their incidence of EA remains substantially lower. These trends have been observed in numerous other westernized countries, including many in western Europe, Australia, and New Zealand. Less dramatic increases in adenocarcinomas of the gastric cardia, which includes tumors arising in the gastroesophageal junction, have also been observed over this same time period. In contrast, the rate of esophageal squamous cell carcinoma (SCC) has been stable or has declined during the same period.

I. INTRODUCTION

Most EAs arise in a columnar metaplastic epithelium termed Barrett's esophagus (BE) that develops in approximately 10% of persons who have chronic gastroesophageal reflux disease (GERD). Furthermore, the relative risk of developing EA increases with the frequency, severity, and duration of reflux symptoms and is specific for esophageal adenocaricnomas compared to those of gastric cardia or to esophageal SCC. The strong association between gastroesophageal reflux and risk of EA has long been noted clinically, but has only recently been quantified. Persons with frequent and long-standing symptoms of reflux, notably heartburn and regurgitation, experience an approximately fivefold increase in EA risk, with a monotonically increasing trend with frequency and duration of reflux symptoms. Reflux is thought to increase the risk of EA by promoting cellular proliferation and by exposing the esophageal epithelium to potentially genotoxic gastric and intestinal contents.

Each year, approximately 1% of persons with BE progress to EA, a rate estimated at 30–40 times higher than the general population. Unfortunately, it remains one of the least survivable cancers, with a median survival of 9 months and a 5-year overall survival of 7.3%. It is only the relatively few patients diagnosed at the *in situ* stage who have a favorable prognosis (approximately 70% 5-year survival). Thus there is ample opportunity for research directed toward prevention and earlier diagnosis to have an important impact on public health.

Although declining in the United States and western Europe, the rates of esophageal SSC mortality in regions of Iran and Northern China are among the highest for any cancer in the world. In addition, isolated pockets of elevated esophageal SCC mortality rates have been reported in parts of France, South Africa, and among African American populations in coastal areas of South Carolina. However, unlike EAs

there are no known premalignant conditions that predispose to esophageal SSCs. Consequently, patients typically present with advanced lesions, making it more difficult to study the events of progression and design effective interventions.

II. RISK FACTORS

A. Tobacco

Studies have elucidated a number of risk factors for esophageal cancers, including the potential role of tobacco use (Table I). It is strongly associated with a risk of both esophageal SCCs and EAs. However, the increase in risk for current smokers (80 or more pack years) compared to nonsmokers is substantially higher in esophageal SCCs than in EAs. For example, studies have consistently demonstrated that current smokers have a $\geq$15-fold risk for ESC but a modest approximately 2-fold increase in risk of EA. Another distinguishing feature of EA is that the risk of cancer remains elevated up to 30 years following smoking cessation. This is in contrast to esophageal SCC and respiratory cancers, in which cessation has a measurable impact within 5 years. This suggests that the major effect of cigarettes must be at a relatively early

TABLE I
Relative Risk of Esophageal Cancer[a]

	Squamous	Adenocarcinoma
Smokers		
Current	5.1 (2.8–9.2)[b]	2.2 (1.4–2.3)
Former	2.8 (1.5–4.9)	2.0 (1.4–2.9)
Alcohol (drinks/week)		
<5	0.8 (0.4–1.6)	0.7 (0.4–1.0)
5–11	1.8 (0.9–3.5)	0.6 (0.4–0.9)
12–30	2.9 (1.5–5.4)	0.7 (0.4–1.1)
>30	7.4 (4.0–13.7)	0.9 (0.5–1.4)
BMI[c]-(quartile)		
I	1.0	1.0
II	0.5 (0.3–0.9)	1.3 (0.8–2.2)
III	0.8 (0.5–1.3)	2.0 (1.3–3.3)
IV	0.6 (0.3–1.0)	2.9 (1.8–4.7)

[a]Data from Blot and McLaughlin (1999).
[b]95% confidence interval.
[c]Body mass index.

stage of neoplastic progression in EA, while affecting a later stage in esophageal SSCs.

B. Alcohol

Alcohol consumption is strongly associated with risk for esophageal SCC. This is strongest for hard liquor consumption. Furthermore, drinking of specific alcoholic beverages has been implicated in several clusters of elevated esophageal cancers in different regions of the world. These include various spirits, including fruit brandies, maize beer, sugar-distilled beverages, and homemade whiskeys. Therefore, other ingredients in these spirits may also be contributing to the overall risk. In addition, the smoking-associated risk of developing ESC was more than doubled among drinkers of any type of alcohol compared to nondrinkers. In contrast, there is at best a weak association between alcohol consumption and EA except perhaps among predominantly hard liquor drinkers and no substantial increase in risk associated with both smoking and alcohol consumption. In fact, there is some suggestion for decreased risk among wine drinkers.

C. Body Mass Index (BMI)

One of the strongest and most consistent risk factor identified for EA is increased BMI. Furthermore, the increase in incidence of esophageal adenocarcinoma has paralleled recent increases in obesity in the United States. In contrast, the risk of squamous cell carcinoma appears to be lower in the higher BMI group. It is not yet clear how being overweight increases EA risk. One hypothesis is that it exacerbates gastroesophageal reflux through increased intraabdominal pressure. Because males who are overweight tend to deposit fat more abdominally than females (so-called male pattern obesity), which results in worse reflux, it is possible that this explains a portion of the gender difference in incidence.

D. Diet

Several studies suggest that a diet high in fat and low in fruits and vegetables increases the risk of esophageal cancer. In a large case-control study of diet and esophageal cancers that included 282 EAs and 206 esophageal SCCs, a higher total fat intake was associated with an approximate doubling of risk of EA with no significant effect on the risk of esophageal SCC (comparing the 75th to the 25th percentile). However, an increased intake of saturated fats was associated with a similar doubling of risk for both types of esophageal cancers. In contrast, a higher intake of fiber and of nutrients found primarily in plant-based foods was associated with a decreased risk of both EA and esophageal SCC. Although an increased consumption of polyunsaturated fats was associated with a deceased risk of both cancers, the effect was significant only for esophageal SCC.

E. Bile

A growing body of evidence in both humans and animals implicates bile reflux in the pathogenesis and progression of Barrett's esophagus. Several studies have suggested that persons whose refluxate contains bile may be at increased risk of BE and subsequent development of cancer. For example, mean esophageal bile exposure has been shown to increase progressively from GERD without mucosal injury ($N = 19$ patients) to erosive esophagitis ($N = 45$) to Barrett's esophagus ($N = 33$) with the highest levels found in early EA ($N = 14$) ($p < 0.01$). In addition, studies using HPLC, a sensitive method for detecting bile acids in gastric fluid that permits identification and quantitation of individual bile acid species, have shown that fasting gastric bile acid concentrations are elevated in patients with BE compared to normal controls, in patients with GERD without mucosal injury, and in patients with erosive esophagitis.

Neoplastic progression occurs in a whole person who has inherited a unique genome and has accumulated a lifetime history of environmental exposures, behaviors, and medical conditions. The identification of environmental exposures and host factors that affect the risk of progression and identifying the stage(s) of progression at which they act will illuminate their mechanism(s) of action and also identify specific interventions that could be tailored to individual patients. To address these questions, it is important to identify objective markers of progression by studying how cancers evolve from early neoplastic lesions.

III. SOMATIC GENETICS OF ESOPHAGEAL CANCER

In 1976, Nowell hypothesized that neoplastic progression develops as a consequence of an acquired genetic instability and the subsequent evolution of clonal populations with accumulated genetic errors. Some clones gain selective proliferative advantages and eventually a subclone evolves that has the capacity for invasion, becoming an early cancer. There is now a substantial body of evidence that most human cancers arise by a process of clonal evolution similar to that postulated by Nowell. For example, cancers and some premalignant lesions typically contain multiple genetic abnormalities not present in the normal tissues from which the cancers arose. Furthermore, studies in different tumors have shown that histologic lesions at different stages of progression have genetic abnormalities consistent with their accumulation over time.

Esophageal cancers, like most solid tissue cancers, contain highly variable populations of neoplastic cells with multiple somatically acquired genetic abnormalities, consistent with Nowell's model. These include DNA content abnormalities, aberrant chromosomes, multiple loss of heterozygosity (LOH) events, and regions of amplification. Studies have also shown that both EAs and esophageal SCCs contain mutations in p53 and p16 tumor suppressor genes, CpG hypermethylation of p16, cell cycle, and flow abnormalities (increased 4N/aneuploidy). Allelotype and comparative genomic hybridization (CGH) studies have identified a number of high-frequency regions of loss and gain in these cancers. For example, multiple regions of highly prevalent LOH (>50%), including 2p, 3p, 5q, 9p, 9q, 13q, 17p, and 18q, have been found in esophageal SCCs, whereas gains of chromosome regions have been found on chromosomes 19, 20q, 22, and 16p in over 60% of cases studied. Furthermore, aneuploid tumors contain higher levels of genetic lesions, including LOH and gene amplification events, when compared to diploid tumors. In addition, patients with aneuploid tumors have a poorer prognosis when compared to those in the diploid group. Similar results, including LOH at 5q, 9p, 13q, 17p, and 18q, and amplifications on 19 and 22 have been reported in EAs. However, there are a number of distinctions in the location of somatic lesions present in each tumor type, suggesting that there are tissue-specific differences in the tumor suppressor and oncogenic pathways that mediate the pathogenesis of esophageal cancers.

The study of advanced neoplasms has been useful in identifying prevalent abnormalities that have accumulated during the progression to cancer. However, the ability of these studies to determine the order in which somatic lesions develop in clonal cell populations during neoplastic progression is limited. Previous *in vivo* models of human neoplastic progression have often relied on the prevalence of genetic lesions at different histologically defined stages of progression. For example, multiple genetic abnormalities, including allelic loss and mutation at the APC locus, activation of k-*ras*, allelic loss at 18q, and inactivation of p53, can be detected in premalignant colonic tissues. However, colonic adenomas are removed by colonoscopic polypectomy when they are detected and cannot be followed during subsequent progression. Consequently, the order in which genetic lesions accumulate during clonal progression to cancer cannot be determined by serial evaluation of the same patient. Furthermore, most human premalignant lesions do not progress to cancer even when highly prevalent somatic lesions are present. For example, only approximately 2.5 adenomatous polyps per 1000 per year progress to colon cancer.

IV. BARRETT'S ESOPHAGUS AS A MODEL FOR HUMAN NEOPLASIA

A. Background

Patients with Barrett's esophagus typically have symptoms of gastroesophageal reflux, such as heartburn or indigestion, and they frequently seek medical attention before they develop cancer. The Barrett's epithelium can be safely visualized and biopsied during upper gastrointestinal endoscopy. At the present time, total removal of Barrett's epithelium requires esophagectomy, a procedure with substantial morbidity and mortality. However, most patients with Barrett's esophagus do not develop cancer. Furthermore, a systematic protocol of endoscopic biopsies that evaluates four-quadrant biopsies from the Barrett's epithelium at a minimum of every 1–2 cm, depending on the presence or absence of high-grade dysplasia, can detect early curable cancers arising in Barrett's esophagus. Therefore, the standard of care for many patients includes endoscopic biopsy surveillance for the early detection of cancer. Thus, intermediate events in neoplastic progression can be evaluated by serial biopsies of the same patient over time and related to progression and to environmental and dietary risk factors. In addition to cancer, esophagectomy specimens frequently contain the surrounding premalignant epithelium in which the cancer arose, permitting the study of multiple stages of neoplastic progression in a single surgical specimen. Thus, BE offers a unique opportunity to investigate interactions among somatic genetic events in human neoplasia and environmental exposures while relating them to progression to validated biomarkers and cancer.

B. Aneuploidy and/or Increased 4N

Biopsies from most patients with BE are diploid, but some patients develop aneuploid and increased 4N (G_2/tetraploid) cell populations. Aneuploid and increased 4N (G_2/tetraploid) cell populations arise in the premalignant epithelium of the esophagus. The prevalence of aneuploid cell populations increases with increasing histological risk of malignancy in BE, and these cells are present in over 95% of esophageal adenocarcinomas. Some clones can spread to involve large regions of esophageal mucosa, persisting for years before the development of a carcinoma. Multiple aneuploid cell populations can evolve in the premalignant epithelium, and typically only one of these aneuploid cell populations acquires the capacity for invasion. This process of clonal evolution can subsequently give rise to multiple ploidies in the cancer itself.

Flow cytometry has also been shown in small studies to predict progression to intermediate end points and cancer, suggesting that it may be an objective aid in identifying patients at increased risk. For example, a small study of 30 dysplasia-free patients followed for 13 years reported that no patient whose biopsies remained diploid progressed to dysplasia or cancer, whereas 6 of 13 patients who had or developed aneuploidy progressed to dysplasia or EA during follow-up ($p < 0.01$). Another study prospectively evaluated 62 patients for a mean of 34 months. Of these 62, 13 had either aneuploidy or increased 4N fractions as their initial flow cytometric abnormality. Nine of these 13 progressed to develop high-grade dysplasia or cancer that was not present at the initial endoscopy. None of 49 patients without aneuploidy or increased 4N fractions progressed to high-grade dysplasia or cancer ($p < 0.0001$). The temporal course of progression from aneuploidy or increased 4N fractions to cancer was variable, ranging from 18 to 84 months. Patients whose biopsies were diploid and had normal 4N fractions did not progress to high-grade dysplasia and cancer during the time course of this study, but 7 of the 49 patients subsequently progressed to develop aneuploid cell populations or increased 4N fractions during prospective follow-up. Furthermore, in a study of 90 patients followed prospectively for a mean of 51.4 months, 11 of 15 patients who had or developed increased 4N during prospective surveillance progressed to aneuploidy compared with 8 of 75 whose 4N fractions remained normal ($p < 0.0001$).

C. p53

p53 mutations and 17p LOH are the most common genetic lesions in EAs, occurring in approximately 90% of cases. Both p53 alleles are typically inactivated (mutation and 17p LOH) in advanced histologic lesions (HGD or cancer). p53 causes cells exposed to genotoxic stress to arrest in the G_1 interval of the cell cycle, leading to terminal cell cycle arrest or apoptosis, both of which prevent transmission of chromosome damage to daughter cells. Loss of p53 function predisposes to genomic instability and the evolution of additional somatic genetic abnormalities. Consistent with its known cell cycle checkpoint function, p53 mutations and 17p LOH develop in diploid cells before increased 4N, aneuploidy, and cancer in BE.

Several studies have reported p53 protein overexpression, a surrogate for p53 mutation, in early histologic grades (negative, indefinite, low-grade dysplasia).

Typically the prevalence of overexpression increases with the histological stage of progression. However, as shown in two reports, up to one-third of p53 mutations in BE are nonsense or frameshifts that would not be detected by immunohistochemistry. Furthermore, it has been shown in multiple studies that p53 overexpression can occur via nonmutagenic mechanisms.

D. p16 (CDKN2a/INK4a)

Approximately 75% of EAs have 9p LOH that include the *INK4a* locus on 9p21. In contrast to p53, the remaining p16 allele is typically inactivated by methylation of its 5' CpG island (>60% cases with 9p21 LOH) or mutation (20–25% cases with 9p21 LOH). Homozygous deletions, which have been reported in other human cancers, have not been detected in EAs. Although two similar genes, p15 and p14^{ARF}, are located near p16^{INK4a} locus on chromosome 9p21, available evidence indicates that p16 is the target of 9p LOH in BE and EA. 9p LOH develops as an early lesion in approximately 60% of Barrett's patients, and mutations can be detected in premalignant diploid cells several years before cancer.

p16 regulates progression through the G_1 interval of the cell cycle by binding and inhibiting cyclin-dependent kinases 4 and 6 and regulating the normal function of the retinoblastoma protein. Protein levels of p16 are increased in senescent cells and are low or undetectable in immortalized cells.

A number of studies in model systems have shown that disruption of the p16/Rb pathway, in combination with loss of normal p53 function, is permissive for the development of immortalized cells and predisposes to the development of cancer. Retrospective studies have shown that diploid cells with lesions in both p53 and p16 are capable of clonal expansion, spreading to large regions of esophageal mucosa. The subsequent evolution of neoplastic progeny from these diploid progenitors involves bifurcating pathways and nonrandom LOH at 5q, 13q, and 18q that occur in no obligate order relative to each other, aneuploidy or cancer (Fig. 1). Therefore, abrogation of these two pathways by a combination of LOH, mutation, and/or methylation events in the early stages of BE is consistent with their proposed role in tumorigenesis. Mapping studies of surgical specimens have shown that esophageal SSCs contain multiple clones consistent with an acquired instability and ongoing evolutionary process.

Advances have shown that reactivation of telomerase, an enzyme that maintains telomere length, cooperates with lesions in the p16/Rb pathway and the p53-dependent cell cycle checkpoint(s) to generate the transformed phenotype. These three somatic events are found in the majority of human cancers, including esophageal cancers. Although the absence of a premalignant *in vivo* model has made it difficult to determine the relationships of the multiple abnormalities present in these tissues to each other and cancer, the high prevalence of similar abnormalities suggests that a similar mechanism may mediate the development of cancer in patients with esophageal SSC.

V. FUTURE DIRECTIONS

The identification of early events, inactivation of p16 and p53, increased cell cycle fractions, and the appearance of aneuploid and increased 4N (G_2/tetraploid) cell populations in Barrett's esophagus have contributed to the understanding of neoplastic progression in esophageal adenocarcinoma, which serves as a model system for other human malignancies, including esophageal SCC. However, there is little information concerning their interactions with each other and with environmental risk and protective factors during human neoplastic progression *in vivo*. Although LOH is a common lesion detected in neoplasias arising in the esophagus and other tissues, it has been difficult to use LOH as a biomarker in large-scaled clinical or epidemiological studies. However, studies have shown that a combination of flow cytometric purification, whole genome amplification, and quantitative fluorescent genotyping can be applied to population-based studies.

Studies have shown a striking heterogeneity in the prevalence and distribution of clones with 9p LOH, 17p LOH, and p53 mutations in patients with HGD in the absence of cancer. For example, 29 of 58 (50%) patients with a maximum diagnosis of HGD had at least one p53 mutant clone in their Barrett's segment.

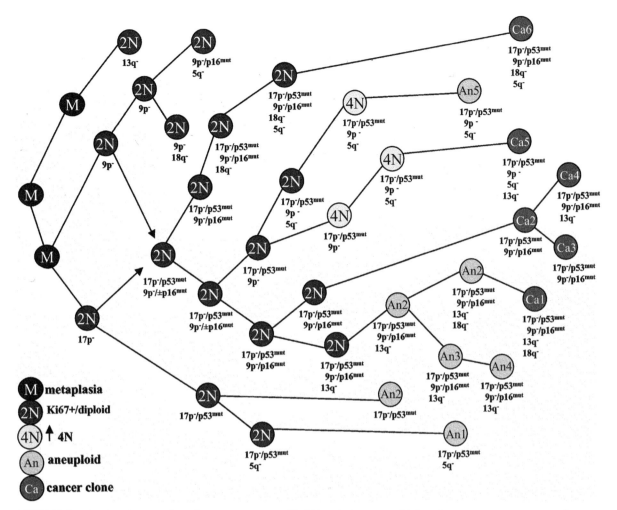

FIGURE 1 Clonal evolution and neoplastic progression in BE. Although there are multiple pathways to cancer, some general patterns appear to be consistent among many patients. LOH events arise in proliferating (Ki67-positive) diploid populations (2N) within Barrett's metaplasia (M). 2N clones with somatic genetic abnormalities involving p53 (17p-/p53^{mut}) and p16 (9p-/p16^{mut}; 9p-) frequently give rise to populations with elevated 4N fractions (4N) that can evolve aneuploid cell populations (An). Methylation of the p16 CpG island was also detected in diploid cells prior to the development of aneuploidy. In some cases the 4N abnormality is not detected, possibly from sampling limitations or failure of a genetically unstable intermediate to persist. In some cases, changes in ploidy may result in a clone with a 2N or near 2N DNA content, yet has multiple genetic abnormalities. 5q, 13q, and 18q LOH have no obligate order relative to aneuploidy, cancer, or each other. During evolution, neoplastic cell lineages may bifurcate, giving rise to mosaics with the same p53 and p16 abnormalities but different ploidies and additional LOHs. Some clones in these mosaics develop into cancer (Ca), whereas others are either delayed in their progression or represent dead ends. Subsequently, multiple malignant clones (Ca) with different ploidies and additional LOHs evolve as the cancer progresses. Reprinted with permission from Barrett *et al.* (1999). Evolution of neoplastic cell lineages in Barrett's oesophagus. *Nat. Genet.* **22**, 106–109.

These p53 mutant clones underwent variable expansion and were more prevalent in patients with abnormal ploidies. Furthermore, the presence of 9p LOH is associated with longer Barrett's segment lengths and the ability to expand in an area within the esophageal mucosa (clonal expansion), consistent with a role for p16 in regulation of the cellular life span and proliferation. Furthermore, the fraction of patients with both 9p LOH and 17p LOH is comparable to the number of patients with HGD who progress to cancer.

Validation of these early biomarkers as predictors of progression, as well as understanding the etiologic mechanisms by which risk and protective factors impact disease progression, could guide surveillance intervals as well as serving as intermediate end points in intervention trials.

See Also the Following Articles

CANCER RISK REDUCTION (DIET/SMOKING CESSATION/ LIFESTYLE CHANGES) • ESOPHAGEAL CANCER: TREATMENT • HEAD AND NECK CANCER • LUNG CANCER: MOLECULAR AND CELLULAR ABNORMALITIES • TOBACCO CARCINOGENESIS • TP53 TUMOR SUPPRESSOR GENE: STRUCTURE AND FUNCTION

Bibliography

Barrett, M. T., et al. (1999). Evolution of neoplastic cell lineages in Barrett oesophagus. Nature Genet. 22(1), 106–109.

Blot, W. J., and McLaughlin, J. K. (1999). The changing epidemiology of esophageal cancer. Semin. Oncol. 26(5 Suppl 15), 2–8.

Brown, L. M., et al. (1995). Adenocarcinoma of the esophagus: Role of obesity and diet. J. Natl. Cancer Inst. 87(2), 104–109.

Devesa, S. S., Blot, W. J., and Fraumeni, J. F. Jr. (1998). Changing patterns in the incidence of esophageal and gastric carcinoma in the United States. Cancer 83(10), 2049–2053.

Eads, C. A., et al. (2000). Fields of aberrant CpG island hypermethylation in Barrett's esophagus and associated adenocarcinoma. Cancer Res. 60(18), 5021–5026.

Galipeau, P. C., et al. (1999). Clonal expansion and loss of heterozygosity at chromosomes 9p and 17p in premalignant esophageal (Barrett's) tissue. J. Natl. Cancer Inst. 91(24), 2087–2095.

Gleeson, C. M., et al. (1995). Base transitions at CpG dinucleotides in the p53 gene are common in esophageal adenocarcinoma. Cancer Res. 55(15), 3406–3411.

Mayne, S. T., et al. (2001). Nutrient intake and risk of adenocarcinomas of the esophagus and gastric cardia. Cancer Epidemiol. Biomark. Prev. 10, 1055–1061.

Nowell, P. C. (1976). The clonal evolution of tumor cell populations. Science 194(4260), 23–28.

Pack, S. D., et al. (1999). Molecular cytogenetic fingerprinting of esophageal squamous cell carcinoma by comparative genomic hybridization reveals a consistent pattern of chromosomal alterations. Genes Chromosomes Cancer 25(2), 160–168.

Prevo, L. J., et al. (1999). p53-mutant clones and field effects in Barrett's esophagus. Cancer Res. 59(19), 4784–4787.

Riegman, P. H., et al. (2001). Genomic alterations in malignant transformation of Barrett's esophagus. Cancer Res. 61(7), 3164–3170.

Roth, M. J., et al. (2001). Genetic progression and heterogeneity associated with the development of esophageal squamous cell carcinoma. Cancer Res. 61(10), 4098–4104.

van Lieshout, E. M., Jansen, J. B., and Peters, W. H. (1998). Biomarkers in Barrett's esophagus. Int. J. Oncol. 13(4), 855–864.

Vaughan, T. L., et al. (1995). Obesity, alcohol, and tobacco as risk factors for cancers of the esophagus and gastric cardia: Adenocarcinoma versus squamous cell carcinoma. Cancer Epidemiol. Biomark. Prev. 4(2), 85–92.

Watanabe, M., et al. (1999). Flow cytometric DNA analysis is useful in detecting multiple genetic alterations in squamous cell carcinoma of the esophagus. Cancer 85(11), 2322–2328.

Esophageal Cancer: Treatment

David H. Ilson
David Kelsen

Memorial Sloan-Kettering Cancer Center and
Cornell University Medical College

GLOSSARY

dysphagia An inability to swallow; pain or difficulty in swallowing food.

esophagectomy The surgical removal of the esophagus (all or in part).

gastroesophageal reflux disease (GERD) A condition marked by an abnormal return flow of the contents of the stomach to the esophagus, causing the presence of acidic gastric fluid in the esophagus, which produces a burning sensation. Association with lack of function of the esophageal sphincter.

Helicobacter pylori A common bacterium residing in the human stomach, affecting a large portion of the world's population and now associated with various gastric disturbances that were previously attributed to other factors, e.g., ulcer disease, certain cancers.

$\mathbf{E}$ sophageal cancer, an uncommon but highly virulent malignancy in the United States, will be diagnosed in 12,300 patients in 2000. More than 90% of patients diagnosed will die of their disease, and esophageal cancer represents the seventh leading cause of cancer death in American men. Although esophageal cancer remains relatively uncommon in the United States, it is a leading worldwide cause of cancer, with a particularly high incidence observed in northern China, the Caspian Littoral, and the Transkei province of South Africa.

I. INTRODUCTION

Epidemiologic factors responsible for geographic variability in the incidence of esophageal cancer, including potential dietary and environmental carcinogens and potential nutritional deficiencies, are under active investigation. In Western countries, an association with abuse of tobacco and alcohol and the development of squamous carcinoma of the esophagus is generally accepted. While the incidence of squamous cell carcinoma of the esophagus has remained relatively constant in the United States, adenocarcinoma of the esophagus is increasing at an epidemic proportion in the United States and Western countries. Adenocarcinoma of the esophagus now exceeds squamous carcinoma in incidence in white male patients, and esophageal adenocarcinoma has had the most rapid rate of increase of any solid tumor malignancy in the past 20 years. One prospective study identified chronic symptoms of esophageal reflux as substantially increasing the risk of esophageal adenocarcinoma and cancer of the gastroesophageal junction, independent of other factors. *Helicobacter pylori*, implicated in gastric ulcer disease and associated with an increased risk in gastric cancer, has not been implicated in the genesis of esophageal adenocarcinoma. Because infection with *H. pylori* may lead to a reduction in gastric acidity in association with atrophic gastritis, there has been speculation that a decline in the prevalence of infection with *Helicobacter* may predispose to an increase in gastroesophageal reflux disease and, potentially, an increase in the incidence of esophageal adenocarcinoma, gastroesophageal junction, and proximal stomach cancer. Epidemiologic studies have also implicated tobacco use and obesity as potential risk factors for the development of esophageal adenocarcinoma. These two lifestyle traits in the United States are characteristic of the latter part of the 20th century and may also predispose patients to gastroesophageal reflux disease.

The prognosis for esophageal cancer patients with locally advanced disease treated with the standard approaches of surgery or radiation therapy is poor. The largest retrospective series of patients treated with either surgery alone or radiotherapy alone reported equally poor 2-year survivals of 6–8% and 5-year survivals of 4–6%. The operative mortality for surgically treated patients in this review was 29%. The significant operative mortality has fueled an ongoing debate regarding the relative efficacy of surgery versus radiation therapy. More recent surgical series from single institutions, however, have reported operative mortalities of 5–15%, including a recent large surgical review with 10% of patients achieving a 5-year survival. Ultimately, the majority of patients treated with either surgery or radiation therapy alone are destined to die of their disease.

The failure of standard surgery or radiation therapy in patients with disease clinically limited to the local/regional area prior to treatment is due both to a high incidence of local regional failure and to early systemic dissemination of disease. Adenocarcinoma of the distal esophagus or gastroesophageal junction appears to have a natural history of disease similar to squamous esophageal carcinoma, with equally poor survival after surgical therapy due to a combination of local and systemic disease recurrence. The clear need to address the early systemic spread of esophageal carcinoma with systemic treatment has led to the development of combined modality therapy with the incorporation of chemotherapy in the surgery and radiation-based management of locally advanced esophageal cancer.

II. CHEMOTHERAPY

Approximately 50% of patients diagnosed with esophageal cancer present with overt metastatic disease, and chemotherapy is the mainstay of palliation in this setting. With the high likelihood of patients with initial local/regional disease developing metastatic disease, systemic chemotherapy will ultimately be used in the majority of patients. The antitumor activity for single agent chemotherapy in esophageal carcinoma is summarized in Table I. Modest antitumor activity for a broad range of chemotherapy drugs is seen in esophageal cancer. The duration of response to single agent chemotherapy is generally brief and on the order of 4–6 months. Trials have included patients with adenocarcinoma, reflecting the increasing incidence of this disease. Active single chemotherapeutic agents in esophageal cancer, including bleomycin, fluorouracil, mitomycin, cisplatin, and etoposide, have response rates ranging from 15 to 25%. Newer chemotherapeutic agents, including paclitaxel, docetaxel, vinorelbine, and irinotecan, also appear to have single agent activity, with response rates in phase II trials ranging from 20 to 35%.

With modest activity demonstrated for single agent chemotherapy, combination chemotherapy has also been extensively studied (see Table II). Cisplatin-based combination chemotherapy has yielded antitumor activity in metastatic squamous carcinoma

TABLE I
Activity of Single Agent Chemotherapy

	Histology[a]	No. patients	No. responses	% response	95% confidence intervals
Antibiotics					
Bleomycin	S	80	12	15	7–23
Mitomycin	S	58	15	26	15–37
Doxorubicin	S	38	7	18	5–31
Antimetabolites					
5-FU	S	26	4	15	1–29
	A + S	13	11	85	60–100
Methotrexate	S	65	23	35	24–47
Plant alkaloids					
Vindesine	S	86	19	22	14–32
Navelabine	S	30	6	20	4–36
Heavy metals					
Cisplatin	S	152	42	28	20–35
	A	12	1	8	0–26
Carboplatin	S	59	3	5	0–11
	A	11	1	9	0–26
Taxanes					
Paclitaxel	S	18	5	28	8–48
	A	32	11	34	15–51
Docetaxel	A	8	2	25	0–55
Topoisomerase inhibitors					
Etoposide	S	26	5	19	4–34
Irinotecan	A	34	5	15	9–21

[a]S, squamous carcinoma; A, adenocarcinoma.

of the esophagus in the range of 25–35%. The response proportion observed in local/regional disease has been consistently higher, on the order of 45–75%. Unfortunately, the higher response rates achieved with cisplatin combinations have not translated into significantly improved response durations or improved survival. In this primarily palliative setting, the greater response rate of combination chemotherapy must be balanced with a frequently higher toxicity and an increasingly complex and time-consuming schedule.

The combination of cisplatin and fluorouracil (5-FU) given by continuous infusion for 4–5 days has been studied extensively. Toxicity observed for the combination of cisplatin and 5-FU, mainly mucositis and myelosuppression, has been substantial but tolerable. In the trials of patients with metastatic or unresectable disease, the response to cisplatin and 5-FU has ranged from 35–40%. Efforts have been made to improve upon this regimen by adding other agents. The addition of doxorubicin, mitomycin, doxorubicin

and etoposide, or etoposide with and without leucovorin has shown no clear advantage. Newer agents have also been combined with cisplatin with the hope of increasing antitumor response rates and improving treatment tolerance. Paclitaxel, which had shown significant promise as a single agent, was added to the cisplatin/5-FU regimen and a response rate of 48% was observed. Similar response rates were seen in patients with adenocarcinoma and patients with squamous cell carcinoma. The median duration of response was 5.7 months and the median survival was 10.8 months. Toxicity was severe, with 48% of patients requiring dose attenuation and half the patients were hospitalized for toxicity. Alternative schedules of cisplatin, 5-FU, and paclitaxel, or cisplatin and paclitaxel without 5-FU have been studied with response rates of 45–50% in metastatic squamous or adenocarcinoma. Carboplatin has also been combined with 3-h paclitaxel every 3 weeks in patients with upper gastrointestinal malignancies, with a 44% response rate reported in a small group of patients.

TABLE II
Activity of Combination Chemotherapy[a]

Combination	Cell type[b]	No. patients	No. responses	%	95% confidence intervals
Bleomycin					
Cisplatin–bleomycin	S	110	28	26	14–37
Cisplatin/methotrexate					
Cisplatin–methotrexate	S	43	32	76	63–89
Cisplatin/etoposide					
Cisplatin–etoposide	S	15	3	20	0–40
	S	65	31	48	36–60
	A	27	13	48	29–67
Cisplatin–etoposide–doxorubicin	A	25	13	52	32–72
Cisplatin/5-FU					
Cisplatin–5-FU	S	238	116	49	43–55
Cisplatin–5-FU–mitomycin	S	33	20	61	47–78
Cisplatin–5-FU–doxorubicin	S	21	7	33	13–53
Cisplatin–5-FU–doxorubicin–etoposide	S	24	17	71	61–81
Cisplatin–5-FU–etoposide	S	20	13	65	47–83
	A	35	17	49	32–66
Cisplatin/paclitaxel					
Cisplatin–paclitaxel–5-FU	A + S	60	29	48	35–61
Cisplatin–paclitaxel–5-FU	S	17	12	71	49–93
Cisplatin–paclitaxel	A + S	32	15	46	26–66
Cisplatin–paclitaxel	A + S	20	11	55	34–76
Cisplatin–paclitaxel	A + S	59	31	52	39–65
Other combinations					
Carboplatin–paclitaxel	A	9	4	44	12–76
Cisplatin–irinotecan	A + S	35	20	57	41–73

[a]Compilation of phase II trials.

[b]S, squamous carcinoma; A, adenocarcinoma.

Based on promising results from Japanese investigators for the new agent irinotecan in colon and gastric cancer, a weekly regimen of irinotecan combined with cisplatin was developed and subsequently studied in metastatic esophageal cancer. A 57% response rate was observed, and response rates for adenocarcinoma (52%) and squamous cell carcinoma (66%) were similar. Toxicity was relatively mild, with tolerable myelosuppression and diarrhea.

The search for effective antitumor agents in the treatment of esophageal cancer continues, given the modest activity of currently available agents and the brief duration of antitumor responses observed. Future strategies in the treatment of esophageal carcinoma will undoubtedly be based on advances in the understanding of the molecular biology of the disease. Ongoing studies indicate a role for numerous oncogenes and tumor suppressor genes in the mechanism of tumorigenesis, and these factors may be potential targets for the development of new antitumor agents as well as biologic prognostic factors. Laboratory studies have revealed evidence of enhanced expression and amplification of the epidermal growth factor (EGF) receptor gene in esophageal squamous carcinoma. Immunohistochemical studies of EGF and EGF receptor protein expression in resected esophageal squamous cancers have shown that an increased degree of expression of EGF or EGF receptor protein correlates with poorer survival. Monoclonal antibodies to the EGF receptor in clinical trial development include the monoclonal antibody C225, which appears to have antitumor activity and may act synergistically when combined with chemotherapy. The enzyme tyrosine kinase, required for signal transduction by the EGF receptor, is another potential target for new drug development. Oral tyrosine kinase inhibitors, including ZD1839, are already in phase I/II clinical trial development and appear to have promising antitumor activity. A high degree of expression of the HER-2 receptor has also been demonstrated in esophageal adenocarcinoma and Barrett's esophagus, and like the EGF receptor, HER-2 is also a tyrosine kinase growth factor receptor. Antibodies to HER-2 are under active clinical investigation, as these agents may lead to tumor growth inhibition and may act synergistically with chemotherapy and possibly with radiotherapy to increase antitumor response. An antibody to HER-2 is now available commercially as the drug herceptin, which when delivered with paclitaxel leads to an enhanced tumor response and increased median patient survival in metastatic breast cancer in patients whose tumors overexpress HER-2. Inhibitors of the enzyme protein kinase C, including flavopiridol and bryostatin, are also the subject of investigation. These agents appear to act synergistically to trigger cellular apoptotic death when coadministered with chemotherapy agents, including paclitaxel. Cell cycle regulatory proteins that also appear to be affected in squamous cell and adenocarcinomas include the tumor suppressor gene p53 and cyclin D, also potential targets for new drug therapeutic intervention. Potential biologic markers of tumor responsiveness or resistance to chemotherapy are also being explored, including the targets of chemotherapeutic agents such as the enzyme thymidylate synthase, the cellular target of 5-FU, and tubulin isoforms, the cellular target of taxanes.

III. PALLIATION

Most chemotherapy trials in metastatic esophageal cancer report on the response rate of single agent or combination therapy. Secondary end points in these trials include median patient survival and toxicity of therapy. Few trials, until recently, have reported on either the symptom palliation or the quality of life achieved on these trials. Studies have, however, included symptomatic relief in response assessment, and quality of life measures are being included in patient assessment on palliative chemotherapy programs. Three chemotherapy trials reported significant palliation of patient dysphagia with chemotherapy alone,

employing cisplatin combination therapy with etoposide, paclitaxel, and irinotecan. Relief of dysphagia on these trials ranged from 80 to 90% and correlated with antitumor response rates ranging from 40 to 50%. The trial of irinotecan plus cisplatin also evaluated quality of life as measured by two quality of life scales, with responding patients showing a statistically significant improvement in quality of life. Given the often substantial toxicity of combination chemotherapy used to palliate metastatic disease, symptom relief and quality of life assessment of patients will play a greater role in the assessment of clinical benefit of systemic chemotherapy programs.

Palliation of dysphagia may also be achieved by local therapies administered endoscopically, including endoscopic dilatation, laser ablation, and photodynamic therapy. Stents placed in the esophagus may also lead to dysphagia palliation, with one trial suggesting superiority for expansile metal stents compared to older prostheses.

IV. NEOADJUVANT CHEMOTHERAPY AND RADIOTHERAPY

Clinical trials of systemic chemotherapy given preoperatively, also termed neoadjuvant or primary chemotherapy, have been undertaken largely because high rates of both local and systemic recurrence of esophageal cancer despite conventional surgery or radiation therapy alone. Such combined modality trials employing chemotherapy have taken one of three different approaches: (1) chemotherapy followed by a planned surgical procedure, (2) chemotherapy given concurrently with radiation therapy, followed by surgery, and (3) chemotherapy and radiation therapy without subsequent surgical intervention. The rationale, both preclinical and clinical, for neoadjuvant chemotherapy has been reviewed. For esophageal cancer patients, the approach of preoperative chemotherapy offers several potential clinical benefits, including enhancing resectability by downstaging the primary tumor. Another potential advantage is the assessment of the response to preoperative chemotherapy directly in the primary tumor, making the end point of adjuvant therapy more precise by identifying patients who respond to chemotherapy and who might therefore benefit from further chemotherapy postoperatively. Administering chemotherapy early on in the course of the disease also has the advantage of treating subclinical but established micrometastatic disease when chemotherapy is likely to have its greatest impact, given the limited effectiveness of systemic therapy to treat clinically apparent metastatic disease. A disadvantage of preoperative chemotherapy is the delay in achieving local control of disease. The rationale for concomitant chemotherapy and radiation therapy has also been reviewed. Concurrent chemoradiotherapy potentially allows the achievement of enhanced local control as well as treating systemic micrometastases.

The use of preoperative chemotherapy in locally advanced esophageal carcinoma has been the subject of numerous trials. Most of these trials have been single arm phase II studies evaluating preoperative chemotherapy given from one to up to six cycles, followed by a definitive surgical procedure. More recent trials, however, have given chemotherapy both pre- and postoperatively. Virtually all preoperative chemotherapy trials in esophageal cancer have employed cisplatin-based combination chemotherapy. While earlier trials included predominantly squamous carcinoma, with the increased incidence of adenocarcinoma, both histologies have been treated on the same preoperative protocols. Pathologic complete responses found at surgery to preoperative chemotherapy are rare, generally less than 5%, and 5-year survivals of up to 20% have been reported in long-term follow-up of patients receiving neoadjuvant chemotherapy.

The recently published American intergroup trial 113 is the most definitive randomized trial to date of preoperative chemotherapy in esophageal cancer. In this trial, patients with adenocarcinoma or squamous carcinoma of the esophagus were randomized to undergo immediate surgery or to receive three cycles of cisplatin and 5-FU followed by surgery followed by two postoperative cycles of cisplatin and 5-FU. The trial failed to show any benefit for neoadjuvant chemotherapy compared to surgery alone (see Fig. 1). The median survival for patients undergoing surgery alone was 16.1 months compared to 14.9 months for patients receiving chemotherapy, not significantly different. Overall survival at 2 years (37% for surgery alone vs 35% for chemotherapy) and 5 years (20% for both treatment

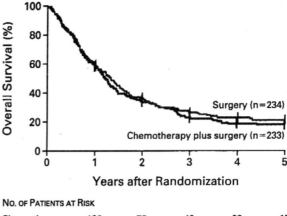

NO. OF PATIENTS AT RISK				
Chemotherapy plus surgery	136	73	42	28	15
Surgery	138	81	45	27	16

FIGURE 1   Patient survival with esophageal carcinoma treated with surgery alone or with chemotherapy and surgery combined. From Kelsen *et al.* (1998). *N. Engl. J. Med.* **339,** 1982, with permission. Copyright © 1998 Massachusetts Medical Society. All rights reserved.

groups) was also not significantly different for the two patient groups, and there was also no difference in 2-year disease-free survival for either group (20%). Curative resections with negative surgical margins (R0 resection) were equivalent in both groups (59% for surgery alone and 62% for preoperative chemotherapy patients), and surgical mortality was also comparable for both groups (6% operative mortality for surgery alone and a 7% operative mortality for preoperative chemotherapy patients). Two percent of patients died of chemotherapy-related complications. Treatment outcomes were comparable for patients with adenocarcinoma or squamous cell carcinoma.

The intensification of radiotherapy with concurrent chemotherapy used as a radiation sensitizer, either in the preoperative setting or as definitive local therapy, has been the subject of numerous phase II studies and, more recently, phase III trials. Overall, in the trials employing preoperative concurrent chemoradiotherapy, consistently 25% or more of patients achieved a pathologic complete response seen at esophagectomy. Five-year survivals of 30–35% have been reported on these trials, and achieving of a pathologic complete response has correlated with an improved survival of up to 60% at 5 years. The contribution of esophagectomy in these trials remains unclear, with some trials indicating long-term survival only in patients achieving a complete response to chemoradiotherapy and other trials indicating that surgery salvages some partial responders to treatment. Toxicity for combined chemotherapy and radiation compared to preoperative chemotherapy alone is greater. Because of the severe gastrointestinal toxicity seen in trials employing infusional 5-FU, cisplatin, and radiotherapy, there is routine use of supplemental enteral or parenteral nutrition during the course of preoperative therapy. Toxicity has been greatest in the trials in which a higher radiotherapy dose or hyperfractionated radiotherapy was given or in which the radiotherapy overlapped all cycles of chemotherapy given preoperatively. Recent trials have combined induction chemotherapy or postoperative adjuvant chemotherapy with preoperative chemoradiotherapy. Other pilot trials have addressed the contribution of additional chemotherapy agents to 5-FU and cisplatin, including etoposide, and leucovorin with or without etoposide. Comparable rates of resectability, pathologic complete responses, and survival have been observed in these studies.

The approach of preoperative concurrent chemotherapy and radiation needs to be validated in the context of a randomized trial comparing combined modality therapy to surgery alone. Results from such trials have drawn conflicting conclusions, with preliminary analysis in some trials failing to show a benefit for preoperative combined modality therapy. A recent trial in esophageal adenocarcinoma comparing surgery alone to preoperative 5-FU/cisplatin/radiotherapy showed a significant survival benefit for combined modality therapy. One hundred thirteen patients were randomized on this trial to receive either surgery alone or one cycle of 5-FU and cisplatin with 40 Gy of concurrent radiotherapy, and a second cycle of 5-FU and cisplatin delivered after completion of the radiotherapy and prior to surgery. A pathologic complete response rate of 25% was observed after preoperative chemoradiotherapy, comparable to reports of other studies. The median survival was 32 months in the chemoradiotherapy group compared to 11 months with surgery alone, and the 3-year survival was 32% for the chemoradiotherapy group compared to 6% for surgery alone, representing a highly significant improvement in survival achieved by combined modality therapy. Despite the indication of a survival

benefit for preoperative chemoradiotherapy on this trial, the poor outcome on the surgical arm, a 6% survival at 3 years, is considerably inferior to other recent trials in which a survival of 15–20% is achieved with surgery alone. Studies are ongoing to better define the role of preoperative chemoradiotherapy and include trials evaluating potential new radiosensitizing agents, including paclitaxel, docetaxel, vinorelbine, and irinotecan.

V. CONCURRENT CHEMORADIATION WITHOUT SURGERY

Concurrent chemotherapy and radiation therapy as definitive therapy without esophagectomy has also been the subject of numerous clinical trials. A nonsurgical, random assignment trial in local/regional esophageal carcinoma comparing radiation therapy alone with radiation given with concurrent 5-FU and cisplatin was conducted by the Radiation Therapy Oncology Group (RTOG). Patients with both squamous and adenocarcinoma were enrolled, although the majority of patients had squamous carcinoma. Patients receiving radiotherapy alone were treated with a total dose of 6400 cGy, delivered over 7 weeks in 200-cGy daily fractions. Patients receiving concurrent chemotherapy and radiation received a total dose of 5000 cGy delivered over 5 weeks; chemotherapy consisted of 5-FU given by continuous intravenous infusion for 4 consecutive days on weeks 1, 5, 8, and 11, with cisplatin given on day 1 of each 5-FU treatment course. Radiation therapy, delivered in 200-cGy daily fractions, overlapped the first two chemotherapy cycles. The chemotherapy design employed two additional cycles of systemic chemotherapy after chemoradiotherapy was completed.

The survival of patients treated with radiotherapy alone or a combination of concurrent chemotherapy and radiotherapy is shown in Fig. 2, and a significant survival benefit was observed for chemoradiation versus radiation therapy alone. A recent update of the survival achieved on this trial indicates a maintenance of survival benefit for the chemoradiotherapy arm at a minimum follow-up of 5 years, with a 5-year

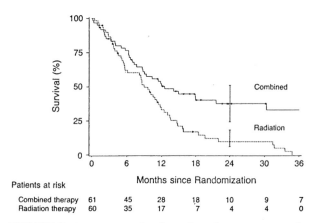

survival of 26% for patients treated with chemoradiotherapy and no survivors treated with radiotherapy alone. A statistically significant reduction in both local and distant recurrence of disease was also noted, favoring combined chemotherapy and radiation. The results strongly indicate that the combination of chemotherapy and radiation is superior to radiation therapy alone. The morbidity of chemoradiotherapy was greater than radiotherapy alone, with 64% of patients treated with chemoradiotherapy versus 28% of patients treated with radiotherapy experiencing severe or life-threatening toxicity (mainly mucositis and myelosuppression). One patient treated with chemoradiotherapy died from treatment-related toxicity (1.6%) and there were no deaths in the radiotherapy arm. Because of toxicity, only one-half of patients treated with combined modality therapy received the final planned two cycles of systemic therapy. Nonetheless, a high percentage of patients treated with combined chemotherapy and radiation (44%), had either persistence or recurrence of local disease at 12 months.

At the present time, in the nonsurgical setting, concurrent chemotherapy and radiation therapy is superior to radiotherapy alone for locally advanced squamous esophageal carcinoma and is now a standard local therapy. The role of this approach remains less well established in adenocarcinoma of the esophagus, although results have indicated a similar treatment

outcome for adenocarcinoma and squamous carcinoma treated with preoperative chemoradiation followed by esophagectomy. Concurrent chemoradiotherapy given prior to an operation remains an investigational approach, and surgery alone remains a standard treatment. The question of whether esophagectomy is an obligate part of local disease control after combined chemotherapy and radiation therapy must ultimately be asked in the context of a random assignment trial comparing surgery or chemoradiotherapy in the treatment of local regional disease.

Two recent trials attempted to intensify the chemoradiotherapy regimen employed in the RTOG 85-01 trial. On Intergroup trial 0122, the duration of chemotherapy was increased from 4 to 5 treatment days, the total number of cycles of chemotherapy was increased from four to five cycles (with the delivery of three induction chemotherapy cycles prior to the start of combined modality therapy), and the radiation dose was increased from 5000 to 6480 cGy. Eligibility was limited to squamous cell carcinoma. This intensive neoadjuvant approach did not appear to offer a benefit compared with conventional doses and techniques of combined modality therapy, and the addition of induction chemotherapy prior to chemoradiotherapy resulted in a significant number of treatment-related deaths. A subsequent RTOG trial compared a higher dose of radiation therapy (6480 cGy) to the standard dose radiotherapy (5040 cGy) and failed to show an improvement in either local disease control or survival for higher dose radiotherapy compared to standard dose radiotherapy. Another approach to the dose intensification of combined modality therapy is to increase the dose of radiation by employing intraluminal esophageal brachytherapy. Intraluminal brachytherapy allows the escalation of the dose to the primary tumor while protecting the surrounding dose-limiting structures such as the lung, heart, and spinal cord. Brachytherapy has been used as primary therapy as well as boost following external beam radiation therapy. As a primary therapy, brachytherapy results in a local control rate of 25–35%. RTOG trial 92-07 treated patients with squamous cell cancer or adenocarcinomas with 5-FU and cisplatin for four cycles with concurrent 5000 cGy of radiotherapy, followed by a boost during cycle 3 of chemotherapy with high-dose rate intraluminal brachytherapy. High-dose rate brachytherapy was delivered in weekly fractions of 500 cGy. Complete response rate, median survival, and local control were no better than historical controls treated with chemoradiotherapy alone. Six tracheosophageal fistulas resulted from the addition of brachytherapy to combined chemoradiotherapy and three were fatal. Given the significant toxicity for this treatment approach, the addition of brachytherapy to combined chemoradiotherapy should be used with caution and should not be given with concurrent chemotherapy.

VI. CONCLUSION

Esophageal cancer remains a significant worldwide health problem, with adenocarcinoma of the esophagus an emerging epidemic in Western countries. The relative merits of surgery versus radiotherapy-based treatments, or a combined chemoradiotherapy/surgery approach, need to be assessed in the context of prospective clinical trials. Given the relatively poor survival achieved with currently available therapy, new systemic therapy, including new chemotherapeutic agents and new drugs targeting more specific tumor growth-promoting pathways, will need to be addressed in combined modality therapy trials.

See Also the Following Articles

CISPLATIN • ESOPHAGEAL CANCER: RISK FACTORS AND SOMATIC GENETICS • GASTRIC CANCER • LUNG, LARYNX, ORAL CAVITY, AND PHARYNX • TP53 TUMOR SUPPRESSOR GENE: STRUCTURE AND FUNCTION

Bibliography

Bosset, J. F., Gignoux, M., Triboulet, J. P., Tiret, E., Mantion, G., Elias, D., Lozach, P., Ollier, J. C., Pavy, J. J. M., and Sahmoud, T. (1997). Chemoradiotherapy followed by surgery compared with surgery alone in squamous-cell cancer of the esophagus. N. Engl. J. Med. 17, 161–167.

Cooper, J. S., Guo, M. D., Herskovic, A., Macdonald, J. S., Martenson, J. A., Al-Sarraf, M., et al. (1999). Chemoradiotherapy of locally advanced esophageal cancer: Long-term follow-up of a prospective randomized trial (RTOG 85-01). J. Am. Med. Assoc. 281(17).

Devesa, S. S., Blot, W. J., and Fraumeni, J. F., Jr. (1998). Changing patterns in the incidence of esophageal and gastric carcinoma in the United States. Cancer 83(10), 2049–2053.

Enzinger, P. C., Ilson, D. H., and Kelsen, D. P. (1999). Chemotherapy in esophageal cancer. Semin. Oncol. 26(5 Suppl. 15), 12–20.

Gaspar, L. E., Winter, K., Kocha, W. I., Coia, L. R., Herskovic, A., and Graham, M. (2000). A phase I/II study of external beam radiation, brachytherapy, and concurrent chemotherapy for patients with localized carcinoma of the esophagus: Radiation Therapy Oncology Group Study 9207, Final Report. Cancer 88(5), 988–995.

Greenlee, R. T., Murray, T., Bolden, S., and Wingo, P. A. (2000). Cancer Statistics, 2000. CA Cancer J. Clin. 50(1), 7–33.

Harris, D. T., and Mastrangelo, M. J. (1991). Theory and application of early systemic therapy. Semin. Oncol. 18, 493–503.

Herskovic, A., Martz, K., Al-Sarraf, M., Leichman, L., Brindle, J., Vaitkevicius, V., et al. (1992). Combined chemotherapy and radiotherapy compared with radiotherapy alone in patients with cancer of the esophagus. N. Engl. J. Med. 326, 1593–1598.

Ilson, D. H., Saltz, L., Enzinger, P., Huang, Y., Kornblith, A., Gollub, M., et al. (1999). A Phase II trial of weekly irinotecan plus cisplatin in advanced esophageal cancer. J. Clin. Oncol. 17(10), 3270–3275.

Kelsen, D. P., Ginsberg, R., Pajak, T. F., Sheahan, D. G., Gunderson, L., Mortimer, J., et al. (1998). Chemotherapy followed by surgery compared with surgery alone for localized esophageal cancer. N. Engl. J. Med. 339(27), 1979–1984.

Lagergren, J., Bergstrom, R., Lindgren, A., and Nyren, O. (1999). Symptomatic gastroesophageal reflux as a risk factor for esophageal adenocarcinoma. N. Engl. J. Med. 340(11), 825–831.

Minsky, B. D., Neuberg, D., Kelsen, D. P., Pisansky, T. M., Ginsberg, R., and Benson, A. (1996). Neoadjuvant chemotherapy plus concurrent chemotherapy and high-dose radiation for squamous cell carcinoma of the esophagus: A preliminary analysis of the phase II Intergroup trial 0122. J. Clin. Oncol. 14(1), 149–155.

Urba, S., Orringer, M., Turrisi, A., Whyte, R., Natale, R., Iannettoni, M., et al. (1995). A randomized trial comparing transhiatal esophagectomy (the) to preoperative concurrent chemoradiation (CT/XRT) followed by esophagectomy in locoregional esophageal carcinoma (CA). Proc. ASCO 14(475), 199.

Vokes, E. E., and Weichselbaum, R. R. (1990). Concomitant chemoradiotherapy: Rationale and clinical experience in patients with solid tumors. J. Clin. Oncol. 8, 911–934.

Walsh, T. N., Noonan, N., Hollywood, D., Kelly, A., Keeling, N., and Hennessy, T. P. J. (1996). A comparison of multimodal therapy and surgery for esophageal adenocarcinoma. N. Engl. J. Med. 335, 462–467.

Estrogens and Antiestrogens

V. Craig Jordan
Northwestern University Medical School

I. Introduction
II. Estrogen Therapy
III. Antiestrogen Therapy for Breast Cancer
IV. Mechanism of Action of Selective Estrogen
    Receptor Modulators (SERMs)
V. Clinical Application of Antiestrogens (SERMs)
VI. Future Development

GLOSSARY

antiestrogen A drug that blocks the estrogen receptor to prevent estrogen action.

aromatase An enzyme that converts steroid precursors into estradiol and estrone.

aromatase inhibitor A drug that reversibly or irreversibly blocks the actions of the aromatase enzyme.

estrogen receptor A nuclear protein that binds natural or synthetic estrogens to form a transcription complex at an estrogen responsive gene.

estrogen target tissue Tissue that contains the estrogen receptor and is therefore responsive to estrogen action.

gene An area of DNA that encodes a message to synthesize a specific protein.

pure antiestrogen A compound that exhibits no estrogen-like actions at any target site and causes the premature destruction of the estrogen receptor.

selective estrogen receptor modulator A compound that can switch on estrogen-like actions of the estrogen receptor at one target site, e.g., bone, but act as an antiestrogen at another, e.g., breast.

transcription complex A combination of two estrogen receptors that assemble a variety of coactivator proteins and enzymes to unwind DNA and transcribe a gene.

Estrogen is important for successful reproduction, the maintenance of bones, and protection from coronary heart disease. However, the finding of a link between estrogen and breast cancer growth has resulted in the successful development of novel strategies for breast cancer treatment and prevention and the development of new multifunctional medicines for postmenopausal women's health. Selective estrogen receptor modulators (SERMs) are nonsteroidal compounds that prevent breast cancer cell replication, maintain bone density, and reduce circulating cholesterol. Tamoxifen is used for breast cancer treatment and prevention, and raloxifene is used for the

Encyclopedia of Cancer, Second Edition
Volume 2

179

prevention of osteoporosis but is being tested for the prevention of breast cancer and coronary heart disease. These pioneering medicines are the first of numerous novel drugs that exploit the estrogen receptor (ER) signal transduction pathway as a therapeutic target.

I. INTRODUCTION

The estrogenic steroids, estrone and estradiol, are synthesized in the ovaries under the cyclical control of gonadotrophins produced by the pituitary gland. When ovarian function stops at menopause, small but significant levels of estrogens are synthesized by the conversion of adrenal precursors to estrone and estradiol. This is accomplished by aromatase enzymes in body fat. Higher levels of body fat are correlated with higher circulating levels of estrogens. This, in turn, has been correlated with a higher incidence of breast and endometrial cancer in postmenopausal women. Thus, increased body fat is a risk factor for breast and endometrial cancer because unopposed estrogen exposure promotes breast and uterine carcinogenesis.

The link between estrogens and breast cancer growth and development has been known throughout the past century. Ablation of the ovaries in premenopausal patients with metastatic breast cancer results in an objective response in about one-third of patients. Similarly, ablation of the pituitary gland or adrenal glands in postmenopausal women results in responses in one-third of patients. However, the reason for the apparently arbitrary responses was not known until the discovery of the estrogen receptor (ER) and the application of the knowledge to predict the responses in breast cancer. The ER is present in estrogen target tissues, e.g., uterus, vagina, and some breast cancers (Fig. 1). Estradiol diffuses into all tissues but binds to the nuclear ER only in its target tissues. The estradiol ER complex then assembles a transcription unit at estrogen responsive genes to orchestrate cell replication (Fig. 2). Thus, it is the presence or absence of the ER that determines the dependence of a breast tumor on estrogen for growth. A breast tumor ER assay is standard medical practice to predict whether a breast cancer patient will or will not respond to any additive or ablative endocrine maneuver. In general terms, a postmenopausal patient with an ER-negative breast cancer will only have a 10% chance of responding to any

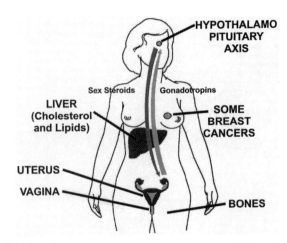

FIGURE 1 Estrogen target tissues around a woman's body. The estrogen receptor in the hypothalamo–pituitary axis orchestrates the cyclical regulation of ovarian estrogen synthesis. Estrogen also causes cell replication in the uterine lining and changes in vaginal histology. The bones are estrogen target tissues, and circulating cholesterol is regulated through estrogen-regulated changes in liver metabolism. Some breast cancers contain the estrogen receptor and are estrogen responsive.

endocrine therapy, but a patient with an ER-positive tumor will have a 60% chance of a response.

II. ESTROGEN THERAPY

The chemistry of steroid hormones is extremely challenging and it was not until the 1940s and 1950s that orally active steroid preparations were available for applications as hormone replacement therapy (sulfated equilin and equilenin from horse urine) or as components of the oral contraceptive (synthetic mestranol or ethinylestradiol). In contrast, discovery of the synthetic nonsteroidal estrogen diethylstilbestrol (DES) in the 1930s provided a simple and inexpensive source of estrogens to use in therapeutics. Although it was clear that physiologic concentrations of estrogen were able to support the growth of breast cancer, pharmacologic doses of DES were, paradoxically, effective in producing tumor regression in one-third of postmenopausal breast cancer patients with advanced disease. Pharmacologic estrogen therapy remained an inexpensive and effective endocrine therapy for about 30 years (1940–1970), but a high incidence of blood clotting was a major side effect that prevented the long-term or widespread use of DES as an adjuvant therapy in early breast cancer. The anti-

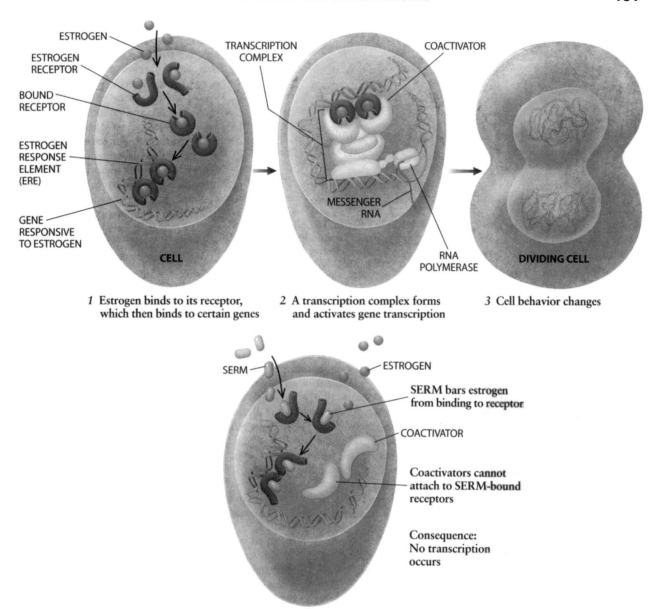

FIGURE 2 (a) How estrogen acts in cells and (b) how SERMs block estrogen action. From *Scientific American*, October 1998, p. 38.

tumor mechanism of pharmacologic estrogen action through the ER is unknown.

III. ANTIESTROGEN THERAPY FOR BREAST CANCER

During the 1960s, ablative or additive endocrine therapies were standard palliative strategies for the treatment of metastatic breast cancer. Discovery of the first nonsteroidal antiestrogen MER-25 (Fig. 3) introduced

a new therapeutic modality for potential applications as a contraceptive, an inducer of ovulation, or breast cancer therapy. Unfortunately, MER-25 was too toxic, but other antiestrogens were successfully developed.

A. Nonsteroidal Antiestrogens

Clomiphene, a mixture of *cis* and *trans* isomers of a substituted triphenylethylene, is used for the induction of ovulation in subfertile women, but has not been pursued as breast cancer treatment. In contrast,

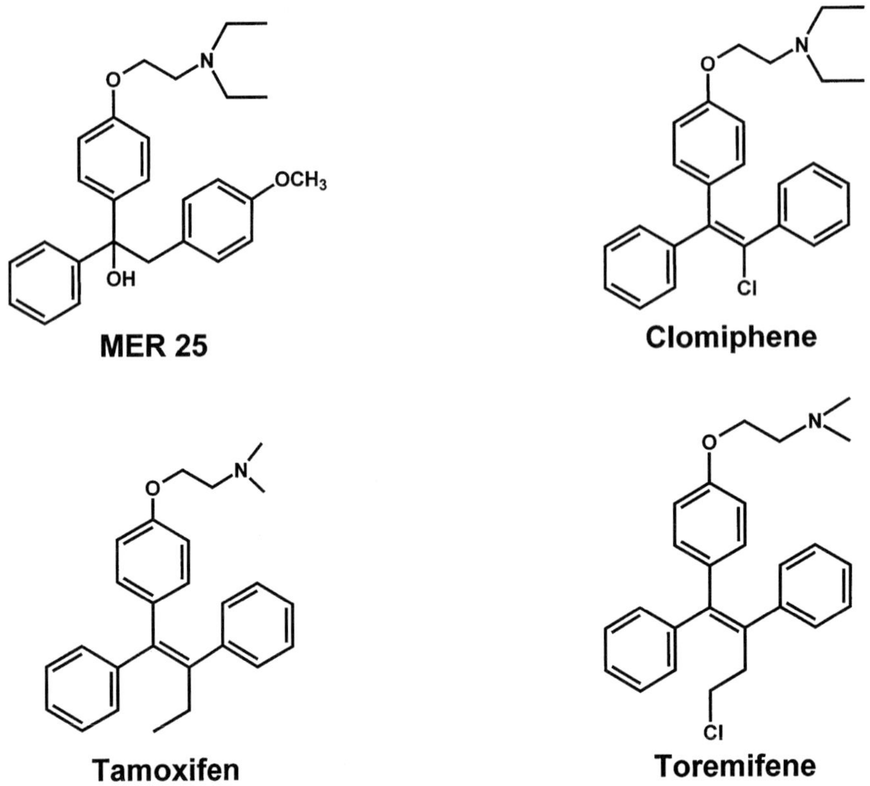

FIGURE 3 Nonsteroidal antiestrogens related to the estrogen triphenylethylene. MER25 was the first nonsteroidal antiestrogen, and clomiphene is used for the induction of ovulation. Tamoxifen is used to treat all stages of breast cancer and for prevention, but toremifene is only used to treat advanced breast cancer in postmenopausal women.

tamoxifen is the antiestrogenic *trans* isomer of a substituted triphenylethylene that is approved as the endocrine treatment for all stages of breast cancer and is the first drug to be shown to reduce the incidence of breast cancer in high-risk women. Tamoxifen is listed as an essential drug for cancer treatment by the World Health Organization.

Several tamoxifen derivatives have been tested, e.g., idoxifene, droloxifene, and toremifene, but only toremifene is available for the treatment of advanced breast cancer in postmenopausal women. The compound produces the same response rates as tamoxifen and because there is cross-resistance, toremifene should not be used after tamoxifen treatment.

B. Selective Estrogen Receptor Modulators (SERMs)

The extensive laboratory and clinical evaluation of tamoxifen has demonstrated that the drug is antiestrogenic in the breast but has estrogen-like properties in bone and circulating cholesterol. Tamoxifen maintains bone density in postmenopausal women and there is evidence that this translates into a reduction in fractures that approaches statistical significance. Tamoxifen has not been tested as a drug to treat or prevent osteoporosis. Tamoxifen reduces low-density lipoprotein (LDL) cholesterol but maintains high-density lipoprotein (HDL) cholesterol in postmenopausal women. Some, but not all, studies suggest that tamoxifen could protect against coronary heart disease (CHD). However, the drug has not been tested prospectively as a preventive for CHD in a clinical trial of high-risk women.

Although tamoxifen possesses a predominantly antiestrogenic effect in the uterus, the drug is sufficiently estrogen-like to increase the risk of endometrial cancer in postmenopausal women. The stage and grade of tumors are the same as those in the general population. It may now be possible to predict patients who are most likely to be at risk. A large epidemiology study has demonstrated that postmenopausal women who are obese or who have a history of taking hormone replacement therapy are most likely to be at risk for endometrial cancer during tamoxifen therapy.

Raloxifene (Fig. 4) is a nonsteroidal antiestrogen in the rodent uterus, but exhibits less uterotropic properties than tamoxifen. Raloxifene is classified as a SERM that maintains bone density and lowers LDL cholesterol in postmenopausal women. The compound significantly reduces spine fractures in elderly women and is being tested prospectively for the reduction of CHD in high-risk women. Because raloxifene is an antiestrogen in the breast and uterus, it is being evaluated as a preventive for breast cancer in high-risk women. A number of SERMs are currently being evaluated in the laboratory to determine low toxicity and safety before

being targeted as agents to prevent osteoporosis, coronary heart disease, and breast and endometrial cancer.

C. Pure Antiestrogens

Tamoxifen is a partial estrogen agonist. Patients taking long-term tamoxifen (>5 years) have the potential to develop drug-stimulated growth of breast and endometrial cancer. It is believed that this form of drug resistance develops because cancer cells that grow in response to tamoxifen are dependent on the estrogen-like properties of the drug, suggesting that compounds that possess no estrogen-like properties would be useful agents to treat breast or endometrial cancer. However, pure antiestrogens are only being tested in patients with advanced disease

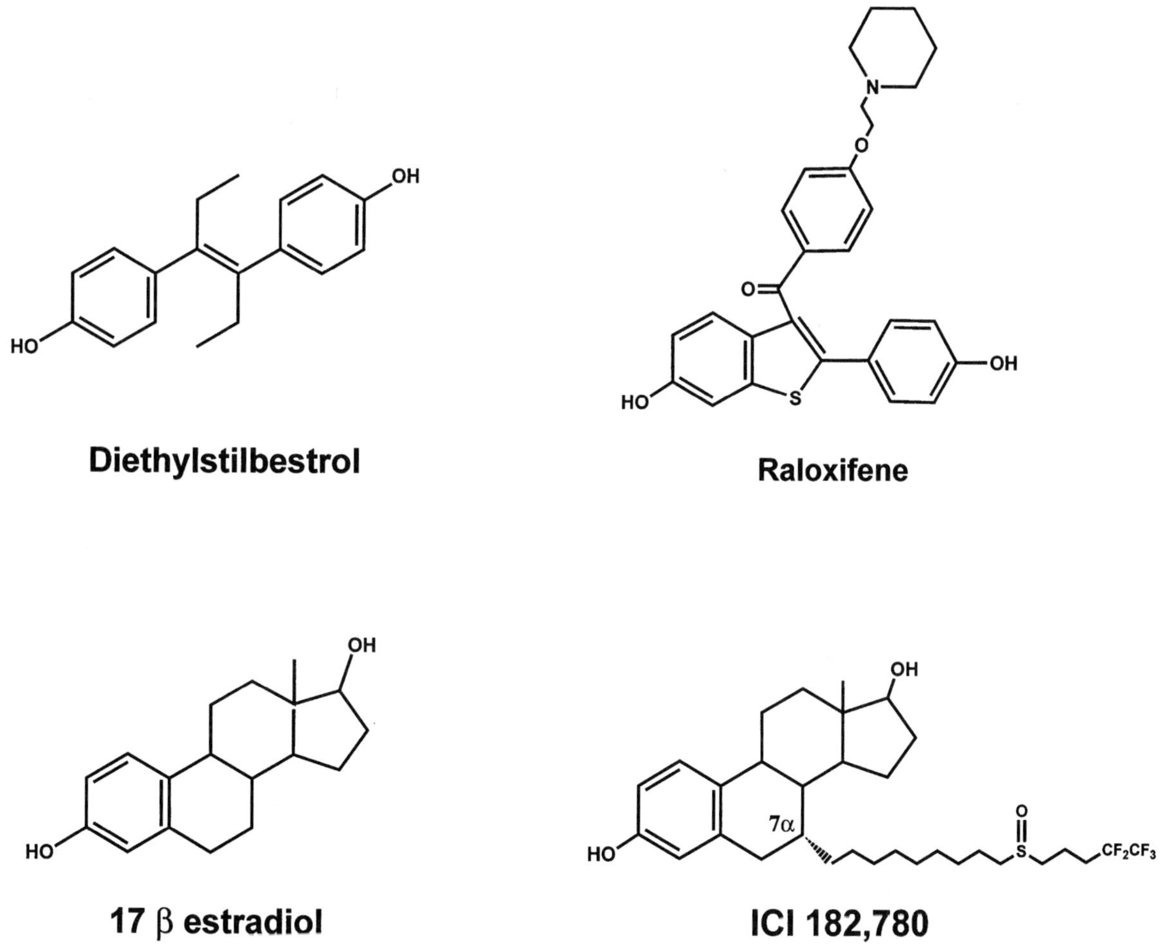

Diethylstilbestrol

Raloxifene

17 β estradiol

ICI 182,780

FIGURE 4 Formulae of estradiol and diethylstilbestrol and the compound raloxifene, which is being tested as a preventive for breast cancer but is approved as an estrogen-like treatment for osteoporosis. The pure antiestrogen ICI 182,780 (Faslodex) is being tested in the treatment of advanced breast cancer.

because of their potential risk of osteoporosis and CHD. The compound ICI 182,780 (Fig. 4) is a derivative of estradiol with a long hydrophobic side chain at the 7α position. ICI 182,780 is an antiestrogen at all target sites. The mechanism of action is unique. Whereas nonsteroidal antiestrogens block estrogen action by changing the shape of the ER complex and preventing the formation of a fully active transcription complex, ICI 182,780 changes the shape of the complex but also enhances the destruction of ER. The loss of the ER as a critical transcription factor for replication results in rapid tumor regression.

The drug ICI 182,780 must be administered by oily injection because depot bioavailablity is poor. Clinical testing of ICI 182,780 shows activity following tamoxifen failure, and the results of trials in advanced breast cancer are being completed.

D. Aromatase Inhibitors

Tamoxifen-resistant tumors often retain the ER, and the tumor can respond to second-line endocrine ther-

apy. One approach is to prevent the synthesis of the small, but significant amounts of circulating estrogen present in the postmenopausal patient. Early studies with aminoglutethimide (Fig. 5), which blocks both adrenal and peripheral steroidogenesis, were successful, but the combination of aminoglutethimide plus hydrocortisone proved too toxic for long-term therapy. A new series of orally active peripherally selective aromatase inhibitors (e.g., letrozole or anastrozole; Fig. 5) prevents the conversion of testosterone and androstenedione to estradiol and estrone, respectively (Fig. 6). At present, anastrozole is used to treat advanced breast cancer and is currently being tested in adjuvant therapy trials.

IV. MECHANISM OF ACTION OF SELECTIVE ESTROGEN RECEPTOR MODULATORS (SERMS)

It is unclear how nonsteroidal antiestrogens produce target site-specific effects. However, with the cloning

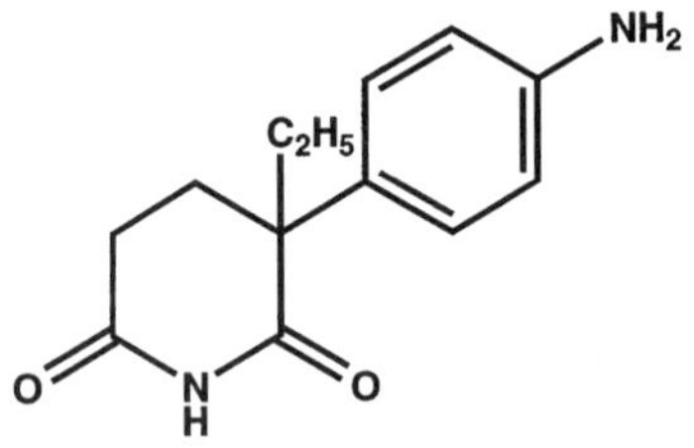

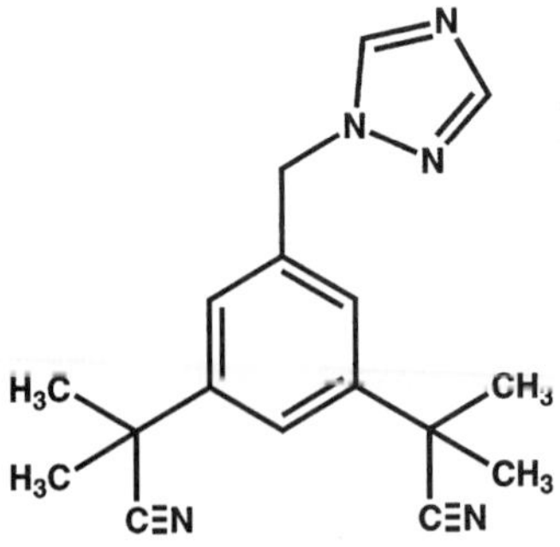

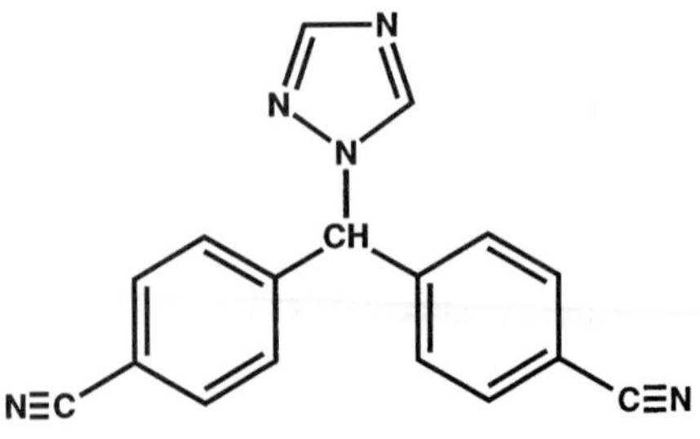

FIGURE 5 Formulae of compounds that block the aromatase enzyme system.

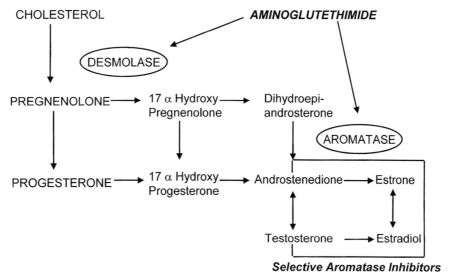

FIGURE 6 The mechanism of action of aromatase of inhibitors.

and sequencing of the ER, it is now possible to describe some of the steps involved in estrogen and antiestrogen action. Two forms of the ER exist: ERα and ERβ. ERα is the classical estrogen receptor that is primarily associated with estrogen action, but ERβ appears to act as a modulator and has a different distribution around the body.

An estrogen binds to the ligand-binding site of the ER and initiates the changes in ER structure necessary to activate the complex as a transcription factor. As a result of tertiary changes in protein structure, the steroid becomes located within a hydrophobic pocket completely surrounded by the protein complex. Two complexes then dimerize and bind to an estrogen response element in the promoter region of an estrogen responsive gene. The complexes then act as a focus to build a transcription unit from numerous coactivator molecules and from proteins that open up the DNA for gene transcription (Fig. 7).

The crystal structure of raloxifene and the ligand-binding domain of ERα show that the antiestrogen binds within the same hydrophobic pocket as estradiol, but a critical section of the protein does not position itself correctly. As a result, coactivators cannot bind to the complex and gene transcription is impaired. The key to the molecular mechanism of action of raloxifene is the location of the antiestrogenic side chain near to amino acid 351 (aspartic acid). Neutralization of this charge clearly has a profound effect on coactivator binding. Mutation at this site to a larger charged amino acid, e.g., tyrosine, results in the reactivation of estrogen-like properties. Modulation of the estrogen-like actions of nonsteroidal antiestrogens is less easy to explain. Some target sites could have an excess of coactivator molecules that permit the antiestrogen ER complex to be more promiscuous or the complex could activate genes through a different signal transduction pathway. One possibility is that antiestrogen ER complexes could activate AP-1 sites by a protein–protein interaction at fos and jun. These possibilities are illustrated in Fig. 8.

V. CLINICAL APPLICATION OF ANTIESTROGENS (SERMS)

Recognition that the nonsteroidal antiestrogen tamoxifen was not only an effective breast cancer therapy in patients with ER-positive disease but also reduced the incidence of contralateral breast cancer encouraged the rigorous evaluation of tamoxifen as a preventive for the disease in high-risk women. Additionally, the finding that tamoxifen could maintain bone density in postmenopausal women led to the concept that a SERM could be used to prevent osteoporosis but potentially reduce the incidence of breast cancer in older, postmenopausal women who

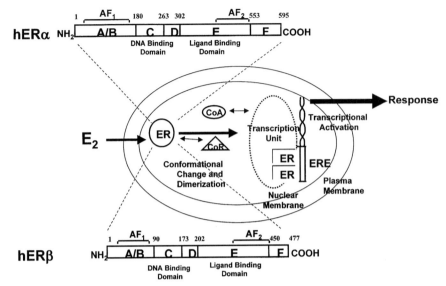

FIGURE 7 Estrogen action in a breast cancer cell containing both ERα and ERβ. Ers are nuclear proteins. Estradiol diffuses in the cell and binds to the ligand-binding domain. This causes the steroid to be surrounded by the protein and sealed within a hydrophobic pocket. Tertiary changes in the receptor complex facilitate dimerization and binding at estrogen response elements (EREs) in the promoter region of estrogen responsive genes. The shape of the complexes facilitates the binding of coactivator molecules that form a transcription unit. ERα and ERβ both an initiate estrogen action at EREs, but ERβ has no constitutive AF-1 activity and can decrease the estrogen-like action of antiestrogen ERα complexes.

have no particular risk factors other than age. Raloxifene is the result.

A. Adjuvant Therapy with Tamoxifen

The Oxford Overview analysis has quantitated the benefits of tamoxifen using data from a large number of randomized clinical trials. Clinical data confirm the laboratory results published in the 1980s. The most important clinical observation is that tamoxifen increases the disease-free and the overall survival of pre- and postmenopausal women with ER-positive node-negative or node-positive breast cancer. Additionally, several important observations are available to guide clinicians in the evaluations of the risks and benefits of tamoxifen. There is no significant advantage for patients by increasing the dose of tamoxifen from the recommended 20 mg daily. Five years of adjuvant tamoxifen are superior to either 1 or 2 years of treatment for survival, disease-free survival, and the reduction of contralateral breast cancer. There is no significant decrease in CHD or increase in liver and colon cancer. However, endometrial cancer increases

two- to threefold from 1 per 1000 woman years to 3 per 1000 woman years. Durations of tamoxifen for longer than 5 years are more likely to increase the risk of endometrial cancer. Nevertheless, the risk of endometrial cancer is much less than the benefits in lives saved from breast cancer recurrence.

B. Raloxifene for the Treatment and Prevention of Osteoporosis

Despite the finding that raloxifene was an antiestrogen with antitumor properties in laboratory models, it has not been tested as a breast cancer therapy in randomized trials. The drug was not pursued as a cancer therapy, but in the 1990s, with the confirmation of SERM action, raloxifene was tested as a preventive for osteoporosis in placebo-controlled trials. Raloxifene at 60 and 120 mg daily increases bone density 2–3% in postmenopausal women and significantly reduces the incidence of spine fractures in high-risk women. Raloxifene lowers LDL cholesterol but does not significantly increase HDL cholesterol or triglycerides. The drug is currently

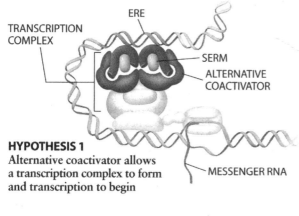

HYPOTHESIS 1
Alternative coactivator allows a transcription complex to form and transcription to begin

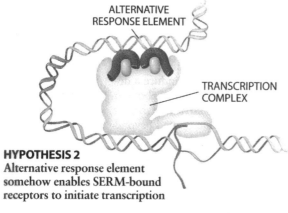

HYPOTHESIS 2
Alternative response element somehow enables SERM-bound receptors to initiate transcription

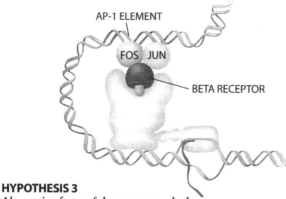

HYPOTHESIS 3
Alternative form of the receptor—the beta receptor—initiates transcription when the standard, alpha type is unable or is absent

FIGURE 8 How SERMs mimic estrogen. From *Scientific American*, October 1998, p. 39.

being tested as a preventive for CHD in a high-risk population.

Women who are participating in the osteoporosis trials have been monitored for their incidence of breast and endometrial cancer. There is a 60–70%

decrease in the incidence of invasive and noninvasive breast cancer overall. The incidence of ER-positive disease is reduced with no significant change in ER-negative disease. Endometrial cancer is rare in the postmenopausal population, but no increase in detection has, as yet, been noted in women taking raloxifene.

C. Prevention of Breast Cancer

Three studies have addressed the question of worth of tamoxifen in the prevention of breast cancer. Two small studies, one from the Royal Marsden Hospital (approximately 2000 women) in England and one from Italy (approximately 5000 women), were unable to show an advantage for tamoxifen. However, the number of patients recruited was small and their risk for breast cancer was low. As a result, the pilot studies were underpowered to show a significant difference. In contrast, the prospective placebo-controlled trial conducted by the National Adjuvant Breast and Bowel Project and sponsored by the National Cancer Institute was designed to recruit more than 13,000 high-risk pre- and postmenopausal women. The trial reached its recruitment goal and was stopped when there was a consistent and established advantage for tamoxifen. The placebo arm could not be justified if the trial had been continued. Tamoxifen produced a 49% reduction in the incidence of breast cancer. The preventive effect was noted in pre- and postmenopausal women for invasive and noninvasive breast cancer. Selective estrogen receptor modulation was noted with a decrease (nonsignificant) in fractures, but a modest increase in early stage low-grade endometrial cancer was seen only in postmenopausal women. Tamoxifen is currently approved for the reduction of breast cancer risk in high-risk pre- and postmenopausal women. A second breast cancer prevention trial is ongoing called the Study of Tamoxifen and Raloxifene (STAR): 22,000 high-risk postmenopausal women are being randomized to tamoxifen (20 mg daily), the approved drug, or raloxifene (60 mg daily), the test drug. Endometrial biopsies are not required, but spotting and bleeding will be followed up rapidly to determine endometrial cancer rates.

VI. FUTURE DEVELOPMENTS

The primary goal of current research is to understand the molecular mechanisms of selective estrogen receptor modulation. Additionally, the development of ERα or ERβ agonists or antagonists will provide important new pharmacologic tools to address clinical issues in prevention. A spectrum of new SERMs is also being advanced from the laboratory to clinical testing that could be applied to the prevention of osteoporosis, coronary heart disease, and breast and endometrial cancer. The key to success from the SERM strategy will be the quality of life during drug administration. The challenge is to develop a novel SERM that provides all the advantages of hormone replacement therapy on well-being, hot flashes, osteoporosis, and coronary heart disease but reduces the risk of breast and endometrial cancer as a beneficial side effect.

See Also the Following Articles

BREAST CANCER • CHEMOTHERAPY: SYNERGISM AND ANTAGONISM • ENDOMETRIAL CANCER • HEREDITARY RISK OF BREAST CANCER AND OVARIAN CANCER • HORMONAL CARCINOGENESIS

Bibliography

Bernstein, L., Deapen, D., Cerhan, J. R., Schwartz, S. M., Liff, J., McGann-Maloney, E., Perlman, J. A., and Ford, L. (1999). Tamoxifen therapy for breast cancer and endometrial cancer risk. *J. Natl. Cancer Inst.* **91,** 1654–1662.

Dodds, E. C., Lawson, W., and Noble, R. L. (1938). Biological effects of the synthetic oestrogenic substance 4:4′-dihydroxy-alpha:beta-diethylstilbene. *Lancet* **1,** 1389–1391.

EBCTCG. (1998). Tamoxifen for early breast cancer: An overview of the randomised trials. *Lancet* **351,** 1451–1467.

Fisher, B., Costantino, J. P., Wickerham, D. L., Redmond, C. K., Kavanah, M., Cronin, W. M., Vogel, V., Robidoux, A., Dimitrov, N., Atkins, J., Daly, M., Wieand, S., Tan-Chiu, E., Ford, L., and Wolmark, N. (1998). Tamoxifen for prevention of breast cancer: Report of the National Surgical Adjuvant Breast and Bowel Project P-1 Study. *J. Natl. Cancer Inst.* **90,** 1371–1388.

Goss, P. E., and Gwyn, K. M. (1994). Current perspectives on aromatase inhibitors in breast cancer. *J. Clin. Oncol.* **12,** 2460–2470.

Jensen, E. V., and Jacobson, H. I. (1962). Basic guides to the mechanism of estrogen action. *Recent Prog. Horm. Res.* **18,** 387–414.

Jensen, E. V., Block, G. E., Smith, S., Kyser, K., and DeSombre, E. R. (1971). Estrogen receptors and breast cancer response to adrenalectomy. *Natl. Cancer Inst. Monogr.* **34,** 55–70.

Jordan, V. C., and Morrow, M. (1999). Tamoxifen, raloxifene, and the prevention of breast cancer. *Endocr. Rev.* **20,** 253–278.

Kennedy, B. J. (1965). Hormone therapy for advanced breast cancer. *Cancer* **18,** 1551–1557.

Lerner, L. J., Holthaus, J. F., and Thompson, C. R. (1958). A non-steroidal estrogen antagonist 1-(p-2-diethylaminoethoxyphenyl)-1-phenyl-2-*p*-methoxyphenylethanol. *Endocrinology* **63,** 295–318.

Levenson, A. S., and Jordan, V. C. (1999). Selective oestrogen receptor modulation: Molecular pharmacology for the millennium. *Eur. J. Cancer* **35,** 1628–1639.

MacGregor, J. I., and Jordan, V. C. (1998). Basic guide to the mechanisms of antiestrogen action. *Pharmacol. Rev.* **50,** 151–196.

Osborne, C. K. (1998). Tamoxifen in the treatment of breast cancer. *N. Engl. J. Med.* **339,** 1609–1618.

Santen, R. J., Manni, A., Harvey, H., and Redmond, C. (1990). Endocrine treatment of breast cancer in women. *Endocr. Rev.* **11,** 221–265.

ETS Family of Transcription Factors

Dennis K. Watson, Runzhao Li, and Victor I. Sementchenko
Medical University of South Carolina

George Mavrothalassitis
University of Crete, Heraklion, Greece

Arun Seth
University of Toronto

I. Conservation
II. Structural/Functional Domains
III. DNA Binding and Transcriptional Activity
IV. Modulation of Activity
V. Oncogenic Activation
VI. ETS Gene Function

GLOSSARY

in vitro Literally, in glass; in a test tube or other artificial setting rather than in a living organism.
in vivo Literally, in life; located or occurring in a living organism.
knockout mice Genetically altered laboratory mice in which a given gene has been deleted ("knocked out") in order to study the effect of this deletion.

E TS is a group of transcription factors, each having a structurally unique DNA-binding domain. Identification of the v-ets oncogene of the avian leukemia virus, E26, in 1983 led to the discovery of a large family of conserved genes consisting of nearly 40 members. ETS transcription factors bind to unique DNA sequences containing GGAA/T and control the expression of genes involved in cellular proliferation, differentiation, development, hematopoiesis, apoptosis, metastasis, angiogenesis, and transformation. Regulation of gene expression is controlled through the action of multiple transcription factors, which function to activate or repress transcription. Identification of functional target genes regulated by a specific transcription factor is critical for understanding the molecular mechanisms that control transcription.

I. CONSERVATION

ETS genes have been characterized from phylogenetically divergent species from sponges, nematodes, and insects to humans and encode a group of evolutionarily conserved transcription factors. All members of the family contain a conserved DNA-binding domain (ETS domain) of approximately 85 amino acids. To date, 25 human family members have been identified (Table I, Fig. 1). Although human ETS genes are dispersed onto 13 different chromosomes, some are closely linked (e.g., ETS1 and FLI1; ETS2 and ERG), possibly suggesting evolutionary duplication. Amino acid sequences of the ETS domain can be used for subclassification of the human proteins into approxi-

mately 11 groups, including ERG, ETS, E4TF1, ERF, ELK, E1AF, PDEF, ELF, TEL, ESX, and SPI (Fig. 2).

II. STRUCTURAL/FUNCTIONAL DOMAINS

A. DNA-Binding Domain

The three-dimensional structure of the DNA-binding domains of FLI1, ETS1, SAP1, and PU.1 have been characterized as a winged helix–turn–helix (wHTH) composed of a three α helix bundle and a four-stranded, antiparallel β sheet. The HTH motif is formed by helices H2 and H3. The current three-

TABLE I
The Human ETS Gene Family[a]

Name	GenBank	Author	Locus	Size	ETS	Pointed
1 ETS1	J04101	Watson 1988	11q23.3	441	331–416	54–135
2 ETS2	J04102	Watson 1988	21q22.3	469	369–443	88–168
3 ERG2	M17254	Rao 1987	21q22.3	462	290–375	120–201
4 ELK1	M25269	Rao 1989	Xp11.2	428	7–92	None
5 SPI1(PU.1)	X52056	Ray 1990	11p11.2	264	168–240	None
6 FLI1(ERGB)	M98833	Watson 1992	11q24.1-q24.3	452	277–361	115–196
7 SAP1(ELK4)	M85165	Dalton 1992	1q32	431	4–89	None
8 ELF1	M82882	Thompson 1992	13q13	619	207–289	None
9 SPIB	X96998	Ray-Gallet 1992	19q13.3-q13.4	262	169–251	None
10 E4TF1(GABP)	D13318	Watanabe 1993	21q21-q22.1	454	318–400	171–249
11 E1AF(PEA3, ETV4)	D12765	Higashino 1993	17q21	462	315–399	None
12 PE1(ETV3)	L16464	Klemsz 1994	1q21-q23	250	56–140	None
13 ERM(ETV5)	X76184	Monte 1994	3q28	510	368–449	None
14 TEL(ETV6)	U11732	Golub 1994	12p13	452	340–419	38–119
15 NET(SAP2, ERP, ELK3)	Z36715	Giovane 1994	12q23	407	5–85	None
16 ERF	U15655	Sguoras 1995	19q13	548	26–106	None
17 ETV1(ER81)	X87175	Monte 1995	7p22	458	314–397	None
18 NERF2(ELF2)	U43188	Oettgen 1996	4q28	581	198–277	None
19 MEF(ELF4, ELFR, ER71)	U32645	Miyazaki 1996	Xq26	663	204–290	None
20 ESX(JEN, ESE1, ERT, ELF3)	AF110184	Chang 1997	1q32.2	371	275–354	47–132
21 FEV	Y08976	Peter 1997	2q23	238	43–126	None
22 EHF(ESE3)	AF170583	Kleinbaum 1999	11p12	300	209–288	42–112
23 ELF5(ESE2)	AF049703	Zhou 1999	11p14	255	165–243	46–115
24 PDEF(ESF,PSE)	AF071538	Oettgen 1999	6p21.3	335	248–332	138–211
25 TREF(TEL2)	AF147782	Smith 1999	6p21	264	149–228	49–114

[a]List of known human ETS genes, including gene name and alternative nomenclature, GenBank accession number, author and year of submission, chromosomal location, size of protein (amino acids), approximate boundaries of the Ets domain (85 amino acids), and approximate boundaries of the pointed domain (65–80 amino acids, if present).

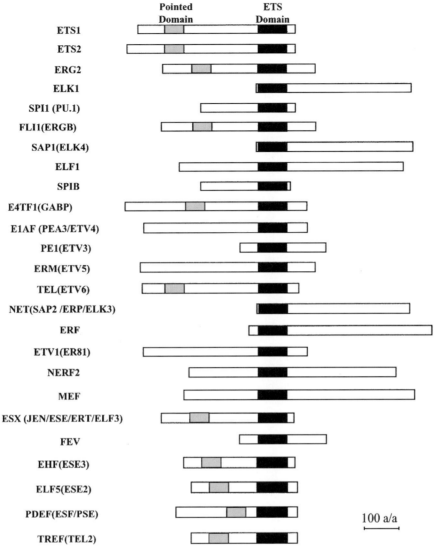

FIGURE 1 Structural organization of human ETS proteins. The ETS domain is indicated by the black box. The pointed domain is indicated by the light gray box.

dimensional models for PU.1 and ETS1 bound to DNA are quite similar. Two invariant arginine residues present in H3 make major groove contacts with the two guanine residues of the EBS (GGAA/T) core.

B. Pointed Domain

The second conserved domain found in a subset of ETS genes is the pointed domain, PNT. This 65–85 amino acid domain is found in 11 of the 25 human ETS genes and may function in protein–protein interaction. Nuclear magnetic resonance spectroscopy

analysis of this domain indicates that it forms an independent structure with the unique architecture of a monomeric five-helix bundle.

C. Autoinhibitory Domain

Deletion analysis demonstrated that DNA binding by the isolated ETS domain was more efficient than the full-length protein for several ETS family members (ETS1, ETS2, SAP1, ELK1, NET, FLI1, and ERM), consistent with a model that sequences present outside the ETS domain were inhibitory to DNA

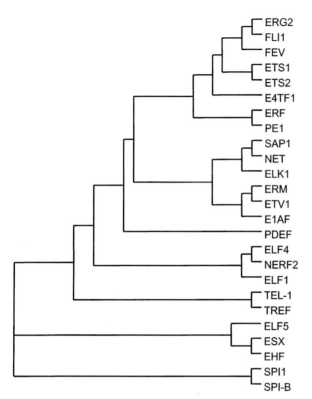

FIGURE 2 Dendrogram of the human ETS gene family. Phylogenetic tree based on multiple sequence alignment of the Ets (DNA-binding) domains of 25 human ETS proteins using CLUSTAL W 1.73 and TreeView 1.5.2.

binding. Structural studies of ETS1 suggest that this autoinhibition of DNA-binding activity is mediated by interactions between three α helixes located N-terminal and C-terminal to the ETS domain and the first helix of the ETS domain. Interestingly, a splice variant of ETS1 does not contain the N-terminal inhibitory domain. Phosphorylation-dependent inhibition of ETS1 DNA binding is mediated in part by stabilization of the inhibitory module.

III. DNA BINDING AND TRANSCRIPTIONAL ACTIVITY

A. Ets-Binding Site (EBS)

ETS proteins bind specific purine-rich DNA sequences with a core motif of 5'-GGAA/T-3'. The DNA consensus recognition sequence for several family members has been determined by *in vitro* selection of randomized oligonucleotides. However, ETS pro-

teins are often shown to interact *in vivo* with EBS sequences that do not conform to the consensus-binding site. Most ETS proteins bind to DNA as monomers; however, it has been shown that the DNA-binding activity is enhanced in the presence of other factors. Indeed, the binding of ETS proteins to subconsensus sequences is facilitated by the binding of other transacting factors to *cis* elements in proximity to the EBS.

B. Activators or Repressors of Transcription

While most ETS proteins function as positive regulators of gene transcription (transcriptional activators), some (e.g., ERF, TEL, NET) have negative effects on gene expression (transcriptional repressors).

IV. MODULATION OF ACTIVITY

A. Protein–Protein Interactions

Transcriptional regulation is dependent on the interactions of nuclear proteins. ETS proteins are able to form complexes with other transcription factors that have their DNA-binding sites adjacent to EBS. Depending on the precise sequence context, binding of an ETS protein near another transcription factor results in higher affinity interaction, synergistic activation, and/or repression of specific target genes. For example, the presence of both ETS1 and CBF proteins enhances the binding affinity for both proteins for the TcR α and β enhancers, resulting in synergistic activation. Similarly, PU.1 and Pip interact to enhance their binding to EBS/Pip sequences. Physical interaction of ETSl with GHF-1 is required for establishing lactotroph-specific PRL gene expression.

Interaction between ETS and other transcription factors also results in gene repression. MafB, an AP1-like protein, interacts with ETS1 in a DNA-dependent manner and inhibits ETS1-mediated transactivation of the transferrin receptor, which is known to be essential for erythroid differentiation. Similarly, ETS1 interacts with the Daxx protein, referred to as EAP1 (ETS1-associated protein 1)/Daxx, and this interaction represses transcriptional activation of model target genes (MMP1 and Bcl2). Interaction between CtBP and NET provides a bridge between NET and the histone deacetylase HDAC1. This recruitment of HDAC1 is a possible mechanism for transcriptional repression.

Multiple ETS proteins can interact with a single regulatory partner. Pax-5 functions as a cell-type-specific docking protein by which ETS1 binds to the early B-cell-specific mb-1 promoter. The functional significance of Pax-5 interaction with NET, ELK1, and FLI1 remains to be determined. Similarly, SRF forms ternary complexes with ELK1, SAP1, NET, EWS/FLI1, and FLI1. Several ETS proteins cooperate with the AP1 transcriptional complex to activate cellular responses by increasing the transcriptional activities of promoters containing AP1–EBS-binding sites. AP1 tethers ETS1 to the TIMP-1 promoter via protein–protein interaction to achieve ETS-dependent transcriptional activation. ETS proteins interact with components of the basal transcription complex. P300/CBP cooperates with ETS1 and ETS2 in the transcriptional activation of the human stromelysin promoter.

ETS family members are able to oligomerize or interact with other family members. GABPβ subunits mediate oligomerization and facilitate GABPα recognition of repeated GGA sequences. TEL is able to self-associate via the PNT domain.

B. Posttranslational Modification

ETS family transcription factors are among the end effector molecules of the signal transduction pathway. Phosphorylation of ETS modulates DNA binding, protein–protein interaction, transcriptional activation, and subcellular localization.

ETS1 is phosphorylated following antigen receptor ligand-induced calcium mobilization. Calcium-induced phosphorylation of ETS1 occurs at serine residues adjacent to the DNA-binding domain (ETS domain) and inhibits ETS1 DNA-binding activity without affecting nuclear localization. For example, in resting T cells, unphosphorylated ETS1 can bind DNA and regulate transcription from ETS-dependent promoters. After T-cell activation, phosphorylated ETS1 no longer can bind to DNA.

PU.1 is phosphorylated *in vitro* by casein kinase II and JNK kinase, but not by ERK1. Lipopolysaccharide activation of casein kinase II in macrophage cell lines leads to phosphorylation of a specific serine residue and increased transcriptional activity.

ERK, JNK, and p38 MAP kinases are downstream components of kinase cascades. ERKs are activated in response to mitogenic signals, whereas JNKs and p38/SAPKs (stress-activated protein kinases) respond to stress signals. Specific ETS factors are substrates for some or all of these signal transduction pathways. For example, ELK1 is a target for all three pathways. MAP kinase phosphorylation of ELK1 in its carboxyl-terminal transactivation domain leads to enhanced DNA binding and TCF transcriptional activity. SAP1, another TCF family member, is preferentially targeted by ERK and p38. ER81 and ERM appear to be targets of the Ras/Raf/MEK/ERK signaling cascade, whereas Spi-B is phosphorylated by ERKs and JNK. Phosphorylation of a mitogen-activated protein (MAP) kinase site adjacent to the PNT domain has been shown to positively regulate transcriptional activities of ETS1 and ETS2. MAP kinase phosphorylation of ETS1 does not affect DNA binding.

Phosphorylation can also affect the subcellular localization of ETS proteins. For example, the subcellular localization and function of ERF are controlled by the Ras/MAP kinase-mediated signal transduction pathway. Upon mitogenic stimulation, ERF is immediately phosphorylated and exported to the cytoplasm. Upon growth factor deprivation, ERF is rapidly dephosphorylated and transported back into the nucleus. Although NET is phosphorylated by ERK and p38, the subcellular localization of NET is controlled by the JNK pathway. In response to stress conditions, NET is excluded from the nucleus. It remains to be determined whether the export of NET is dependent on its own phosphorylation.

V. ONCOGENIC ACTIVATION

The involvement of ETS genes in cancer was first demonstrated by the presence of the Ets sequence in the oncogenic virus, E26. Their importance in human carcinogenesis is supported by the observations that ETS genes are located at translocation breakpoints, are chromosomally amplified or deleted, or have altered expression patterns in leukemias and solid tumors. Furthermore, ETS target genes (e.g., metallo-protease genes) contribute to oncogenesis and promote tumor invasiveness, cell migration, and metastasis, as well as angiogenesis.

A. Translocations

ETS genes can be translocated to new chromosomal positions in the absence of any apparent gene rearrangement. However, several chromosomal breakpoints result in hybrid ETS proteins that may be expressed in the wrong cell type, allowing for clonal expansion and tumor formation.

1. EWS/ETS Fusions

The t(11;22)(q24;q12) chromosomal translocation, detected in the majority of Ewing's sarcoma (ES) and primitive neuroectodermal tumors (PNET), fuses the amino terminus of the EWS gene to the carboxyl terminus of the FLI1 gene. In other ES and PNET tumors, translocations fuse the EWS gene to other members of the ETS family, including ERG [t(21;22)], ETV1 [t(7,22)], E1AF [t(17;22)], and FEV [t(2;22)]. These translocations result in the fusion of the promoter and transactivation domain of the EWS gene to the DNA-binding domain of an ETS gene. The EWS–FLI1 fusion protein is a more potent transcriptional activator than the FLI1 protein and, in contrast to FLI1, is a transforming gene. Both the transactivation domain of EWS and the ETS (DNA-binding) domain are required for transformation, and the transforming phenotype can be suppressed by blocking EWS–FLI1 production.

2. ERG/TLS

The t(16,21)(p11;q22) translocation fuses TLS-derived seqences to the carboxy-terminal half of ERG2 and is associated with several types of myeloid leukemias, including chronic myeloid leukemia (CML).

3. TEL Fusions

Either the PNT domain or the ETS domain of TEL, or both domains have been identified in specific translocations observed in cancer. Fusions involving the PNT domain of TEL often lead to oligomerization, which is necessary for the constitutive activation of kinase activity (e.g., PDGFRβ, ABL) and resultant transformation.

a. t(5;12)(q33;p13) results in the fusion of the PNT domain of TEL to PDGFRβ; associated with chronic myelomonocytic leukemias (CMML).

b. t(9;15;12) fusion of the PNT domain of TEL to JAK2; associated with CML.

c. Translocations that result in the fusion of the PNT domain of TEL to ABL [t(9;12)], JAK2 [t(9;12)], or AML1B [t(12;21)] are each associated with acute lymphoblastic leukemia (ALL).

d. t(4;12)(q11-q12;p13) has been associated with acute myeloid leukemia (AML-MO) and results in the expression of chimeric protein fusing BTL to both PNT and ETS domains of TEL.

e. t(12;22) fusion of the ets domain of TEL to MN1; associated with myeloid malignancy.

B. Chromosomal Amplification or Deletions

ETS family members have been amplified or deleted as the result of specific chromosomal changes. ETS1 and FLI1 are amplified in acute myeloid leukemia presenting with multiple abnormal and double minute chromosomes. ETS2 amplification has been observed in acute nonlymphoblastic leukemia [t(6;21;18)]. Congenital megakaryocytic maturation defects, as well as a mild hemorrhagic phenotype, have been found in individuals heterozygous for a chromosomal deletion that removes FLI1 and ETS1.

C. Elevated ETS Expression in Cancer

Elevated ETS1 expression has been observed in pancreatic cancer and thyroid tumors. ETS2 is expressed at elevated levels in hepatic, cervical, prostate, and breast cancer. ESX and PEA3 family members also have elevated expression in breast cancer. Significantly, ETS2 function is necessary for the transformed state in breast and prostate cancer cells. Furthermore, a single targeted Ets2 allele has been shown to restrict the development of mammary tumors in transgenic mice. Invasive and metastatic tissues express high levels of ETS1.

D. Altered Expression in Other Diseases

FLI1 and ETS1 have elevated expression in lymphocytes of patients with systemic lupus erythematosus, and ETS2 has elevated expression in rheumatoid arthritis.

VI. ETS GENE FUNCTION

Several approaches have been or can be used to define target genes that are unique to specific ETS proteins. Generation of transgenic, knockout, and mutant mice provides a means to determine the biological functions of specific ETS proteins and to identify target genes that are critical for these functions. They may also provide model systems for human diseases.

A. Identification of EBS Sequences in Target Genes

Identification of ETS targets is often initially based on the identification of GGAA/T core sequences in the promoters/enhancers of various cellular or viral regulatory regions. Subsequently, synthetic oligonucleotides containing potential EBS are used in electrophoretic mobility shift assays (EMSAs). Incubation of nuclear extracts with ETS antibodies (specific to a unique family member) is used to identify the ETS factor that potentially functions *in vivo*. Candidate ETS factors are also evaluated using transactivation assays using different ETS expression constructs together with reporter genes containing the prospective target genes EBS. Collectively, these studies demonstrate that ETS genes control the expression of genes associated with the following.

1. Cellular proliferation: p21, cyclins, and cyclin-dependent kinase.
2. Differentiation and development: homeobox genes and prolactin.
3. Hematopoiesis: cytokines and lineage-specific receptors.
4. Apoptosis: Bcl2 and caspase 1.
5. Metastasis and angiogenesis: MMPs, TIMP1, MET, PTHrP, VEGFR, and TIE2.
6. Transformation: viral promoters and enhancers.

B. Coexpression Studies

Identifying the specific ETS protein that controls specific ETS target genes can be accomplished by experimentally blocking or enhancing the expression of a specific gene and looking for genes that are suppressed or activated.

1. Loss of Function

For example, antisense block of ETS1 in T cells results in the increased production of IL-2, indicating that the ETS1 protein may be a negative regulator of this gene. The antisense approach has been used to demonstrate the importance of ETS1 in VEGF-induced endothelial cell migration, manifested by the upregulation of ETS target genes, including the urokinase plasminogen activator. Another approach for blocking ETS function is the expression of dominant interference vectors (express the ETS DNA-binding domain without the activation domain).

2. Gain of Function

Inducible expression of specific ETS genes allows correlation with altered expression of presumptive targets. ETS1, when expressed in model colon cancer cells, suppresses tumor formation and induces apoptosis.

C. Transgenic Mice

Overexpression of Ets2 in transgenic mice has been shown to cause skeletal abnormalities similar to those seen in Down's syndrome. This hypothesis is consistent with the location of human ETS2 on chromosome 21. Overexpression of Fli1 in all tissues of transgenic mice results in death from progressive immunological renal disease associated with an increased number of autoreactive T and B lymphocytes. PU.1 transgenic mice develop erythroleukemia, similar to that associated with retroviral activation of PU.1/Spi1.

D. Knockout Mice

Another experimental approach for identifying ETS targets is the creation of conditional null or mutant mice (knockout mice) lacking the function of a single or multiple family members. Analysis of these mice will allow for the identification of genes whose expression or repression is dependent on an ETS family member. To date, six Ets genes (PU.1, SpiB, Ets1, Ets2, Tel, and Fli1) have been targeted by homologous recombination. These gene-targeting studies demonstrate important roles for Ets genes in embryogenesis and hematopoiesis.

PU.1 $-/-$ mice die at embryonic day (E) 16.5, lacking lymphoid and myeloid cells, demonstrating that PU.1 has a role in the development of these lineages. SpiB $-/-$ mice are viable, but have defective B- and T-cell functions. Ets1$-/-$ mice are viable; the most dramatic phenotype is a marked reduction in natural killer (NK) and NK T cells, along with a moderate reduction in thymocyte number. T and B cells from Ets1-deficient mice display functional defects. Ets2$-/-$ mice die before E8.5, with extraembryonic defects. Tel $-/-$ mice die between E10.5 and E11.5 with defective yolk sac angiogenesis and intraembryonic apoptosis. Two different Fli1 mice have been generated by homologous recombination. One disruption of Fli1 resulted in a nonlethal phenotype, consisting of a reduced thymus size and a reduction in the total number of thymocytes. A second targeted disruption of Fli1 results in lethality before E12.5 with hemorrhage and impaired hematopoiesis.

In cases of embryonic lethality, targeted cell lines can be used for *in vitro* differentiation studies and for the generation of chimeric mice. For example, studies using Tel/chimeric mice demonstrated that Tel is required for hematopoiesis of all lineages in the bone marrow. The ability to rescue the phenotype of a specific knockout mouse by expression of the targeted gene can be used to test the function of specific domains of Ets proteins. For example, analyses of *in vitro* differentiation following the transgenic expression of PU.1 and PU.1 mutants in targeted PU.1 -/- ES cells allowed for the identification of specific domains required for myeloid development. In the future, a similar experimental approach can be used with the existing or new targeted cells.

See Also the Following Articles

Ewing's Sarcoma (Ewing's Family Tumors)

Bibliography

Ascione, R., Watson, D. K., and Papas, T. S. (1993). "Family of ETS Genes as Transcriptional Regulatory Factors." Academic Press, San Diego.

Bhat, N. K., Fischinger, P. F., Seth, A., Watson, D. K., and Papas, T. (1996). Pleiotropic functions of ETS-1. *Int. J. Oncol.* **8,** 841–846.

Crepieux, P., Coll, J., and Stehelin, D. (1994). The Ets family of proteins: Weak modulators of gene expression in quest for transcriptional partners. *Crit. Rev. Oncogen.* **5,** 615–638.

Dittmer, J., and Nordheim, A. (1998). Ets transcription factors and human disease. *Biochim. Biophys. Acta* **1377,** F1–F11.

Ghysdael, J., and Boureux, A. (1997). The ETS family of transcriptional regulators. *In* "Oncogenes as Transcriptional Regulators" (M. Yaniv and J. Ghysdael, eds., Vol. 1, pp. 29–88. Birkhauser Verlag, Basel.

Graves, B. J., and Petersen, J. M. (1998). Specificity within the ets family of transcription factors. *Adv. Cancer Res.* **75,** 1–55.

Janknecht, R., and Nordheim, A. (1993). Gene regulation by Ets proteins. *Biochim. Biophys. Acta* **1155,** 346–356.

Papas, T. S., Bhat, N. K., Spyropoulos, D. D., Mjaatvedt, A. E., Vournakis, J., Seth, A., and Watson, D. K. (1997). Functional relationships among ETS gene family members. *Leukemia* **11,** 557–566.

Sharrocks, A. D., Brown, A. L., Ling, Y., and Yates, P. R. (1997). The ETS-domain transcription factor family. *Int. J. Biochem. Cell Biol.* **29,** 1371–1387.

Wasylyk, B., Hagman, J., and Gutierrez-Hartmann, A. (1998). Ets transcription factors: nuclear effectors of the Ras-MAP-kinase signaling pathway. *Trends Biochem. Sci.* **23,** 213–216.

Watson, D. K., and Seth, A. (2000). Ets gene family. *Oncogene Rev.* **19,** 6393–6548.

Watson, D. K., Ascione, R., and Papas, T. S. (1990). Molecular analysis of the ets genes and their products. *Crit. Rev. Oncog.* **1,** 409–436.

Ewing's Sarcoma (Ewing's Family Tumors)

Timothy J. Triche

Keck School of Medicine at the University of Southern California

I. Introduction
II. Historical Aspects
III. Unique Clinical Behavior
IV. Biologic and Genetic Character
V. Current Understanding
VI. Future Directions

GLOSSARY

adult neuroblastoma A historical term used to describe Ewing's tumors of soft tissue with marked neural differentiation.

Askin tumor A pPNET of chest wall originally thought to be distinct from Ewing's, now recognized as a member of the same family of EFTs.

ERG The other major ets family gene commonly translocated (10+%) to EWS in EFTs.

EWS Unique gene cloned from the Ewing's fusion gene, now implicated in multiple malignancies.

ETS A family of oncogenes, including ERG and FLI-1, both of which are involved in the Ewing's translocation.

ETS domain The downstream (3′) region of highly conserved sequence homology in ETS family oncogenes, found in all Ewing's translocations.

FLI-1 The most common gene (85% of cases) fused with the Ewing's EWS gene in Ewing's tumors. Originally described as the genomic integration site for the Friend erythroleukemia virus.

gene translocation The physical union of two normally separate chromosomal fragments often resulting in the disruption or creation of novel genes.

peripheral neuroepithelioma Alternative term for neurally differentiated Ewing's tumors. No longer commonly used.

PNET Generic term for any undifferentiated tumor of brain or elsewhere with some degree of neural differentiation.

peripheral primitive neuroectodermal tumor (pPNET) An alternate term to describe all members of the Ewing's family of tumors.

transcription factor The ability of a gene, such as the Ewing's chimeric gene, EWS-FLI1, to control gene expression by physical binding to DNA.

Unique among human malignancies, Ewing's sarcoma is in fact an eponym attributed to James Ewing for his description in 1921 of a unique, nonosteogenic bone tumor of unknown histogenesis that displayed uncommon sensitivity to radiation therapy. The term is now only of historical interest but is retained to define what is now known to be a family of tumors with common molecular genetic and clinical characteristics. Retention of the term for over 80 years can be attributed to the historical confusion as to the nature of this tumor. The historical methods of diagnosing cancer, based largely on microscopic morphology, are of limited value in this seemingly undifferentiated malignancy. Advances in tumor biology, especially the advent of molecular genetic analysis, have clarified the origin, etiology, and relationships of this enigmatic tumor. Instead of an unusual, radiosensitive bone tumor as originally described, it is now recognized that Ewing's sarcoma is just one of a number of malignancies of bone and soft tissue occurring in almost any anatomic location that all share a common genetic abnormality and treatment responsiveness. For that reason, current opinion groups all these tumors of diverse historical name under the all-encompassing term Ewing's family tumors (EFTs). As a result, optimized, uniform therapy and objective distinction from other morphologically undifferentiated "round cell tumors" are now possible. Recognition that these tumors are all to a greater or lesser degree neuroectodermal in character gave rise to the alternative nomenclature, peripheral primitive neuroectodermal tumor (pPNET), originally intended to distinguish these primitive neuroectodermal tumors from the fundamentally distinct PNETs of the central nervous system. To both recognize the historical origins of this tumor, while recognizing its diverse clinical and pathologic presentations, the overarching term Ewing's family tumors enjoys broad acceptance as the preferred terminology to describe this tumor entity.

I. INTRODUCTION

All common human malignancies are now described on the basis of the presumed normal tissue counterpart thought to have undergone malignant degeneration. Thus, almost all adult cancer is carcinoma, or epithelially derived. This, coupled with an organ or tissue origin, leads to the common nomenclature "breast carcinoma," or "ductal carcinoma of breast," true of almost all adult malignancies. In childhood

cancer, a few eponyms survive, such as Wilms' tumor, although the equivalent diagnosis, nephroblastoma, correctly describing this as a tumor of renal developmental origin, is universally recognized. Ewing's tumor, or Ewing's sarcoma (connoting a belief that the tumor arises from mesoderm, like other sarcomas), is the rare if not sole exception to this trend of incorporating developmental or tissue origin terms in the diagnostic terminology used to categorize human tumors. This ambiguity reflects the fact that until recently there has been insufficient knowledge of the origins and character of this tumor to invoke a comparably specific diagnosis. This has now changed, as all EFTs are believed to derive from mesenchymal cells and can occur in virtually any anatomic site where such mesenchymal tissues are found, including bone and soft tissue. As such, the term "sarcoma" would be suitable, but the now documented neuroectodermal character of this tumor family encourages the term "Ewing's family tumor" instead. This appears to be widely accepted and is the preferred inclusive term used to encompass the various members of the tumor group, discussed in some detail later.

II. HISTORICAL ASPECTS

In 1921, the eminent pathologist James Ewing published the first known paper describing a unique bone tumor that showed little if any evidence of morphologic differentiation (Fig. 1a).

Ewing described this tumor as an endothelioma of bone, but 8 years later published a second paper describing the tumor as an "endothelial myeloma," a somewhat mystifying concept now but entirely acceptable then, as a distinction between vascular structures (endothelial cells) and hematopoietic cells (myeloid and lymphoid cells) was unclear. From the outset this tumor entity has been marked by ambiguity and confusion, as noted rather outspokenly in 1940 by Rupert Willis, a contemporary and critic of Ewing, who claimed that all Ewing's tumors were in fact only metastatic neuroblastoma, creating thereby a "Ewing's syndrome." Although incorrect in his assertion, Willis was the first to draw attention to the neural or neuroepithelial character of the tumor (Fig. 1b), a point that was unappreciated for the next

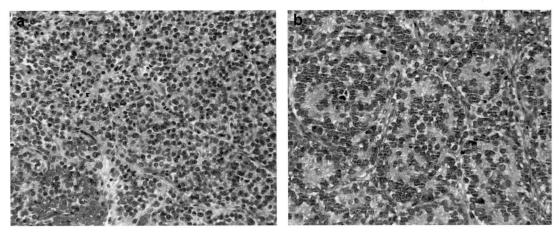

FIGURE 1 (a) Typical undifferentiated histology of Ewing's tumor. Note the lack of any identifying histology or unique cytology. Prominent vascularity is evident. Hematoxylin and eosin. Nominal magnification: ×250. (b) "Neural" histology area of the same tumor. Note the obvious pseudo-rosettes responsible for the various neural eponyms ascribed to this tumor. Hematoxylin and eosin stain. Nominal magnification: ×250.

50 years. At about the same time, Arthur Purdy Stout, working with Margaret Murray, described a "neuroepithelioma" of the ulnar nerve that grew in tissue culture with characteristics of neural cells, but which Stout believed represented something apart from conventional neuroblastoma. This concept was in fact correct, and only 40 years later was it united with the neuroectodermal character of Ewing's "endothelioma of bone" and Willis' "Ewing's syndrome" of metastatic neuroblastoma.

Unfortunately, from the 1940s until the 1980s, little progress in the understanding of the basic biology of this unusual tumor was made, although a uniquely abundant content of glycogen, detectable by a conventional PAS stain, was noted by Schajowicz, a prominent bone pathologist, in 1959. Even the advent of diagnostic electron microscopy, which promised to elucidate the tissue origins of virtually all human tumors, failed to detect any fine structural evidence of cell or tissue differentiation in this highly undifferentiated tumor. As a result, most authors resorted to a diagnosis of exclusion: if no features of a known tumor entity could be found, the tumor by default became a Ewing's tumor of bone. This ambiguity was further extended in 1975, when Angervall and Enzinger described a soft tissue counterpart to Ewing's of bone, soon to be known as "extraosseous Ewing's."

The situation became even more confusing with the description in 1979 of the "malignant small cell tumor of the thoracopulmonary region in childhood," commonly termed "Askin tumor," based on the last name of the first author. This tumor, initially described as distinct from Ewing's tumor of bone, was in fact morphologically indistinguishable from Ewing's, but was reported to lack the PAS positivity (due to large cytoplasmic pools of glycogen) normally found in conventional Ewing's tumor of bone. Further, a female predominance and chest wall predilection were also noted. In an interesting observation, three cases were noted to have electron microscopic features suggestive of neural differentiation. Thus, for the first time, variable evidence of neural differentiation was noted in a tumor otherwise indistinguishable from Ewing's sarcoma of bone. Further, a bone versus soft tissue origin was not even certain, given the large size of the tumor at diagnosis in most cases, coupled with a combined bone and soft tissue involvement. Thus, a common theme true of bone and soft tissue versions of a seemingly identical tumor, with suspected neural differentiation, was becoming apparent. This same time frame witnessed the widespread adoption of immunohistochemistry as a diagnostic tool in pathology. When a quite specific marker for Ewing's was described, the MIC2 gene product (now termed CD99), it quickly became apparent that all suspected members of the family were in fact positive for CD99, adding further substance to the suspicion that all shared a common character if not origin.

Biologic studies of ordinary Ewing's tumors from bone in the 1980s clearly established the potential for any Ewing's tumor to undergo spontaneous or induced neural differentiation *in vitro*. Thus, a tissue character could now be reliably ascribed to all Ewing's tumors. Further analysis revealed in addition, however, that certain fundamental differences between this neural differentiation and that found in primitive brain tumors (where neuronal and glial differentiation are commonly observed) or common sympathetic nervous system tumors in children (e.g., neuroblastoma) were uniformly present, thus distinguishing Ewing's tumors from neuroblastoma. Thus, Willis' contention was clearly refuted (although in fact by the 1980s the unique, nonmetastatic origin of Ewing's was well established) and a separate category for these tumors was identified. To distinguish these neural tumors from the common neuroblastoma, various terms were introduced, such as "adult neuroblastoma," "peripheral neuroblastoma," and "peripheral neuroepithelioma," used in deference to Stout's original description of a peripheral nerve tumor he felt was distinct from neuroblastoma. In reality, the Ewing's group of tumors is not known to occur as peripheral nerve sheath tumors, but the nomenclature did serve to create a separate treatment category, itself an important event, as discussed later.

III. UNIQUE CLINICAL BEHAVIOR

From the outset, as illustrated in Ewing's original paper, it was recognized that Ewing's sarcoma, unlike its more common bone tumor counterpart, osteosarcoma, was inordinately radiosensitive. Impressive reductions in tumor mass, if not apparent complete ablation, were routinely obtained, yet the patients almost invariably recurred and died. The net effect for over 40 years was an overall survival rate approximating 9%.

This dismal prognosis spurred great interest in the potential use of systemic chemotherapy once its success in another dreary childhood malignancy, leukemia, was demonstrated in the 1960s and early 1970s. Commencing in the 1970s at the National Cancer Institute and subsequently in trials sponsored by national cooperative group studies (Intergroup Ewing's Sarcoma Study, IESS), systemic chemotherapy

(e.g., vincristine, dactinomycin, cytoxan, and, in some cases, doxorubicin) was added to radiation therapy of the primary lesion as front-line, multimodality treatment of this disease, with remarkable success; 5-year survivals for patients with localized disease rose to 50% or better. In particular, in the intergroup studies it was noted that the addition of doxorubicin to VAC therapy conferred a significant survival advantage. Notably, the role of surgery was limited to biopsy for confirmation of diagnosis. Subsequent refinements in treatment protocols, including the introduction of intermittent high-dose therapy (IESS II) and the agents etoposide + ifosfamide (IESS III) have improved 5-year survival for patients with localized disease (>70%), but long-term survival remains close to 50% for patients overall due to the lack of any improvement in survival among patients with metastatic disease (~20% 5-year relapse-free survival).

Ewing's remains the most clearly radiosensitive tumor of children and young adolescents, yet it is also by definition "micrometastatic" (i.e., nonlocalized) at presentation in virtually all cases (otherwise, surgery or localized radiation therapy should be curative, but are not). Given this clinical presentation and situation, it clearly becomes desirable to be able to assess the persistence of disease and overall tumor burden. Fortunately, this is now possible due to the existence of a highly specific gene translocation virtually unique to this tumor, to be discussed later. At the same time, this chimeric gene, EWS-FLI1 or equivalent, may offer new immunotherapy opportunities, a possibility now being evaluated in clinical trials.

IV. BIOLOGIC AND GENETIC CHARACTER

Unraveling the enigma of Ewing's "sarcoma" has benefited greatly from advances in cytogenetics, molecular biology, and the elucidation of the human genome. Seventy years of intense scrutiny by other methods failed to elucidate the origins of this tumor, yet in just the past 20 years cytogenetic and molecular genetic analyses have largely resolved the issue. It is now apparent that the Ewing's family of tumors nearly always results from a critical gene fusion, and the resulting chimeric tumor gene is likely responsible, in the proper setting, for both malignant transformation and tumor phenotype.

A. Cytogenetic Studies

In 1983, two groups, headed by Turc-Carel and Aurias, described a recurring cytogenetic abnormality in Ewing's tumors. This previously undescribed translocation resulted from chromosomal breakage and fusion involving the long arms of chromosomes 11 and 22. The t(11;22)(q24;q12) translocation was noted in about 85% of cases by Turc-Carel and subsequently confirmed by many other authors. A detailed example of chromosomes 11 and 22 is seen in Fig. 2.

Cytogenetic and molecular genetic studies of apparently related tumors (as discussed previously) confirmed a putative relationship, at least based on a common, unique t(11;22) translocation that results in the fusion of a novel gene on chromosome 22, termed EWS, to a known gene, FLI1, on chromosome 11. In fact, virtually all of the suspected relatives have subsequently been shown to have the identical translocation in the majority of cases, like Ewing's itself.

Subsequent to detailed molecular genetic analyses described later, and inspired thereby, four additional Ewing's translocations have been described: (1) the t(21;22), which fuses the EWS gene to ERG, another ETS gene family member; (2) an uncommon t(7;22) that fuses EWS to another Ets domain-containing gene, ETV1; (3) a very uncommon variant t(17;22) that fuses EWS to E1AF (also known as ETV4 or

PEA3); and (4) a rare t(2;22) that fuses EWS to yet another ETS family member, FEV (albeit with a truncated carboxy-terminal domain). Even greater complexity arises at the genomic level due to variable exon usage by even the common EWS-FLI1 chimeric gene, resulting in many variants, depending on which exons of EWS 3′ to exon 7 are used in conjunction with exon 5′ to exon 9 of FLI1, which encodes the mandatory ETS domain.

All variants of the EWS-ETS gene are thought to be functionally similar, as all result in a similar structural motif: the 5′ amino-terminal portion of EWS fused to the 3′ carboxy-terminal portion of an Ets family member, always containing an intact 85 amino acid ETS DNA-binding domain encoded by the particular ETS family member involved in the translocation. This generic structure is illustrated in Fig. 3 using combinatorial variants of EWS and the most common partner, FLI1, as an example. The resultant chimeric protein is known to be a potent transactivating transcription factor, although the specific targets and mechanism of control of gene expression are only incompletely understood.

B. Molecular Genetics

The most significant event in the definition and understanding of this tumor family has been the initial cloning of the EWS-FLI1 fusion gene by DeLattre

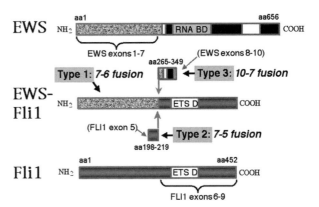

FIGURE 3 Schematic diagram of the common EWS and FLI1 fusion variants found in all Ewing's tumors. Note that EWS always includes the 5′ transactivation domain (black) and may include some 3′ RNA-binding domain (e.g., type 3). Fli1 always contributes an intact ETS DNA-binding domain, required for transforming activity of the chimeric gene.

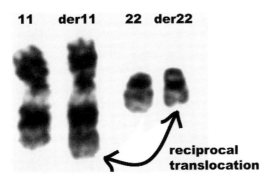

FIGURE 2 Chromosome pairs 11 and 22 from an Ewing's tumor. The left of each is normal; the right is the derivative (e.g., translocated) partner. Note additional chromosomal material on the long arm of 11 and the loss of the same on der22.

and co-workers. This singular event has served to define this tumor family based on its molecular genetic character, with consequences for its diagnosis, prognosis, therapy, and basic understanding of oncogenesis, at least as it relates to this tumor system.

The EWS gene remains enigmatic, despite years of study. Although a member of a family of RNA-binding genes, the RNA-binding region (RBD) of the normal EWS protein is substituted by an ETS gene DNA-binding domain in the resultant chimeric gene (as illustrated in Fig. 3). This suggests that the normal RNA-binding function of EWS is not relevant to its role in the malignant transformation in Ewing's tumors. The ubiquitous expression of EWS in virtually all cells may be the more important factor, as EWS is fused 5′ to the ETS gene in all tumors, thereby leading to ubiquitous expression of the chimeric gene. Further, the included 5′ region contains a potent transcriptional transactivation domain, EAD, which is necessary for transformation. Recently, however, it has been noted that the 3′ RBD not only binds RNA, but *cis* represses the *trans*-activating function of the 5′ EAD, therein providing a clue to the oncogenicity of EWS-FLI1 compared to EWS alone. However, it would be incorrect to assume that this alone explains the role of EWS in Ewing's tumors, especially since numerous other functions, including interference of the chimeric gene with RNA polymerase II-mediated RNA splicing and even cell surface (as opposed to nuclear localization), have been documented.

Both the chimeric EWS-ETS gene and the normal EWS gene appear to be expressed at high levels in virtually all tissues. Thus, high levels of expression of the tumor-specific EWS-FLI1 or equivalent gene are expected and observed. It is reasonable to expect that overexpression of the chimeric gene might likely result in oncogenic conversion of the host cell, but simple expression of the chimeric gene against a normal cellular background is not sufficient, as demonstrated by many authors. Further, apparent loss of the chimeric gene in some tumors has not necessarily resulted in curtailed malignancy, although enhanced neural differentiation has been observed.

Prior to its association with Ewing's tumors, FLI1 had been known primarily as a somewhat obscure gene that appeared to provide a preferred integration site for the Friend erythroleukemia virus, leading to the development of erythroleukemia in mice. No role in human cancer had been identified until DeLattre's work, although ongoing work had identified normal FLI1 as a naturally occurring member of the large ETS family of oncogenes. The ETS oncogenes were historically well known in human cancer due to the association of ETS-1 on chromosome 11 with the t(4;11) translocation found in acute myelogenous leukemia. As noted earlier, all members of the ETS family possess a conserved sequence, 3′ or downstream of the usual translocation breakpoint, termed the ETS domain. ETS proteins uniformly include this sequence, which imparts DNA-binding ability in a sequence-specific manner (i.e., NNNNGGAANNNN). These genes as a group are known to be nuclear transcription factors; the chimeric EWS-FLI1 gene likewise is known to be a potent transcription factor. Many potential target sequences for normal ETS genes have been identified, but to date the full complex of genes affected by the Ewing's chimeric EWS-ETS chimeric transcription factor and, more importantly, the pathways by which it induces malignant transformation have yet to be identified, although some unusual patterns of gene activation have been documented. None appear to be directly responsible for the oncogenesis uniformly associated with the presence of an expressed EWS-ETS chimeric transcription factor in tumors, but intriguing mechanisms of transformation via signal transduction pathways have been postulated.

C. Biologic Studies

Although the exact pathway by which the chimeric EWS-ETS protein elicits malignant transformation of a cell remains unknown, there is nonetheless compelling biologic evidence that expression of the chimeric gene is fundamentally important to the etiology of Ewing's tumors. Evidence for this comes from at least three sets of observations.

In the first, transfection of normal NIH/3T3 cells with an EWS-FLI1 gene construct results in loss of substrate adherence, a transformed phenotype, and formation of large tumors in nude mouse xenografts, all accepted evidence of malignant transformation. Unfortunately, efforts to replicate these results in normal human cells have been unsuccessful.

The second line of evidence for the transforming ability of the usual chimeric gene derives from parallel studies. When the ETS domain of FLI1 is deleted from the construct, no transformation is observed. Thus, evidence to date indicates that the ETS DNA-binding domain is mandatory for tumorigenesis. These results are of particular interest, as they provide a logical explanation for the fact that although breakpoints are highly variable and transcript sizes are accordingly variable (resulting in at least six common transcripts and corresponding chimeric proteins), *all* occur upstream of the ETS domain. This results in the incorporation of an intact ETS domain in the resultant chimeric genes and their protein translation products.

Evidence for a causal role of the chimeric EWS-ETS gene and its expressed protein also comes from studies in which RNA antisense inhibition of EWS-FLI1 transcription in Ewing's cells, but not control neuroblastoma cells, resulted in markedly diminished EWS-FLI1 expression and cell mitotic activity. The effect on tumorigenesis remains undefined, however.

D. Specificity of the EWS-ETS Gene Translocation to Ewing's

The apparent specificity of EWS-ETS to Ewing's tumors has led to its widespread use as the mandatory minimum requirement for a diagnosis. Various methods have been employed, including polymerase chain reaction (PCR) amplification of complementary DNA transcripts generated from expressed mRNA (e.g., RT-PCR) and fluorescent *in situ* hybridization (FISH). An example of the latter is illustrated in Fig. 4. Any tumor lacking confirmation of an EWS-ETS chimeric gene is highly suspect as a EFT. Only rare exceptions to this rule, if they exist at all, have been reported.

Although rearrangement of the EWS gene with a member of the ETS family of oncogenes was initially uniquely associated with Ewing's tumors, rearrangement of the EWS gene with other genes is widely recognized in diverse sarcomas, and even the occasional leukemia. On the contrary, at least five other variants have now been described in melanoma of soft parts, the desmoplastic round cell tumor of peritoneum, liposarcoma, chondrosarcoma, and leukemia, always between EWS or its equivalent, TLS (for translocated

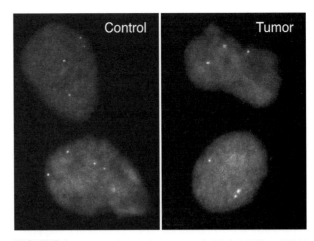

FIGURE 4 FISH analysis with fluorescently labeled EWS and FLI1 DNA probes. The two control nuclei show two red and two green signals, as expected. The tumor nuclei show one red, one green, and one fused red–green pair, indicative of an EWS-FLI1 fusion in both nuclei. DAPI-stained nuclei. Digitally enlarged images from 35-mm slide originals. Nominal magnification: >3000.

in liposarcoma) fused 5′ to a known oncogene, and thereby replacing the normal EWS RBD with a DNA BD derived from the 3′-fused oncogene partner. Liposarcoma has been found to have translocations involving both TLS and EWS. This is summarized in Table I, where EWS or TLS is listed with its partner, along with the associated tumor name and description.

Ideally, the EWS-ETS translocation effectively serves to diagnose Ewing's/pPNETs. However, although all members of this family of tumors possess this chimeric gene, it may not be limited to this group of tumors only. Recent observations of the EWS-ETS

TABLE I

Tumor	Fusion gene	Description
Ewing's tumors	EWS-ETS	Neuroectodermal tumor
Melanoma of soft parts	EWS-ATF1	Melanoma (deep soft tissue)
Desmoplastic small cell tumor	EWS-WT1	Rare polyphenotypic tumor
Myxoid liposarcoma	EWS or TLS-CHOP	Sarcoma of adipose tissue
Myxoid chondrosarcoma	EWS-CHN	Extraskeletal cartilage
Myelogenous leukemia	TLS-ERG	t(16;21) + leukemia

translocation in tumors, which at least appear to be unrelated to Ewing's tumors in general, mandate a broader purview. Studies by several authors have now confirmed the presence of the EWS-ETS fusion gene in rhabdomyogenic tumors, most diagnosed as either embryonal or alveolar rhabdomyosarcoma, or occasionally as polyphenotypic tumors with rhabdomyogenic and neurogenic phenotype, generally termed malignant ectomesenchymoma historically but "biphenotypic tumor" in current terminology.

If one accepts the thesis that the specific gene translocations here as elsewhere are strongly correlated with specific tumor phenotypes, then the presence of the Ewing's translocation in a tumor morphologically distinct from Ewing's does not necessarily convey nonspecificity, particularly if the tumor in question displays a neuroectodermal phenotype similar to that found in Ewing's as one component of the tumor's phenotype. Such has been the case to date with all tumors carrying an EWS-ETS fusion gene. Various morphologic, biochemical, and gene expression analyses have demonstrated at least a minimal neuroectodermal phenotype in each. Thus, the more correct interpretation may be that Ewing's is neural in character in part *because* of the EWS-ETS translocation, although this remains to be confirmed.

E. Genetic Determinants of Prognosis

Although localized versus disseminated disease is the strongest single predictor or outcome in Ewing's patients, there is a clear-cut need for more precise determinants of likely outcome among even non-metastatic patients, who currently enjoy an estimated 70+% survival rate; conversely, nearly one-third still die. The recent advances in our understanding of the molecular genetic basis of this disease, coupled with an appreciation of a unifying theme underlain by remarkable molecular genetic heterogeneity, have suggested that differential clinical behavior might be related to specific molecular genotypes.

The primary focus of studies in both Europe and the United States to date has been the relationship, if any, between fusion type and outcome. Although there seems to be no significant difference between EWS-FLI1 and EWS-ERG fusions, there is a statistically significant difference in outcome among sub-

groups of EWS-FLI1 patients. As noted previously, variable exon usage leads to various genotypes of the EWS-F:I1 fusion gene; the most common, type 1, fuses exon 7 of EWS with exon 6 of FLI1. The next most common, type 2, includes an additional exon, 5, from FLI1. When compared for their transactivational potency, type 1 fusions are weaker. Clinically, patients with type 1 chimeric genes show improved survival when compared to nontype 1 chimeric genes.

Additional genetic determinants of prognosis have also been studied, with lesser prognostic import. Notably, although INK4A (p16), ARF(p14), INK4B, and p53 homozygous deletions or mutations are associated with poor outcome, the predictive power of these alterations is often dependent on covariates such as type of therapy. Nonetheless, larger prospective studies may yet validate these preliminary observations.

V. CURRENT UNDERSTANDING

The current state of knowledge with regard to the Ewing's family of tumors has clearly advanced markedly in the past several years, from an enigmatic, ill-understood eponymic entity to a surprisingly common malignancy of children, adolescents, and young adults. In the process, it has emerged as a genetically defined malignancy, rare (until recently) among human malignancies. It has also offered thereby an unprecedented opportunity to study and understand the basic mechanisms of malignant transformation in a well-defined tumor system. Despite this, the mechanisms, although better understood, still defy simple explanation. For example, simple transfection of normal human cells with the EWS-FLI1 gene fails to induce malignant transformation; in fact, progressive cell death is observed instead. Clearly, fundamental understanding of the process whereby this gene induces cancer remains to be determined.

Concomitant with this progress, reliable objective critera to define the tumor have been defined: at this point, it appears that a putative Ewing's family tumor *must* display rearrangement of the EWS gene and demonstrate fusion with a known or novel member of the ETS family of oncogenes. Beyond this, other less homogeneous and undifferentiated tumors may also show rearrangement of EWS, but when this occurs with another gene than ETS, a distinctly different tumor results, as noted in Table I. Conversely, when EWS-ETS occurs within a more differentiated tumor, such as rhabdomyosarcoma, it appears that the tumor will routinely demonstrate neuroectodermal as well as rhabdomyogenic differentiation.

These points lead to a simplistic but reasonable conclusion, commensurate with the data presented earlier: Ewing's tumors in general are defined by the EWS-ETS fusion gene, but this gene may occur in other malignancies as well. This still allows for the use of EWS-ETS fusion as a necessary criterion for the diagnosis of Ewing's tumors, but also implies that the tumor must be morphologically commensurate with that diagnosis, as illustrated in Fig. 1. Given these criteria, it is possible to rule out a diagnosis as well as rule in (with suitable morphologic and immunochemical confirmation) any suspected case of Ewing's family tumor.

VI. FUTURE DIRECTIONS

The availability of a ubiquitous tumor-specific marker in EFTs allows for several specific tools to diagnose and therefore treat the malignancy. At a bare minimum, molecular diagnostic methods can identify and confirm the presence of the tumor-specific gene translocation, thereby establishing a diagnosis beyond any reasonable doubt. This has already led to remarkable reproducibility of diagnosis for a tumor that historically had an abysmal misdiagnosis rate.

Beyond diagnosis, PCR can be beneficially used to identify and quantify residual tumor in bone marrow or circulating blood cells, using quantitative PCR. Studies of peripheral blood have readily detected tumor cells, but have not necessarily predicted metastasis or outcome. Bone marrow studies appear to be more reliable predictors of future course, but this will require more definitive study. If valid, such information could allow more rational decisions regarding continuation or cessation of therapy, not to mention occult relapse during apparent clinical remission.

In the future, it appears likely that the reliable presence of such tumor-specific abnormalities may be used

to therapeutic advantage in several ways. For example, because tumor cells have been shown to present EWS-ETS fusion protein on their cell surface, specific cell-mediated immunotherapy, as is currently being evaluated, might be efficacious. Further, specific gene targets of the EWS-ETS chimeric gene may be targeted for therapy, or EWS-ETS itself may be manipulated. Perhaps most likely, the downstream targets that represent approachable targets, such as signal transduction pathways, known to be widely used by ETS family genes to affect their biological activity, may represent practical therapeutic targets. Finally, the increasing evidence that Ewing's tumors display and utilize a variety of growth factors and their receptors may represent the most practical targets, analogous to HER2 in breast cancer. In this regard, it is interesting to note that Ewing's tumor cells allegedly express high levels of HER2 protein and that downregulation of HER2 greatly increases their sensitivity to topoisomerase II-targeted drugs, such as VP-16 and adriamycin, both known to be highly efficacious in this disease.

Regardless of the specific gene targeted or the specific mechanism to be interdicted, it seems likely that future advances in the therapy of this disease will be based on a better understanding of the fundamental biologic processes whereby the chimeric gene unique to this tumor eventuates in malignancy. As such, Ewing's family tumors are a paradigm of the widespread belief that tumors in the future will be classified based on their molecular characteristics and that this information will be used to tailor therapy, often directed at specific gene targets, likely in parallel with conventional therapy. Improvement in the outcome for patients with localized disease will be desirable; it remains to be seen whether this will favorably impact the currently dismal outcome for those with metastatic disease.

See Also the Following Articles

Ataxia Telangiectasia Syndrome • Bone Tumors • Brain Tumors: Epidemiology and Molecular and Cellular Abnormalities • ETS Family of Transcription Factors • Genetic Alterations in Brain Tumors • Neuroblastoma • Pediatric Cancers, Molecular Features • Sarcomas of Soft Tissue • Wilms Tumor: Epidemiology

Bibliography

Angervall, L., and Enzinger, F. (1975). Extraskeletal neoplasm resembling Ewing's sarcoma. *Cancer* **36,** 240–251.

Arndt, C. A., and Crist, W. M. (1999). Common musculoskeletal tumors of childhood and adolescence. *N. Engl. J. Med.* **341,** 342–352.

Askin, F. B., Rosai, J., Sibley, R. K., Dehner, L. P., and McAlister, W. H. (1979). Malignant small cell tumor of the thoracopulmonary region in childhood. *Cancer* **43,** 2438–2451.

Aurias, A., Rimbaut, C., Buffe, D., Dubousset, J., and Mazabraud, A. (1983). Chromosomal translocations in Ewing's sarcoma. *N. Engl. J. Med.* **309,** 496–497.

Belyanskaya, L. L., Gehrig, P. M., and Gehring, H. (2001). Exposure on cell surface and extensive arginine methylation of ewing sarcoma (EWS) protein. *J. Biol. Chem.* **276,** 18681–18687.

Cavazzana, A. O., Miser, J. S., Jefferson, J., and Triche, T. J. (1987). Experimental evidence for a neural origin of Ewing's sarcoma of bone. *Am. J. Pathol.* **127,** 507–518.

Dahlin, D. C., Coventry, M. B., and Scanlon, P. W. (1961). Ewing's sarcoma: A critical analysis of 165 Cases. *J. Bone Joint Surg.* **43-A,** 185–192.

de Alava, E., and Gerald, W. L. (2000). Molecular biology of the Ewing's sarcoma/primitive neuroectodermal tumor family. *J. Clin. Oncol.* **18,** 204–213.

Dehner, L. P. (1986). Peripheral and central primitive neuroectodermal tumors: A nosologic concept seeking a consensus. *Arch. Pathol. Lab. Med.* **110,** 997–1004.

Delattre, O., Zucman, J., Melot, T., Garau, X. S., Zucker, J.-M., Lenoir, G. M., Ambros, P. F., Sheer, D., Turc-Carel, C., Triche, T. J., Aurias, A., and Thomas, G. (1994). The Ewing family of tumors: A subgroup of small-round-cell tumors defined by specific chimeric transcripts. *N. Engl. J. Med.* **331,** 294–299.

Delattre, O., Zucman, J., Ploustagel, B., Desmaze, C., Melot, T., Peter, M., Kovar, H., Joubert, I., de Jong, P., Rouleau, G., Aurias, A., and Thomas, G. (1992). Gene fusion with an ETS DNA binding domain caused by chromosome translocation in human cancers. *Nature* **359,** 162–165.

Ewing, J. (1921). Diffuse endothelioma of bone. *Proc. N. Y. Pathol. Soc.* **21,** 17–24.

Ewing, J., (1924). Further report on endothelial myeloma of bone. *Proc. N. Y. Pathol. Soc.* **24,** 17–24.

Glaubiger, D., Makuch, R., and Schwartz, J. (1981). Influence of prognostic factors on survival in Ewing's sarcoma. *In* "Sarcomas of Soft Tissue and Bone in Childhood," Vol. 56, pp. 285–288. NCI, Bethesda.

Jeon, I.-S., Davis, J. N., Braun, B. S., Sublett, J. E., Roussel, M. F., Denny, C. T., and Shapiro, D. N. (1995). A variant Ewing's sarcoma translocation (7;22) fuses the EWS gene to the ETS gene *ETV1. Oncogene* **10,** 1229–1234.

Knezevich, S. R., Hendson, G., Mathers, J. A., Carpenter, B., Lopez-Terrada, D., Brown, K. L., and Sorensen, P. H. (1998). Absence of detectable EWS/FLI1 expression after therapy-induced neural differentiation in Ewing sarcoma. *Hum. Pathol.* **29,** 289–294.

Li, K. K., and Lee, K. A. (2000). Transcriptional activation by the Ewing's sarcoma (EWS) oncogene can be cis-repressed by the EWS RNA-binding domain. *J. Biol. Chem.* **275,** 23053–23058.

Mackall, C., Berzofsky, J., and Helman, L. J. (2000). Targeting tumor specific translocations in sarcomas in pediatric patients for immunotherapy. *Clin. Orthop.* 25–31.

May, W. A., Gishizky, M. L., Lessnick, S. L., Lunsford, L. B., Lewis, B. C., Delattre, O., Zucman, J., Thomas, G., and Denny, C. T. (1993). Ewing sarcoma 11;22 translocation produces a chimeric transcription factor that requires the DNA-binding domain encoded by FLI1 for transformation. *Proc. Natl. Acad. Sci. USA* **90,** 5752–5756.

Nesbit, M. E., Jr., Gehan, E. A., Burgert, E. O., Jr., Vietti, T. J., Cangir, A., Tefft, M., Evans, R., Thomas, P., Askin, F. B., Kissane, J. M., *et al.* (1990). Multimodal therapy for the management of primary, nonmetastatic Ewing's sarcoma of bone: A long-term follow-up of the first intergroup study. *J. Clin. Oncol.* **8,** 1664–1674.

Peter, M., Couturier, J., Pacquement, H., Michon, J., Thomas, G., Magdelenat, H., and Delattre, O. (1997). A new member of the ETS family fused to EWS in Ewing tumors. *Oncogene* **14,** 1159–1164.

Schajowicz, F. (1959). Ewing's sarcoma and reticulum-cell sarcoma of bone. *J. Bone Joint Surg.* **41-A,** 349–356.

Sorensen, P. H. B., Lessnick, S. L., Lopez-Terrada, D., Liu, X. F., Triche, T. J., and Denny, C. T. (1994). A second Ewing's sarcoma translocation, t(21;22), fuses the EWS gene to another ETS-family transcription factor, ERG. *Nature Genet.* **6,** 146–151.

Stout, A. P., and Murray, M. R. (1942). Neuroepithelioma of the radial nerve with a study of its behavior in vitro. *Rev. Can. Biol.* **1,** 651–659.

Teitell, M. A., Thompson, A. D., Sorensen, P. H., Shimada, H., Triche, T. J., and Denny, C. T. (1999). EWS/ETS fusion genes induce epithelial and neuroectodermal differentiation in NIH 3T3 fibroblasts. *Lab. Invest.* **79,** 1535–1543.

Triche, T. J., and Sorensen, P. (2001). Molecular pathology of pediatric malignancies. *In* "Principles and Practice of Pediatric Oncology" (P. A. Pizzo and D. G. Poplack, eds.), 4th Ed. Lippincott, Philadelphia.

Turc-Carel, C., Philip, I., Berger, M. P., Philip, T., and Lenoir, G. M. (1983). Chromosomal translocation in Ewing's sarcoma. *N. Engl. J. Med.* **309,** 497–498.

Urano, F., Umezawa, A., Hong, W., Kikuchi, H., and Hata, J. (1996). A novel chimera gene between EWS and E1A-F, encoding the adenovirus E1A enhancer-binding protein, in extraosseous Ewing's sarcoma. *Biochem. Biophys. Res. Commun.* **219,** 608–612.

Whang-Peng, J., Triche, T. J., Knutsen, T., Miser, J., Douglass, E. C., and Israel, M. A. (1984). Chromosome translocation in peripheral neuroepithelioma. *N. Engl. J. Med.* **311,** 584–585.

Whang-Peng, J., Triche, T. J., Knutsen, T., Miser, J., Kao-Shan, A., Tsai, S., and Israel, M. A. (1986). Cytogenetic characterization of selected small round cell tumors of childhood. *Cancer Genet. Cytogenet.* **21,** 185–208.

Willis, R. A. (1940). Metastatic neuroblastoma in bone presenting the Ewing's syndrome, with a discussion of "Ewing's sarcoma." *Am. J. Pathol.* **16,** 317–331.

Yang, L., Chansky, H. A., and Hickstein, D. D. (2000). EWS.Fli-1 fusion protein interacts with hyperphosphorylated RNA polymerase II and interferes with serine-arginine protein-mediated RNA splicing. *J. Biol. Chem.* **275,** 37612–37618.

Zhou, Z., Jia, S. F., Hung, M. C., and Kleinerman, E. S. (2001). E1A sensitizes HER2/neu-overexpressing Ewing's sarcoma cells to topoisomerase II-targeting anticancer drugs. *Cancer Res.* **61,** 3394–3398.

EWS/ETS Fusion Genes

Christopher Denny

UCLA School of Medicine

I. EWS/ETS Genes Are Found in Ewing's
   Family Tumors
II. Chromosomal Translocation Fuses the N Terminus
   of EWS to the C Termini of ETS
   Transcription Factors
III. EWS/ETS Fusions Are Dominant-Acting
   Oncoproteins
IV. EWS/ETS Fusions Have Biochemical Features of
   Aberrant Transcription Factors

GLOSSARY

cellular transformation The process of changing cells to
display growth and/or morphologic behaviors similar to
those seen in malignancy.

chromosomal translocation A physical rearrangement of
the genome where two normally distinct chromosomes are
fused.

dominant negative A mutant construct of a particular gene
that antagonizes the effect of the corresponding unmodified
gene product.

fusion point Molecular location marking an abnormal
junction between nucleotide sequences from two different
chromosomes.

transcription factor A protein whose major biologic function is to regulate the expression of specific target genes at
an mRNA level.

EWS/ETS fusion genes are the direct result of
tumor-associated chromosomal translocations that are
found in the Ewing's family of tumors. These genomic
rearrangements fuse the amino terminus of the EWS
gene to the carboxyl terminus of one of five potential
ETS transcription factors. Resultant chimeric products can act as dominant oncoproteins and promote
abnormal cellular growth. EWS/ETS fusions have biochemical characteristics of aberrant transcription factors suggesting that their oncogenic effects are mediated by transcriptionally modulating target genes.
Recent data suggests that EWS/ETS fusions may also
have effects on RNA processing.

I. EWS/ETS GENES ARE FOUND IN EWING'S FAMILY TUMORS

EWS/ETS fusion genes result from specific chromosomal translocations that are found in Ewing's family of tumors (EFTs). As a group, EFTs include Ewing's sarcomas and primitive neuroectodermal tumors and afflict young adults in their first and second decade of life. EFTs typically present as destructive masses associated with bone, although about 15% of patients show only soft tissue masses without apparent bone involvement.

A fundamental impediment to basic understanding of EFTs is that the cell of origin is unknown. The current majority opinion is that EFTs arise from neural crest-derived progenitors. This hypothesis is based on particular cellular features observed in some EFTs, including (i) expression of catachol acetyl transferase, an enzyme involved in neurotransmitter biosynthesis in cholinergic nerves; (ii) expression of neuron-specific enolase; and (iii) propensity for certain EFT tumor-derived cell lines form primitive dendrites and express neural associated proteins in response to differentiating agents.

Because of their uncertain lineage and nonspecific histology, the diagnosis of EFTs had been one of a process of elimination. If a particular tumor displayed a small round cell histology but lacked specific markers, it was deemed an EFT. Recognition of a specific 11;22 chromosomal translocation associated with EFTs represented the first step toward prospective defining EFTs as a distinct clinicopathologic entity.

II. CHROMOSOMAL TRANSLOCATION FUSES THE N TERMINUS OF EWS TO THE C TERMINI OF ETS TRANSCRIPTION FACTORS

Approximately 85% of EFTs carry a tumor-associated t(11;22)(q24;q12) rearrangement that is detectable on karyotypic analysis. This results in juxtaposition of the EWS gene on chromosome 22 with FLI1 on chromosome 11. As a consequence, chimeric transcripts and proteins are produced that consist of the N terminus of EWS fused to the C-terminal portion of FLI1 (Fig. 1). Variant EFT translocations have been also described that join EWS to one of four additional ETS family transcription factors (Table I). The observation that individual EFTs have only a single EWS fusion suggests that despite their structural differences, all five EWS/ETS fusions play similar oncogenic roles.

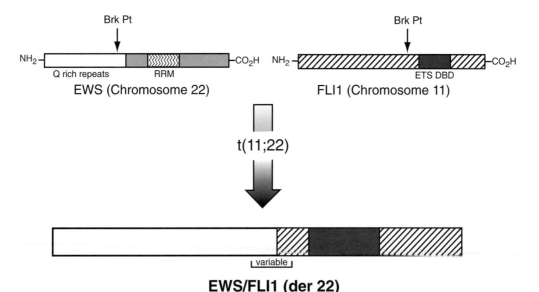

EWS/FLI1 (der 22)

FIGURE 1 Schematic depicting EWS/FLI1 fusion resulting from t(11;22). Structural elements of normal EWS (glutamine-rich N terminus, clear box; RNA-binding RRM domain, vertical stripe) and FLI1 (ETS DNA-binding domain, gray box) genes are shown. The region of variability among different EWS/FLI1 fusions caused by translocation breakpoint heterogeneity is shown in brackets.

TABLE I
EFT EWS Fusion Genes

Translocation	EWS/ETS fusion	Reference
t(11;22)(q24;q12)	EWS/FLI1	Delattre (1992)
t(21;22)(q22;q12)	EWS/ERG	Sorensen (1994)
t(7;22)(p22;q12)	EWS/ETV1	Jeon (1995)
t(2;21;22)(q33;q22;q12)	EWS/FEV	Peter (1997)
t(17;22)(q12;q12)	EWS/E1AF	Urano (1996)

EWS was discovered in the context of being an EFT translocation partner and its normal functions are still being defined. It is one of three members of the TET family that also includes TLS/FUS, a gene involved in a tumor-associated chromosomal translocation in mixoid liposarcoma, and TAFII68, a TBP-associated factor present in some transcription complexes. Full-length EWS contains an N-terminal domain consisting of glutamine-rich degenerate repeats and an RRM motif located near the C terminus that is thought to mediate RNA binding.

As a result of chromosomal translocation the glutamine-rich N terminus of EWS minus the RRM domain is fused to one of five possible ETS proteins. ETS proteins form a well-characterized family of transcription factors. ETS members have previously been associated with carcinogenesis in lower mammals either by being transcriptionally deregulated via retroviral insertion or through direct incorporation into oncogenic retroviruses. ETS factors are defined by an 87 amino acid motif that is frequently located near the C terminus and that is both necessary and sufficient for site-specific DNA binding *in vitro*. This ETS DNA-binding domain (DBD) is invariably present and intact in all EFT EWS/ETS fusions.

Not only can there be five different ETS partners in EFT EWS rearrangements, but there is also molecular variability in translocation breakpoints within a single EWS/ETS fusion type. This results in slightly different EWS and ETS exons being incorporated into the fusion genes. There have been nine different EWS/FLI1 fusions described, each with variable combinations of exons flanking the fusion point. Two retrospective studies suggest that structurally different EWS/FLI1 fusions may have prognostic significance. It appears that patients with EFTs harboring a type 1 fusion (EWS exon 7 juxtaposed to FLI1 exon 6) have an increased chance of survival over those EFT pa-

tients with alternate EWS/FLI1 fusions. These observations are currently being confirmed in prospective studies but suggest that different EWS/FLI1 fusion proteins may have different biologic potencies.

III. EWS/ETS FUSIONS ARE DOMINANT-ACTING ONCOPROTEINS

The high prevalence of EWS/ETS fusions in EFTs suggested that these chimeric products were important to the genesis and perhaps maintenance of these tumors. Work in animal model systems supports the view that EWS/ETS fusions act as dominant oncogenes. Forced expression of EWS/FLI1 promotes anchorage-independent growth of NIH 3T3 murine fibroblasts. Polyclonal NIH 3T3 populations stably expressing EWS/ETS fusion genes form tumors in immunodeficient mice at an accelerated rate. Instead of displaying spindle cell histology that is typical for transformed fibroblasts, EWS/ETS NIH 3T3 tumors have a small round cell morphology that is reminiscent of that seen in human EFTs. These data suggest that in addition to actively promoting oncogenesis, EWS/ETS fusions also appear to dictate some of the histologic characteristics found in EFTs.

Studies in human EFT tumor-derived cell lines also indicate that EWS/ETS fusions play crucial biologic roles. Transduction of antisense or dominant-negative constructs into EFT cell lines results in growth inhibition. Treatment of EFT cell lines with antisense oligonucleotides directed at the EWS/FLI1 fusion results in decreased *in vivo* tumor growth in immunodeficient mice. These data indicate that continued expression of EWS/ETS fusion genes is necessary for maintaining tumor growth.

IV. EWS/ETS FUSIONS HAVE BIOCHEMICAL FEATURES OF ABERRANT TRANSCRIPTION FACTORS

Considering that EWS/ETS oncoproteins are fusions between a putative RNA-processing molecule and members of a known family of transcription factors, the current hypothesis is that the resulting fusions are themselves transcription factors. EWS/ETS proteins display several biochemical attributes supporting this theory: (i) in both EFT cell lines and transduced NIH 3T3 cells, EWS/ETS proteins localize to the nucleus; (ii) EWS/ETS fusions can bind DNA in a site-specific manner; and (iii) the N-terminal EWS domain present in EWS/ETS fusions can act as a potent transcriptional activation domain in model reporter assays.

Sequence analysis of EFT fusions and mutagenesis studies also indicate that EWS/ETS proteins can act as aberrant transcription factors. Despite their structural heterogeneity across different tumors, all EWS/ETS fusions contain an intact ETS DNA-binding domain. Site-directed mutagenesis within the ETS DBD results in EWS/ETS proteins with reduced or absent transformation potential. Similarly, deletion of EWS transcriptional activation domains reduces the biological potency of EWS/ETS proteins. These data indicate that both EWS and ETS portions of the fusion are necessary for full biologic activity.

Two major inherent biochemical properties dictate the specificity of transcription factors: (i) protein–DNA interaction specificity defined in the case of EWS/ETS fusions by the ETS DBD and (ii) protein–protein interaction specificity at transcriptional activation domains. Through somatic genomic rearrangement, normal ETS transcriptional activation domains are replaced with the EWS N terminus, thereby generating transcription factors with novel biochemical and genetic specificities. It therefore appears that a major mechanism through which EWS/ETS fusions promote oncogenesis is by transcriptionally modulating a repertoire of target genes that is qualitatively and/or quantitatively different than the normal ETS gene partners.

A number of strategies, including microarray analysis and polymerase chain reaction-based differential expression screens, have been used to identify EWS/ETS target genes. By comparing gene expression patterns in NIH 3T3 populations with and without EWS/ETS fusions, a number of putative target genes have been identified. While some appear to encode signaling and regulatory proteins, assessing the importance of individual EWS/ETS target genes in EFT biology has been difficult. For example, *manic fringe (m-FNG)*, a gene coding for a glycosyltransferase important in normal limb development, is upregulated by EWS/ETS genes. Furthermore, forced

expression of *m-FNG* accelerates NIH 3T3 tumorigenesis in immunodeficient mice. However, m-FNG NIH 3T3 tumors do not display the small round cell histology that is invariably seen in tumors derived from EWS/ETS NIH 3T3 cells and EFT tumor-derived cell lines. This and similar findings demonstrate that while some EWS/ETS target genes may themselves demonstrate oncogenic potential when overexpressed, none have recapitulated the complete EWS/ETS phenotype. This suggests that EWS/ETS fusions promote oncogenesis through a gene network where the modulation of multiple target genes is necessary for complete biologic impact.

In addition to acting as an aberrant transcription factor, recent data suggest that EWS/ETS genes may be able to modulate gene expression through mechanisms other than simply binding promoter/enhancer sites at specific target genes. This was prompted by the finding that an artificial EWS/FLI1 DBD mutant that has no apparent *in vitro* DNA-binding activity still retains some transformation potency. It has been shown that EWS/FLI1 binds the U1C RNA splicing factor and that EWS/FLI1 is able to alter the splicing patterns of model RNA constructs. This suggests that EWS/ETS proteins may modulate gene expression at both the transcription initiation—acting as a transcription factor—and the RNA processing stages of transcription control. The relative contributions of each biochemical mechanism to EWS/ETS biologic activity are currently being investigated.

See Also the Following Articles

ALL • PAX3–FKHR AND PAX7–FKHR GENE FUSIONS IN ALVEOLAR RHABDOMYOSARCOMA • RUNX/CBF TRANSCRIPTION FACTORS • TLS-CHOP

Bibliography

Bertolotti, A., Lutz, Y., Heard, D. J., Chambon, P., and Tora, L. (1996). hTAF(II)68, a novel RNA/ssDNA-binding protein with homology to the pro-oncoproteins TLS/FUS and EWS is associated with both TFIID and RNA polymerase II. *EMBO J.* **15**, 5022–5031.

Braun, B. S., Freiden, R., Lessnick, S. L., May, W. A., and Denny, C. T. (1995). Identification of target genes to the Ewing's sarcoma EWS/FLI fusion protein by representational difference analysis. *Mol. Cell. Biol.* **15**, 4623–4630.

Cavazzana, A. O., Ninfo, V., Roberts, J., and Triche, T. J. (1992). Peripheral neuroepithelioma: A light microscopic, immunocytochemical, and ultrastructural study. *Mod. Pathol.* **5,** 71–78.

Delattre, O., *et al.* (1992). Gene fusion with an ETS DNA-binding domain caused by chromosome translocation in human tumours. *Nature* **359,** 162–165.

Jeon, I. S., Davis, J. N., Braun, B. S., Sublett, J. E., Roussel, M. F., Denny, C. T., and Shapiro, D. N. (1995). A variant Ewing's sarcoma translocation (7;22) fuses the EWS gene to the ETS gene ETV1. *Oncogene* **10,** 1229–1234.

Knoop, L. L., and Baker, S. J. (2000). The splicing factor U1C represses EWS/FLI1-mediated transactivation. *J. Biol. Chem.* **275,** 24865–24871.

Kovar, H., Aryee, D. N., Jug, G., Henockl, C., Schemper, M., Delattre, O., Thomas, G., and Gadner, H. (1996). EWS/FLI-1 antagonists induce growth inhibition of Ewing tumor cells in vitro. *Cell Growth Differ.* **7,** 429–437.

May, W. A., Arvand, A., Thompson, A. D., Braun, B. S., Wright, M., and Denny, C. T. (1997). EWS/FLI1-induced Manic Fringe renders NIH 3T3 cells tumorigenic. *Nature Genet.* **17,** 495–497.

May, W. A., Gishizky, M. L., Lessnick, S. L., Lunsford, L. B., Lewis, B. C., Delattre, O., Zucman, J., Thomas, G., and Denny, C. T. (1993). Ewing sarcoma 11;22 translocation produces a chimeric transcription factor that requires the DNA-binding domain encoded by FLI1 for transformation. *Proc. Natl. Acad. Sci. USA* **90,** 5752–5756.

Peter, M., Couturier, J., Pacquement, H., Michon, J., Thomas, G., Magdelenat, H., and Delattre, O. (1997). A new member of the ETS family fused to EWS in Ewing tumors. *Oncogene* **14,** 1159–1164.

Sorensen, P. H., Lessnick, S. L., Lopez-Terrada, D., Liu, X. F., Triche, T. J., and Denny, C. T. (1994). A second Ewing's sarcoma translocation, t(21;22), fuses the EWS gene to another ETS-family transcription factor, ERG. *Nat. Genet.* **6,** 146–151.

Tanaka, K., Iwakuma, T., Harimaya, K., Sato, H., and Iwamoto, Y. (1997). EWS-Fli1 antisense oligodeoxynucleotide inhibits proliferation of human Ewing's sarcoma and primitive neuroectodermal tumor cells. *J. Clin. Invest.* **99,** 239–247.

Turc-Carel, C., Aurias, A., Mugneret, F., Lizard, S., Sidaner, I., Volk, C., Thiery, J. P., Olschwang, S., Philip, I., and Berger, M. P. (1988). Chromosomes in Ewing's sarcoma. I. An evaluation of 85 cases demonstrates remarkable consistency of t(11;22)(q24;q12). *Can. Genet. Cytogenet.* **32,** 229–238.

Urano, F., Umezawa, A., Hong, W., Kikuchi, H., and Hata, J. (1996). A novel chimera gene between EWS and E1A-F, encoding the adenovirus E1A enhancer-binding protein, in extraosseous Ewing's sarcoma. *Biochem. Biophys. Res. Commun.* **219,** 608–612.

Zoubek, A., Dockhorn-Dworniczak, B., Delattre, O., Christiansen, H., Niggli, F., Gatterer-Menz, I., Smith, T. L., Jürgens, H., Gadner, H., and Kovar, H. (1996). Does expression of different EWS chimeric transcripts define clinically distinct risk groups of Ewing tumor patients? *J. Clin. Oncol.* **14,** 1245–1251.

Zucman, J., Melot, T., Desmaze, C., Ghysdael, J., Plougastel, B., Peter, M., Zucker, J. M., Triche, T. J., Sheer, D., Turc-Carel, C., Ambros, P., Combaret, V., Lenoir, G., Aurias, A., Thomas, G., and Delattre, O. (1993). Combinatorial generation of variable fusion proteins in Ewing family tumors. *EMBO J.* **12,** 4481–4487.

Extracellular Matrix and Matrix Receptors: Alterations during Tumor Progression

Lloyd A. Culp
Raymond Judware
Priit Kogerman
Julianne L. Holleran
Carson J. Miller
Case Western Reserve University School of Medicine

GLOSSARY

adhesion Cell attachment and subsequent responses with inert natural matrices or artificial substrata.

bone metastasis Colonization of the bone matrix and/or bone marrow by highly selected tumor cells.

extracellular matrix Insoluble supramolecular complexes composed of several classes of macromolecules with specific binding interactions that span large two- or three-dimensional distances in tissues.

integrin receptors Dimeric complexes of α and β subunits that span the plasma membrane and bind with considerable specificity and coordinately to extracellular matrix molecules and to intracellular signaling elements.

oncogene An "activated" protooncogene in tumor cells that participates in malignant conversion of cells and alleviation of normal growth control and matrix regulatory mechanisms.

progression-related genes Genes that participate in promoting tumor cell movement and establishment from their primary site of residence to distant target sites where metastatic growth becomes established.

proteoglycans Complex glycoconjugates bound to the matrix and to the cell surface that contain a carbohydrate chain(s) of acidic glycosaminoglycans covalently linked to a core protein.

transmembrane signaling Ability of certain integral plasma membrane-spanning receptors to bind a ligand at the cell's exterior and, via this binding, to communicate one or more signals to the interior of the cell via its transmembrane and cytosolic protein domains.

tumor progression Competence for malignantly converted cells to expand into a large primary tumor population and evolve variants competent for metastatic spread to one or more target organs at great distance from the primary tumor.

The extracellular matrix is an elaborate array of proteins and carbohydrates responsible for the organization of cells into complex organs. Matrix components are assembled into various combinations, producing specific environments within tissues. Signals are transduced from the matrix into cells from cellular receptors binding to specific components of the matrix, regulating many intracellular physiological events. Tumor cells exhibit many alterations in the composition of their matrices, matrix receptors, and the cellular constituents necessary for signaling from the matrix. This article reviews (i) properties of the extracellular matrix (ECM), (ii) mechanisms underlying the regulation of cellular functions by the matrix, and (iii) alterations in cell:matrix interactions observed in a variety of cancerous tissues.

I. INTRODUCTION

Mechanisms of ECM adhesion reflect not only a passive adhesion of cells to ECMs, but also a complex network of signals from the organizational framework of the ECM, through ECM receptors spanning the plasma membrane, and into the interior of the cell, subsequently regulating many physiological and gene transcriptional events. Using untransformed cells, analyses have begun to decipher how these mechanisms go awry upon oncogene activation and during tumor progression in highly selected clonal populations; how they evolve as a consequence of the genetic instability in tumor cell populations; and how clonal selections take advantage of this diversity during metastatic spread. Our attention is focused on

a few of the best-studied normal cell/malignant cell systems.

II. CELLULAR INTERACTIONS WITH EXTRACELLULAR MATRICES

A. Overview of Adhesion Biology

At the leading edge of the moving cell, newly synthesized cell surface molecules, including ECM receptors, are accumulated into an actively ruffling plasma membrane. Finger-like processes, filopodia, emanate from this ruffling membrane to "feel" the ECM. Filopodia contain high concentrations of ECM receptors and are packed with microfilament bundles to be organized in response to receptor:ECM binding. Two classes of adhesions can be formed in nonepithelial cells depending on the availability of ECM receptors and the molecular organization of the ECM itself. Close contacts, of spacing distance 20–25 nm between the plasma membrane and ECM, are formed by many ECM receptors acting singly or collectively without cytoskeletal participation. It is not clear whether close contacts are merely adhesion sites that do not participate in signaling to the inside of the cell or whether they send their own set of signals. The second class of adhesions, the focal contact of spacing distance 5–10 nm, is a footpad-like structure at the undersurface of the cell where a very precise array of ECM receptors must organize (and not all receptors permit focal contact formation). These contacts are the end points of F-actin stress fibers, appear to be the principal sites of signaling to the inside of the cell, and are composed of hundreds to thousands of receptor:ECM-binding events. A typical connective tissue cell may have 50–100 of these focal contacts. Their half-lives can vary from 15–20 min, for an actively migrating cell, to greater than 24 h for a stationary cell. Epithelial cells generate two different adhesion classes on basal lamina—hemidesmosomes and focal contacts—with the latter class resembling the focal contacts of connective tissue cells in both molecular architecture and supramolecular organization.

Cell migration raises the critical issue as to how cells "break" their contacts. The paradox between the making of new contacts and the breaking of old contacts is particularly relevant for tumor cells and is reviewed in some detail in Section IV.A. There is no evidence that the degradation of ECM receptor: ligand complexes is responsible in adhesion breakage; this would require degradation of hundreds to thousands of the individual molecular-binding reactions in each focal adhesion site. Instead, cells leave their focal contacts behind on the ECM as "footprints" by complex events that are not well understood at the molecular level (in contrast to our better understanding of how new adhesions are made!). These footprints evolve from a combination of two interrelated processes: (1) the disorganization of the cytoskeleton by mechanisms that operate entirely within the cell (a model is provided by cytochalasin D-mediated breakdown of F-actin stress fibers) and (2) disorganization of receptor complexes at the edges of adhesive contacts with elastic retraction fibers generated at adjacent plasma membrane. Culmination of these processes is the breakage of retraction fibers by fluid motion near the cell so that "footprints" are left bound to the ECM while the cell is liberated along the matrix. While these biological events have been best studied in tissue culture model systems, considerable evidence has been obtained that these same processes occur *in vivo* in the developing embryo, where very active cell migration events are occurring, and in certain pathogenic conditons

(e.g., migration and invasion of tumor cells into foreign tissues).

B. Classes of Extracellular Matrix Molecules

1. Collagens

The largest group of ECM molecules is represented by the collagen family (Table I), large glycoproteins (on the order of 300 kDa) that comprise 30% of the total protein mass (6% of total body weight) in humans. Collagens maintain the three-dimensional shape of tissues and are secreted from cells as procollagen molecules, which are processed in the extracellular space to give rise to the mature protein.

There are at least 15 different types of collagen encoded by at least 27 distinct genes on 11 different chromosomes. This diversity is further enhanced by alternative splicing of pre-mRNA transcripts. For example, the gene for collagen type XIII can give rise to at least 12 different mRNA species generated through alternative splicing. Expression of the various collagens is both spatially and temporally regulated during development, as well as in various pathogenic states in the adult.

The 15 collagens are designated by roman numerals I–XV. Each chain of collagen is termed an α chain,

TABLE I
Features of the Major Components Involved in Adhesion to Extracellular Matrices

Component	Number of genes[a]	Number of different protein subunits[a]	Structure of mature protein	Number of protein isotypes[a]	Molecular mass of mature protein (kDa)
Collagen	27	27 (+) α	Homo- or heterotrimers	15 (+)	300
Fibronectin	1		Heterodimers	20	500
Laminin	5	2 A, 1 B, 2B1	Heterotrimers	3	1000
Vitronectin	1	1	Monomer	1	75
Tenascin	6	6	Hexamer	1	1000
Proteoglycans	10 (+)	10 (+)	Monomers	10 (+)	20–210
Serine proteases	6 (+)	6 (+)	Monomers	6 (+)	33–90
MMPs[b]	9	9	Monomers	9	42–83
TIMPs[c]	2	2	Monomer	2	21–28
Integrins	22	14 α, 8 β (+)	Heterodimers	20	200–300

[a]A (plus sign) indicates that more forms of this particular component may be discovered in the future.
[b]Matrix metallo proteinases, which include collagenases and stromelysins.
[c]Tissue inhibitors of MMPs.

and each of the 15 forms is composed of different α chains. Collagens can be made up of a single type of α chain, giving rise to a homotrimer, or of multiple chains, generating a heterotrimer. For example, collagen type II of cartilages is a homotrimer $[\alpha1(II)]_3$. Collagen type I $\{[\alpha1(I)]_2[\alpha2(I)]\}$ is a heterotrimer composed of two identical chains of a single type (α1) and one chain of another type (α2).

The most common form of collagen is type I (Fig. 1A), a fibrillar collagen that makes up 90% of the to-

tal collagen found in humans. Collagenous domains (found in the fibrillar collagens I, II, III, V, and XI) are characterized by a distinctive tripeptide repeat structure, gly-X-Y, where X/Y is usually lys/hydroxy-lys and/or pro/hydroxy-pro. Lys and hydroxy-lys residues are utilized for covalent cross-linking between collagen trimers after incorporation into the three-dimensional matrix. Cross-linking confers great rigidity to the collagen fibrils, which associate into networks necessary for the support of tissues and or-

A. Fibrillar Collagen

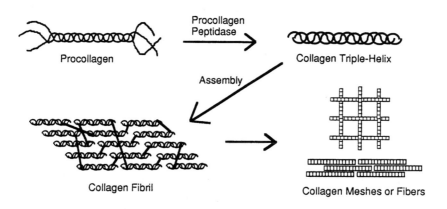

B. Non-Fibrillar Collagen

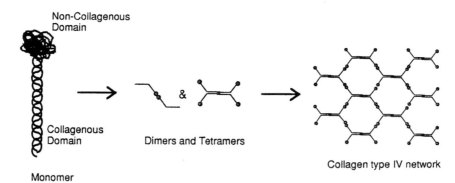

FIGURE 1 Assembly of collagen matrices. (A) Fibrillar procollagen is secreted from connective tissue cells as a triple helix and processed extracellularly into the mature collagen (CN) monomer by procollagen peptidases. Monomers organize into fibrils with a four monomer overlap, creating a characteristic "quarter-stagger" arrangement. The fibril is held together by covalent cross-links between monomers through the hydroxylysine residues. Collagen fibrils associate into the wickerwork meshes or linear fibers. (B) Nonfibrillar collagens, composed of type IV collagen and other minor collagens and forming basal laminae in all tissues, are also triple helical; however, noncollagenous domains at one end of the molecule are retained to form a globular head. Monomers associate through head-to-head and tail-to-tail interactions to form dimers and tetramers, which are then arranged into the "chicken-wire" arrays typical of two-dimensional basal lamina matrices.

gans and fibers that are basic components of tendons and ligaments.

Nonfibrillar forms of collagen also exist that contain both collagenous and noncollagenous domains (Fig. 1B). These collagens (types IV, VII, VIII, IX, and X) form networks providing elasticity to tissues. Nonfibrillar collagens are more easily removed from the ECM by proteolysis than fibrillar collagens. Of particular note, collagen type IV is the prominent component of all basal laminae in the body underlying all epithelia and endothelia and forms a selective filter in the kidney as the glomerular basement membrane.

2. Fibronectins (FNs)

FNs are another important constituent of the ECM and form an adhesion link between the collagenous matrix and adherent mesenchymal cells and select other cell types. Mature FNs are a 500-kDa dimeric glycoproteins encoded by a single gene, which through alternative splicing of the primary transcripts gives rise to 20 distinct variants in the human (Table I). These FN isoforms are produced in cell-type-specific and developmentally regulated manners.

The FN protein (Fig. 2A) contains multiple repeats of three types of homologous domains (types I, II, or III repeats), which are, for the most part, encoded by discrete exons in the FN gene. Alternative splicing is carefully regulated to include 45 invariant exons and to include or exclude exons encoding type III repeat regions ED_A and ED_B (for "extra domain"; also referred to as EIIIA and EIIIB, respectively) and all or part of the IIICS region (a type III repeat "connecting segment"; also referred to as the V region). There are two biological classes of FN, cellular (cFN) and plasma (pFN), which differ in the inclusion/exclusion of ED/IIICS regions. pFN, which circulates freely in the blood plasma, does not contain ED regions and lacks or includes one chain each of the entire IIICS type III repeat. cFN, which is associated with cells, may contain or lack all of these regions of diversity, depending on the class of cells that produced the cFN in question.

A complex pattern of disulfide bond formation appears to hold the FN molecule in a conformation that gives rise to discrete functional domains. These moderate the complex cell and matrix-binding properties

of FN. Two FN monomers are joined through disulfide bond formation near the carboxyl-terminal ends to give rise to the 500-kDa functional protein. Multiple cFN dimers can also associate to form very large insoluble aggregates at the cell surface.

FNs exhibit a wide variety of cell and ECM binding properties (Fig. 2A). In general, cell-binding domains are localized in the central portion of FN within various type III repeats, whereas matrix-binding domains are found on the ends of the molecule in type I and II repeats. The principle cell-binding domain of FN (cell$_1$) contains the three amino acid region gly-arg-asp (RGD), which is a recognition site for some integrin receptors (see later). There are also proteoglycan-binding domains at several locations, as well as cell-binding domains whose receptors have not been characterized.

3. Other Matrix Proteins

Laminins (LNs) are glycoproteins found in the ECM, which promote the adhesion of epithelial and certain neuronal cells to matrices. LNs are larger (>800 kDa) and more complex than FNs (Fig. 2B). LNs are encoded by at least five genes, which produce three distinct subunits, designated A, B1, and B2 chains. These chains interact to form a triple helix on the carboxyl-terminal end of the molecule, while the amino-terminal ends of the LN chains remain in a globular form. Diversity in the LN gene family gives rise to distinct protein isoforms. Merosin is a form of LN with an alternate A chain, whereas S-LN contains an alternate B1 chain.

Tenascin is a very large (1000 kDa) matrix protein with a characteristic hexabrachion structure. The six arms of tenascin are individual proteins of 190–250 kDa, linked through disulfide bonds to form the mature tenascin complex. This protein exhibits weak cell-adhering properties but also exhibits antiadhesive properties in many situations. Tenascin is normally expressed at high levels during development and in some tumors, but poorly in adult tissues.

4. Proteoglycans (PGs)

The ECM and cell surfaces also contain a variety of carbohydrate–protein moieties, which are known as proteoglycans (PGs). PGs (Fig. 2C) are composed of a protein core covalently linked to chains of

A. Fibronectin

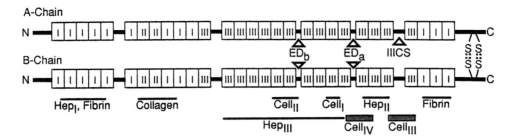

B. Laminin

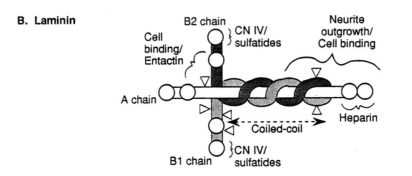

C. Proteoglycan

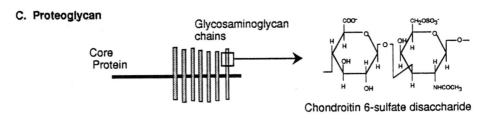

D. Integrin

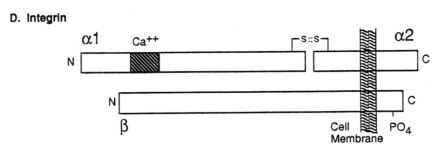

FIGURE 2 Other cell adhesion participants. (A) Fibronectin (FN) is a dimer of two chains connected on the C-terminal ends by disulfide bonds. Each chain is composed of three types of homology repeats (types I, II, and III, as defined in boxes and numbered from left to right) linked by a flexible peptide sequence. Generic domains of all FNs are shown; however, "extra domains" may be spliced into the A chain (ED_a or $_b$ and IIICS) or B chain (ED_a or ED_b only) at the indicated locations. Cell/matrix-binding domains have been localized to several regions of FN as indicated. The cell$_{II}$ or $_{IV}$ binding sites are located in "extra domains" or neighboring type III repeats; receptors to these cell-binding domains have not been defined. Cell$_I$ recognizes the RGDS (arg-gly-asp-ser) sequence in III$_{10}$ and sequences in repeats III$_8$ and III$_9$. Cell$_{III}$ contains a CS1 peptide sequence in an alternatively spliced IIICS region, which is recognized by integrin $\alpha_4\beta_1$. Three domains have been described for binding heparan sulfate proteoglycans (Hep$_{I,II,III}$), as well as domains for binding to fibrin and collagen in matrices. (B) LN is composed of three chains (A, B1, B2) arranged into a triple-helical coiled-coil, with globular domains located at the end of each individual chain. Binding domains to other matrix components (e.g., collagen type IV, entactin, and heparin/heparan sulfate) are found within these globular domains. Cell attachment to LN is mediated through several cell-binding domains (which recognize integrins $\alpha_6\beta_1$ and $\alpha_b\beta_4$), indicated by the open arrows. Binding domains have also been described for glycolipid sulfatides on the cell surface. (C) PGs are composed of a central protein core to which are attached GAG chains made up of repeating units of disaccharides. The disaccharide found in chondroitin-sulfate (glucuronic acid linked to N-acetylgalactosamine-sulfate) is depicted. Other PGs are composed only of heparan sulfate or dermatan sulfate chains, while some rare PGs can contain two different GAG classes. (D) Integrins are dimeric glycoproteins of one α and one β chain. The large N-terminal extracellular domains confer noncovalent α/β association, Ca^{2+}-binding, and Ca^{2+}-dependent matrix ligand binding to these receptors. In many, but not all, cases, the α subunit is cleaved into two pieces, which are joined by a disulfide bond. The intracellular domain of the β subunit associates with talin in focal contacts and may be phosphorylated in some circumstances.

carbohydrates known as glycosaminoglycans (GAGs). These chains contain multiple repeats of disaccharides, which typically contain a uronic-acid sugar alternating with an aminosugar, which can be sulfated. Common GAGs include keratan sulfate (KS), dermatan sulfate (DS), heparan sulfate (HS), heparin (Hep), and nonsulfated hyaluronic acid (also called hyaluronan). With the exception of hyaluronic acid, GAGs are covalently linked to a protein core, which range from 20 to >300 kDa. Better-studied PGs include aggrecan of cartilage (KS, CS), decorin of skin and cartilage (CS, DS), biglycan of skin and cartilage (CS, DS), and perlecan of many tissues (HS).

PGs bind to each other, to specific binding proteins such as FNs and LNs, and to cells. HS-PGs on the cell surface bind to matrix components such as collagen, FN, and LN and can function as an ECM receptor because they span the plasma membrane via a hydrophobic protein sequence. They communicate with the interior of the cell via a cytosolic domain to affect cytoskeletal rearrangements. In addition, CS- and DS-PGs can, in some cases, block adhesion of cells to FN either by binding to FN and sterically hindering the association of FN with integrin or by binding to cell surface "receptors" for PGs and perturbing adhesion-promoting events. PGs and hyaluronan provide viscoelastic properties necessary in joints and for tissue deformation, as occurs in the eye during vision correction by contact lenses.

5. Matrix Proteases

Certain matrix molecules must be deposited to ensure the appropriate development of tissue-specific cell types; in other cases, matrices must be degraded for the proper developmental sequence. This regulation of matrix assembly is controlled by the modulation of the expression of matrix molecules. In many cases, old matrix must be removed to make way for new matrix and partly to prevent the old matrix from interfering with signals imparted by the new matrix. Matrix turnover is the responsibility of matrix proteases, which degrade matrix molecules.

Four broad classes of ECM proteases have been identified, based on the type of active site in the protease. (a) Serine proteases utilize a ser residue in their active sites and include plasminogen activator, plasmin, and elastase. (b) Cysteine proteases contain a catalytically active free sulfhydryl group and include

most of the cathepsin family of proteases. (c) Matrix metalloproteinases (MMPs) include collagenases and stromelysins. (d) Some proteases, such as cathepsin D, make use of an asp residue in the active site.

ECM proteases can be highly specific or quite general in their preference for a substrate. For example, interstitial collagenases are specific for collagen I, whereas type IV collagenase is specific for collagen IV. In contrast, stromelysins are more general, degrading FN, LN, or the protein core of PGs. Specific proteases, such as type IV collagenase, are not only limited to a single molecular target, but often cleave their target only at a single or a very few locations. This tends to "activate" the substrate for more rapid and less specific degradation by other general proteases.

MMPs, with their roles in tumor progression (see Section IV.B), are a well-studied family of matrix proteases that use a Cys sulfhydryl group in their active site. MMPs are produced and secreted from cells as an inactive zymogen. The enzyme is held in an inactive state due to its association with the divalent metal Zn^{2+}. In the zymogen, the cys-SH group is associated with the Zn^{2+} in the active site.

Cells also produce specific inhibitors of matrix proteases. These inhibitors include proteins such as tissue inhibitors of MMPs (TIMPs) or plasminogen activator inhibitors (PAIs). TIMP-1 is a 28-kDa glycoprotein that binds to procollagenases with a 1:1 stoichiometry, maintaining the enzyme in its inactive form.

C. Cell Surface Receptors for Extracellular Matrix Molecules

1. Integrins

The largest family of ECM receptors on cells are the dimeric integrins composed of one α and one β subunit. At least 22 integrin genes have been identified encoding 14 α and 8 β subunits (Table II). Further diversity is achieved through alternative splicing of the primary transcripts for several of the subunits.

In general, α subunits range from 120 to 180 kDa, and β subunits are slightly smaller, ranging from 90 to 110 kDa. Each subunit has three discrete regions: a small carboxyl-terminal intracellular domain, a transmembrane helix, and a large extracellular

β subfamily	α subunit	Ligands[a]	Recognition peptide[b]	Special properties
β$_1$[c]; also VLA subfamily; universal distribution	α$_1$	Col, LN		
	α$_2$	Col, LN	DGEA (Col)	Matrix contraction
	α$_3$[c]	Col, FN, LN	RGD±	
	α$_4$	FN, V-CAM-1	EILDV (FN-IIICS)	Adhesion to endothelial cells; on leukocytes and melanoma cells
	α$_5$	FN	RGD	FNR; matrix assembly
	α$_6$[c]	LN		
	α$_7$	LN		
	α$_8$	?		
	α$_v$	Col, FB, FN, vWF, VN	RGD	
β$_2$, cell–cell adhesion receptors	α$_L$	I-CAM-1, ICAM-2		Cell–cell adhesion; located on leukocytes
	α$_M$	C3i, factor X, FB, I-CAM		Cell–cell adhesion; located on leukocytes
	α$_X$	C3i, FB	GPRP	Cell–cell adhesion; located on leukocytes
β$_3$[c], universal distribution	α$_V$	BSP, FB, FN, LN, TSP, VN, vWF	RGD	
	α$_{IIb}$[c]	FB, FN, TSP, VN, vWF	RGD, KQAGDV(FB)	Platelet-specific integrin -GPIIb-IIIa
β$_4$[c]	α$_6$	LN		Epithelial cell integrin; hemidesmosomes
β$_5$	α$_V$	FB, FN, VN	RGD	
β$_6$	α$_V$	FN	RGD	Epithelial cell integrin
β$_7$	α$_4$	FN, V-CAM-1	EILDV (FN IIICS)	Located on mucosal lymphocytes
	α$_{IEL}$	?		Located on mucosal lymphocytes
β$_8$	α$_V$	?		

[a]BSP, bone sialoprotein; C3i, complement component; Col, collagen; FB, fibrinogen; FN, fibronectin; FNR, classical fibronectin receptor; LN, laminin; I-CAM, intercellular adhesion molecule; TSP, thrombospondin; VN, vitronectin; vWF, von Willebrand factor; V-CAM-1, vascular cell adhesion molecule-1.

[b]Single letter amino acid codes indicate the peptide sequence in the ligand recognized by integrin.

[c]Modifications through alternative splicing of pre-mRNAs have been noted.

amino-terminal domain. A functional receptor (Fig. 2D) of one α and one β subunit has a molecular mass ranging from 200 to 300 kDa. Extracellular domains are responsible for α/β association, binding of divalent metals, and adherence to ECM components. Intracellular domains of α subunits are essential for signal transduction into the cell's interior mediated by integrin binding to ECM. The β subunit intracellular domain is involved in association with the cytoskeleton in focal contacts (see Section II.D.3). Integrins are "activated" for signaling and/or cytoskeletal association by outside/in mechanisms subsequent to ECM binding or by inside/out mechanisms based on cytosolic events via binding of nonintegrin proteins.

Although the large numbers of α/β pairs could conceivably give rise to 100 or more possible receptors, there is apparently some restriction on the association of the subunits, as only 20 combinations have been identified thus far (Table II). This determines the pre-cise specificity of the integrin for one or more ECM component(s). A single α/β pair can be specific for a single ECM molecule or it can recognize several matrix components. Several α/β pairs can recognize a single ECM component, either utilizing distinct sites on the matrix molecule or the same site. This apparent multiple and overlapping recognition scheme of integrins for the matrix allows precise modulation of adhesion of cells to the specific matrix environment in a tissue.

2. Nonintegrin Receptors

HS-PGs as integral membrane components can function as cellular receptors for the ECM components FN, collagen, LN, and tenascin. That HS-PGs can participate in signal transduction across the plasma membrane was demonstrated by the reorganization of F-actin when cells adhere to HS-binding substrata. Whether they participate in other signaling events awaits experimental testing.

A number of other nonintegrin proteins have been identified that bind other matrix components. Entactin is a 170-kDa sulfated glycoprotein that binds LN and collagen IV. A family of LN-binding proteins ranging from 67 to 100 kDa have also been identified; however, these have not been well characterized as to form and function.

D. Receptor: Matrix Interaction and Signal Transduction

In untransformed cells, there is a direct relationship between adhesion to a matrix and cell division/ differentiation. Cells must be attached to a compatible surface for cell division to occur. The ECM provides signals to cells in much the same way as do the well-known growth factors. Adhesion signals are transmitted into the cell via integrins and HS-PGs. Once inside the cell, signal transduction mechanisms pass the message from the matrix to the nucleus, where specific transcriptional events occur in response to adhesion to specific matrices. The following is a discussion of the relationship between adhesion and cellular responses to adhesion. Receptor signaling is also reviewed in other articles of this volume.

1. Organization of the Matrix

ECM deposition of matrix components is highly specific. Matrices are laid down in spatially and temporally regulated patterns that are crucial for the ordered development of every tissue type in the body. Cells may regulate matrix composition by modulating either the type and/or the amount of specific components secreted into the matrix.

The most evident example of ordered matrix composition is found in collagen. Collagen fibrils, composed of bundles of individual collagen triple helical molecules, exhibit a characteristic pattern due to the quarter-stagger alignment of individual molecules (Fig. 1A). Fibrils, in turn, are ordered into complex meshes or parallel bundles. Meshes, similar to that found in woven cloth or wicker furniture, are commonly found in skin and around organs and provide strength in two dimensions, forming a "bag" to hold components in. Bundles provide a linear, elastic strength that is necessary for tendon function.

Collagen arrays then provide a foundation upon which other components of the matrix are deposited.

FNs are also deposited by cells in layered arrays. Collagen-binding sites have been identified in the amino-terminal regions of FN. The association of FN with collagen leaves the central and carboxyl-terminal portions of FN free to associate with other matrix molecules or cells. Thus, arrays of FN form a bridge between the collagen foundation and cells. LN and vitronectin are also woven into some collagen layers. LN seems to be enriched in matrices deposited by epithelial and certain neuronal cells. In addition, specialized forms of LN include merosin and S-LN (see Section II.B.3), are localized in nervous tissue, and may have specific neurological functions.

2. Organization of Receptors by the Matrix: Focal Contacts

Many parallels can be drawn between the actions of ECM receptors and well-characterized growth factor receptors. In many cell types, there is a prerequisite of receptor expression for the deposition of ECM components into the matrix, suggesting that cells will only make matrices for which they have existing receptors. For example, in fibroblasts, cell attachment induces collagen expression. In other cells, FN was only expressed from cells that had a functional FN receptor ($\alpha_5\beta_1$ integrin) prior to FN adhesion. This implies that receptor expression may be a fundamental property of a cell and that once the receptors are present an appropriate matrix will form.

Cell adhesion to the ECM is not a randomly distributed process but is a localized event that occurs in focal contacts (also, focal adhesions). These sites serve as "feet" through which the cell contacts the matrix and within which are concentrated the matrix receptors. Because of the interrelationships between receptor and matrix expression, matrix molecules for which the cells express functional receptors are concentrated in focal contacts.

3. Organization of Cytoskeletal Components at Focal Contacts

Extension of receptors through the cell membrane mediates intracellular transduction of the extracellular signal. Integrin cytoplasmic domains are in general small to contain intrinsic enzymatic activity, such as the tyrosine kinase activity associated with growth factor receptors. However, clustering of many different ECM-recognizing integrins within focal adhesions may generate a supramolecular complex that has some intrinsic and additive activity. Alternatively, clustering of integrin cytoplasmic domains within a focal contact may merely form a superstructure with which freely circulating cellular enzymes may associate to form the signal transduction apparatus.

The cytoplasmic domains of integrins within focal contacts form a base upon which the cellular cytoskeleton forms. It has been demonstrated that the actin filament base plate components, talin and vinculin, associate with integrin cytoplasmic domains, with talin forming a bridge between the β integrin subunits and actin. After recruitment of talin and vinculin by integrin, actin monomers polymerize into actin filaments (F-actin), which extend into the cytosol to form the cytoskeleton.

4. Signal Transduction from the Focal Contact

A wide variety of signal transduction mechanisms have been implicated in passing an ECM signal from focal contacts to the cell nucleus. Some of these mechanisms have previously been implicated in signal transduction from growth factor receptors.

Intracellular pH is a critical factor for cell survival and cells expend much effort in acid/base balance. Adhesion induces an increase in intracellular pH by integrin-mediated recognition of FN or by antibody-mediated clustering of integrins. Cell attachment activates a Na^+- H^+ antiport, resulting in an increased intracellular pH due to removal of H^+ from the cell. Many growth factor/receptor interactions have a similar effect mediated by receptor clustering.

Ca^{2+} fluxes are well-recognized mediators of intracellular signal transduction and modulate a number of signal-transducing protein kinase systems. In platelets, attachment to collagen induces a rapid influx of extracellular Ca^{2+} and activation of the Ca^{2+}/calmodulin-dependent myosin light chain kinase. This kinase is involved in the regulation of actin–myosin-related contractility necessary for granule release, a platelet function in response to adhesion. In addition, Ca^{2+}/calmodulin-dependent kinase inhibitors prevent adhesion to several matrix proteins, including LN, FN, and collagen IV.

Another important Ca^{2+}- modulated kinase is protein kinase C (PKC). It has been implicated in a number of adhesion-related activities. PKC stimulates FN but not LN-mediated adhesion; PKC phosphorylates integrin, vinculin, and talin. Phosphorylation of integrins $\alpha_6\beta_1$ or $\alpha_5\beta_1$ enhanced the attachment of microvascular endothelial cells to LN or FN, respectively.

Tyrosine phosphorylation is a hallmark of the initial signal transmitted by growth factor receptors. Tyrosine phosphorylation is also involved in attachment to the ECM. The principle kinase involved is a 125-kDa protein termed the focal adhesion kinase (FAK, also known as pp125[fak]). FAK is an essential component in focal contacts and, if phosphorylation is an indicator of activation, FAK activation is an immediate-early event in virtually all integrin-mediated adhesion on FN, LN, vitronectin, and collagen matrices. Antibody-mediated clustering of integrins also induces FAK phosphorylation. The identification of FAK in focal contacts provides further evidence that (a) adhesion promotes signal transduction events and (b) the integrin receptors functionally resemble growth factor receptors.

5. Nuclear Responses to ECM Adhesion

Gene expression responses to cell adhesion are slowly being characterized. Adhesion-specific promoters and enhancers have been identified in a few genes. Cultured mammary cells will only produce the milk protein β-casein when they are attached to a matrix. In these cells, an enhancer of 161 bp in length has been identified 5' of the casein gene. This enhancer conveys ECM responsive expression for the casein gene.

An excellent model for the study of gene expression in response to adhesion is provided by the monocyte. These cells adhere to the endothelial cell basement membrane prior to differentiation into mature tissue macrophages. Circulating monocytes are undifferentiated cells and express few of the inflammatory proteins expressed by macrophages. Attachment to tissue culture plastic induces the expression of a number of genes, including IL-1, CSF-1, c-fos, c-jun, IκB, and various, as yet unidentified, monocyte adherence (MAD) proteins. In addition, the expression of c-fms, lysozyme, and CD-4 genes declines upon attachment. Under these same conditions, the expression of HLA-DR and β-actin are unaffected by adherence. Interestingly, adherence to different matrices induces different panels of gene expression. Attachment to collagen induces expression of MAD-5, -6, and -7, whereas attachment to FN induces IL-1 and CSF-1. These effects on gene expression can be reproduced by the artificial clustering of integrin receptors with monoclonal antibodies, indicating that these effects are a response to attachment.

Examination of upstream elements of these genes, which are up- or downregulated by adhesion, revealed some possible mechanisms. A binding site for the transcription factor NF-κB was present in all genes whose transcription was enhanced by adhesion. NF-κB is known to be mobilized from an inactive cytoplasmic pool to an active nuclear transcription factor when monocytes adhere. Transcriptional regulatory elements were also observed in genes that were downregulated by attachment. Binding sites for c-*myb* and HLH factors were present upstream of downregulated, but not most upregulated, genes.

E. Cell-Type Specificity in Adhesion

Cell-type specificity can be provided at several levels of molecular composition of adhesion sites: integrin receptor specificity, cytoskeletal organization within the cell in response to specific receptors, and the array of genes being expressed in cells. There are many examples of how integrins provide cell-type specificity for adhesion. The β_1 subunit is a common player in adhesion events for many cell types. When β_1 is associated with α_2, connective tissue cells adhere specifically to collagen types I or III. When β_1 is associated with α_4, lymphoid cells can adhere to FN matrices and to a target ligand on endothelial cells. When the same β_1 is associated with α_6, epithelial cells generate focal adhesions, resulting in F-actin polymerization into stress fibers. Clearly, these differentiated cells control their ECM adhesion processes by regulation of which α integrin subunits are being expressed at specific times. Keratinocytes do not normally express the prominent FN receptor, $\alpha_5\beta_1$, unless they initiate migration upon a FN matrix, providing an example as to how the molecular nature of the ECM regulates which integrin genes the cell expresses.

The second level of specificity is provided by the cytoskeleton and its association with specialized adhesions. Epithelial cells are highly polar, with a basal surface in adhesive contact with the basal lamina, whereas the apical surface interfaces the medium or lumenal space of an organ. Two classes of adhesions are observed in contact with the basal lamina. Focal contacts are generated by $\alpha_3\beta_1$ and $\alpha_6\beta_1$ integrins binding to LN or collagen IV of the basal lamina; these integrins then organize F-actin into stress fibers. In addition, the $\alpha_6\beta_4$ integrin plays a critical role in organizing hemidesmosomal contacts with the same basal lamina. This particular integrin is unique in having a very long cytoplasmic domain on the β_4 subunit (1000 amino acids). It is likely that this amount of genetic information is critical in several signaling events that result in keratin filament association with hemidesmosomes and the participation of bullous pemphigoid antigens (detected by antibodies in humans displaying autoimmune responses to their own epithelial cell adhesions) in these same contacts.

III. MODULATION OF MATRIX ADHESION MECHANISMS BY TUMOR CELLS

In order for tumor progression to occur, malignant cells must (a) detach from the primary tumor, (b) invade surrounding tissue, (c) intravasate into the circulatory system, (d) adhere to vascular endothelial cells at distant sites, and (e) extravasate through the endothelial basement membrane and colonize new tissues. All of these steps must include alterations in the various matrix/receptor-regulated events discussed earlier. Alterations in the components of adhesion may render tumor cells more mobile, contributing to the metastatic potential of select subsets of tumor cells. The notorious genetic instability of tumor cell populations also provides a diversity of matrix molecule and ECM receptor expressions within that population that provide a highly selective advantage for a small subset of tumor cells to undergo one of these steps and subsequently expand to provide further diversity in adhesion mechanisms at the target site.

A. Alterations in Matrix Molecules

It is becoming clear that every type of tumor cell is different in how interactions with ECM are mediated, how much diversity in ECM receptor expression can be found within tumor cell populations isolated either from the primary tumor or from metastases, and how this diversity guarantees successful selective advantage for tumor cell migration to distant sites. Consequently, examples can be found for alterations of each type of matrix molecule discussed in Section II.B.

1. Collagens

Collagen expression may either be increased or decreased in tumors. Transformation of murine 3T3 cells with v-mos caused a decrease in collagen type I gene transcription. In colorectal cancer, deficiencies in collagen expression at the edge of the tumor may contribute to the invasive characteristic of this disease. Enhanced expression of collagen types I and III has been observed in malignant gliomas compared with normal brain tissue. Whether altered collagen gene expression plays some critical role in the progression of any tumor system remains to be proven.

2. Fibronectins

Modulation of FN expression occurs in many types of tumor cells. Transformation of mammary epithelial cells consistently resulted in the complete loss of FN expression. FN is also lost from the surface of glioblastomas and ras-transformed 3T3 cells. Studies have demonstrated that ras-induced transformation results in a four- to eightfold decrease in the level of FN gene transcription in some metastasizing, as compared with nonmetastasizing, cells. Rous sarcoma virus (RSV)-transformed chick embryo fibroblasts exhibited a seven- to eightfold reduction in FN gene transcription, whereas RSV transformation of rat hepatocytes resulted in decreased FN expression and a decreased ability to adhere to exogenously supplied FN. In these cells the FN integrin receptor $\alpha_5\beta_1$ was no longer being expressed. This may not be surprising because FN and integrin $\alpha_5\beta_1$ expressions are interrelated (see Section II.D.2).

Other tumor cells overexpress FN or express rare alternatively spliced variants. FN was expressed at a 10-fold higher level in c-sis-transformed fibroblasts, whereas enhanced FN synthesis was also observed in the malignant glioma cell lines BT4A and BT4An. Analysis of the composition of FN isoforms from a variety of normal and transformed cells indicated that transformed cells express a significantly higher percentage of IIICS-containing FNs than normal cells. In addition, ED_A-containing FNs were produced by transformed liver cells, which normally produce only pFN lacking the ED domains.

3. Tenascins

Tenascins are normally expressed with tissue remodeling during development. It is not surprising therefore that enhanced expression of these matrix molecules may play some role in tumor progression. Tenascin is expressed in the stroma of many malignant tumors, where its antiadhesive properties may serve to liberate malignant cells from the primary tumor mass. Tenascin expression was found to be 10-fold higher in invasive breast carcinomas than in normal breast tissue. It was very highly elevated in gliomas, where this molecule was originally discovered, and in colonic adenocarcinomas.

B. Alterations in Matrix Receptor Molecules

1. Integrins

Integrins are a primary target for the modulation of ECM receptors in tumor cells. Expression for some integrins decreases, whereas for others (usually novel or unexpressed variants) expression is enhanced. As with the expression of the ECM components themselves, there is no clear pattern for the effects of transformation on ECM receptor expression. Differences are as prevalent as are the types of tumor cells investigated. In general, the tumor cells have a much greater diversity of integrin expression than their normal cell counterparts, particularly for promiscuous receptors such as $\alpha_3\beta_1$ and $\alpha_v\beta_3$, which recognize many different matrices and which provide versatility for tumor cell populations that must now face "uncommon" matrices.

Integrin receptor modulation has been observed in a number of tumorigenic cell types. $\alpha_4\beta_6$ integrin expression is reduced in breast carcinoma, whereas overexpression of $\alpha_4\beta_1$ (to FN) correlated with progression of melanoma. Chinese hamster ovary cells, which lack $\alpha_5\beta_1$ (to FN), are more tumorigenic than clones that have this receptor; conversely, overexpression of this receptor reduced tumorigenicity in these cells.

$\alpha_5\beta_1$ (to FN) integrin is lost after transformation of NRK cells by *ras*, whereas $\alpha_3\beta_1$ (to LN, FN, collagen) was retained. Coincident with loss of the principal FN receptor in these cells was the loss of ability to adhere to FN, implying that the remaining $\alpha_3\beta_1$ receptor was not very active in promoting adhesion to FN. Alterations in integrin expression profiles have also been reported on neuroblastoma cells (see Section IV,A).

Adhesion to LN is also altered in some transformed cells. LN binding is important in the metastatic process, as fragments of LN that are recognized by integrin receptors reduce experimental metastatic ability when coinjected with tumor cells into the tail veins of nude mice. In a number of instances, altered expression of the nonintegrin LN receptor has been reported. The 67-kDa LN receptor is strongly expressed in invasive carcinomas, whereas benign or normal cells express this protein at low levels.

Tumor cells can modulate LN-specific integrins as well. Chemical transformation increases the expression of $\alpha_1\beta_1$ and $\alpha_6\beta_1$ receptors, while having no effect on $\alpha_3\beta_1$ and $\alpha_5\beta_1$ receptors. Integrin receptors were examined on 41 renal carcinoma cell lines. All lines expressed the poly-specific $\alpha_3\beta_1$ receptor; however, only the more metastatic lines expressed the $\alpha_6\beta_1$ (LN) receptor.

Vitronectin receptors seem to be another commonly altered receptor in transformed cells. Overexpression of the vitronectin receptor $\alpha_v\beta_3$ correlates with progression (i.e., of vertical growth phase) of malignant melanoma. Several carcinomas express novel vitronectin receptors not normally seen on untransformed cells.

2. CD44

CD44 includes a large family of transmembrane glycoproteins whose primary RNA transcript can be spliced into a very complex pattern of mature mRNAs, resulting in many cell type- and tumor type-specific patterns of expression. Its simplest form in lymphoid cells and some connective tissue cells has a cytoplasmic domain that binds to the cytoskeleton in response to hyaluronan binding to its most external domain. Near and external to the plasma membrane lies a domain responsible for lymphocyte homing whose receptor has yet to be identified. In epithelial cells, the lymphocyte-homing domain is frequently spliced out and these variants may bind hyaluronan.

Two types of experiments suggest that CD44 may be a critical player during tumor progression and metastasis. First, screening of many human primary tumors and their metastases reveal that (a) primary tumors frequently have reduced or elevated patterns of specific CD44 isoforms as compared to the patterns in untransformed cell counterparts. (b) Metastatic tumor populations frequently have a different pattern of isoform expression from that of the primary tumor, in some cases with very high levels of these isoforms and in other cases fairly low levels. Second, an experimental model of fibrosarcoma in nude mice has demonstrated very high expression levels of the simplest isoform of CD44 in newly formed primary tumors followed by loss of its expression as the primary tumor population grows rapidly into a large mass; in parallel, very high levels of CD44 are observed in the earliest micrometastases of lung and other organs but are lost as these populations grow rapidly into overt metastases. This plasticity of expression suggests that CD44 is an important player in the early steps of colonization of the lung but is antagonistic to the rapid outgrowth of tumor cell populations. That CD44 plays an important role in lung colonization is also supported by experimental metastasis studies in this same system.

C. Consequences for Signal Transduction

The development of malignancy is a multistep process. Initial events relieve normal regulation of growth, leading to clonal expansion of the newly mutated cell. Rapid proliferation and genetic instability allow for the generation of further mutations. Final events involve loss of anchorage-dependent growth, resulting in a cell that can migrate from the primary tumor and initiate a metastatic lesion at a distant site.

A number of observations indicate that transformation induces the disassembly of the adhesion apparatus, from the ECM through focal contacts and to the cytoskeleton. Loss of FN from the surface of *ras*-transformed cells correlates with loss of focal contacts and F-actin stress fibers. Addition of FN to transformed cells promotes adhesion and cell spreading and reorganization of F-actin microfilaments.

However, this does not restore regulation of growth, suggesting that altered morphology and loss of growth control are independent events.

Transformation with RSV, with its active v-src oncogene, produces many effects on focal contact components. In RSV-transformed cells, v-src tyrosine kinase becomes localized in focal contacts concomitant with the phosphorylation of integrins and vinculin. Talin and vinculin become diffuse throughout the cell and F-actin depolymerizes into its individual actin monomers. Subsequently, cells reduce expression of FN, round up, and lose their adhesive properties. Cells transformed with an RSV that encodes a mutant v-src that does not localize to focal contacts display none of these effects. As with ras-transformed cells, when exogenous FN is supplied, focal contacts reorganize.

Many oncogenes, including ras and src, promote anchorage-independent growth. Early in the transformation process with these oncogenes, intracellular events occur, such as alkalinization of the cytoplasm, which also occurs as a consequence of adhesion. Integrin phosphorylation, PKC activation, and NFκB mobilization—all of which occur during adhesion—are also observed in transformed cells capable of anchorage-independent growth. If adhesion is a requirement for cell growth, then oncogenes that mimic the signals sent to the nucleus by adhesion may "short-circuit" adhesion signals and allow cells to grow in the absence of adhesion. Disassembly of the adhesion apparatus and reduced expression of adhesion-related proteins may be merely the result of cellular housekeeping; cells do not necessarily produce components that they do not need or use, i.e., those with no function requirement or selective advantage.

IV. TUMOR PROGRESSION AND METASTASIS

A. Overview and Paradoxes

Consideration of the adhesion mechanisms described in Section II led to several paradoxes that tumor cells must overcome during the complete sequence of progression from the initially transformed cell, through all stages of primary tumor formation, and finally through the events leading to metastatic spread to highly foreign tissue sites. We will consider some of these paradoxes from a biological perspective, as little insight has been gleaned on their molecular mechanisms thus far.

The most common paradox is that of adhesion to a matrix versus the concept of deadhesion (or detachment) from that same matrix. Clearly, tumor cells must be versatile in both aspects of behavior if they are to be successful. As examples, tumor cells must detach from surrounding matrices in the primary tumor in order to extravasate into neighboring blood vessels or lymphatic vessels. Similarly, intravasation of tumor cells at metastatic target sites must include adherence of tumor cells to endothelial cells, migration between endothelial cells to gain access to blood vessel basal lamina, adherence to the basal lamina, destruction of the basal lamina, and finally movement into the tissue architecture. It is increasingly clear that these events require the expression of many different genes in various arrays at each of these steps. This is where clonal and genetic diversity of tumor cell populations come into play by providing small subsets of tumor cells at some unknown frequency, which are successful at executing these events.

Probably the most complex events of tumor progression must occur at the basal lamina of blood vessels where intravasation and extravasation must both occur, as well as the destruction of the integrity of the basal lamina providing penetrability of tumor cells. Selective expression of type IV collagenase appears critical for the destruction of basal lamina integrity. In addition, expression of matrix metalloproteases may complement the activity of type IV collagenase. When the organizational integrity of the matrix is destroyed by these degradative enzymes, the cell may become a wandering entity, searching for another class of matrix to adhere to without expressing degradative enzymes for that particular matrix class.

Some consideration should be given to the different classes of molecules that facilitate the adhesion of tumor cells versus those that facilitate detachment of cells. It has become clear over many years of investigation that hyaluronan mediates the detachment of cells (and possibly motility, although this latter point has not been addressed adequately) by binding to hyaluronan-binding proteins on the cell surface whose expression is tightly regulated. One class of such hyaluronan binding "receptors" are the CD-44 antigens as described in Section III.B.2. CD44 receptors are integral membrane proteins, which, upon binding of hyaluronan, act as a counteradhesion receptor. It appears likely that hyaluronan-complexed CD-44 transmits countersignals into the cell that countermand the adhesion-promoting signals of integrins and other ECM receptors. How this occurs remains to be determined. In light of this evidence, many tumor cell classes have elevated levels of synthesis of the GAG hyaluronan and of hyaluronan-binding proteins, consistent with their proposed functions in facilitating tumor cell detachment by mechanisms that may be shared with specific migrating cells in the developing embryo.

In addition to hyaluronan, two other classes of molecules appear to promote detachment of cells. Tenascin, as reviewed in Section II.B, neutralizes adhesion to FN matrices by unknown mechanisms and its expression is highly elevated on glioblastoma and select other tumor cells. Dermatan sulfate and/or chondroitin sulfate proteoglycans have also been implicated in cell detachment and their expression has been elevated on several tumor cell classes at the very stages when metastatic spread is optimized. How counteradhesion mechanisms would operate to facilitate tumor cell detachment remains for detailed investigation *in vivo* at the single-cell level.

As summarized in Section III, very little study has been dedicated to altered expression of ECM receptors that may be causative in the tumor-progressing characteristics of specific tumor classes. This is particularly true for *in vivo* analyses in animal model systems, in contrast to the better-studied tissue culture model systems. However, some insight has been gained into the different integrin expression patterns during the progression of human melanoma in a nude mouse model system. In this case, radial growth phase melanoma cells, prior to invasive spread in the skin, express a wide array of integrins that more or less reflect the expression pattern observed in human melanocytes. However, once vertical growth phase has been inititated, two integrins become prominent as if they are contributing factors in invasion: $\alpha_4\beta_1$, which recognizes the IIICS-binding site in FNs and V-CAM-1 on endothelial cells, and members of the

β_3 family of integrin adhesion receptors commonly observed on platelets (this latter point suggests that invasive melanoma cells may share some common mechanisms with adhering and activated platelets).

Expression of integrin subunits has also been examined in human neuroblastoma systems. Neuroblastoma is a pediatric cancer; aggressive and metastatic forms of the disease are characterized by amplification and overexpression of the N-*myc* oncogene. Examination of neuroblastoma cell lines with or without N-*myc* amplification/overexpression has revealed that overexpression of N-*myc* results in the downregulation of several common integrins (e.g., $\alpha_2\beta_1$ to collagen and LN and $\alpha_3\beta_1$ to FN) normally found on cell lines that do not express N-*myc*. In contrast, expression of $\alpha_1\beta_1$ is unaffected. These downregulations occur by both transcriptional and posttranscriptional mechanisms. Transfection of the N-*myc* gene into cells that do not normally express the protein results in decreased integrin expression and altered adhesion.

It appears likely that each tumor cell class may have distinctively different patterns of integrin and antiadhesive molecule patterns of expression that provide cell-type-specific versatility in the progression of each tumor type. This may not be surprising, as embryonic cells have very different and exclusive mechanisms for adhering, responding, and detaching from their specific matrices. This raises the critical issue whether tumor cells use an adhesion/deadhesion mechanism that is different from their normal cell counterpart and that could be the target of antimetastasis clinical therapy. Much more basic science must be learned about these molecular events before such considerations can be taken seriously.

B. Enhanced Turnover of Matrix and Receptors

Tumor cells may accelerate the turnover of matrix molecules by either increasing the expression of matrix proteases or decreasing the expression of protease inhibitors such as TIMPs or PAIs. Both mechanisms are utilized in specific tumor types. Altered ECM protease activity may be an intrinsic trait of the cell line in question. In some tumors, however, the primary site of the tumor may affect protease expression. When colon carcinoma cell lines were injected into nude mice, it was found that only cells implanted in the abdominal wall (orthotopic injection), as compared to cells injected subcutaneously (ectopic injection), expressed high levels of MMPs. It was also observed that MMP expression correlated with metastatic potential.

MMPs have been observed to be overexpressed in a number of tumor cell types, including melanoma, adenocarcinoma, invasive breast carcinoma, and squamous carcinoma. Benign or nonmetastatic cells produce normal levels of MMPs. Interestingly, the expression of MMPs is enhanced when cells are exposed to fragmented, but not whole, FN. The urokinase-type plasminogen activator, which is expressed at high levels by B16 melanoma cells, ras-transformed 3T3 cells, and squamous carcinoma cell lines, behaves in a similar manner. This implies that once initial matrix degradation occurs, a cascade is activated that further increases the extent of matrix turnover. Enhanced MMP activity was also observed in the metastatic gastric cancer cell line KKLC. In this instance, MMP activity was not the result of enhanced MMP gene expression but was found to be due to reduced expression of TIMP-1. Cells transfected with a plasmid expressing TIMP-1 from the SV40 promoter exhibited reduced MMP activity and lost their metastatic potential.

Plasticity of expression of the CD44 gene in progressing and metastasizing tumor cell subsets may play critical roles during specific steps of these events. Examples of these reversible expressions were provided in Section III.B.2.

C. Metastasis to Bone: Special Case

Metastasis to bone is a special case because of the relative simplicity of bone structure and its rigid framework of collagen:calcium phosphate complexes. This ECM may require special rules by which very select tumor cells adhere and grow on this inert matrix, rules that differ from the "classical" ECMs that support tumor metastasis in virtually all other organs of the body (including the bone marrow). [In this context, metastases to brain must also encounter a highly unique ECM environment.] Micrometastases of human prostate carcinoma CWR22R cells, tagged with

the histochemical marker gene *lacZ*, are shown in Fig. 3. These micrometastases have colonized bones of the spinal column and the long bones of athymic nude mice. Whether these micrometastases require expression of bone-specific proteins, such as osteopontin or osteonectin, remains to be seen. Metastasis to bone is probably the most understudied area of tumor biology, yet proves so very important in human breast cancer, prostate cancer, lung cancer, and select other cancers. For patients with symptom-expressing bone cancer, some of these metastases are osteolytic, whereas others synthesize new bone.

V. CONSIDERATIONS FOR THE FUTURE

A. Summary of Current Findings

Analyses of matrix adhesion mechanisms of normal mammalian cells over the past two decades have revealed both complexity and versatility by which cells can execute their adhesion-dependent functions. Several classes of molecules at the cell surface can function as matrix receptors, whereas each matrix ligand has numerous binding sites for two or more receptors on cells and binding sites for other matrix molecules, providing complex "cross-linking" mechanisms among these molecules. To some extent, this complexity may reflect redundancy of mechanisms operating in any one cell. However, it remains to be shown whether each adhesion mechanism is linked to differing and/or overlapping transmembrane signaling mechanisms; if the former is the case, then redundancy may not be as extensive as currently thought. It has also become clear that embryonic cell populations and certain cell types in the adult, in response to pathogenic conditions, can modulate their matrix adhesion mechanisms in carefully orchestrated patterns to respond to environmental cues.

Matrix adhesion mechanisms operating in the many different classes of tumor cells have not been as well studied as those of their untransformed cell counterparts, particularly in a concerted fashion with regard to their significance for tumor progression *in vivo*. There is indication that upon transformation, specialized adhesion mechanisms are downregulated in tumor cells, whereas other promiscuous adhesion mechanisms become more prominent, probably providing versatility for tumor cells in encountering the very different matrices in blood vessels and in target organs that they do not "normally" associate with.

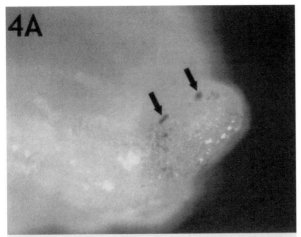

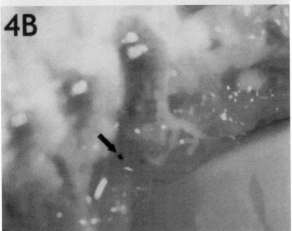

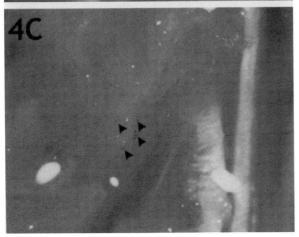

Because of the genetic and phenotypic instability in tumor cells, it is likely that small subsets of tumor cells may express a unique class of matrix receptors, allowing this subset to invade and metastasize to a particular target organ. Once this small subset is established in that organ site, the specialized adhesion mechanism would be lost in the diluted cell population because it does not provide selective growth advantage from that point forward. Many similar possibilities will require detailed and careful analysis of the expression of both matrix molecules and matrix receptors at the single-cell level during tumor progression *in vivo*.

B. Future Directions for Research

Better understanding of the matrix adhesion mechanisms of primary tumor cells and their metastatic counterparts will require much more detailed information on structures and functions of receptor molecules, such as integrins and membrane-intercalated proteoglycans, as well as the many regulatory elements in their gene promoters (particularly whether related families of receptors are under coordinate control). Only limited information is currently known about synthesis regulation of these receptor classes. Receptors for other sites in adhesion molecules FN, laminin, and others remain to be identified and characterized. Aberration of transmembrane signaling mechanisms from matrix receptors must be deciphered for the many different classes of tumor cells and their metastatic counterparts to determine if any general patterns emerge. In contrast, promoter studies of matrix genes are being thoroughly analyzed in some cases

FIGURE 3 Micrometastasis to bone. Human prostate carcinoma cells (CWR22R clone H, tagged with bacterial *lacZ*) after culturing were injected into athymic nude mice subcutaneously in PBS or Matrigel vehicles. When primary tumors had become large, the animals were sacrificed for excision of many bones, followed by bone fixation and X-gal staining. Control animals (no tumor cells injected) failed to yield any X-gal staining of their bones. (A) Micrometastases (small arrowheads) in the long bone of the leg 17 days post-PBS injection. Original magnification, ×42. (B) Micrometastases (e.g., small arrow) along the spinal column 113 days post-PBS injection. Original magnification, ×13. (C) Micrometastases (small arrows) along the spinal column 44 days post-Matrigel injection. Original magnification, ×34. From J. L. Holleran, C. J. Miller, and L. A. Culp, *J. Histochem. Cytochem.* **48,** 643–651 (2000), with permission.

but not well in other cases. It will also be essential to determine if there is coordinate regulation in cells for synthesis of a particular matrix molecule and receptors targeted for that molecule.

There has been little investigation of the cell-to-cell diversity in matrix adhesion mechanisms that operate in one cell type in a particular tissue; this issue is critical for clonal expansion or contraction of specialized cell types in tissues. There is relatively poor understanding of the heterologous interactions of two or more cell types in the same tissue environment, how these interactions alter the expression of matrix molecules and their receptors, and how these mechanisms are ablated for advantage of by malignantly converted cells of one of these classes.

C. Potential Clinical Significance

We are rapidly approaching the point in time when basic science information on tumor cell adhesion mechanisms can be applied to the human patient bearing cancer. Perhaps this point is best illustrated with the finding that RGDS and other synthetic peptides, as well as certain proteolytic fragments of FNs or laminin, which mimic specific matrix-binding mechanisms, can inhibit experimental metastasis of some tumor cells in the lung in mouse model systems when tumor cells and peptide are coinjected (but not subsequently, indicating that inhibition operates at the time of endothelial cell binding and/or intravasation). There is some optimism that these synthetic peptides could be administered topically and intravenously during the surgical removal of tumors in humans in order to prevent labilization and reestablishment of tumor cells during surgical intervention over a limited span of time. In contrast, it is unlikely that these synthetic peptides could be administered over long periods of time to inhibit *natural metastatic spread* of human tumors because of serious toxic effects on the critical adhesion mechanisms necessary for normal cell functions in so many tissues.

Another approach would be the implantation of a capsule in or neighboring a tumor site. This capsule would contain synthetic peptides that interfere with the matrix adhesion mechanism(s) and that would be released over a long period of time, inhibiting tumor cell association with neighboring matrices and possi-

bly lead to tumor regression because apotosis (programmed cell death) would be invoked in such tumor cells. This approach may prove of special benefit in brain tumors, which, in many cases, cannot be removed surgically because of their intertwining patterns with normal brain tissue. Clearly these synthetic peptides would have to be targeted specifically to tumor cell adhesion mechanisms while having minimal effects on normal brain neuron or glial cell functions.

As more information becomes available on environmental cues that regulate matrix receptor gene expression, it is likely that pharmacological intervention in receptor gene expression will provide another approach for regulating tumor cell growth. Again, specificity of the intervention must be maximized against possible regulation of the same receptor class in neighboring normal host tissue cells. Tumor cells may provide a unique mechanism by which the pharmacological agent could be selectively introduced into that population of cells. Alternatively and in light of the expanding use of gene therapy, antisense genes could be introduced into tumor cells specifically to interfere with expression of a matrix ligand and/or a matrix receptor that these tumor cells require for successful growth and expansion of the population. The next decade of research should provide a variety of approaches for regulating matrix adhesion mechanisms in specific classes of tumor cells to the benefit of the human patient.

Acknowledgments

The authors acknowledge support for their studies from the National Institutes of Health to LAC (Research Grants CA27755 and NS17139), training grant support to RJ (T32-AG00105), and a U.S. Army grant to LAC (DAMD17-98-1-8587). Pilot studies were supported by the Ireland Cancer Center of Case Western Reserve University (NCI-supported P30-CA43703). They extend appreciation to Kathleen O'Connor for some of the models in Figs. 1 and 2 and data of Table II and to Daniel Ling for computer-based literature searches.

See Also the Following Articles

BIBLIOGRAPHY

Albelda, S. M. (1993). Role of integrins and other cell adhesion molecules in tumor progression and metastasis. *Lab. Invest.* **68,** 4–17.

Clarke, E. A., and Brugge, J. S. (1995). Integrins and signal transduction pathways: The road taken. *Science* **268,** 233–239.

Culp, L. A., Radinsky, R., and Lin, W.-C. (1991). Extracellular matrix interactions with neoplastic cells: Tumor- vs. cell type-specific mechanisms. *In* "Aspects of the Biochemistry and Molecular Biology of Tumors" (T. G. Pretlow II and T. P. Pretlow, eds.), pp. 99–149. Academic Press, Orlando, FL.

Giancotti, F. G. (1997). Integrin signaling: Specificity and control of cell survival and cell cycle progression. *Curr. Opin. Cell Biol.* **9,** 691–700.

Hay, E. D. (1991). "Cell Biology of Extracellular Matrix," 2nd Ed. Plenum Press, New York.

Hynes, R. O. (1990). "Fibronectins." Springer-Verlag, New York.

Judware, R., and Culp, L. A. (1997). Concomitant downregulation of expression of integrin subunits by N-*myc* in human neuroblastoma cells: Differential regulation for α2, α3, and β1. *Oncogene* **14,** 1341–1350.

Juliano, R. L., and Haskill, S. (1993). Signal transduction from the extracellular matrix. *J. Cell Biol.* **3,** 577–585.

Kjellen, L., and Lindahl, U. (1991). Proteoglycans: Structures and interactions. *Annu. Rev. Biochem.* **60,** 443–475.

Kogerman, P., Sy, M.-S., and Culp, L. A. (1997). Overexpressed human CD44 promotes lung colonization during micrometastasis of murine fibrosarcoma cells: Facilitated retention in the lung vasculature. *Proc. Natl. Acad. Sci. USA* **94,** 13233–13238.

Miyamoto, S., Katz, B. Z., Lafrenie, R. M., and Yamada, K. M. (1998). Fibronectin and integrins in cell adhesion, signaling, and morphogenesis. *Ann. N.Y. Acad. Sci.* **857,** 119–129.

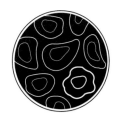

Folate Antagonists

Barton A. Kamen
Peter Cole

Cancer Institute of New Jersey and
Robert Wood Johnson Medical School

I. Folate Homeostasis
II. Methotrexate
III. Trimetrexate
IV. Folate Analogs as Inhibitors of Thymidylate
   Synthase and *de novo* Purine Pathways
V. Summary

GLOSSARY

aminoimidazole carboxamide ribonucleotide trans-formylase Enzyme that catalyzes a formyl-tetrahydrofolate-dependent step in the completion of the second ring during purine synthesis.

dihydrofolate reductase (DHFR) Presumed target of methotrexate. DHFR maintains the intracellular pool of tetrahydrofolate necessary for pyrimidine synthesis by catalyzing the reduction of dihydrofolate.

folate A generic term used to define a family of compounds made up of the reduced forms of folic acid. The fully reduced form, tetrahydrofolic acid, is the one carbon donor for the biosynthesis of purines, thymidine, and some amino acids. Some members of the family include 5-methyltetrahydrofolic acid, 10-formyltetrahydrofolic acid and 5,10-methylenetetrahydrofolic acid. Folate (folic acid) is a water-soluble vitamin.

folate analog A drug that is structurally related to folic acid and that interferes with folate metabolism or folate-dependent reactions.

folylpolyglutamate A unique peptide in which a number of glutamates are coupled to the glutamate in folate via the γ carboxy and α amino moieties. The predominant intracellular folates in humans are folylpenta through folylhepataglutamate, i.e., folate with a total of five to seven glutamates.

glycinamide ribonucleotide transformylase Enzyme responsible for catalyzing one of the early steps in purine synthesis: the transfer of a formyl group from N-10-formyltetrahydrofolate to glycinamide ribonucleotide.

thymidylate synthase Enzyme that catalyzes the rate-limiting, tetrahydrofolate-dependent step in thymidylate synthesis: the conversion of deoxyuridine monophosphate to deoxythymidine monophosphate.

Folic acid is a water-soluble vitamin associated with the other B vitamins. In its fully reduced form (tetrahydrofolate), folate serves as a one-carbon donor of synthesis of purines and thymidines, as well as in the remethylation cycle of homocysteine to methionine. Therefore, it is not surprising that folate analogs are useful as antibiotics and cytotoxic drugs in the treatment of cancer, autoimmune diseases, psoriasis, and bacterial and protozoal infections. Since the 1950s, many of the enzymes requiring folate as a cofactor (e.g., thymidylate synthase, dihydrofolic acid reductase) and molecules critical in folate homeostasis (e.g., the reduced folate carrier, folylpolyglutamate synthase and the folate receptor) have been purified and even crystallized. The genes have been cloned, sequenced, and mapped, providing detailed knowledge of their regulation and three-dimensional structure. This has, in part, led to the rational synthesis of a large number of folate analogs that differ from methotrexate (MTX), the "classical antifolate," in transport, metabolism, and intracellular targets. This article highlights the similarities and differences between natural folate and antifolates with respect to biochemistry and metabolism and presents the pharmacology of methotrexate and some representative "next-generation" folate antagonists. There are more than 25,000 Medline citations for MTX alone so the reader is referred to citations in the bibliography for more detailed information about specific topics and other experimental folate analogs.

I. FOLATE HOMEOSTASIS

A basic understanding of the pharmacokinetics and pharmacodynamics of folate analogs can be best appreciated within the context of folate metabolism, including such parameters as absorption, transport, metabolism, clearance, and folate-mediated reactions. Moreover, the effects of these drugs can be more completely understood and appreciated when considered in light of their effects on normal folate metabolism. Some of the important reactions in the cellular pharmacology of folate are shown in Fig. 1.

In humans, plasma folate is 5-methyltetrahydrofolate. The concentration is in the range of 0.01–0.03 μM; thus, the total plasma folate in the average 60- to 70-kg person is only 10 to 20 μg. Folate deficiency can lead to increased plasma homocysteine or aberrant DNA synthesis, with the latter resulting in megaloblastic anemia. Because folate is a vitamin, its overall conservation by the body is great. There is little folate lost in the urine because of specific receptors on the brush border of the kidney proximal tubules. High-affinity receptors also ensure that there is an appropriate accumulation of folate by the fetus (fetal blood

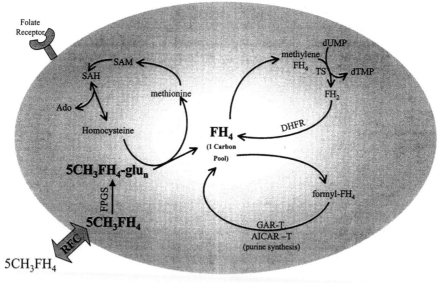

FIGURE 1 Schematic pathway of some folate-mediated reactions and transport highlighting folate antagonists' sites of action and/or drug resistance. 5CH$_3$FH$_4$, 5-methyltetrahydrofolate; FH$_4$, tetrahydrofolate; FH$_2$, dihydrofolate; SAM, S-adenosylmethionine; SAH, S-adenosylhomocysteine; Ado, adenosine; FPGS, folate polyglutamate synthetase; DHFR, dihydrofolate reductase; TS, thymidylate synthase; GAR-T, glycinamide ribonucleotide transformylase; AICAR-T, aminoimidazole carboxamide ribonucleotide transformylase.

has three to four times the folate of maternal blood), and the cerebrospinal fluid has two to three times the concentration of a matched plasma sample. The initial step in folate accumulation from plasma by most cells is via the reduced folate carrier (RFC), a nonconcentrative, bidirectional process with a Michaelis–Menten dissociation constant (K_m) for folate in the 1–10 μM range. Because plasma folate concentration is only 0.01–0.03 μM and intracellular folate concentration is $\cong 1$–$10 \cdot M$, it seems intuitively correct that there must be an intracellular trap, such as high-affinity binding to enzymes, an anabolic process, or both. Thus, it is not surprising that most folate exists in cells in the form of a folylpolyglutamate (Fig. 2). This is a unique peptide in that the terminal glutamates are linked via the γ not the usual α carboxy group in the glutamyl moiety. The enzyme catalyzing this reaction is folylpoly-glutamate synthetase (FPGS). Folylpolyglutamates are retained by the cell and are better substrates than monoglutamates [i.e., they generally have a lower K_m and a greater maximal velocity (V_{max})] for the various folate-requiring enzymes. Human FPGS is a growth-regulated enzyme and the gene maps to the long arm of chromosome 9.

Folic Acid

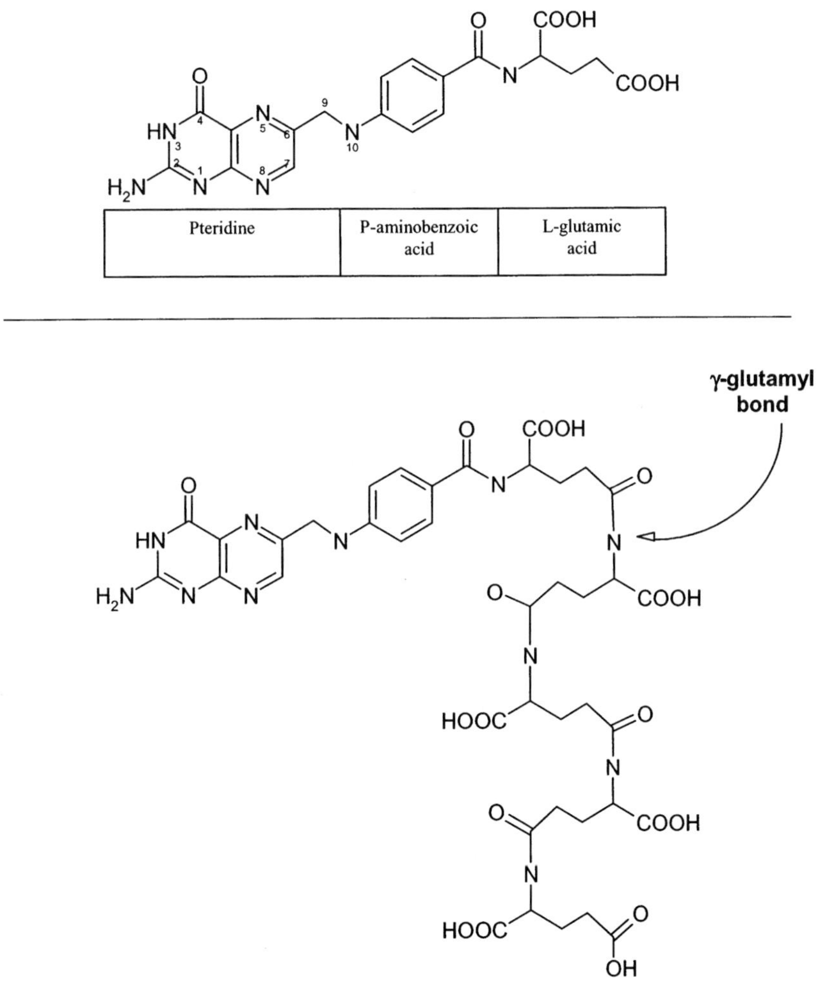

| Pteridine | P-aminobenzoic acid | L-glutamic acid |

Folate pentaglutamate

FIGURE 2 Structure of folic acid mono- and polyglutamate highlighting the component structures of folic acid and the unique γ-glutamyl bond in the polyglutamate form.

II. METHOTREXATE

Methotrexate is a "classical" 4-amino-substituted folate (Fig. 3) that is a tight binding inhibitor of dihydrofolate reductase (DHFR). It has been used clinically since the early 1950s and remains a mainstay in the treatment of patients with a number of malignant and nonmalignant disorders. MTX enters mammalian cells via at least two different transport systems: the RFC and the folate receptor (Fig. 1). The RFC has a K_m 1 to 10 μM for MTX and reduced folates. The folate receptor, which is present in the choroid plexus and the proximal tubules of the kidney, has a K_m of approximately 1 nM for 5-methyltetrahydrofolate and 20 to 50 nM for MTX. These differences may account for the increased accumulation of folate compared with MTX in the cerebro-spinal fluid. Once inside the cell, MTX will either bind to DHFR [in the presence of nicotinamide adenine dinucleotide phosphate (NADPH), the dissociation constant (K_d) is 1–10 pM] or be metabolized to a polyglutamate and then bind to DHFR or other enzymes. MTX polyglutamation increases its intracellular half-life and results in inhibition of additional enzymes involved in the *de novo* synthesis of purines. Compared with natural folates, MTX is a relatively poor substrate for FPGS.

A. Pharmacokinetics

Until high drug concentrations are attained (>10 μM), MTX is principally cleared by the kidneys. At conventional doses of 20 to 500 mg/m^2, 70 to 90% of the drug is found unchanged in the urine. As a polyanion, MTX will be taken up at the basolateral surface of tubule cells by an organic anion transporter that is likely in the same superfamily of transporters as the RFC. In transfected cells, this transporter mediates basolateral uptake of MTX but not taurocholate, *p*-aminohippurate, prostaglandin E$_2$, or leukotriene C$_4$. Folic acid, sulfobromophthalein, and 4,4'-diisothiocyanostilbene-2,2'-disulfonic acid inhibit MTX accumulation. The organic anion transporter (multiorganic anion transporter, i.e., a MOAT) was found to be identical to the multidrug-related protein MRP2, the protein deficient in Dubin–Johnson syndrome. A MOAT is important in the clearance of MTX by both the liver and the kidney.

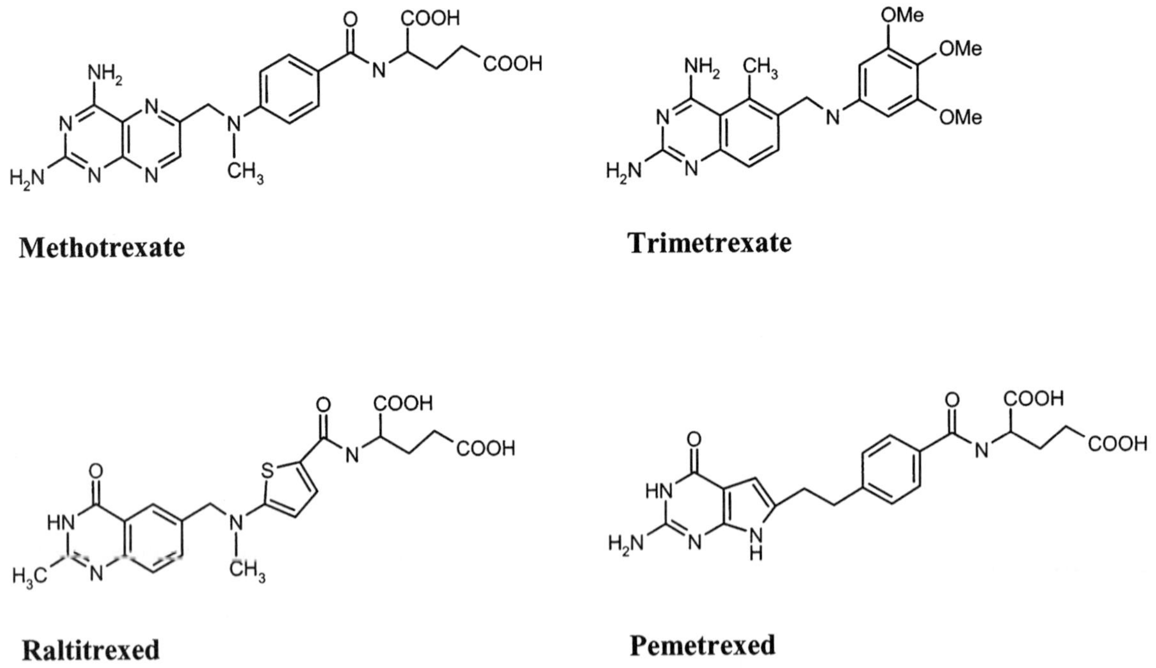

Methotrexate

Trimetrexate

Raltitrexed

Pemetrexed

FIGURE 3 Four antifolate analogs: methotrexate, trimetrexate, raltitrexed, and pemetrexed.

When high-dose MTX (>5 g/m^2) is administered such that plasma MTX exceeds 10 μM, as much as 20 to 50% of MTX is renally excreted as the 7-OH metabolite formed by aldehyde oxidase in the liver. The 7-OH metabolite is a weak inhibitor of DHFR, but 7-OHMTX polyglutamates have been reported to be potent inhibitors of thymidylate synthase and aminoimidazole carboxamide ribonucleotide transformylase. Although 7-OH is not generally considered a significantly toxic antimetabolite, it has a very long terminal plasma half-life ($T_{1/2}$ β) and, because of its insolubility, may play a role in the renal failure associated with high-dose MTX therapy.

B. Resistance

As may be expected, resistance to MTX can be multifactorial. Two primary mechanisms are decreased metabolism (transport and polyglutamylation) or mutations or overproduction of enzymes such as DHFR.

III. TRIMETREXATE

Trimetrexate (TMTX) is a lipophilic folate analog (Fig. 3), which is a tight-binding inhibitor of DHFR, not a substrate for FPGS, and does not require the RFC or the folate receptor for cellular uptake. It was initially developed as an antimalarial agent and is approved for the treatment of *Pneumocystis carinii* pneumonia and is also active against *Toxoplasma gondii*. A number of clinical trials in patients with refractory malignancies, using daily and weekly schedules of TMTX, have also shown TMTX to have anticancer activity. If tumors are resistant to MTX by virtue of decreased folate transport, then the same pharmacologic principles that allow large doses of TMTX to be administered concurrently with folate rescue to treat patients with *P. carinii* should allow high-dose TMTX to be administered with low-dose folate to treat patients with cancer. This strategy is an example of selective protection of normal cells. All cells accumulate TMTX, but only normal cells take up the antidote (folate) when minimal doses of the latter are used.

TMTX, like MTX, seems to be an S phase or at least a cell cycle-dependent drug because it interferes with nucleotide synthesis. Based on *in vitro* studies, there seems to be a threshold concentration (approximately 0.01 to 0.1 μM) above which time becomes the more critical variable in determining the degree of cytotoxicity. For example, an increase from 3 h of drug exposure to 26 h was associated with a 1000-fold increase in cytotoxicity, whereas a 3 log increase in concentration over only a 3-h time period only attained a 50% increase.

A. Pharmacokinetics

Pharmacokinetic data have been obtained in patients infected with the human immunodeficiency virus who suffer from *P. carinii* and in oncology patients with malignancies refractory to standard chemotherapy. In humans, approximately 25% of TMTX is excreted unchanged; the majority is metabolized before excretion. Hepatic metabolism consists of oxidative demethylation, likely via cytochrome P$_{450}$ 3A. Pharmacokinetic data are consistent with either a two- or a three-exponent model. Large protein binding (>95%) of TMTX may be in part responsible for the calculated $T_{1/2}$β of 7 to 10 h and a γ phase up to 16 h. In patients with the human immunodeficiency virus receiving 30 mg/m^2 intravenous (iv) TMTX, the $T_{1/2}$β was approximately 8 h and the bioavailability was 44%, with a range of 19 to 67%. The area under the curve of oral TMTX can be normalized to the iv dose in the postdistribution phase when the oral dose was doubled.

B. Resistance

Although TMTX does not require a specialized transport system (i.e., the RFC or folate receptor), cells resistant to TMTX have been found to have impaired influx and/or expression of the multidrug resistance protein, P-glycoprotein. Giving TMTX with agents designed to neutralize a P-glycoprotein-mediated drug efflux has not yet been reported. Alternatively, increased activity of the salvage pathways for nucleotide synthesis would result in resistance to folate antagonists and use of nucleoside transport inhibitors such as dipyridamole may be synergistic.

IV. FOLATE ANALOGS AS INHIBITORS OF THYMIDYLATE SYNTHASE AND *de novo* PURINE PATHWAYS

Several newer antifolates are currently in preclinical and clinical trials. Some of these drugs inhibit TS, DHFR, or one of the two steps in *de novo* synthesis of purines that require folate. Two representative drugs are pemetrexed (multitargeted antifolate, MTA, LY231514, Alimta) and raltitrexed (ZD 1694; Tomudex), both of which are transported into cells by the RFC, are bound by the folate receptor, and are rapidly metabolized to a polyglutamate species.

A. Raltitrexed

Raltitrexed is a highly selective inhibitor of TS (Fig. 3). Rescue experiments have shown that thymidine alone prevents drug-mediated cytotoxicity, suggesting that TS is the only enzyme affected *in vitro*. Raltitrexed is a good substrate for the RFC, the folate receptor, and FPGS. Polyglutamylation of raltitrexed increases its intracellular retention, and the polyglutamate forms are more than 100 times more potent inhibitors of TS then the monoglutamate. Because raltitrexed is an excellent substrate for the folate receptor, it is conserved just as if it were folate. Clinical trials showed that a dose of only 3–5 mg/m^2 (about 10 times the daily requirement for folate) once every 3 weeks seems to be an effective dose and schedule for patients with colon cancer.

1. Pharmacokinetics

Raltitrexed had linear kinetics [i.e., the area under the concentration times time curve (AUC) is proportional to the dose] and catabolism is primarily in the liver followed by biliary excretion. There is a triexponential decay with $T_{1/2}$ β of 1.3–2.6 h and a $T_{1/2}$ γ of 50–100 h.

2. Resistance

Because the raltitrexed target is TS and the drug needs to be metabolized to a polyglutamate form for maximum potency, screening of tumor lines *in vitro* has re-vealed that decreased FPGS and increased TS both account for drug resistance.

B. Pemetrexed

Although pemetrexed (Fig. 3) is primarily an inhibitor of thymidylate synthase, the drug also inhibits dihydrofolate reductase and glycinamide ribonucleotide formyl transferase, hence its original name of "multitargeted antifolate." The latter is one of the two folate-mediated steps in the *de novo* synthesis of purine nucleotides. Thus, unlike raltitrexed cytotoxicity, which can be circumvented with thymidine, rescue from pemetrexed requires both hypoxanthine and thymidine. Pemetrexed is an excellent substrate for RFC, the folate receptor, and FPGS. The pentaglutamate species predominates intracellularly and is a very potent inhibitor of thymidylate synthase.

1. Pharmacokinetics

Pemetrexed clearance appears to be primarily renal with >80% of the drug recovered in the urine during the first 24 h. The mean plasma half-life is 3.1 h with a range of 2.2–7.2 h. Clearance and steady state volume of distribution were found to be 40 ml/min/m^2 and 7.0 liter/m^2, respectively. Like raltitrexed, the schedule most explored in clinical trials was once every 3 weeks. Because the drug interferes with folate metabolism at many levels, plasma homocysteine was found to be a very strong predictor of drug toxicity.

2. Resistance

As for other antifolates, resistance to pemetrexed appears to be multifactorial. Increased TS is a primary mechanism for cellular resistance. However, some cell lines highly resistant to pemetrexed are only modestly resistant to MTX. Moreover, a pemetrexed-resistant cell line known to overproduce TS has cytotoxicity of the drug reversed or prevented with hypoxanthine only. Thus the activity of both *de novo* thymidine and purine pathways must be important in determining the effect of the drug on nucleotide synthesis and may vary from cell to cell. Analysis of the mechanism for biochemical resistance should allow the development of combination drug therapy to overcome these problems.

V. SUMMARY

Folate metabolism and folate-mediated reactions remain a focus of intense study because of their central role in the biochemistry of nucleic acids. The large amount of work that has been done with MTX to decipher its mechanism of action, pharmacology, and mechanisms of cellular resistance has led to the development of a large number of new folate analogs, each with theoretical and often laboratory-proven advantages over MTX. The new analogs may be transported differently, they may be better or worse substrates for FPGS, and they may have different enzyme targets than MTX. While these new antifolates are moving onto the proving ground of clinical trials, they also afford us the opportunity to dissect various metabolic reactions by nature of their inherent specificity. This should allow the circumventing of drug resistance and, indeed, may even take advantage of it (e.g., selective protection of normal cells and synthesis of drugs that bypass usual transport mechanisms).

Folate antagonists have served medical science well and should continue to do so as biochemical probes, all the while remaining clinically important drugs in the treatment of patients with neoplastic and nonneoplastic diseases.

See Also the Following Articles

AKYLATING AGENTS • ANTHRACYCLINES • BLEOMYCIN • CAMPTOTHECINS • CISPLATIN AND RELATED DRUGS • HYPOXIA AND DRUG RESISTANCE • L-ASPARAGINASE • PURINE ANTIMETABOLITES • PYRIMIDINE ANTIMETABOLITES

Bibliography

Blakely, R. L., and Benkovic, S. J. (eds.) (1984). "Chemistry and Biochemistry of Folates," Vol. 1. Wiley, New York.

Farber, S., Diamond, L., Mercer, R., et al. (1948). Temporary remissions in acute leukemia in children produced by folic acid antagonist, 4 amino-pteroyl-glyutamic acid (aminopterin). N. Engl. J. Med. **238,** 787–793.

Kamen, B. A., Cole, P., and Bertino, J. R. (2000). Chemotherapeutic agents: Folic acid antagonists. In "Cancer Medicine" (J. F. Holland, E. Frei, R. C. Bast, D. W. Kufe, D. L. Morton, and R. R. Weichselbaum, eds.), pp. 612–625. Williams and Wilkins.

Peters, G. J., and Ackland, S. P. (1996). New antimetabolites in preclinical and clinical development. Exp. Opin. Invest. Drugs **5,** 637–679.

Quinn, C. T., and Kamen, B. A. (1996). A biochemical perspective of methotrexate neurotoxicity with insight on nonfolate rescue modalities. J. Invest. Med. **44,** 522–530.

Stryer, L. (1995). Biosynthesis of nucleotides. In "Biochemistry," pp. 739–762. Freeman, New York.

Weitman, S., Anderson, R., and Kamen, B. (1994). Folate binding proteins. In "Vitamin Receptors: Vitamins as Ligands in Cell Communication" (K. Dakshinamurti, ed.), pp. 106–136. Cambridge Univ. Press, New York.

fos Oncogene

Tom Curran

St. Jude Children's Research Hospital, Memphis, Tennessee

GLOSSARY

bZIP Two parallel α helices, brought together in a coiled-coil structure, that extend into the major groove of DNA.

c-*jun* Cellular gene whose product is a component, along with c-*fos*, of the AP transcription factor involved in signal transduction pathways for DNA repair and cell proliferation.

fos Oncogenic transcription factor that functions as a component of dimeric leucine zipper protein complexes, known as activator protein 1 (AP1), that bind to DNA and regulate gene expression.

oncogene Any of a heterogeneous group of genes that influence cell proliferation at various levels.

transcription factor A protein that binds to a specific DNA sequence and regulates the transcription of the adjacent gene from DNA to mRNA.

Fos is an oncogenic transcription factor that functions as a component of dimeric leucine zipper protein complexes, known as activator protein 1 (AP1), that bind to DNA and regulate gene expression. It was originally derived from the Finkel–Biskis–Jinkins murine osteogenic sarcoma virus (FBJ-MSV), which induces bone tumors in mice. The cellular homolog of the viral gene, c-*fos*, is a founding member of the class known as cellular immediate-early genes. It is expressed continuously in several tissues, including skin and hair follicle cells, but in many cell types it can be induced rapidly and transiently by a great variety of extracellular stimuli associated with mitogenesis, differentiation, cell death, and depolarization of neurons. Fos is thought to function in coupling short-term signals, elicited by cell surface stimuli, to long-term alterations in the cell phenotype by regulating the expression of specific target genes. Gene disruption studies have indicated that c-*fos* plays a particular role in bone development by regulating the maturation of osteoclasts.

I. ORIGIN

FBJ-MSV was isolated from a bone tumor that arose spontaneously in a laboratory mouse at the Argonne National Laboratories, Illinois, in 1966. A continuous cell-free passage of tumor extracts gave rise to a virulent strain of virus that induced cell transformation in tissue culture and produced bone tumors in as little as 3 weeks when inoculated into newborn mice. The *fos* oncogene was first uncovered as a transformation-specific protein encoded by FBJ-MSV that was identified using antisera from rats inoculated with *fos*-transformed fibroblasts. Molecular characterization of FBJ-MSV revealed a unique sequence specifying a Fos protein of 381 amino acids. The cellular *fos* gene (c-*fos*) is highly related to v-*fos* with the exception of the replacement of 49 C-terminal amino acids with 48 novel amino acids as a consequence of an out-of-frame fusion in the viral gene. The existence of a family of *fos*-related genes was first suggested by the identification of several Fos-related proteins using anti-Fos antibodies. A total of four family members have now been described: *fos*, *fos*-related antigen-1 *(fra1)*, *fos*-related antigen 2 *(fra2)*, and *fosB*. These genes have similar properties: they are all inducible immediate-early genes and they encode proteins that bind to DNA as components of AP1 leucine zipper dimers formed with Jun and members of the set of transcription factors known as ATF/CREB.

II. REGULATION OF c-*fos* EXPRESSION

The c-*fos* gene is a founding member of the set of genes known as cellular immediate-early genes (Fig. 1). The salient characteristic of this class of genes is that their transcription rate increases dramatically following the treatment of cells with a variety of stimuli, even in the presence of protein synthesis inhibitors. The increase in c-*fos* mRNA and protein is transient, lasting only a few hours. Although the induction was initially characterized in cells treated with mitogenic growth factors, it is now clear that the same stereotypic response can be triggered by agents that provoke proliferation, differentiation,

cell death, and even depolarization of neurons. Thus, rather than considering the cellular immediate-early response in a specific biological context, it should be regarded as a signaling mechanism that is tailored to specific purposes in each cell type in response to particular stimuli. All of the Fos-related proteins and most of the leucine zipper partners of Fos are cellular immediate-early genes. However, the extent and the time course of induction of *fos*-related genes vary considerably. In most circumstances, c-*fos* activation follows a proscribed time course: rapid activation of transcription occurs within 5 to 10 min, peak mRNA expression within 30 to 60 min, and maximal protein expression at 2 to 3 h. However, prolonged periods of c-*fos* expression have been observed in situations associated with cell death signaling. The c-*fos* promoter has proved to be of great utility as a model system for studying gene regulation. Analyses of the molecular events involved in c-*fos* activation have led to numerous insights into the mechanisms responsible for the selective regulation of gene expression in mammalian cells. Several regulatory elements in the c-*fos* promoter control transcription in response to extracellular stimuli. The first of these to be characterized was the serum response element (SRE). The SRE plays a critical role in regulating the basal and inducible levels of c-*fos* expression and has been found in many promoters of genes regulated by growth factors. A region of DNA, including the SRE and an adjacent Ets motif, is bound by protein complexes formed among the serum response factor (SRF) and the ternary complex factor (TCF). Together these elements increase transcription in response to the activation of several major signaling pathways, including the ubiquitous Ras-Raf-MapK cascade and increases in intracellular calcium. Several members of the Ets family of transcription factors can function as TCFs.

In addition to the SRE, many regulatory elements in c-*fos* cooperate in the physiological regulation of the promoter, including the cyclic AMP response element (CRE), an element first described as Sis-inducible element (SIE), now known to be a sequence that binds STATs (signal transducers and activators of transcription), and an AP1 site. Additional regulatory sequences that influence the rate

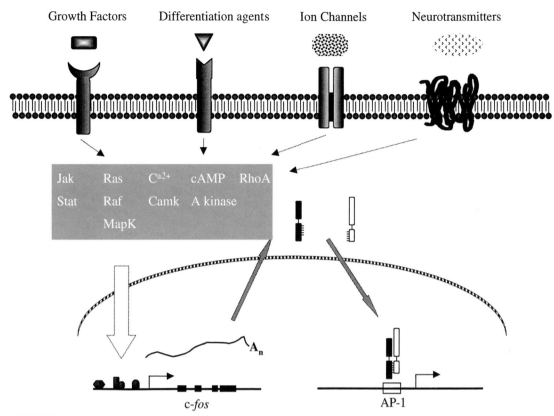

FIGURE 1 Induction of c-*fos* expression. Expression of c-*fos* is induced rapidly and transiently by a variety of extracellular stimuli, including growth factors, differentiation stimuli, voltage-gated calcium fluxes, and neurotransmitters. Signals transduced through a complex network of second messenger pathways and protein kinase cascades impinge on transcription control elements in the c-*fos* promoter. c-*fos* mRNA and protein are relatively short-lived. Fos is produced as a monomer in the cytoplasm and then is transported to the nucleus where it forms dimers with Jun family proteins that bind to AP1 sites and regulate the expression of target genes.

of transcription initiation or elongation have also been shown to contribute to the control of c-*fos* expression. Studies in transgenic mice indicate that all of these regulatory elements function in conjunction to trigger the rapid synthesis of c-*fos* mRNA in response to a very broad range of physiological signals. In the majority of situations, the period of transcription activation is short-lived, and following induction, c-*fos* mRNA and Fos protein are rapidly degraded. A common theme among these regulatory pathways is that they lead to the phosphorylation of specific amino acids on the respective transcription factors. This results in recruitment of coactivators with histone acetylase activity (HAT), acetylatation of lysine residues on histones, and increased access of the transcriptional machinery to DNA.

III. BIOCHEMICAL PROPERTIES OF Fos

The protein product of the *fos* gene (Fos) is a nuclear protein that associates with chromatin *in vivo* and binds to DNA *in vitro*. Fos undergoes extensive posttranslational modification. It can be phosphorylated on many sites by protein kinases, it is subject to redox regulation, and it is degraded by ubiquitin-dependent proteolysis mechanisms. Fos was first identified as a stable nuclear protein complexed with a 39-kDa protein (p39) that was subsequently identified as Jun, the protein encoded by the *jun* oncogene. Fos and Jun form dimeric complexes in the nucleus that bind to AP1 elements and regulate gene transcription. Dimerization is mediated by a structure known as the leucine zipper that juxtaposes regions of each protein rich in basic amino acids to form a bipartite DNA-binding domain (Fig. 2). This so-called bZip motif comprises two parallel α helices, brought together in a coiled-coil structure, that extend into the major groove of DNA. Although other regions of Fos and Jun contribute to DNA binding indirectly, the bZip domain is sufficient for sequence-specific DNA binding. This motif is shared among a broad class of transcription factors, including all members of the Fos, Jun, and CREB families. Jun family members can bind to DNA as homodimers, however, Fos family members do not form stable homodimers; Fos–Jun heterodimers are more stable than Jun homodimers and bind to DNA with a higher apparent affinity. Numerous bZip complexes are capable of binding to DNA sequences related to the AP1 and CRE motifs. The choice of binding partner influences the specificity of site selection,

the affinity of the interaction, effects on DNA bending, and the consequences for gene transcription. Fos–Jun dimerization has served as a paradigm for the generation of transcriptional complexity by the formation of protein complexes among subunits that cooperate in DNA binding. Fos also contains a C-terminal region that can repress the function of SRE elements in transient transfection assays. However, this effect may only be apparent in overexpression assays.

Fos may play several roles in the control of gene transcription. Fos–Jun dimers can interact with complex regulatory elements in association with other transcription factors, such as NFAT and SMADs. Furthermore, Fos and Jun can bind to components of the basal transcription machinery and to several coactivator proteins. The prevailing view is that transcription initiation involves the assembly of many proteins into higher order complexes on DNA. In certain cases, Fos may be critical for the formation of such complexes. However, the family of Fos-related proteins also can fulfill similar biochemical functions. Thus, it may be best to consider Fos as a component of a complex network of transcription factors that function together to regulate target gene expression in a temporal-, tissue-, and stimulus-specific manner.

IV. BIOLOGICAL ROLE OF Fos

The major biochemical function of Fos is the regulation of gene transcription through protein–protein and protein–DNA interactions. However, the biological consequences of this function have been more difficult to pin down for a number of reasons. Fos is expressed continuously in several tissues and can be induced transiently under a very broad range of circumstances in almost all cell types examined. There is a widespread misconception that Fos and AP1 are involved in cell proliferation. However, *in vivo* Fos expression is more closely associated with differentiation and even cell death signaling than with proliferation. The most critical question is the identity of the target genes regulated by Fos in each situation. Several target genes have been described, but it is likely that there are many others and that each target gene is regulated by a host of other transcription factors as well as Fos. Among the genes shown to be reg-

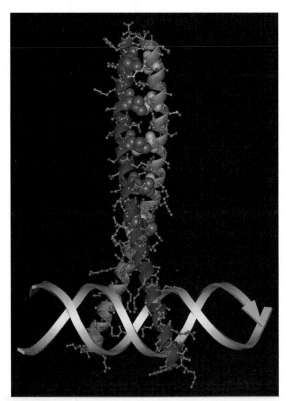

FIGURE 2 Crystal structure of Fos–Jun complex with DNA. A ribbon model represents the α helices of Fos (red) and Jun (green). The DNA helix is depicted in yellow. The leucines of the zipper are depicted in a space-filling model, whereas the other amino acid side chains are represented in a ball-and-stick model. The side chains of the basic amino acids in the DNA-binding domain are colored blue. See color insert in Volume 1.

ulated by Fos are transin, collagenase1, vimentin, and even the *fos*-related gene *fra*-1. However, it has not yet been possible to explain any of the biological functions of Fos based on the properties of the known target genes.

Some of the most revealing clues about the biological function of Fos have been obtained through gene disruption studies. Targeted disruption of c-*fos* in mice is associated with a variety of abnormalities, including osteopetrosis, delayed gametogenesis, reduced lymphocyte populations, and resistance to tumor promoters. The bone defect is a consequence of a failure to generate mature osteoclasts. Thus, Fos functions as a key regulator of osteoclast development, although the target genes responsible for this effect are not yet known. Mice deficient in c-*fos* are also resistant to light-induced apoptosis of photoreceptor cells in the retina. This implies that Fos plays a critical role in cell death signaling in this cell type. It is also possible that Fos contributes to many other biological processes that are not revealed in c-*fos*$^{-/-}$ mice because of compensation by other family members.

In cell culture, transient induction of c-*fos* expression can be linked to numerous cellular responses. However, enforced expression of c-*fos* does not necessarily induce the same effects. Therefore, Fos should be viewed as just one component of a complex cascade of events that is initiated by activation of cell surface receptors or ion channels. The classic induction system for Fos, serum stimulation of fibroblasts, which has been used as a model for growth factor-induced mitogenesis *in vitro*, does not have a clear parallel *in vivo*. The most dramatic examples of c-*fos* induction *in vivo* occur in response to tissue damage or to insults such as seizure activity in the brain. In these cases, broad areas of Fos induction can be detected that are not just restricted to directly stimulated cells or, in the case of tissue damage, to dying cells. In fact, in some circumstances, Fos may be viewed as proapoptotic, whereas in others it may provide an antiapoptotic function. Thus, in a generic sense, c-*fos* induction can be regarded as part of a global response to various kinds of stress. Together with many other inducible transcription factors, it contributes to alterations in gene expression provoked by the initiating event.

V. MECHANISM OF ONCOGENESIS

The unusual characteristic that first drew attention to the *fos* oncogene was its unique association with bone tumors. Virus-induced tumors on the long bones arise from the periosteum and they spread by local invasion. They are nonvascularized, rich in collagen, and often contain areas of differentiated cartilage and bone tissue. It seems that *fos* transforms a connective tissue precursor cell that has the capacity to differentiate into both osteoid and chondroid tissues. Transgenic mice expressing c-*fos* also develop bone tumors that can be either osteoblastic or chondroblastic. In transformed cells, Fos exists primarily as a dimeric complex with Jun. Dimerization and DNA-binding functions of Fos are required for transformation. The role of transcription activation and repression regions present in Fos in cell transformation, is less clear. Some of these regions contribute to transformation, although a truncated Fos protein lacking activation or repression regions can still induce transformation. However, Fos proteins that lack transcription activation domains still function in transcription regulation by binding to Jun, which also contains activation domains.

In tissue culture, *fos* can induce the morphological transformation of fibroblast cell lines and extended self-renewal of primary embryo cells. Although v-*fos* genes are more efficient at inducing transformation, continuous expression c-*fos* also results in cell transformation. Enforced expression of *fos* does not stimulate cell proliferation, and *fos* is capable of inducing morphological transformation of growth-arrested cells maintained in low serum. Thus, it appears that *fos* does not induce oncogenesis by directly deregulating cell proliferation.

Several Fos target genes have been shown to be expressed at higher levels in *fos*-transformed cells. However, only one of these, DNA methyl transferase-1 (*dnmt1*), has been shown to be both necessary and sufficient for transformation. Fos transformation is associated with an elevated expression of *dnmt1* and an increase in the 5-methylcytosine content of DNA. Methylated sites on DNA bind protein complexes that have histone deacetylase activity. These complexes reduce the level of histone acetylation, resulting in a compact chromatin structure and repression of gene expression. Thus, induction of oncogenesis by

Fos may result from a combination of direct gene activation and indirect gene repression through altered methylation patterns as a result of increased *dnmt1* expression. The critical question now facing the field is to identify and characterize the function of these genes. Targeted disruption of c-*fos* in mice reduces the ability of tumor promoters to induce malignant disease. It is possible that this effect is mediated by the ability of Fos to regulate the expression of secreted proteases and other proteins that influence the spread of tumor cells.

There have been many reports of altered Fos expression in human tumors. However, these studies are difficult to interpret. In many cases it is not clear if Fos is present in tumor cells, stromal cells, or cells of the immune system. The procedure used to collect the tumor tissue can also influence the result. Surgical trauma is sufficient to induce c-*fos* expression. This will result in high levels of c-*fos* expression if it takes longer than a few minutes to harvest and freeze the tissue. Based on existing studies, it appears that c-*fos* is not frequently mutated in human tumors. However, it is possible that the altered regulation of Fos contributes to tumor formation, particularly considering its potential role in apoptotic signaling.

Acknowledgments

This work was supported in part by NIH Cancer Center Support CORE Grant P30 CA21765, by National Cancer Institute Grant R01 CA84139, and by the American Lebanese Syrian Associated Charities (ALSAC).

See Also the Following Articles

Bcl-2 Family Proteins and the Dysregulation of Programmed Cell Death • c-mos Protooncogene • ETS Family of Transcription factors • Insulin-like Growth Factors • myb • Ras Protein • STAT Proteins in Growth Control • Wnt Signaling

Bibliography

Bakin, A. V., and Curran, T. (1999). Role of DNA 5-methylcytosine transferase in cell transformation by *fos*. *Science* **283,** 387–390.

Curran, T. (1988). The fos ongogene. *In* "The Oncogene Handbook" (E. P. Reddy, A. M. Skalka, and T. Curran, eds.), p. 307. Elsevier Science, Amsterdam.

Curran, T., and Franza, B. R., Jr. (1988). Fos and Jun: The AP-1 connection. *Cell* **55,** 395–397.

Curran, T., and Vogt, P. K. (1992). Dangerous liaisons: Fos and Jun, oncogenic transcription factors. *In* "Transcriptional Regulation" (S. L. McKnight and K. R. Yamamoto, eds.), p. 797. Cold Spring Harbor Laboratory Press, Cold Spring Harbor, NY.

Ginty, D. D. (1997). Calcium regulation of gene expression: Isn't that spatial? *Cell* **18,** 183–186.

Grigoriadis, A. E., Wang, Z.-Q., and Wagner, E. F. (1995). Fos and bone cell development: Lessons from a nuclear oncogene. *Trends Genet.* **11,** 436–441.

Morgan, J. I., and Curran, T. (1991). Stimulus-transcription coupling in neurons: Involvement of the inducible proto-oncogenes *fos* and *jun*. *Annu. Rev. Neurosci.* **14,** 421–451.

Price, M. A., Hill, C., and Treisman, R. (1996). Integration of growth factor signals at the c-fos serum response element. *Phil. Trans. R. Soc. Lond. B* **351,** 551–559.

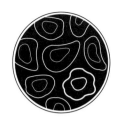

Gastric Cancer: Epidemiology and Therapy

Jaffer A. Ajani
University of Texas M. D. Anderson Cancer Center

GLOSSARY

adjuvant therapy The use of an agent that increases the specific immune response to antigens.

chemotherapy The use of a chemical agent to destroy or inhibit cancer cells.

Gastric cancer, although rare in North America, is a frequent malignancy in many countries around the world. In many endemic areas, because there are no programs in place for early detection, this cancer is often diagnosed in advanced stages. Diagnosis is made only when patients have developed symptoms. Thus, the 5-year survival rate is often less than 20% for all patients. Nearly half of the patients have metastatic disease at diagnosis, and even in patients with local-regional cancer, curative surgery is often possible in only 50% of cases. Statistics are still disappointing in patients who have had a curative (R0) resection: their 5-year survival rate after surgery is only 30 to 35%. Until recently, postoperative adjuvant chemotherapy, chemoimmunotherapy, or radiation therapy had not resulted in survival benefit for treated patients compared with those patients who were simply observed after surgery. However, the recent intergroup trial (INT 0116) has demonstrated statistically significant advantage in disease-free and overall survival durations for patients who received postoperative chemoradiation than those who were observed after surgery. Therefore, postoperative chemoradiotherapy should now be considered standard for patients who have had a node positive resected gastric carcinoma. Advanced gastric carcinoma remains an incurable condition; although combination chemotherapy, when compared to best supportive care, may increase survival duration, it has only a palliative impact. A number of new agents are on the horizon. Several trials are now underway to investigate the impact of new combinations. The field of gastric cancer research continues to be interesting and promising.

I. INTRODUCTION

By some estimates, gastric carcinoma is the second most frequent malignancy worldwide. Despite its continued decline in incidence worldwide since the 1950s, more than 800,000 new cases of gastric carcinoma and more than 630,000 deaths were estimated in the year 2000. The incidence of gastric cancer varies substantially not only by various world regions, but also among ethnic groups and by gender. In endemic and nonendemic areas, men develop gastric cancer almost twice as frequently as women. The reason for this striking difference is not clear. Rates are highest in Japan, Korea, eastern Asia, eastern Europe, parts of Latin America, and certain countries of the previous Soviet Union. United States and many industrialized nations have among the lowest incidence of gastric cancer in the world. In the United States, Koreans, Vietnamese, Japanese, Alaska natives, and Hawaiians tend to have the highest incidence of gastric carcinoma than the other ethnic groups. Hispanic, Chinese, and African populations have an intermediate incidence, whereas Filipinos and Caucasians have the lowest rates. In addition, there is proximal migration of gastric carcinoma; this is especially striking among men of Caucasian origin.

For patients with local-regional cancer, the potential curative treatment is surgery. However, recurrences are common. In the Western world, approximately 35% of patients having undergone a curative resection (R0) are expected to be cured. The cure rates are much higher in Japan, where 70% of patients can undergo an R0 resection (this excludes the increasing number of patients undergoing endoscopic mucosal resection) because the diagnosis is made at an earlier stage and possibly as a result of a more extended lymphadenectomy. In the United States, a recent postoperative adjuvant chemoradiotherapy study was reported to be positive. However, this approach of postoperative chemoradiotherapy has not yet been widely accepted abroad.

II. NATURAL HISTORY OF GASTRIC CANCER AND PATTERN OF RECURRENCE

Gastric cancer commonly results in weight loss, anemia, and abdominal pain. In addition, cancer is far advanced and beyond surgery in nearly 50% of patients. In countries where no effort is made for the early detection of gastric carcinoma, the R0 resection rates are approximately $\leq$ 50% for patients with local-regional disease.

The overall survival for patients with gastric cancer correlates well with the stage at diagnosis. In addition, the level of resection achieved also correlates with patient survival. The survival of patients also depends on the ratio of involved and removed lymph nodes.

Local relapse rate may be as high as 40% in clinical series and up to 80% in the autopsy series. Distal gastric cancer is more likely to result in peritoneal spread, and proximal cancer is more likely to result in liver metastases.

III. ADJUVANT THERAPY

There have been many adjuvant studies in Asia, Europe, and North America since the 1970s. The results have been mixed and often not considered positive by the oncology community. However, a recent postoperative adjuvant therapy trial that examined the value of postoperative chemoradiotherapy has demonstrated a benefit for patients treated with postoperative therapy compared to observation following surgery. A previous study investigating the role of postoperative radiotherapy alone did not demonstrate any benefit; however, the addition of chemotherapy to radiotherapy has at least a theoretical advantage. 5-Fluorouracil, being the most frequently studied agent with radiotherapy in gastrointestinal malignancies, was chosen along with folinic acid in the Intergroup trial 0116. In this trial, patients with stage Ib through IV M0 gastric cancer, who have had an R0 resection, were randomized to adjuvant chemoradiation or observation alone. A total of 603 patients were accrued to this study. The majority of them (85%) had lymph node metastasis and T3 or T4 primary (70%). Chemotherapy consisted of one cycle of 5-fluorouracil/leucovorin daily for 5 days prior to the initiation of chemoradiation therapy. Patients also received two cycles of the same chemotherapy during and after chemoradiotherapy. The 3-year overall survival rate was 52% for the treatment arm and 41% for the control arm. The disease-free survival was 49% for the treatment arm versus 32% for the control arm. The frequency of grade 3 and 4 toxic effects was 41% in the treatment arm and 32% in the control arm. One drawback of this study was the lack of uniformity in the type of surgery performed. However, no particular surgical procedure was specified, as surgery was not part of this protocol and the eligibility requirement was to have an R0 resection. Less than 50% of patients had even a traditional D1 dissection of the lymph nodes. In addition, the use of postoperative radiotherapy of the gastric bed will require substantial education of the radiation oncology community to minimize inaccuracies. Although, in North America, this is accepted as standard postoperative adjuvant therapy, its value continues to be debated in Europe and Asia. Follow-up studies are already being planned in the United States.

IV. PREOPERATIVE THERAPY

The preoperative approach to local-regional gastric carcinoma has a number of theoretical advantages; however, to date, data do not exist to support the routine use of any preoperative therapy in patients with a potentially respectable gastric carcinoma. The preoperative approach affords an excellent model for studying the biologic effect of various therapies, as one often has access to the surgical specimen following therapy. Thus it is possible to study the pathologic response but also, if one desires, to study molecular markers.

A number of phase II studies have demonstrated that a multimodality approach is feasible. One of the approaches that has interested investigators at the University of Texas M. D. Anderson Cancer Center includes the use of preoperative chemoradiotherapy. Preliminary results suggest that there are no excessive early toxic effects and a number of patients achieve a pathologic complete response. With the

advent of laparoscopic staging and endoscopic ultrasonography, it is now possible to select patients properly for this type of approach. There is interest in mounting a phase III study that would compare preoperative chemoradiotherapy to postoperative chemoradiotherapy.

In addition, there are currently studies underway (phase II and III designs) to establish the value of a preoperative approach in this group of patients.

V. ADVANCED GASTRIC CARCINOMA

Advanced gastric carcinoma is an incurable disease. The median survival duration of patients afflicted with metastatic gastric carcinoma varies from 6 to 9 months. Patients with liver involvement have a shorter survival than those with only nodal metastases. Chemotherapy is palliative and does seem to prolong survival when compared to best supportive care; however, all four randomized studies that made such comparisons had very small number of patients. In addition, combination chemotherapy results in a higher response rate but not in a statistically significant survival advantage compared to single agent chemotherapy with 5-fluorouracil. The combination of 5-fluorouracil plus folinic acid or 5-fluorouracil and cisplatin is widely used as the standard regimen in most of the world. However, there is no universal agreement regarding a standard. It should be noted that a number of new agents have been found active against advanced gastric carcinoma, and combination regimens that incorporate new agents also result in intriguingly high response rates.

The classes of agents that seem to have activity against gastric carcinoma include taxanes, camptothecins, and oral fluoropyrimidines. In addition, there is a lot of interest in newer classes of agents, such as vaccines, antineoangiogenic agents, anti-EGFR (epidermal growth factor receptor), and similar agents.

Future prospects of developing a better classification, standardizing the surgical approach, more effective combination chemotherapy, vaccine therapy, antigrowth agents, and better defining molecular biology, including predictors of response, are excellent.

Acknowledgments

This work was supported by grants from the Cantu and Caporella Families and from Rivercreek Foundation.

See Also the Following Articles

BLADDER CANCER: ANATOMY AND EVALUATION • COLORECTAL CANCER: EPIDEMIOLOGY AND TREATMENT • ESOPHAGEAL CANCER: TREATMENT • KIDNEY, EPIDEMIOLOGY • LIVER CANCER: ETIOLOGY AND PREVENTION • LUNG, LARYNX, ORAL CAVITY, AND PHARYNX • PANCREATIC CANCER: CELLULAR AND MOLECULAR MECHANISMS • PROSTATE CANCER

Bibliography

Ajani, J. A., Fairweather, J., Dumas, P., et al. (1998). Phase II study of Taxol in patients with gastric carcinoma. *Cancer J. Sci. Am. Cancer J. Sci. Am.* **4**, 269–274.

Ajani, J. A., Mansfield, P. F., and Ota, D. M. (1995). Potentially resectable gastric carcinoma: Current approaches to staging and preoperative therapy. *World J. Surg.* **19**, 216–220.

Ajani, J. A., Mayer, R. J., Ota, D. M., et al. (1993). Preoperative and postoperative chemotherapy for potentially resectable gastric carcinoma. *JNCI* **85**, 1839–1844.

Ajani, J. A., Ota, D. M., Jessup, J. M., et al. (1991). Resectable gastric cancer: An evaluation of preoperative and postoperative chemotherapy. *Cancer* **68**, 1501–1506.

Boku, N., Ohtsu, A., Shimada, Y., et al. (1999). Phase II study of a combination of Irinotecan and cisplatin against metastatic gastric cancer. *J. Clin. Oncol.* **17**, 319–323.

Eingzig, A. I., Lipsitz, S., Wiernik, P. H., and Benson, A. (1995). Phase II trial of Taxol in patients with adenocarcinoma of the upper gastrointestinal tract: The Eastern Cooperative Oncology Group (ECOG) Results. *Invest. New Drugs* **13**, 223–227.

Einzig, A. I., Newberg, D., Remick, S. C., et al. (1996). Phase II trial of docetaxel (Taxotere) in patients with adenocarcinoma of the upper gastrointestinal tract previously untreated with cytotoxic chemotherapy: The Eastern Cooperative Oncology Group (ECOG) results of protocol E1293. *Med. Oncol.* **13**, 87–93.

Greenlee, R. T., Murray, T., Bolden, S., and Wingo, P. A. (2000). Cancer statistics, 2000. *CA Cancer J. Clin.* **50**, 7–33.

Hundahl, S. A., Menck, H. R., Mansour, E. G., and Winchester, D. P. (1997). The national cancer data base report on gastric carcinoma. *Cancer* **80**, 2333–2341.

Lawrence, W., Menck, H. R., Steele, G. D., and Winchester, D. P. (1995). The national cancer data base report on gastric cancer. *Cancer* **75**, 1734–1744.

Macdonald, J. S., Smalley, S., Benedetti, J., et al. (2000). Postoperative combined radiation and chemotherapy improves disease-free survival (DFS) and overall survival (OS) in resected adenocarcinoma of the stomach and G.E. junction: Results of intergroup study INT-0116 (SWOG 9008). *Proc. ASCO* **19**, 1a.

Macdonald, J. S., Schein, P. S., Woolley, P. V., et al. (1980). 5-Florouracil, doxorubicin and mitomycin (FAM) combination chemotherapy for advanced gastric cancer. *Ann. Intern. Med.* **93**, 533–536.

Miller, B. A., Kolonel, L. N., Berstein, L., et al. (1996). "Racial/Ethnic Patterns of Cancer in the United States 1988–1992." National Cancer Institute, Bethesda, MD.

Ohtsu, A., Sakata, M., Horikoshi, N., et al. (1998). A phase II study of S-1 in patients with advanced gastric cancer. *Proc. Am. Soc. Clin. Oncol.* **17**, 262. [Abstract 1005]

Roth, A. D., Maibach, R., Martinelli, G., et al. (1998). Taxotere-cisplatin in advanced gastric carcinoma: An active drug combination. *Proc ASCO* **17**, 283a. [Abstract 1088]

Shimada, K., and Ajani, J. A. (1999). Adjuvant therapy for gastric carcinoma patients in the past 15 years: A review of western and oriental trials. *Cancer* **86**, 1657–1668.

Siewet, J. R., Bottcher, K., Stein, H. J., et al. (1998). Relevant prognostic factors in gastric cancer: Ten-year results of the German gastric cancer study. *Ann. Surg.* **228**, 449–461.

Sulkes, A., Smyth, J., Sessa, C., et al. (1994). Docetaxel in advanced gastric cancer: Results of a phase II clinical trial. EORTC Early Clinical Trials Group. *Br. J. Cancer* **70**, 380–383.

Taguchi, T. (1997). A late phase II study of docetaxel in patients with gastric cancer. *Proc ASCO* **16**, 263a.

Takiuchi, H., and Ajani, J. A. (1998). UFT in gastric cancer: A comprehensive review. *J. Clin. Oncol.* **16**(8), 2877–2885.

Tamura, F., Ohtsu, A., Boku, N., et al. (1997). Three-hour infusion of paclitaxel for advanced gastric cancer. *Proc ASCO* **16**, 307a.

Wanebo, H. J., Kennedy, B. J., Chmiel, J., et al. (1993). Cancer of the stomach: A patient care study by the American College of Surgeons. *Ann. Surg.* **218**, 583–592.

Wisbeck, W. M., Becher, E. M., and Russell, A. H. (1986). Adenocarcinoma of the stomach: Autopsy observations with therapeutic implications for the radiation oncologist. *Radiother. Oncol.* **7**, 13–18.

Yao, J. C., Shimada, K., and Ajani, J. A. (1999). Adjuvant therapy for gastric carcinoma: Closing out the century. *Oncology* **13**, 1485–1505.

Gastric Cancer: Inherited Predisposition

Anita K. Dunbier
Parry J. Guilford
University of Otago, Dunedin, New Zealand

I. Familial Inheritance
II. Predisposition Genes
III. Gastric Cancer and Other Predisposition Syndromes
IV. Genetic Susceptibility to Environmental Damage

GLOSSARY

diffuse type gastric tumor Poorly differentiated tumor, characterized by highly invasive, infiltrative growth.

gastrointestinal stromal tumor Submucosal tumor of the gastrointestinal tract: 60% occur in the stomach, 30% in the small intestine, and 10% elsewhere.

hereditary diffuse gastric cancer syndrome Inherited cancer syndrome defined by germline mutations in the E-cadherin gene (CDH-1)

intestinal type gastric tumor Differentiated tumor characterized by intestinal metaplasia and usually associated with severe atrophic gastritis.

mixed type gastric tumor Tumor with mixed diffuse and intestinal patterns.

Wide variation is observed in the rates of gastric cancer amongst different populations. In some Asian countries the incidence is as high as 80 per 100,000 males while most European countries have incidence rates of between 20 and 40 per 100,000. These figures, together with studies of cancer incidence in Asian migrants to North America, support the theory that environmental factors play an important role in the aetiology of gastric cancer. However, within the last decade increasing documentation of familial aggregation has highlighted the importance of inherited predisposition to the incidence of gastric cancer.

I. FAMILIAL INHERITANCE

History's most famous report of gastric cancer clustering occurred in the Bonaparte family, in which Emperor Napoleon, his father, his grandfather, four sisters, and a brother are all thought to have died from the cancer. Their pedigree (Fig. 1) alludes strongly to the presence of an autosomal-dominant predisposition gene, with approximately half of Napoleon's generation affected by gastric cancer.

More recently, epidemiological studies have confirmed that familial clustering of gastric cancer occurs in patients from a range of ethnic backgrounds and geographical locations. Two comprehensive studies from Italy and Japan have demonstrated a threefold increased risk of the disease in the first-degree relatives of affected individuals. Overall, studies suggest that approximately 10% of gastric cancers show familial clustering.

II. PREDISPOSITION GENES

Despite the apparent high incidence of familial clusters, discovery of the genes predisposing to gastric cancer has been slow. To date, only germline mutation of the E-cadherin gene has been shown to predispose predominantly to gastric cancer. However, mutation of a second gene, *KIT*, may predispose to tumors of the gastric stroma.

A. E-cadherin

A genetic linkage analysis on a large New Zealand Maori family led to the description of a familial gastric cancer syndrome designated hereditary diffuse gastric cancer (HDGC). HDGC is an autosomal dominant cancer syndrome caused by inactivating germline mutations in the gene for the cell-to-cell adhesion protein E-cadherin (*CDH*-1). E-cadherin is a member of the cadherin family of homophilic cell adhesion proteins that are central to the processes of development, cell differentiation, and the maintenance of tissue integrity. It is the predominant cadherin family member expressed in epithelial tissue and is localized at the adherens junctions on the basolateral surface of the cell (Fig. 2).

Germline *CDH*-1 mutations have now been identified in numerous HDGC families from diverse ethnic groups. HDGC families are predisposed predominantly to diffuse-type gastric cancer and linitis plastica. A small number of patients with germline *CDH*-1 mutations have the mixed type of gastric tumor, but there is no association with the pure intestinal type. Affected families may also have an elevated risk of lobular breast cancer and possibly colorectal cancer. Histologically, gastric tumors are highly invasive, poorly differentiated, and display occasional signet ring cells. The lifetime penetrance of HDGC is about 65%, and its age of onset shows marked variation between and within families, ranging from 14 years upward with a median age in the late thirties.

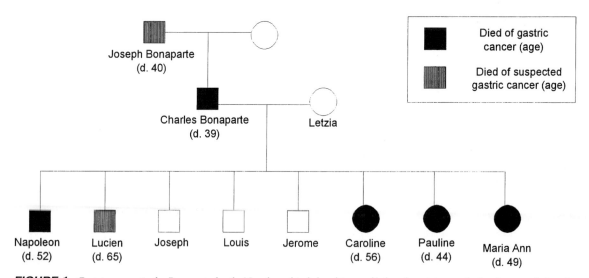

FIGURE 1 Gastric cancer in the Bonaparte family. Napoleon, his father, his grandfather, four sisters, and a brother are all thought to have died from gastric cancer.

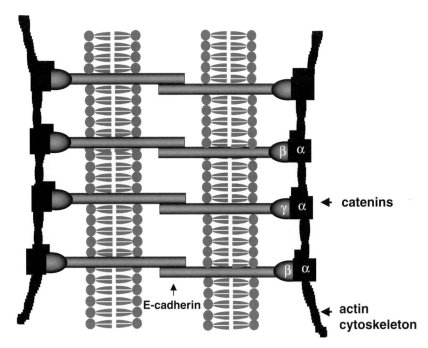

FIGURE 2 Cellular localization of E-cadherin. E-cadherin is a homophilic transmembrane protein localized at adherens junctions on the basolateral surface of an epithelial cell. It effectively forms a bridge between the actin cytoskeletons of adjacent cells.

1. Mutations in CDH-1

The CDH-1 coding sequence is 2.6 kb in length and is divided over 16 exons. The CDH-1 germline mutations identified in HDGC families consist predominantly of frameshift mutations, premature termination codons, and exon/intron splice site mutations that are distributed throughout the gene without any apparent hot spots. Missense CDH-1 mutations have also been observed in some families and would be predicted to be responsible for gastric cancer predisposition if they disrupted critical functional domains of the protein.

Somatic CDH-1 mutations occur in at least 50% of sporadic diffuse gastric tumors and lobular breast cancers, but occur very rarely in other tumors, including intestinal type gastric cancers. Thus, the range of sporadic tumors carrying somatic CDH-1 mutations resembles the spectrum of tumors observed in HDGC families.

Immunohistochemical staining of HDGC tumors with anti-E-cadherin antibodies has shown that the second CDH-1 allele is inactivated somatically. HDGC therefore resembles other inherited cancer syndromes caused by germline mutation of tumor suppressor genes in requiring somatic inactivation of the wild-type allele to enable tumor progression. However, unlike other cancer syndromes, loss of heterozygosity (LOH) does not appear to be frequent in HDGC. In contrast, the second CDH-1 allele may be vulnerable to inactivation by promoter hypermethylation.

2. Molecular Mechanism of HDGC Predisposition

The invasive phenotype of malignant epithelial tumor cells can be reversed in model systems by transfection with E-cadherin cDNA. Perl and colleagues have also demonstrated that downregulation of E-cadherin coincides with the transition from well-differentiated adenoma to invasive carcinoma in a mouse model of pancreatic β-cell tumorigenesis. These observations have led to CDH-1 being described as a tumor invasion suppressor gene.

The close relationship between cell proliferation and cell migration during development, wound repair, and stem cell proliferation would imply that there is considerable cross-talk between the molecular pathways for cell adhesion and cell proliferation. E-cadherin loss in the gastric epithelium would therefore be predicted to contribute to tumorigenesis not only by enhancing tumor invasion, but also by stimulating cell proliferative pathways. One such pathway is the *Wnt* signaling pathway, which is implicated in the majority of human gastrointestinal tumors. The cytoplasmic domain of E-cadherin interacts with a complex of proteins at the adherens junction, including the key mediator of *Wnt* signaling, β catenin. There is some evidence that loss of functional E-cadherin may shift the cellular equilibrium of β catenin away from the adherens junction toward the pool of free β catenin. Increased free β catenin would activate the transcriptional targets of the *Wnt* pathway, which include the oncogene c-*myc*, the regulator of cell proliferation *CCND1* and components of the AP1 transcription complex. In this way, *CDH-1* would act as a classic tumor suppressor gene.

3. Clinical Criteria and Management of HDGC

The distinction between the histological subtypes of gastric cancer occurring in HDGC is a key feature of the clinical criteria used as a screen for HDGC families. Currently, the following criteria are used: (1) Two or more documented cases of diffuse gastric cancer in first/second-degree relatives, with at least one diagnosed before the age of 50 years or (2) three or more cases of documented diffuse gastric cancer in first/second-degree relatives, independent of age of onset. About 50% of families meeting these criteria have identifiable germline mutations in the *CDH-1* coding region. The remainder of families may have undetected mutations in *CDH-1* regulatory sequences or germline mutations in unidentified genes that also contribute to a diffuse, poorly differentiated phenotype. Alternatively, families lacking *CDH-1* mutations may simply represent chance clusters of sporadic cancer.

Five-year survival rates of gastric cancer patients following complete gastrectomy are approximately 90% for stage Ia cancers but fall to about 15% for stage IV. Intensive clinical surveillance of germline *CDH-1* mutation carriers therefore provides an opportunity to improve outcome. Diffuse gastric cancer can be difficult to detect due to a tendency to spread submucosally; nevertheless, regular endoscopy (every 6–12 months) currently provides the best method for early detection of HDGC. *Helicobacter pylori* infection, gastric ulceration, and inflammation are likely to add to the risk of cancer onset in *CDH-1* mutation carriers.

Prophylactic total gastrectomy may constitute an appropriate preventative strategy for gastric cancer in HDGC families. However, the decision to carry out a prophylactic gastrectomy must take into account the 1–2% risk of mortality following surgery, the 100% long-term morbidity, the incomplete penetrance of HDGC, and the unknown risk of later development of extragastric tumors.

B. KIT

While the majority of primary gastric tumors develop in the stomach epithelium, stromal tumors, which arise predominantly within the gastric wall, make up a small portion of gastric cancers. Likewise, stromal tumors comprise a small subset of familial gastric tumor clusters. The *KIT* protooncogene, which encodes a receptor tyrosine kinase, is mutated in sporadic gastrointestinal stromal tumors (GISTs), the most common mesenchymal neoplasms of the human digestive tract. A germline gain-of-function mutation in the *KIT* gene, which resulted in constitutive activation of the receptor, has been found in a large kindred with GIST. This mutation segregated with the GISTs over four generations, implicating the gene in inherited stromal gastric cancer.

III. GASTRIC CANCER AND OTHER PREDISPOSITION SYNDROMES

While gastric cancer is the predominant consequence of germline CDH-1 mutations, it may also form a minor component of the tumor spectrum of other inherited cancer predisposition syndromes.

A. Hereditary Nonpolyposis Colorectal Cancer (HNPCC) Syndrome

A 1913 report by Warthin detailed a cancer-prone kindred with aggregation of cancer of the colon, stomach, and endometrium. The predominant lesion in this initial report was gastric cancer. Follow-up of the same family in the 1960s found that the incidence of colorectal cancer had increased, but gastric cancer had decreased in accordance with the cancer's decline in developed nations.

The syndrome exhibited by this family, now known as hereditary nonpolyposis colorectal cancer (HNPCC), is caused by germline mutations in any of five DNA mismatch repair genes: *MSH2, MLH1, PMS1, PMS2,* or *MSH6.* The discovery of the genes responsible for this syndrome has enabled analysis of gastric cancer risk among mutation carriers. Comprehensive studies of gastric cancer in HNPCC patients have been conducted using clinical data and tumor samples relating to patients from the Finnish HNPCC registry. In one study, a total of 50 families, including 360 *MLH1* or *MSH2* mutation carriers, were examined. It was found that mutation carriers had a cumulative gastric cancer incidence of 13% by 70 years of age, a rate 16 times greater than that seen in the general Finnish population.

The predominant histological type of gastric cancer in HNPCC is the intestinal form. Examination of gastric tumor samples from 24 HNPCC patients showed that 19 of the tumors were of the intestinal type and only 3 were classified as diffuse. In support of this association, a number of studies on sporadic gastric cancer have demonstrated that of the tumors that display microsatellite instability, a hallmark of the mutation of mismatch repair genes, approximately 90% are of the intestinal type.

B. Familial Adenomatous Polyposis

Familial adenomatous polyposis (FAP) is an autosomal-dominant, precancerous condition of the colon caused by mutations in the APC tumor suppressor gene. FAP is characterized by the appearance of adenomatous polyps throughout the large bowel and a virtually 100% chance of malignant degeneration unless the colon is prophylactically removed. However, after colectomy, a number of FAP patients develop other related cancers, including gastric cancer. Approximately 60% of APC mutation carriers develop multiple gastric polyps and 12% have true gastric adenomas. Fundic gland polyps are the most common gastric lesion in FAP and undergo malignant transformation at low frequency. Inactivation of the APC gene is seen in about 20% of early sporadic gastric cancer, suggesting that the APC gene may play a key role in the initiation of a subset of gastric cancers.

C. Li–Fraumeni Syndrome

Families with Li–Fraumeni Syndrome caused by germline mutation of *TP53* or *hCHK2* exhibit a broad range of malignancies, including sarcomas, breast cancer, brain tumors, and adrenal cortical carcinomas. Gastric cancers appear to make up a small subset of the tumors affecting Li–Fraumeni families.

D. Other Associated Syndromes

A number of reports have been published in which gastric cancer cases appear occasionally as part of other defined cancer syndromes. In such reports, it is difficult to establish whether gastric cancer has developed as a consequence of the cancer predisposition gene or whether it simply reflects a chance clustering of sporadic gastric cancers with the cancer syndrome.

A number of families affected by Peutz–Jeghers syndrome (PJS), a rare autosomal-dominant disorder characterized by hamartomatous polyposis of the gastrointestinal tract, appear to have elevated levels of gastric cancer. The frequency of the cancer in these kindreds, and whether it reflects a role for the PJS gene in gastric carcinogenesis, is not known.

The orocutaneous hamartomas and disseminated gastrointestinal polyposis characteristic of Cowden's disease are thought to relate to the malignant predisposition observed in the disease. Gastric polyps are frequently present and there is some evidence to suggest that these have the potential to undergo transformation to form tumors. A small number of gastric carcinomas have been observed in association with Cowden's disease, and it is possible that the syndrome may be responsible for a small proportion of hereditary gastric cancers.

The breast cancer susceptibility gene BRCA2 may also make a small contribution to the incidence of inherited gastric cancer. The 999del5 BRCA2 founder mutation identified in the Icelandic population has been found in individuals with different cancers, including cancer of the prostate, pancreas, ovary, colon, stomach, thyroid, cervix, and endometrium. However, current data suggest that the rate of gastric cancer in 999del5 mutation carriers is only slightly above that of the general population.

IV. GENETIC SUSCEPTIBILITY TO ENVIRONMENTAL DAMAGE

While most cancer predisposition genes play a direct role in promoting tumorigenesis, genes that alter response to environmental stimuli may also affect susceptibility to gastric cancer. *H. pylori* infects half the world's population with a variety of clinical outcomes, including gastric and duodenal ulcer disease and occasional gastric cancer. The reasons behind this variable outcome are not clear, but the gastric physiological response appears to be influenced by the severity and anatomical distribution of gastritis induced by *H. pylori*. It has been suggested that specific polymorphisms in the interleukin-1 gene cluster may enable increased expression of the proinflammatory cytokine IL-1β, favoring the initiation of a set of responses to *H. pylori* that result in hypochlorhydria, corpus atrophy, and increased risk of gastric cancer.

It is likely that other genes that modulate individual response to environmental damage also affect susceptibility to gastric cancer. Although data linking gastric cancer risk to detoxifying enzyme polymorphisms are limited, the influence of such genetic variation cannot be excluded. As our knowledge of human genetic variation grows, it is probable that the number of genes known to be associated with response to environmental influences will also increase. Such background genetic factors will both influence an individual's risk of "sporadic" gastric cancer and affect the penetrance of defined inherited gastric cancer syndromes.

See Also the Following Articles

GASTRIC CANCER: EPIDEMIOLOGY AND THERAPY • GENETIC ALTERATIONS IN BRAIN TUMORS • GENETIC PREDISPOSITION TO PROSTATE CANCER • HEREDITARY RISK OF BREAST CANCER AND OVARIAN CANCER • HEREDITARY COLON CANCER AND DNA MISMATCH REPAIR • HER2/NEU • LI–FRAUMENI SYNDROME

Bibliography

Caldas, C., Carneiro, F., Lynch, H. T., Yokota, J., Wiesner, G. L., Powell, S. M., Lewis, F. R., Huntsman, D. G., Pharoah, P. D., Jankowski, J. A., MacLeod, P., Vogelsang, H., Keller, G., Park, K. G., Richards, F. M., Maher, E. R., Gayther, S. A., Oliveira, C., Grehan, N., Wight, D., Seruca, R., Roviello, F., Ponder, B. A., and Jackson, C. E. (1999). Familial gastric cancer: overview and guidelines for management. *J. Med. Genet.* **36,** 873–880.
Guilford, P. (1999). E-cadherin downregulation in cancer: Fuel on the fire? *Mol. Med. Today* **5,** 172–177.
Frixen, E. H., Behrens, J., Sachs, M., Eberle, G., Voss, B., Warda, A., Lochner, D., and Birchmeier, W. (1991). E-cadherin-mediated cell-cell adhesion prevents invasiveness of human carcinoma cells. *J. Cell Biol.* **113,** 173–185.
Grady, W. M., Willis, J., Guilford, P. J., Dunbier, A. K., Toro, T. T., Lynch, H., Wiesner, G., Ferguson, K., Eng, C., Park, J. G., Kim, S. J., and Markowitz, S. (2000). Methylation of the *CDH1* promoter as the second genetic hit in hereditary diffuse gastric cancer. *Nature Genet* **26,** 16–17.
Guilford, P., Hopkins, J., Grady, W., Markowitz, S., Willis, J., Lynch, H., Rajput, A., Wiesner, G., Lindor, N., Burgart, L., Toro, T., Lee, D., Limacher, J.-M., Shaw, D., Findlay, M., and Reeve, A. (1999). E-cadherin germline mutations define an inherited cancer syndrome dominated by diffuse gastric cancer. *Hum. Mutat.* **14,** 249–255.
Guilford, P., Hopkins, J., Harraway, J., McLeod, M., McLeod, N., Harawira, P., Taite, H., Scoular, R., Miller, A., and Reeve, A. E. (1998). E-cadherin germline mutations in familial gastric cancer. *Nature* **392,** 402–405.
Lynch, H., and Smyrk, T. (1996). Hereditary nonpolyposis colorectal cancer (Lynch syndrome): An updated review. *Cancer* **78,** 1149–1167.
Nishida, T., Hirota, S., Taniguchi, M., Hashimoto, K., Isozaki, K., Makamura, H., Kanakura, Y., Tanaka, T., Takabayashi, A., Matsuda, H., and Kitamura, Y. (1998). Familial gastrointestinal stromal tumours with germline mutation of the *KIT* gene. *Nature Genet.* **19,** 323–324.
Perl, A.-K., Wilgenbus, P., Dahl, U., Semb, H., and Christofori, G. (1998). A causal role for E-cadherin in the transition from adenoma to carcinoma. *Nature* **392,** 190–193.
Vleminckx, K., Vakaet, L., Mareel, M., Fiers, W., and van Roy, F. (1991). Genetic manipulation of E-cadherin expression by epithelial tumor cells reveals an invasion suppressor role. *Cell* **66,** 107–119.

Gene Therapy Vectors: Safety Considerations

Eda T. Bloom
Alexander E. Kuta
Philip D. Noguchi

U.S. Food and Drug Administration, Bethesda, Maryland

I. Background
II. Gene Therapy Products Are Biologics
III. Safety Considerations

GLOSSARY

biologic product or biologic "Any virus, therapeutic serum, toxin, antitoxin, vaccine, blood, blood component or derivative, allergenic product, or analogous product, or arsphenamine or its derivatives (or any other trivalent organic arsenic compound), applicable to the prevention, treatment, or cure of diseases or injuries of man" (from the Public Health Service Act of 1944).

drug "Articles intended for use in the diagnosis, cure, mitigation, treatment, or prevention of disease in man or other animals" (from the Federal Food Drug and Cosmetic Act of 1938; partial definition).

gene therapy The use of products containing genetic material, administered to modify or manipulate the expression of genetic material, or to alter the biological properties of living cells.

investigational new drug (IND) A clearance status granted by the FDA, in response to a satisfactory application by a sponsor, to exempt an investigational drug from the premarketing approval requirements and allow it to be shipped lawfully interstate for the purpose of conducting clinical investigations.

license The approval by FDA to market a biologic, granted after the product is proved to meet standards of safety, purity, and potency, and efficacy in appropriate clinical trials. Licenses must be obtained for the product (Product License) and for the establishment(s) in which the product is manufactured (Establishment License).

somatic cell therapy Autologous (self), allogeneic (intraspecies), or xenogeneic (interspecies) cells that have been propagated, expanded, selected, pharmacologically treated, or with otherwise *ex vivo* altered biological characteristics, to be administered to humans for the prevention, treatment, cure, diagnosis, or mitigation of disease or injury.

Gene therapy, a medical intervention that is based on modification of the genetic material of living cells, offers a potentially promising approach to the therapy of many serious and life-threatening diseases. The Center for Biologics Evaluation and Research (CBER) of the U.S. Food and Drug Administration (FDA) has been charged with ensuring that gene therapy products are safe and effective. This article addresses the regulatory policy for these products, the background and rationale underlying the regulatory approach at the time of writing, as well as recommendations for appropriate safety testing.

I. BACKGROUND

A. Rationale for Regulation of Biologics

To appreciate the approach used by the FDA to assure the safety of gene therapy in humans, certain background information is important and instructive. The need for regulation of the production of biologic products dates to the clinical applications of scientific breakthroughs of the late nineteenth century. These advances, particularly in the areas of bacteriology and immunology, led to novel approaches, such as antiserums, to the prevention and treatment of some of the most devastating diseases of the era. However, the safety, purity, and potency of these early antiserums and related products varied widely. After a series of events, including the deaths of 13 children from tetanus following injection with contaminated diphtheria antitoxin, the Biologics Control Act of 1902 was passed. Also known as the Virus, Serum, and Toxin Act, it mandated the federal regulation of biologic products, requiring manufacturers to obtain licensure from the Hygienic Laboratory within the Public Health and Marine Hospital Service, both for the product itself and for the manufacturing facilities. The Public Health Service (PHS) Act of 1944 recodified and updated existing laws. In 1986 the National Childhood Vaccine Injury Act specifically amended section 351 of the PHS Act to provide recall authority if it is determined that a biologic product presents an imminent or substantial hazard to the public health.

The food and drug legislation relevant to biologics has also undergone a series of modifications beginning with the initial passage of the Pure Food and Drugs Act in 1906. The Federal Food Drug and Cosmetic (FD&C) Act of 1938, which established premarket review, was passed in response to the more than 100 deaths associated with sulfanilamide elixir, and the 1962 Kefauver–Harris Amendments in response to the thalidomide tragedy mandated that clinical efficacy be demonstrated before allowing marketing of a drug. Subsequently, there was general agreement that biologic products were also subject to relevant provisions of the act, and its implementing regulations. The act was amended in 1976, and the Safe Medical Devices Act of 1990 instituted a system for regulating medical devices, thus further strengthening FDA regulatory controls over medical devices.

Since 1902, the responsibility for regulating biologic products has remained within the Public Health Service, and today resides within the Center for Biologics Evaluation and Research (CBER). Table I lists certain documents relevant to the regulation of biologic products, with an emphasis on gene therapy products.

B. Safety of Biologic Products: Quality Control

In general, since biologics are also drugs, their manufacture is expected to comply with current Good Man-

---

TABLE I
Documents Relevant to Gene Therapy and
Related Biologic Products

Federal Laws
   Biologics Control Act of 1902, (1902) 32 Stat. 728.
   Food, Drug and Cosmetic Act, (1938), 21 U.S.C. 321(g), sect. 201(g).
   Public Health Service Act, July 1, 1944, ch. 373, Title III, 351, 58 Stat. 702, currently codified at 42 U.S.C. 262.
Federal Register Notice
   Application of current statutory authorities to human somatic cell therapy products and gene therapy products. Docket No. 93-N-0173, *The Federal Register* 58(197): 53248–53251, October 14, 1993.
Points to Consider[a]
   Points to Consider in the Collection, Processing and Testing of *Ex-Vivo*-Activated Mononuclear Leukocytes for Administration to Humans (8/22/89)
   Points to Consider in Human Somatic Cell Therapy and Gene Therapy (8/27/91)
   Points to Consider—Characterization of Cell Lines Used to Produce Biologicals (7/12/93)

[a]Available through the CBER, Division of Congressional and Public Affairs.

ufacturing Practice Regulations (GMPR) as defined in Title 21 of the Code of Federal Regulations, part 211. In addition, the concept of control of the production of biologic products in particular has been progressively revised since the 1902 act, and relies on three central principles: (a) control of the biological source(s); (b) control of the production process; and (c) control of the bulk and final product.

The assurance of product safety requires that biological sources be well characterized, uniform, distinguishable from similar materials, and free from contaminating hazardous adventitious agents. Earliest control of source materials involved microbiological testing and control of animal husbandry; the soundness of the approach was verified when foot-and-mouth disease occurred in animals used to produce smallpox vaccine, necessitating license revocation. More recently developed technologies, starting with tissue culture-based vaccine production, have required commensurate innovative measures to ensure product safety. For example, viral seed lot systems, involving limiting passage of a well-characterized parent virus stock, were developed to control the potential reversion of attenuated strains to virulent phenotypes. The concept of production cell substrate, that is, a defined cellular source material used to produce a biologic product, was developed along with procedures to evaluate identity, tumorigenicity, and freedom from contaminants developed. In one case, simian virus 50 (SV40) was found in the monkey kidney cell cultures used for the production of polio vaccine. This collective experience has resulted in the cell banking and testing recommendations that are used today to qualify cell substrates used in the production of biologics including vaccines, monoclonal antibodies, recombinant DNA products, and certain cellular and gene therapy products.

Some biologic products, including somatic cell and gene therapy products, utilize cells that have been removed directly from humans or other species. The regulation of these types of source materials present a unique challenge to CBER. The need for safety assurances for fresh cells was first appreciated with blood transfusions during World War II. Because of the inability to sterilize blood, new strategies, concentrating on donor screening, became essential for assuring the safety of blood cells. As new viruses, such as hepati-

tis B virus and human immunodeficiency virus, have been discovered, new tests have been successfully incorporated into the current donor screening program.

The second principle for assuring the safety of biologic products involves the control of the manufacturing process. This is extremely important because of the variability of biologic products derived from nonuniform source materials such as blood, cells, or viruses. Moreover, experience has shown that apparently minor changes in such production segments as culture conditions or purification processes can significantly alter the biological properties of the final product. Testing of only the final product, whether it consists of cells, microorganisms, or macromolecules, cannot be relied on to detect or control for product variability. In addition, the frequently small lot sizes of certain biologic products, in particular somatic cell or gene therapy products, can severely limit the amount of testing possible on the final product. Therefore, reliance on process control is important for ensuring production of a uniform and safe product.

The third mechanism by which safety of biologic products is achieved involves control of the bulk and final product. Tests for sterility are relatively straightforward, whereas complete chemical characterization of biologic products is often more problematic. Therefore, proper testing for, and control of, biological potency has become a prominent issue, although the choice of appropriate measurements to assess potency of some of the newer products, such as those used for gene therapy, remains a challenge.

II. GENE THERAPY PRODUCTS ARE BIOLOGICS

A. Definition

Gene therapy is a medical intervention based on modification of the genetic material of living cells. Cells may be modified *ex vivo* for subsequent administration to humans, or they may be altered *in vivo* by gene therapy products given directly to the subject. When genetic manipulation is performed *ex vivo* on cells that are then administered to the patient, this is also a form of somatic cell therapy. The genetic manipulation may be intended to produce a therapeutic or prophylactic effect, or it may provide a way of marking cells for later identification.

Section 201(g)(1) of the FD&C Act, 1938 [21 U.S. C. 321(g)(1)] defines the term drug as meaning, in part, "articles intended for use in the diagnosis, cure, mitigation, treatment, or prevention of disease in man or other animals." Section 351(a) of the Public Health Service Act of 1944 [42 U.S. C. 262(a)] identifies a biologic product as "any virus, therapeutic serum, toxin, antitoxin, vaccine, blood, blood component or derivative, allergenic product, or analogous product, or arsphenamine or its derivatives (or any other trivalent organic arsenic compound), applicable to the prevention, treatment, or cure of diseases or injuries of man."

B. Ongoing Evolution of Gene Therapy

The reality of gene therapy has emerged because of remarkable advances in the science of molecular biology. The ability to manipulate genetic material *ex vivo*, and to identify and isolate genes, has provided the scientific environment enabling the practicality of gene therapy. In addition, extensive efforts in research and development of viral vectors and chemically mediated transduction procedures have provided scientists with several systems by which to deliver genetic material to a new host.

Changes within the science and clinical practice of gene therapy continue to occur rapidly. In 1988, the first gene therapy protocol was reviewed by the Recombinant DNA Advisory Committee (RAC) of the National Institutes of Health and the clinical trial initiated subsequent to review of an application for an Investigational New Drug (IND) exemption by FDA. By 1995, more than 100 protocols had been approved by the NIH RAC.

Three basic rationales exist for introducing genes into humans: (a) to replace dysfunctional but necessary genes, (b) to supply an internal, perhaps localized source of a molecule thought to be useful for direct or indirect induction of a therapeutic effect, or (c) to provide a stable means by which to mark and thereby detect transferred cells in order to trace their traffic and survival or understand their biology. All of these approaches have proved feasible in model systems both in experimental animals and *in vitro*. A notable example of replacement gene therapy can be found in the attempt to deliver the gene encoding human adenosine deaminase to children who congenitally lack the functional gene. Clinical trials have also involved the *ex vivo* insertion of cytokine genes into autologous or allogeneic tumor cells or lymphocytes, and delivery of these transduced cells to patients with advanced malignancies. Examples of gene marking studies can be found in experiments to mark bone marrow cells from cancer patients, prior to redelivering the autologous bone marrow, with the bacterial gene conferring the neomycin-resistant phenotype.

C. Components and Production of Gene Therapy Products: Vectors in Gene Therapy

Because the transfer of genetic information with high efficiency is a major concern for the application of gene therapy to humans, the use of viral vectors emerged early as one potentially productive approach. The two types of viral vectors that have been most frequently utilized are those constructed from retrovirus or adenovirus backbones. Although these viral vectors are engineered to minimize the possibility of viral replication, the use of potentially pathogenic viruses still poses many theoretical and real risks to human patients. Although other types of vectors (e.g., liposomes) and even direct administration of DNA are options in gene therapy, these have not found as wide an application to date as have viral vectors.

Potentially serious and severe adverse events have been noted in nonhuman primates receiving either retroviral or adenoviral vectors. Regarding retroviruses, for example, T-cell lymphomas were induced in immunosuppressed nonhuman primates following injection with bone marrow stem cells transduced with retroviral vectors contaminated with replication-competent virus. Moreover, Khan and co-workers (in preparation) found that retroviremia could be detected for 6 months following injection of immunocompetent monkeys with retroviral vectors. In the case of adenovirus vectors, various portions of the viral genome are generally removed in order to reduce the possibility of infection in patients. Nevertheless, inflammatory responses were documented in nonhuman primates following intrapulmonary administration of adenoviral vectors containing the Cystic Fibrosis Transductance Regulator (CFTR) gene intended for therapeutic administration to humans. The need for ensuring safety of viral vectors prior to their administration to humans, either directly or by administration of cells transduced *ex vivo,* has therefore been well established. Taking into account what is known about vector production and about the potential for adverse events, the CBER has developed a series of recommendations for safety tests to be performed throughout the production process. The current recommendations are discussed in principle in Section III; however, it should be remembered that these recommendations will undergo revision as new evidence, methods, and vectors emerge. The use of such tests adheres to the principles described earlier, that is, ensuring the safety of biologic products through the control and monitoring of source materials and the production process.

Finally, it is noteworthy that although the control of the manufacturing process is important for the production of all biologic products, it is absolutely crucial for the production of certain gene therapy products, especially those which involve the administration of viable cells as the final product. Such products, by their very nature, will not be amenable to standard postlicense lot release evaluation by the CBER, and therefore will present new challenges for the development of criteria for assuring product safety, purity, and potency.

D. Ancillary Products: Other Components Used for Manufacture of Gene Therapy Products

The manufacture of gene therapy products is usually quite complex and can involve a number of ancillary products used as part of the manufacturing process. Ancillary products include, for example, such components as cytokines, other growth factors, and monoclonal antibodies. These ancillary products may not be intended to be present in the final gene therapy product, but nevertheless they have a potential impact on the safety, purity, and potency of the final product. Occasionally the manufacturer of a gene therapy product may intentionally retain ancillary products in the final formulation, that is, produce a

combination product. In still other cases, intermediates of the final gene therapy products may be produced by one manufacturer and shipped to another as a biologic product intended for further manufacture. Situations in which ancillary products are used, or in which the production of a final gene therapy product involves more than one manufacturer, introduce additional challenges to maintaining the safety of the final product. For example, it may be necessary to determine the residual amount of ancillary product (e.g., cytokine) in the final product and to demonstrate its potential biological effect. In the case of shared manufacturing, each participating manufacturer bears the responsibility for assuring safety for its segment of the process.

III. SAFETY CONSIDERATIONS

A. Rationale

The nature of gene therapy, as with certain other drugs and biologics, makes it impossible to exclude the potential for adverse events, not only those directly affecting the patient receiving the experimental therapy, but also those affecting individuals with direct or indirect patient contact, future generations, and the environment. Because of these prospects, in response to studies outlined earlier that clearly demonstrate the potential pathogenic effects of viral vectors, and in consideration of what is known about the manufacturing processes, the CBER has taken a conservative approach to the assessment of potential risks. Current recommendations are based on the general principles for testing of biologic products. However, they also incorporate additional features based on the scientific experience of the CBER staff, information gained through the review of relevant IND submissions, and recommendations of FDA Advisory Committees and the National Institutes of Health Recombinant DNA Advisory Committee. It should be emphasized that the recommendations outlined below represent the prevailing knowledge in the area and are expected to change as that body of knowledge expands. Because an IND must provide sufficient information on product manufacturing and testing to ensure that human subjects are not exposed to unreasonable and major risks, each potential sponsor or manufacturer of a gene therapy product should consult the CBER at the appropriate time before filing an IND application, generally as early in the development phase as is feasible, to obtain descriptions of the current recommended procedures.

B. Current Recommendations

1. Manufacturing

A significant amount of information regarding the manufacture of retroviral vectors for gene therapy has been gained over the past few years. Though clearly much remains to be learned, the CBER has developed a series of specific recommendations for testing for replication-competent retrovirus (RCR) at various stages during the manufacturing process. Basically, the recommendations follow the basic principles of cell banking, about which *Points to Consider* documents are available from the CBER Office of Consumer and Public Affairs. These recommendations were first presented and endorsed at a meeting of the Viral Vaccines and Related Biological Products FDA Advisory Committee in October of 1993.

Though specific details for recommended testing may evolve, a sponsor can always obtain such details directly from the CBER at the appropriate time. As of 1995, recommendations include a single testing each of the supernatant and cells of the producer Master Cell Bank for RCR. The current recommendation includes testing of the supernatant by amplification on a permissive cell line (e.g., *Mus dunni*) followed by the S + L − assay for RCR on PG4 cells. The producer cells should be tested by coculture with the permissive cell line, and the resulting supernatant tested on PG4 cells as above. The manufacturer's Working Cell Bank should also be tested once using at least one of the two tests (i.e., supernatant or cells) recommended for the Master Cell Bank. A qualification run in which cells of the representative target population is transduced and subsequently tested for RCR at high multiplicity of infection is optional. Vector-containing supernatants should be tested for RCR after each production run. Both the clinical grade supernatant and the producer cells at the end of production should be tested as indicated for the

Master Cell Bank. In addition, it is recommended that samples of the producer cells be retained and archived in case future clinical or development data indicate that further testing would be useful. Extended culture of postproduction cells might be useful for producer/vector systems that do not exhibit receptor interference, and should be considered on a case-by-case basis.

In some cases the final gene therapy product administered to the patient consists of cells that have been transduced *ex vivo*. Such cellular products should be examined for RCR using the same assays and samples recommended for testing the Master Cell Bank. In still other cases, the gene therapy product may consist of cells producing the retroviral vector. Testing for these products is identical to the lot testing of vector supernatants. Samples should also be archived at the end of production for potential follow-up tests, and extended culture should be considered if appropriate. In general, tests should be complete prior to administration to human subjects if vector supernatants, producer cells, or transduced cells can remain in culture or be cryopreserved. Even if it is not possible to complete tests before treatment, tests should still be performed. In general, manufacturers or sponsors should contact the CBER regarding special testing needs or modifications that may be necessary for their specific products.

In the case of adenovirus vectors, little is yet known regarding the relationship between the inflammatory response they elicit and the relative proportion of defective virions in the vector preparation. Therefore, a conservative approach to limiting the amount of defective virions is being employed. Again, FDA recommendations emerge in response to the expanding information base, and specific current advice should be sought from the CBER as products are developed for clinical testing.

2. Patient Monitoring

Clearly the fundamental principle in all attempts to assess and control safety of biologic products, including gene therapy products, is protection of the patients receiving these products. Therefore, in addition to testing product source materials, monitoring the manufacturing process, and screening the final product, the CBER believes that it is imperative that individual patients be monitored not only for potential adverse events, but also for early evidence of potential problems.

In September of 1993 the CBER issued a letter to all sponsors of INDs involving gene therapy using retroviral vectors. It addressed the current CBER recommendation for the monitoring of patients receiving such gene therapy products. The letter recommended that periodic monitoring of experimental subjects should include serological assays for evidence of antibody to retroviral envelope proteins, assays for reverse transcriptase, and direct assays for viral nucleic acid in peripheral blood leukocytes using a polymerase chain reaction technique. The recommended frequency of monitoring was at least monthly during treatment, monthly for the first 3 months following completion of therapy, every 3 months for the remainder of the year following completion of treatment, and then at least yearly thereafter. In addition, sera and peripheral blood leukocytes should be obtained and archived indefinitely for each time point during the monitoring period. For patients exhibiting any positive response, the CBER further recommended that attempts be made to identify the infectious retrovirus using coculture techniques. In certain situations not all of these recommendations may be appropriate or feasible to apply. Sponsors are encouraged to discuss these unique situations with the CBER.

The use of adenovirus or certain other viral vectors might at first appear to present somewhat fewer risks than those presented by potentially oncogenic viruses. However, application of such vectors has been more limited, and our knowledge is therefore restricted. Thus, although specific recommendations for patient monitoring have not yet evolved, a cautious approach would seem prudent. There is even less collective experience with other nonviral vectors and other gene delivery systems. The FDA will continue to apply standards for safety evaluation that have proved useful for other biologics and gene therapies, and will proceed to apply current scientific knowledge to address unique issues as the needs arise.

See Also the Following Articles

CATIONIC LIPID-MEDIATED GENE THERAPY • CYTOKINE GENE THERAPY • P53 GENE THERAPY • RETROVIRAL VECTORS • TARGETED VECTORS FOR CANCER GENE THERAPY

Bibliography

Blaese, R. M. (1991). Progress toward gene therapy. *Clin. Immunol. Immunopathol.* **61**, S47.

Brenner, M. K., Rill, D. R., Moen, R. C., Krance, R. A., Mirro, J., Jr., Anderson, W. F., and Ihle, J. N. (1993). Gene-marking to trace origin of relapse after autologous bone-marrow transplantation. *Lancet* **341**, 85.

Colombo, M. P., and Forni, G. (1994). Cytokine gene transfer in tumor inhibition and tumor therapy: Where are we now? *Immunol. Today* **15**, 48.

Donahue, R. E., Kessler, S. W., Bodine, D., McDonagh, K., Dunbar, C., Goodman, S., Agricola, B., Byrne, E., Raffeld, M., Moen, R., Bacher, J., Zsebo, K. M., and Nienhuis, A. W. (1993). Helper virus induced T cell lymphoma in nonhuman primates after retroviral mediated gene transfer. *J. Exp. Med.* **176**, 1125.

Kessler, D. A., Siegel, J. P., Noguchi, P. D., Zoon, K. C., Feiden, K. L., and Woodcock, J. (1993). Regulation of somatic-cell therapy and gene therapy by the food and drug administration. *N. Engl. J. Med.* **329**, 1169.

Miller, A. D. (1990). Retrovirus packaging cells. *Hum. Gene Ther.* **1**, 5.

O'Shaughnessy, J. A., Cowan, K. H., Wilson, W., Bryant, G., Goldspiel, B., Gress, R., Nienhuis, A. W., Dunbar, C., Sorrentino, B., Stewart, F. M., Moen, R., Fox, M., and Leitman, S. (1993). Pilot study of high dose ICE (ifosfamide, carboplatin, etoposide) chemotherapy and autologous bone marrow transplant (ABMT) with neo^R-transduced bone marrow and peripheral blood stem cells in patients with metastatic breast cancer. *Hum. Gene Ther.* **4**, 331.

Pittman, M. (1987). The regulation of biologic products, 1902–1972. In "National Institute of Allergy and Infectious Diseases. Intramural Contributions, 1887–1987" (H. R. Greenwald and V. A. Harder, eds.), pp. 61–70. U. S. Department of Health and Human Services, Washington, D.C.

Simon, R. H., Engelhardt, J. F., Yang, Y., Zepeda, M., Weber-Pendleton, S., Grossman, M., and Wilson, J. M. (1993). Adenovirus-mediated transfer of the CFTR gene to lung of nonhuman primates: Toxicity study. *Hum. Gene Ther.* **4**, 771.

Vega, M. A. (1992). Adenosine deaminase deficiency: A model system for human somatic cell gene correction therapy. *Biochim. Biophys. Acta* **1138**, 253.

Wilson, J. M. (1993). Vehicles for gene therapy. *Nature (London)* **365**, 691.

Genetic Alterations in Brain Tumors

Thomas J. Cummings
Sandra H. Bigner
Duke University Medical Center

I. Astrocytomas
II. Oligodendrogliomas
III. Ependymomas
IV. Medulloblastomas
V. Atypical Teratoid/Rhabdoid Tumors
VI. Meningiomas and Schwannomas
VII. Hereditary Brain Tumor Syndromes

GLOSSARY

amplification The production of multiple copies of certain genes. The amplified sequence of DNA is recognized by the presence of small extra chromosomes known as double-minute chromosomes.

comparative genomic hybridization A technique whereby DNA from neoplastic tissue is analyzed and discerns a genetic profile including chromosomal gains and losses and gene amplification.

double-minute chromosomes Short double-stranded DNA elements that reside as independent elements in karyotypic spreads or homogeneously staining elongated regions of repeated DNA sequences that exhibit monospectral staining on karyotypic spreads.

fluorescent *in situ* hybridization A technique whereby fluorochromes are attached to DNA probes and hybridized with chromosome or cell preparations.

isochromosomes A chromosomal aberration resulting in duplication of either long or short chromosomal arms. The two arms of an isochromosome are of equal length and contain the same set of genes.

loss of heterozygosity Loss of a normal allele through somatic mutation or chromosomal rearrangement at a tumor suppressor locus removes constraints on growth-promoting genes in the tissue and allows the tissue to become neoplastic due to the remaining abnormal allele.

monosomy Loss of one member of a homologous pair of chromosomes resulting in one less than the diploid number of chromosomes.

mutation A change in genetic material, either in a single gene or in chromosome number or structure.

Recent advances in molecular pathology have discovered stereotypical genetic abnormalities in primary brain tumors of neuroepithelial origin (Table I). Molecular studies have also provided the foundation for the association of certain brain tumors among

TABLE I
Characteristic Chromosomal and Genetic Alterations in Specific Brain Tumors

Tumor/WHO grade	Chromosomal abnormality	Genetic alteration
Pilocytic astrocytoma/I	+7, +8	Unknown
Diffuse astrocytoma/II	−17p	TP53 mutation
Anaplastic astrocytoma/III	−9p	CDKN2A deletion
	−13q	RB1 mutation
	−17p	TP53 mutation
Primary glioblastoma/IV	+7	Unknown
	−9p	CDKN2A, CDKN2B deletion
	−10q	PTEN mutation
	Dmins	EGFR amplification and rearrangement
Secondary glioblastoma/IV	−17p	TP53 mutation
	−10q	PTEN mutation (rare)
	−19q	Unknown
Oligodendroglioma/II	−1p, −19q	Unknown
Anaplastic oligodendroglioma/III	−1p, −19q	Unknown
	−9p	CDKN2A, deletion
	−10q	PTEN mutation (rare)
Ependymoma/II	−22q	NF2 mutation?
Anaplastic ependymoma/III	−22q	NF2 mutation?
Medulloblastoma/IV	−17p	Unknown/HIC-1 hypermethylation?
	−9q	PTCH mutation (Gorlin syndrome)
	5q	APC mutation (Turcot syndrome)
	Dmins	C-MYC, N-MYC amplification
Atypical teratoid/rhabdoid/IV	−22q	hSNF5/INI1 deletion, mutation
Meningioma/I	−22q	NF2 mutation
Schwannoma/I	−22q	NF2 mutation

distinct familial tumor syndromes and diseases (Table II). This article outlines neoplasms of the central nervous sysyem known to contain distinctive cytogenetic and molecular features.

I. ASTROCYTOMAS

Astrocytomas are glial neoplasms derived from astrocytes and are known to occur in all areas of the brain and spinal cord in children and adults. The World Health Organization (WHO) classification categorizes astrocytomas into grades I through IV.

A. Pilocytic Astrocytoma

Pilocytic astrocytomas are grade I astrocytomas that occur mainly in children and young adults. They are typically circumscribed, slow-growing, cystic neoplasms. Fluorescence *in situ* hybridization (FISH) studies have shown gains on chromosomes 7 and 8, whereas cytogenetics have shown either similar abnormalities or normal karyotypes. Comparative genomic hybridization (CGH) studies have shown gains and deletions involving multiple chromosomes, but none in a consistent fashion. Unlike diffuse astrocytomas, mutations of the TP53 gene do not appear to play a significant role in pilocytic astrocytoma, as they never or rarely show TP53 mutations.

B. Well-Differentiated Diffuse Infiltrating Astrocytoma

Grade II astrocytomas are slow growing, diffusely infiltrating, well-differentiated fibrillary astrocytomas that typically affect young adults. CGH studies have

TABLE II
Familial Brain Tumor Syndromes

Syndrome/disease	Chromosome	Gene	Protein	Typical brain tumor
Neurofibromatosis 1	17q11	NF1	Neurofibromin	Astrocytoma
Neurofibromatosis 2	22q12	NF2	Merlin (schwannomin)	Schwannoma, meningioma, glioma
Li–Fraumeni	17p13	TP53	TP53 protein	Astrocytoma, PNET
Tuberous sclerosis	9p34	TSC1	Hamartin	Subependymal giant cell astrocytoma,
	16p13	TSC2	Tuberin	cortical tuber
Nevoid basal cell carcinoma (Gorlin)	9p31	PTCH	Ptch	Medulloblastoma
Turcot	5q21	APC	—[a]	Medulloblastoma
	3p21	hMLH1	—[a]	Glioblastoma
	7p22	hPMS2	—[a]	Glioblastoma
Trilateral retinoblastoma	13q14	RB1	RB	Retinoblastoma, pineoblastoma
Von Hippel–Lindau	3p25	VHL	VHL protein	Hemangioblastoma
Cowden	10q23	PTEN	—[a]	Dysplastic gangliocytoma of the cerebellum

[a]A common name for the protein is not described.

reported gain, or amplification, of chromosomes 7q and 8q. Other abnormalities include loss of chromosome 10p and 17p loss associated with *TP53* mutations. *TP53* mutations have been seen in greater than 60% of grade II astrocytomas that progress to glioblastoma, including the gemistocytic variant with its tendency toward rapid progression to glioblastoma.

C. Anaplastic Astrocytoma

Anaplastic astrocytomas (AA) are WHO grade III tumors. They diffusely infiltrate surrounding brain parenchyma and have an intrinsic tendency for malignant progression to glioblastoma. The genotype of the AA is not well delineated; it may contain changes found in either the low-grade diffuse astrocytoma or its higher grade counterpart, glioblastoma. Losses of 9p, 13q, and 17p are common and affect the known tumor suppressor genes *CDKN2A*, *RB1*, and *TP53*, respectively. Loss of heterozygosity (LOH) on 19q and chromosome 10 deletions have been reported in AAs. Unlike glioblastoma, genetic amplification is observed in less than 10% of cases of AAs; if present, one should consider the diagnosis of glioblastoma rather than AA.

D. Glioblastoma

The most common primary malignant brain tumor of adults is the glioblastoma multiforme (GBM), a grade

IV astrocytoma in the WHO classification. There are two subtypes of GBM: the *de novo* or primary type and the progressive or secondary type. Primary GBMs typically occur in patients older than 50 years of age and show loss of chromosome 10q with mutation of the *PTEN/MMAC1* (phosphatase and tensin homolog deleted on chromosome 10) / (mutated in multiple advanced cancers) gene, gain of chromosome 7, loss of chromosome 9p with deletion of *CDKN2A* and *CDKN2B* genes, and amplification or overexpression of the epidermal growth factor receptor gene (*EGFR*). Amplification of DNA sequences results in hyperexpression of oncogenes and is manifest cytogenetically as dmins. In many GBMs, the amplified *EGFR* gene is truncated, resulting in autonomous growth stimulation of the cell independent of receptor binding. Progressive GBMs tend to occur in patients younger than 50 years of age, contain 19q losses with an interstitial deletion of the 19q13.3 region, are likely to contain *TP53* mutations, and seldom contain amplification of *EGFR*. The high rate of *TP53* mutations in diffuse astrocytomas and secondary GBMs indicates that *TP53* gene mutations are an early event in the genesis of progressive malignant astrocytomas. Losses involving chromosome 10 occur in progressive GBMs, but they rarely contain *PTEN/MMAC1* mutations. Regulators of the cell cycle include protein p16, which is encoded by the *CDKN2* gene located at chromosome 9p21 and appears to be more common in primary GBMs. Alterations involving the *RB1* tumor suppressor gene located on chromosome 13q have been described in both primary and secondary high-grade astrocytomas.

II. OLIGODENDROGLIOMAS

Oligodendrogliomas are infiltrating gliomas that occur mainly in the cerebral hemispheres of adults and are derived from oligodendrocytes. The WHO subtypes oligodendrogliomas into well-differentiated oligodendrogliomas (WDO) (WHO grade II) and anaplastic oligodendrogliomas (AO) (WHO grade III).

A. Well-Differentiated Oligodendroglioma

Although most cytogenetic analyses of oligodendrogliomas have failed to demonstrate consistent findings, LOH studies have shown that complete allelic loss of one p arm of chromosome 1 and/or complete allelic loss of one q arm of chromosome 19, with retention of both alleles of the 1q and 19p arms, occurs commonly in these tumors. In contrast, astrocytic tumors are more likely to show varied patterns of chromosome 1 and 19 abnormalities, such as partial loss of 19p alleles and distal losses on the 1 p arm. Other findings in WDOs have shown LOH for chromosome 10, 9p, and 17p. *EGFR* gene amplification, homozygous deletion of the *CDKN2A* gene, and *PTEN* gene mutations do not occur in WDOs.

B. Anaplastic Oligodendroglioma

AOs share many molecular features with WDOs, including LOH for 1p, 19q, or both. In contrast to WDOs, AOs show allelic loss of 9p, homozygous deletion of the *CDKN2A* gene, and losses involving chromosomes 4, 14, 15, and 18. The histologic distinction of AO from GBM is not always readily apparent. However, the identification of AO is important because of its typically good response to chemotherapeutic agents in contrast to the GBM. Genetic studies can help distinguish between AO and GBM. Although AOs and GBMs may both contain 9p loss, 19q loss, and deletion of the *CDKN2A* gene, AOs do not contain mutations of the *PTEN* gene, *EGFR* gene amplification, or the characteristic +7, −10 CGH pattern of GBM.

III. EPENDYMOMAS

Ependymomas are tumors of neoplastic ependymal cells that typically originate from the wall of the cerebral ventricles or from the spinal canal in children and young adults. The WHO classifies ependymal neoplasms into two groups: ependymoma (WHO grade II) and anaplastic ependymoma (WHO grade III). Subependymoma and myxopapillary ependymoma are WHO grade I tumors without consistent cytogenetic or molecular alterations and are not further discussed.

The most common cytogenetic abnormalities of grade II ependymomas include monosomy 22 and translocations involving 22q. Despite the association of ependymomas with neurofibromatosis type 2 and the location of the *NF2* gene on chromosome 22q, evidence implicating *NF2* as a candidate gene in ependymomas has been speculative. Cytogenetics and molecular studies in grade III anaplastic ependymomas have not yielded any consistent features.

IV. MEDULLOBLASTOMAS

Medulloblastomas are the most common malignant primary brain tumors of childhood. They are embryonal neoplasms that arise in the cerebellar vermis or hemispheres and are WHO grade IV tumors.

Karyotype and LOH studies have shown that the most common specific chromosomal abnormality in medulloblastomas is loss of 17p through formation of isochromosome 17q [i(17q)] or by unbalanced translocations. The site of the breakpoint is controversial and appears to involve either 17p11.2 or 17p13.1-13.3. Resolution of the precise site of the breakpoint may eventually uncover the 17p gene or genes responsible for the 17p abnormalities. Despite the location of the *TP53* gene on 17p, *TP53* gene mutations occur in only about 5% of medulloblastomas, further suggesting that an undescribed gene is responsible for the 17p loss in these tumors. *HIC-1* (hypermethylated in cancer) is a candidate tumor suppressor gene located at 17p13.3. Hypermethylation of *HIC-1* and loss of *HIC-1* expression are common in primary breast cancer and appear to be present in a high percentage of medulloblastomas. However, the independent significance of hypermethylation affecting *HIC-1* in medulloblastomas remains to be determined. Although supratentorial primitive neuroectodermal tumors (S-PNET) histologically resemble medulloblastoma, S-PNETs do not show 17p loss or i(17q).

Dmins are seen in about 5% of medulloblastoma biopsies, but can be identified in a majority of permanent cultured cell lines and xenografts derived from these. In most samples with Dmins, genomic amplification maps to chromosome 8q24 (C-MYC gene), or less often to chromosome 2p23-24 (N-MYC gene). Molecular analysis of childhood PNETs has shown that medulloblastomas with MYC amplification are aggressive tumors that are resistant to therapy and have rapidly fatal outcomes.

Medulloblastomas are associated with two familial brain tumor syndromes (Table II). The first is the nevoid basal cell carcinoma syndrome (NBCCS), also known as Gorlin syndrome. The gene responsible for NBCCS was identified as *PTCH*, the human homologue of the *Drosophila patched* gene, and was mapped to chromosome 9q22.3. In addition to multiple basal cell carcinomas of the skin, patients with NBCCS are predisposed to develop medulloblastomas, predominantly of the desmoplastic variant. The other familial brain tumor syndrome that predisposes to medulloblastoma is Turcot syndrome. Turcot syndrome comprises two syndromes. Turcot type 1 is associated with hereditary nonpolyposis colorectal carcinoma (HNPCC) syndrome and GBMs and contains germline mutations in the DNA mismatch repair genes located at 3p21 and 7p22. Turcot type 2 is characterized by familial adenomatous polyposis (FAP), colon carcinoma, and medulloblastoma. The *APC* (adenomatous polyposis coli) gene is responsible for Turcot type 2 and maps to chromosome 5q21. The *APC* protein regulates β-catenin and the Wnt signaling pathway. In the absence of Turcot syndrome, *APC* mutations rarely occur in sporadic brain tumors.

V. ATYPICAL TERATOID/RHABDOID TUMORS

The atypical teratoid/rhabdoid (AT/RT) tumor is a WHO grade IV tumor of infancy and childhood that is frequently mistaken for medulloblastoma. These tumors typically occur in the posterior fossa and have a mean postoperative survival of 11 months. Cytogenetic and molecular observations that characterize AT/RT include monosomy for chromosome 22. LOH studies have identified a common region of deletion at 22q11.2-22q12.2. *hSNF5/INI1* is a gene that maps to chromosome 22q11.2 and is apparently responsible for the monosomy/deletions involving chromosome 22. Studies have suggested that *INI1* functions as a tumor suppressor gene and that their mutations are a predisposing factor for AT/RTs.

VI. MENINGIOMAS AND SCHWANNOMAS

Meningiomas and schwannomas are typically extraaxial neoplasms that may involve the intracranial or intraspinal compartments. They are derived from meningothelium and schwann cells, respectively. The common genetic alteration in both of these neoplasms is allelic losses of chromosome 22q, and mutations in the *NF2* gene have been reported in approximately 60% of sporadic cases.

VII. HEREDITARY BRAIN TUMOR SYNDROMES

Genetic studies have been instrumental in the characterization of brain tumors and other central nervous system manifestations in certain inherited cancer syndromes and diseases. The responsible genes, chromosomal loci, and affected proteins have been identified and named in many of these disorders (Table II). They include neurofibromatosis type 1, neurofibromatosis type 2, Li–Fraumeni syndrome, tuberous sclerosis complex, nevoid basal cell carcinoma syndrome (Gorlin syndrome), Turcot syndrome, trilateral retinoblastoma (*RB1* deletion syndrome associated with bilateral retinoblastomas and pineoblastoma), von Hippel–Lindau disease, and Cowden disease.

Acknowledgments

The authors greatly appreciate the contributions of Darell D. Bigner, Roger E. McLendon, Henry Friedman, and Allan Friedman for providing information on the material provided here.

See Also the Following Articles

Bibliography

Aldosari, N., Rasheed, B. K. A., McLendon, R. E., *et al.* (2000). Characterization of chromosome 17 abnormalities in medulloblastomas. *Acta Neuropathol.* **99,** 345–351.

Biegel, J. A., Zhou, J.-Y., Rorke, L. B., *et al.* (1999). Germ-line and acquired mutations of INI1 in atypical teratoid and rhabdoid tumors. *Cancer Res.* **59,** 74–79.

Bigner, S. H., Matthews, M. R., Rasheed, B. K. A., *et al.* (1999). Molecular genetic aspects of oligodendrogliomas including analysis by comparative genomic hybridization. *Am. J. Pathol.* **155,** 375–386.

Bigner, D. D., McLendon, R. E., and Bruner, J. M. (eds.) (1998). "Russell and Rubinstein's Pathology of Tumors of the Nervous System," 6th Ed. Arnold, London.

Cairncross, J. G., Ueki, K., Zlatescu, M. C., *et al.* (1998). Specific genetic predictors of chemotherapeutic response and survival in patients with anaplastic oligodendrogliomas. *J. Natl. Cancer Inst.* **90,** 1473–1479.

Fujii, H., Biel, M. A., Zhou, W., *et al.* (1998). Methylation of the HIC-1 candidate tumor suppressor gene in human breast cancer. *Oncogene* **16,** 2159–2164.

Graham, D. I., and Lantos, P. L. (eds.) (1997). "Greenfield's Neuropathology," 6th Ed. Arnold, London.

Kleihues, P., and Cavenee, W. K. (2000). "Pathology and Genetics: Tumours of the Nervous System." World Health Organization Classification of Tumors. IARC Press, Lyon.

Pietsch, T. (2000). Genetics of medulloblastomas. *Brain Pathol.* S08–02, **10,** 614.

Reifenberger, J., Reifenberger, G., Liu, L., *et al.* (1994). Molecular genetic analysis of oligodendroglial tumors shows preferential allelic deletions on 19q and 1p. *Am. J. Pathol.* **145,** 1175–1190.

Watanabe, K., Tachibana, O., Sata, K., *et al.* (1996). Overexpression of the EGF receptor and p53 mutations are mutually exclusive in the evolution of primary and secondary glioblastomas. *Brain Pathol.* **6,** 217–223.

Genetic Basis for Quantitative and Qualitative Changes in Drug Targets

Amelia M. Wall
John D. Schuetz

St. Jude Children's Research Hospital, Memphis, Tennessee

GLOSSARY

ABC A large family of ATP-binding cassette transporters; one member is MDR1, whose gene product, P-glycoprotein, encodes a multisubstrate cellular efflux pump.

amplicon The unit-repeating sequence that is amplified.

DNA amplification Process in which the copy number of a subchromasomal length of DNA is selectively increased relative to flanking DNA sequences.

double minute chromosome Small chromosome-like DNA that lacks a centromere and consists of multiple tandem amplicons.

MRP1 (multidrug resistance protein) Member of the ABC transporters associated with drug resistance in cancer; effluxes organic anions such as methotrexate and daunorubicin.

nondisjunction Process in which a replicated chromosome, or a part thereof, fails to separate at mitosis so that both copies are distributed to one daughter cell.

p53 Nuclear transcription factor that can activate or repress gene transcription, a tumor suppressor gene that is deleted or mutated in approximately half of all cancers, and a central regulatory gene involved in cell proliferation, DNA repair, and apoptosis.

p-glycoprotein Member of the ATP-binding cassette transporters that effluxes hydrophobic cytotoxic drugs such as adriamycin, vincristine, etoposide, and taxol.

Cancer chemotherapy frequently initiates a series of pleiotropic changes within tumor cells that lead to the emergence of tumors refractory to chemotherapy. These cellular changes evolve because of the unique properties of the tumor cell, i.e., a cell that has lost the ability, in many cases, to appropriately stop replication in the presence of DNA damage. DNA damage to the cell facilitates the engagement of cellular mechanisms to evade chemotherapy and acquire chemotherapeutic resistance. The acquired phenotypes of these chemotherapy-resistant cancer cells are alterations in the ability to accumulate drugs, as well as changes in either the amount or the ability of a target protein to bind the chemotherapeutic agent. Mechanistically, these changes include increased gene copy, mutations, altered transcription, and epigenetic changes, such as an alteration in methylation status. Knowledge of the different mechanisms by which tumors evade chemotherapy is the first step toward increasing therapeutic efficacy. This article discusses these genetic alterations in drug targets that affect tumor response to therapy.

I. GENETIC ALTERATION

The genomic instability of tumor cells predisposes them to higher rates of genetic alteration than normal cells. An intact p53 signaling pathway is critical for the maintenance of genomic stability and allows a cell to stop DNA replication after damage and engage repair processes after DNA damage. Because over 50% of human cancers have mutations in the p53 gene, this pathway is disabled and renders the genome unstable. Studies by Tlsty and co-workers demonstrated that genetic deletion of p53 rendered cells that were normally refractory to gene amplification, highly prone to gene amplification. Further studies by Stark and co-workers have provided evidence that DNA damage is critical for gene amplification. Moreover, the absence or loss of p53 function leads to a cell replicating damaged, unrepaired DNA. Thus, replication after DNA damage, in the presence of the appropriate cytotoxic drug selective pressure, facilitates increased copy number of a gene that will cause the tumor cell to acquire, in many cases, resistance to the cytotoxic drug.

A. Amplification

Gene amplification is the selective duplication of DNA. While the region of amplified DNA is large, it usually contains a gene or genes that provide the tumor cell with a survival advantage in the presence of

a chemotherapeutic agent (specific examples are mentioned later). Nevertheless, in the early stage, the amplified DNA is unstable and essentially remains as an extrachromsomal element called a double minute. However, the double minute is unstable due to absence of a centromere and, without the appropriate drug selective pressure, is lost because they segregate unevenly during mitosis. Notably, sustained cytotoxic drug exposure facilitates chromosomal integration into the normal chromosomal locus. Moreover, as the drug concentration increases, multiple copies form at this locus and are referred to as homogenous staining regions (HSRs). After chromosomal integration, a stable dominant phenotypic change has occurred in the cancer cell. Specific examples of gene amplification follow.

1. ATP-Binding Cassette (ABC) Transporters

a. MDR1   The multidrug resistance gene (*MDR1*) encodes a protein, P-glycoprotein (Pgp), that confers resistance to the cytotoxic effects of a broad range of structurally unrelated compounds (Table I). Pgp is found in the plasma membrane and, as a member of the ABC transporter family, requires ATP as an energy source to transport drugs out (efflux) of cells. Pgp was first functionally identified in cells that acquired resistance to the cytotoxic effects of either vinca alkaloids or anthracyclines. Unexpectedly, cells with acquired resistance to this drug were also resistant to multiple drugs, without prior exposure. This phenotype was re-

TABLE I
Selected Substrates of Pgp

Actinomycin D
Anthracyclines
Colchicine
Epipodophyllotoxins
Ethidium bromide
Hoechst 33342
Mitomycin C
Paclitaxel
Rhodamine 123
Steroids
Topotecan
Vinca alkaloids

ferred to as pleiotropic drug resistance. The pleiotropic drug resistance phenotype was characterized by a biochemical change of decreased drug accumulation. Notably, decreasing cellular ATP led to increased drug accumulation, a finding that facilitated the understanding that Pgp is an ATP-dependent efflux transporter. Subsequent studies have demonstrated that high levels of resistance can be achieved in tumor cells by amplification of the MDR1 gene, leading to Pgp overexpression and resistance to multiple drugs (see Table I).

b. MRP1 and Related Genes The multidrug resistance related protein cDNA was originally isolated from a small cell lung cancer cell line that acquired drug efflux-mediated resistance, but was not due to increased Pgp expression. Using differential hybridization, an overexpressed mRNA was identified in the resistant cells, and DNA sequence analysis revealed that it belonged to the ABC transporter superfamily. This new gene was named multidrug resistance related protein. MRP1 transports anionic compounds (e.g., methotrexate) (see Table II), but can also transport some cationic compounds (e.g., vincristine) in the presence of glutathione. An increased expression of MRP1 has been correlated with increased gene transcription, secondary to gene amplification. MRP1 is expressed in lung, testis, nasal respiratory mucosa, liver, and peripheral blood mononuclear cells and has been demonstrated to be expressed in tumors derived

from these tissues (see Table II). Notably, MRP1 was the first member described in this rapidly expanding gene subfamily, and additional members of the MRP subfamily also have been shown to be capable of transporting and conferring resistance to anticancer antiretroviral drugs (see Table III).

c. BCRP To uncover resistance mechanisms independent of Pgp, cells were treated with a chemical inhibitor of Pgp (verapamil) and a known Pgp substrate (doxorubicin). Subsequently, utilizing a screening technique to identify differentially expressed genes, the gene encoding the ABC transporter, BCRP (breast cancer-resistance protein, a.k.a. ABCP, MXR, ABCG2), was isolated. BCRP is an ABC "half molecule," which means it contains only a single ATP-binding domain and a single transmembrane domain. Currently, there is no direct evidence for an ABC transporter to function with a single ATP-binding domain, it has been assumed BCRP either homo- or heterodimerizes. Nevertheless, BCRP overexpression can confer resistance to many compounds, including mitoxantrone, camptothecins, and, in some cases, anthracyclines (see Table III).

2. Non-ABC Transporter Mechanisms of Resistance

Dihydrofolate reductase (DHFR) is required to maintain the reduced folates necessary for donating carbon atoms, which are essential for the *de novo* synthesis of purines, pyrimidines, and amino acids, and is the intracellular target of four amino analogs of folic acid (i.e., antifolates). Inhibition of DHFR by antifolates (e.g., methotrexate) causes purine and or pyrimidine

TABLE II
Cancers Expressing Drug-Resistant
ABC Transporters

Acute myeloid leukemia	MDR1, MRP1, BCRP
Acute lymphocytic leukemia	MDR1, MRP4, MRP5
Breast	BCRP, MDR1, MRP1
Ovarian	MDR1
Bladder	MRP1
Lymphoma	MDR1, MRP1
Adult sarcoma	MDR1
Non-small cell lung cancer	MDR1, MRP1
Prostate	MRP1, MRP4
Neuroblastoma	MDR1, MRP1
Gastrointestinal tumors	MDR1, MRP1, MRP4
Esophageal	MDR1, MRP1

TABLE III
Chemotherapy Substrates of ABC Transporters

MDR-1	Vinca alkaloids, anthracyclines, taxanes, actinomycin D, epipodophyllotoxins, steroids
MRP-1	Doxorubicin, daunomycin, vincristine, etoposide, methotrexate
MRP-2	Vinca alkaloids, cisplatin, CPT-11, methotrexate
MRP-3	Etoposide, teniposide, methotrexate, vincristine
MRP-4	Methotrexate, purine antimetabolites, antivirals
MRP-5	Purine antimetabolites
BCRP	Mitoxantrone, camptothecins, anthracyclines

starvation. Tumor cell lines with acquired resistance to methotrexate have increased DHFR expression, which correlates with both increased DHFR gene copy and degree of resistance. Clinical reports suggest that increased DHFR expression is related to changes in gene copy.

BCR/ABL is an oncogenic fusion protein isolated from chronic myelogenous and acute lymphocytic leukemias. A chromosomal translocation between chromosomes 9 and 22 produces this chimeric molecule, bcr/abl, which possesses tyrosine kinase activity. A unique tyrosine kinase inhibitor, STI571, was developed to inhibit bcr/abl and appears very successful in eradicating chronic myelogenous leukemic cells in vivo. However, cells in culture can develop resistance due to the amplification and/or mutation of bcr/abl after chronic exposure to STI571; these promising results should be interpreted with caution.

The reduced folate carrier (RFC) is primarily responsible for the accumulation of reduced folates and antifolates (e.g., methotrexate) in the cell. Cells grown under conditions of folate deprivation can amplify the RFC gene. These cells with amplified and overexpressed RFC can more effectively accumulate natural folates, thus providing them the means to accumulate folates and override antifolate-induced cytotoxicity.

B. Mutation/Loss of Function/Deletion

Alterations of a gene encoding a drug target have been shown in vitro and in vivo to contribute to drug resistance and may be secondary to either a loss or a gain of function.

1. Mutation of DHFR has been documented in some cell lines with acquired methotrexate resistance. Mutations have been described that result in catalytically less active DHFR, which poorly binds antifolates.

2. RFC is the major carrier protein for transporting reduced folates and antifolates into the cell, and RFC mutations have been discovered in human and rodent cells with an acquired resistance to methotrexate. Thus, lack of antifolate accumulation via RFC mutants can limit its antitumor activity.

3. In some cell lines, resistance to a lipophilic an-

tifolate (pyrimethamine) was caused by a loss of folate efflux. This loss of folic acid efflux was sufficient to maintain the cellular uptake of folate cofactors and allowed subsequent survival on picomolar concentrations of folate.

C. Methylation

DNA methylation occurs in eukaryotes and is characterized by the transfer of a methyl group by DNA methyltransferase to the carbon 5 position of the cytosine ring in the context of a 5'-CG-3' sequence. Methylation of a gene silences its expression, whereas demethylation activates expression.

Hypermethylation in the promoters of tumor suppressor genes has been documented (e.g., p16INK4a, BRCA1, p73, Apaf-1). Although it is a possible mechanism of decreased expression of tumor suppressors, it has not yet been unequivocally demonstrated as a mechanism affecting expression of a drug target (e.g., MDR1).

II. ROLE OF TRANSCRIPTION FACTORS

Another mechanism by which the levels of a drug target can change is by alterations in transcription. Normally, transcription factors are tightly balanced to control gene transcription, such that alterations in either the amount or the composition of any of one factor could change expression of the gene. In cells, transcription factors might increase or decrease secondary to cellular stresses (e.g., irradiation, hypoxia, or chemotherapy). These alterations in transcription factors change patterns of gene expression that can alter drug sensitivity. In addition, transcription factors may be mutated or form novel chimeras that acquire the ability to interact with different transcription factors. The following discussion, using the MDR1 gene as a model, illustrates some of these issues.

The MDR1 promoter contains multiple DNA elements that control transcription and it can be regulated by multiple transcription factors. This explains the differential tissue expression of MDR1. MDR1 is highly expressed in colon, liver, intestinal epithelium, and kidney, and this high expression undoubtedly contributes to the intrinsic insensitivity to the chemotherapy of cancers that arise in these tissues. This gene, which encodes the efflux transporter, Pgp, renders tumor cells resistant to multiple, structurally diverse, amphipathic, cationic drugs (see Table III).

One transcription factor demonstrated to affect MDR1 transcription is p53. p53 can either activate or repress transcription. p53 is mutated in greater than 50% of human cancers, with most of the mutations causing a loss in the ability to bind DNA as well as to repress transcription. p53 was demonstrated to repress transcription because direct inactivation of endogenous wild-type p53 caused increased MDR1 expression. These findings provided direct experimental evidence that loss of p53 repression upregulates *MDR1*. This provides a basis for the clinical observations showing mutation of p53 in several tumors (e.g., breast, colon, esophageal) highly correlates with increased MDR1 expression.

Clearly, mutation of p53 leads to a loss of repression. Notably, mutant p53s also acquire unique transcription function; however, it is unknown if mutant p53 upregulates endogenous *MDR1*. Certainly if mutant p53 can upregulate the endogenous MDR1 gene, then one can envision the possibility of a mutant p53 causing a "double whammy," i.e., p53 mutation can lead to both loss of repression and activation of *MDR1* transcription by the mutant p53. This would undoubtedly lead to highly drug-resistant tumors. Future studies are needed to address this issue.

NF-Y is a transcription factor that binds to the inverted CCAAT box of the *MDR1* promoter and regulates the constitutive expression of MDR1 in some cells. NF-Y recruits P/CAF, a coactivator with histone acetyltransferase activity, to activate *MDR1* transcription by inducing the hyperacetylation of promoter-associated histones. Thus, the use of agents that inhibit histone deacetylases (e.g., trichostatin) may lead to an increase in MDR1 expression and therefore drug resistance.

Some chimeric transcription factors affect *MDR1* transcription. Myeloid leukemias frequently have translocations in the AML-1 gene, a gene that is one of the most frequently mutated genes in human leukemia. It has been shown that the chimeric transcription factor AML/ETO, created by a translocation between the AML and the ETO genes [t(8;21)], represses MDR1 gene transcription. This finding provides a molecular explanation for why some adult AML patients with the t(8;21) translocation do not express MDR1 and respond favorably to a chemotherapeutic regimen that includes Pgp substrates (see Table I).

III. IMPLICATIONS/CONCLUSIONS

Genetic and epigenetic changes in either the chemotherapeutic drug target or the transporters mediating cellular accumulation permit an "escape" mechanism for tumor cells to evade therapy by either preventing the cell from achieving the concentration of drug sufficient to produce cytotoxicity or increasing the amount of drug required to inhibit an intracellular enzyme. Mechanistically, this can occur through either gene amplification or alteration in expression by changes in transcription factors. It is hoped that further studies in these areas will lead researchers to exploit pathways within tumor cells that will ultimately lead to better anticancer therapies.

See Also the Following Articles

BCR-ABL • DNA METHYLATION AND CANCER • MULTIDRUG RESISTANCE I: P-GLYCOPROTEIN • MULTIDRUG RESISTANCE II: MRP AND RELATED PROTEINS

Bibliography

Ling, V. (1997). Multidrug resistance: Molecular mechanisms and clinical relevance. *Cancer Chemother. Pharmacol.* **40**, S3–S8.

Tlsty, T. D. (1998). Cell-adhesion-dependent influences on genomic instability and carcinogenesis. *Curr. Opin. Cell. Biol.* **10**(5), 647–653.

Genetic Predisposition to Prostate Cancer

Ellen L. Goode
Gail P. Jarvik

Fred Hutchinson Cancer Research Center
University of Washington

I. Does Prostate Cancer Cluster in Families?
II. Is the Familial Clustering of Prostate Cancer Due to Genetics?
III. What Specific Genetic Factors Are Involved with Prostate Cancer?
IV. Difficulties in the Search for Major Susceptibility Genes
V. Summary and Future Considerations

GLOSSARY

allele Alternate form of a gene.

association study A study seeking to identify disease alleles by examining whether allele frequencies differ between affected and unaffected individuals in a population.

complex segregation analysis A method to assess the presence of, and Mendelian pattern of, disease transmission in families.

fully penetrant gene All individuals with the disease genotype are affected.

linkage analysis A method to localize disease genes by examining the transmission of disease with genetic markers in families.

locus The position of the gene on the chromosome.

locus heterogeneity More than one genetic locus causes the disease.

phenocopy An affected individual who does not carry the disease-causing genotype.

P rostate cancer is a significant public health problem in the United States. In 2002, 189,000 new prostate cancer cases and 30,200 deaths due to the disease were expected in the United States. Prostate cancer incidence increases with age and varies by race: Asian males have a lower incidence, whereas North American, European, and Australian males have a higher incidence. African-American males have the highest incidence of prostate cancer in the world. Epidemiologic studies of environmental variables have not identified consistent risk factors other than diet, particularly a low intake of cruciferous vegetables. This article reviews evidence for genetic predisposition to prostate cancer in the context of three questions that the field of genetic epidemiology seeks to address. The article then discusses difficulties in the search for major susceptibility genes and considers possible directions for future research.

I. DOES PROSTATE CANCER CLUSTER IN FAMILIES?

One of the first clues as to whether genetic predisposition exists for any disease is that the disease runs in families. Comparisons of men affected with prostate cancer and unaffected men show that affected men are more likely to have a previously affected relative. Similarly, studies of men with and without a family history of prostate cancer show that men with an affected relative are more likely to develop the disease. A multitude of these studies have consistently suggested that having an affected first-degree relative increases the risk of developing prostate cancer two- to threefold. Several studies further indicate that if an affected relative is diagnosed at a young age (less than 65 years) or if there are several affected men in a family, the risk of prostate cancer is increased as much as 6 or 11 times. Interestingly, some studies have also shown that the risk of prostate cancer is increased more among men with affected brothers than among men with affected fathers, suggesting an X-linked or autosomal recessive mode of inheritance. The observed familial clustering of any disease may be due to genetic or nongenetic factors (shared environment or diet); therefore, further studies have been conducted to evaluate the relative importance of genetic and nongenetic factors.

II. IS THE FAMILIAL CLUSTERING OF PROSTATE CANCER DUE TO GENETICS?

Twin studies, migrant studies, and complex segregation analyses (CSAs) all address the role that genetic factors play in the observed clustering of prostate cancer in families. Research on identical and fraternal twins has shown that identical twins more often share the same disease state (both affected or both unaffected). Although identical twins may share more environmental or *in utero* factors, as well as more genetic material, these results suggest a genetic influence on prostate cancer. Studies of recent migrants from Asia to the United States show a moderate incidence of prostate cancer compared to the lower incidence in Asia and the higher incidence in the United States. Because the incidence of prostate cancer among recent migrants is less than that of native-born U.S. males, a suggestion of a genetic influence is made. However, interpretation of migrant studies is also limited because of continuation of diet and other cultural practices by migrants.

CSAs are another type of study that aims to assess the relative influence of genes and environment in disease. In a CSA, the transmission pattern of affected men in families is analyzed. The relative likelihoods of the observed patterns of inheritance are compared when different genetic and nongenetic components are assumed; if a genetic component is supported, tests of specific Mendelian patterns may be made. Several CSAs of families with prostate cancer support the existence of one or more major susceptibility genes that are inherited in a Mendelian fashion. Most of the CSAs suggest autosomal-dominant inheritance; however, one also shows support for recessive or X-linked inheritance of a major gene or genes. CSAs also provide descriptions of the proposed prostate cancer susceptibility genes; risk alleles are thought to be rare (frequency of 0.003 to 0.0167) and highly penetrant (63 to 100% of allele carriers will become affected). Such studies have inspired searches for prostate cancer susceptibility genes in the human genome.

III. WHAT SPECIFIC GENETIC FACTORS ARE INVOLVED WITH PROSTATE CANCER?

Much work has been done to identify and understand the particular genetic factors involved in prostate cancer. Techniques in molecular genetics and histochemistry have highlighted certain chromosomal regions and genes that may be candidates; epidemiologic population-based studies have attempted to determine which alleles confer an increased risk in the general population; and linkage analyses of families with multiple cases have tried to localize novel susceptibility genes.

A. Candidate Genes: Clues from *in Vitro* Studies

Candidate prostate cancer susceptibility genes may be identified through the observation of chromosomal alterations (deletions, amplifications, or DNA copy number gains) or genetic changes occurring in prostate cancer tumor tissue that do not occur in normal tissue. Chromosomal alterations have been observed in prostate tumor tissue and most often are deletions, suggesting a role of the deleted region in tumor suppression. The most common regions of loss occur on chromosomes 8p and 13q; because known genes in these regions [including *BRCA2* and the retinoblastoma gene *(RB1)*] do not appear to be mutated in prostate cancer, as yet unidentified tumor suppressor genes may reside here. In advanced-stage (hormone-refractory) tumors, DNA copy number gains or amplification is observed more often than deletions, and the most common alteration is gain of the entire chromosome 8q, a region including MYC, eukaryotic initiation factor-3 subunit 3 *(EIF3S3)*, and prostate stem cell antigen *(PSCA)*. Other *in vitro* work has attempted to characterize the involvement of particular genes in these and other regions, such as hypermethylation of glutathione *S*-transferase pi *(GSTP1)* and E-cadherin *(CDH1)*, mutation in p53, reduced expression of mismatch repair genes, and overexpression of ERBB2 and the androgen receptor gene *(AR)*. Molecular genetic analysis of these and other genes involved in possibly pathways to prostate cancer may help in our understanding of genetic predisposition to prostate cancer.

B. Association Studies: Common Alleles with Low Penetrance

Variants of several hormone metabolism genes have been shown to be associated with hormone metabolic activity and have been studied for associations with prostate cancer risk in population-based studies (see Table I). An association could indicate that the variant itself confers increased risk or that it is in linkage disequilibrium with another variant involved in pathway to disease. Polymorphisms in the steroid 5α-reductase type II gene *(SRD5A2)* have been associated with a twofold risk of prostate cancer in Caucasian men. AR contains several polymorphic repeat regions, including a CAG repeat in exon 1. Several epidemiological studies have shown that longer CAG repeats (≤ 18 bp versus ≥ 26 bp) are associated with an increased risk of prostate cancer, although some studies have not confirmed this. One study has reported an interaction between *AR* genotypes and genotypes of the prostate-specific antigen gene *(PSA)*. A variant of the vitamin D receptor gene *(VDR)* has been shown to confer about a two- to threefold increased risk of prostate cancer in some North American and Japanese populations. Polymorphism in several other genes, including the 17-hydroxylase cytochrome P450 gene *(CYP17)*, *GSTP1*, and E-cadherin *(CDH1)*, have been examined for an association with prostate cancer risk; results have not been consistent. Larger population-based epidemiologic studies are needed to further characterize the involvement of common variants in candidate genes.

TABLE I

Common Variants of Hormone and Carcinogen Metabolism Genes and Risk of Prostate Cancer

Gene	Function	Polymorphism	Variant frequency, Caucasian controls	Relative risk (range)
SRD5A2	Catalytic enzyme converts testosterone to DHT	V89L	~0.28	1.0–2.5
AR	Mediates action of androgens in prostate	(CAG)$_n$	~0.27 (<20 repeats)	1.3–3.0
PSA	Target of AR	G/A in promoter at −158	~0.50	1.0–2.9
VDR	Mediates action of the active form of vitamin D	*BsmI, ApaI,* and *TaqI,* restriction enzyme sites	~0.35	1.0–3.3
CYP17	Catalytic enzyme in steroid hormone biosynthesis	T/C in 5′ UTR	~0.35	1.0–2.8
GSTP1	Carcinogen metabolism	I105V	~0.33	0.2–1.0

C. Linkage Studies: Rare Alleles with High Penetrance

Reports from CSAs, in particular, have fueled the search for highly penetrant susceptibility genes in families with multiple cases of prostate cancer. Linkage analysis (using lod score and other methods) is a powerful statistical tool to identify particular chromosomal regions that might contain these genes. The chromosomal regions are suggested by the coinheritance in a family of disease and known genetic markers in the region. The disease genes themselves can then be isolated by positional cloning methods using the known genetic markers as signposts. Numerous scans of the human genome for prostate cancer loci have been conducted in this way, and many have identified multiple genetics regions that may contain a highly penetrant prostate cancer locus.

To date, one gene has been identified through the analysis of prostate cancer families and clone: *HPC2/ELAC2* at chromosome 17p. In the original finding, two families had high lod scores and a critical region was found. The gene was identified and *HPC2/ELAC2* mutations were identified in two families. Subsequent studies, however, have shown that the importance of this gene in hereditary prostate cancers may be small (only a small percentage of hereditary prostate cancers share linkage or mutations). The function of *HPC2/ELAC2* is still unknown.

Five other putative loci have been identified that have not been cloned. The first was *HPC1* in the 1q24-25 chromosomal region. A significant linkage result was seen in a collection of 96 prostate cancer families, and 34% of families were estimated to be linked. Later a combined dataset of 772 families estimated that prostate cancer was linked to *HPC1* in 6% of the families studied. Evidence for additional susceptibility loci has been observed in other datasets: *PCaP* at chromosome 1q42.2-43, particularly among younger-onset families; *HPCX* at chromosome Xq27-28; *CAPB* at chromosome 1p36 among prostate cancer families with a history of brain cancer; *HPC20* at chromosome 20q13 and *PG1* at 8p22-23. Confirmation studies at *HPC1*, *PCaP*, *HPCX*, *CAPB*, and *HPC20* have produced disparate results (discussed later); a smaller proportion of families than estimated

by original linkage findings are expected to be linked to each of these loci.

In addition, genomic scans in prostate cancer families have identified "regions of interests" that have not satisfied significance thresholds, but may nonetheless contain susceptibility loci. These regions include chromosomes 2q, 4q, 8p, 8q, 10q, 12p, 12q, 14q, 15q, 16p, 16q, and 21q. Regions detected by multiple groups are of particular interest.

IV. DIFFICULTIES IN THE SEARCH FOR MAJOR SUSCEPTIBILITY GENES

As described earlier, there is a wealth of evidence for genetic predisposition to prostate cancer. Numerous research groups are currently conducting linkage analyses for prostate cancer; although evidence has been seen for several loci, confirmation of each has been difficult, and only one putative major susceptibility gene (*HPC2/ELAC2*) has been cloned. Reasons for the difficulties encountered involve heterogeneity within and among families.

Even within a family that passes down a susceptibility gene, nongenetic cases of prostate cancer among older men (phenocopies) are likely to occur by chance because prostate cancer is a common disease. This problem is particularly difficult because the increased use of screening for prostate cancer by PSA testing has increased the incidence of disease. In the search for the susceptibility gene, the nongenetic case would give evidence against linkage (not sharing allele with affected relatives). Additionally, because prostate cancer is an age-dependant disease and the susceptibility genes are not expected to be fully penetrant, men may carry a mutation but not be affected (nonpenetrance). The presence of genetic and nongenetic cases and affected and unaffected carriers leads to misclassification and decrease of power to detect linkage.

It is clear that locus heterogeneity exists among families with prostate cancer, i.e., that different susceptibility genes may be responsible for disease in different families. In the search for the susceptibility genes, grouping families linked to different genes decreases the power to detect linkage to any particular gene. If some other characteristic can indicate linkage to a certain gene, then families with this characteristic may be examined separately. Characteristics such as mean age at onset, presence of other cancers, and disease severity have been used to define family subgroups and may have been useful in identifying linked subsets. For instance, *HPC1* may be most important among families with more advanced prostate cancer, and *CAPB* may be particularly important among prostate cancer families with brain cancer. The strategy of grouping families, however, does create smaller sets of families, which decreases power.

Difficulties in the confirmation of loci may also occur because the picture of inherited prostate cancer susceptibility is complex. The number of major loci may be larger than expected from the breast cancer linkage experience: *BRCA1* and *BRCA2* together account for >80% of inherited breast cancers, whereas the six putative prostate cancer loci are expected to account for not more than 30% of inherited prostate cancers. Additionally, although CSAs predicted autosomal-dominant inheritance, an X-linked locus has been identified, and recessive models have been useful in finding regions of interest from genomic scans. It is also possible that multiple risk-conferring alleles act within a family or that gene–environment interactions are involved in a cascade of pathways leading to inherited prostate cancer.

Several strategies may assist in the identification and confirmation of prostate cancer loci. As was done for *HPC1*, analyses using data combined from many research groups would have increased power and allowed for subgroup analysis. Additionally, the use of novel regression-based methods to incorporate clinical characteristics without having to stratify may be a powerful approach. Approaches to deal with the inheritance of multiple loci, such as Markov Chain Monte Carlo methods, may be useful, as well as approaches that combine linkage and association methods.

V. SUMMARY AND FUTURE CONSIDERATIONS

From evidence gathered to date, prostate cancer appears to cluster in families, and genetic factors are likely to be involved. We now need to clarify our understanding of the suspected genetic factors and learn how they work with each other and with other factors in predisposing to prostate cancer. Because of the complexity of prostate cancer genetics, research will be greatly enhanced by the continued collaboration of scientists from multiple disciplines. As we have learned from research on other cancers, an interdisciplinary approach will be increasingly important.

Continued work in molecular biology and histochemistry will help us understand possible pathways involved in prostate carcinogenesis. In addition, molecular genetic analysis may facilitate the development of chemoprevention strategies. Molecular epidemiology will continue to play a role in understanding how candidate genes and pathways, such as androgen metabolism and cell growth, affect the risk of prostate cancer in the population. In addition, potential interactions of genes with diet and environmental exposures can be identified. The fields of statistical genetics and genetic epidemiology will develop and apply methods to facilitate the identification of major susceptibility genes for prostate cancer.

After major susceptibility genes are cloned, their importance to familial prostate cancer must be assessed by mutation detection. Additional molecular work will be needed to understand how these genes affect prostate cancer. Epidemiologic studies can also assess the importance of these genes for men with and without prostate cancer family history, particularly if genetic testing is a consideration. Presymptomatic genetic testing will be of limited use until methods to delay or prevent onset of disease exist. With the goals of eventual treatment and prevention, understanding how highly penetrant susceptibility genes work and how they may interact with less penetrant genetic and environmental factors will help clarify the complex picture of genetic predisposition to prostate cancer.

See Also the Following Articles

Bibliography

Cannon, L., Bishop, D. T., Skolnick, M., Hunt, S., Lyon, J. L., and Smart, C. R. (1982). Genetic epidemiology of prostate cancer in the Utah Mormon genealogy. *In* "Inheritance of Susceptibility to Cancer in Man" (W. F. Bodmer, ed.), pp. 47–69. Oxford Univ. Press, New York.

Carter, B. S., Beaty, T. H., Steinberg, G. D., Childs, B., and Walsh, P. C. (1992). Mendelian inheritance of familial prostate cancer. *Proc. Natl. Acad. Sci. USA* **89**, 3367–3371.

Cui, J., Staples, M. P., Hopper, J. L., English, D. R., Mc-Credie, M. R., and Giles, G. G. (2001). Segregation analyses of 1,476 population-based Australian families affected by prostate cancer. *Am. J. Hum. Genet.* **68**, 1207–1218.

Elo, J. P., and Visakorpi, T. (2001). Molecular genetics of prostate cancer. *Ann. Med.* **33**, 130–141.

Gibbs, M., Stanford, J. L., McIndoe, R. A., Jarvik, G. P., Kolb, S., Goode, E. L., Chakrabarti, L., Schuster, E. F., Buckley, V. A., Miller, E. L., Brandzel, S., Li, S., Hood, L., and Ostrander, E. A. (1999). Evidence for a rare prostate cancer-susceptibility locus at chromosome 1p36. *Am. J. Hum. Genet.* **64**, 776–787.

Giovannucci, E., Stampfer, M. J., Krithivas, K., Brown, M., Brufsky, A., Talcott, J., Hennekens, C. H., and Kantoff, P. W. (1997). The CAG repeat within the androgen receptor gene and its relationship to prostate cancer. *Proc. Natl. Acad. Sci. USA* **94**, 3320–3323.

Goddard, K. A., Witte, J. S., Suarez, B. K., Catalona, W. J., and Olson, J. M. (2001). Model-free linkage analysis with covariates confirms linkage of prostate cancer to chromosomes 1 and 4. *Am. J. Hum. Genet.* **68**, 1197–1206.

Goldgar, D., Easton, D. F., Cannon Albright, L. A., and Skolnick, M. H. (1994). Systematic population-based assessment of cancer risk in first-degree relatives of cancer probands. *J. Natl. Cancer Inst.* **86**, 1600–1608.

Goode, E. L., Stanford, J. L., Chakrabarti, L., Gibbs, M., Kolb, S., McIndoe, R. A., Buckley, V. A., Schuster, E. F., Neal, C. L., Miller, E. L., Brandzel, S., Hood, L., Ostrander, E. A., and Jarvik, G. P. (2001). Clinical characteristics of prostate cancer in an analysis of linkage to four putative susceptibility loci. *Clin. Cancer Res.* **7**, 2739–2749.

Habuchi, T., Suzuki, T., Sasaki, R., Wang, L., Sato, K., Satoh, S., Akao, T., Tsuchiya, N., Shimoda, N., Wada, Y., Koizumi, A., Chihara, J., Ogawa, O., and Kato, T. (2000). Association of vitamin D receptor gene polymorphism with prostate cancer and benign prostatic hyperplasia in a Japanese population. *Cancer Res.* **60**, 305–308.

Haenszel, W., and Kurihara, M. (1968). Studies of Japanese migrants. I. Mortality from cancer and other diseases among Japanese in the United States. *J. Natl. Cancer Inst.* **40**, 43–68.

Ingles, S. A., Coetzze, G. A., Ross, R. K., Henderson, B. E., Kolonel, L. N., Crocitto, L., Wang, W., and Haile, R. W. (1998). Association of prostate cancer with vitamin D receptor haplotypes in African-Americans. *Cancer Res.* **58**, 1620–1623.

Irvine, R. A., Yu, M. C., Ross, R. K., and Coetzee, G. A. (1995). The CAG and GGC microsatellites of the androgen receptor gene are in linkage disequilibrium in men with prostate cancer. *Cancer Res.* **55**, 1937–1940.

Jarvik, G. P. (1998). Complex segregation analysis: Uses and limitations. *Am. J. Hum. Genet.* **63**, 942–946.

Jemal, A., Thomas, A., Murray, T., and Thun M. (2002). Cancer statistics, 2002. *Ca-A Cancer J. Clin.* **52**, 23–47.

King, M. C., Lee, G. M., Spinner, N. B., Thomson, G., and Wrensch, M. R. (1984). Genetic epidemiology. *Annu. Rev. Public Health* **5**, 1–52.

Monroe, K. R., Yu, M. C., Kolonel, L. N., Coetzee, G. A., Wilkens, L. R., Ross, R. K., and Henderson, B. E. (1995). Evidence of an X-linked or recessive genetic component to prostate cancer risk. *Nature Med.* **1**, 827–829.

Nam, R. K., Toi, A., Vesprini, D., Ho, M., Chu, W., Harvie, S., Sweet, J., Trachtenberg, J., Jewett, M. A., and Narod, S. A. (2001). V89L polymorphism of type-2, 5-alpha reductase enzyme gene predicts prostate cancer presence and progression. *Urology* **57**, 199–204.

Ostrander, E. A., and Stanford, J. L. (2000). Genetics of prostate cancer: Too many loci, too few genes. *Am. J. Hum. Genet.* **67**, 1367–1375.

Page, W. F., Braun, M. M., Partin, A. W., Caporaso, N., and Walsh, P. (1997). Heredity and prostate cancer: A study of World War II veteran twins. *Prostate* **33**, 240–245.

Parkin, D. M., Muir, C. S., Whelan, S. L., Gao, Y. T., Ferlay, J., and Powell, J. (1992). Cancer Incidence in Five Continents. World Health Organization, International Agency for Research on Cancer, Lyon, France.

Potter, J. D. (2001). At the interfaces of epidemiology, genetics and genomics. *Nature Rev. Genet.* **2**, 142–147.

Ross, R. K. (2001). The role of molecular genetics in chemoprevention studies of prostate cancer. *IARC Sci. Publ.* **154**, 207–213.

Schaid, D. J., McDonnell, S. K., Thibodeau, S. N. (2001). Regression models for linkage heterogeneity applied to familial prostate cancer. *Am. J. Hum. Genet.* **68**, 1189–1196.

Steinberg, G. D., Carter, B. S., Beaty, T. H., Childs, B., Walsh, P. C. (1990). Family history and the risk of prostate cancer. *Prostate* **17**, 337–347.

Tavtigian, S. V., Simard, J., Teng, D. H., Abtin, V., Baumgard, M., Beck, A., Camp, N. J., *et al.* (2001). A candidate prostate cancer susceptibility gene at chromosome 17p. *Nature Genet.* **27**, 172–180.

Visakorpi, T., Kallioniemi, A. H., Syvänen, A.-C., Hyytinen, E. R., Karhu, R., Tammela, T., Isola, J. J., and Kallioniemi, O.-P. (1995). Genetic changes in primary and recurrent prostate cancer by comparative genomic hybridization. *Cancer Res.* **55**, 342–347.

Whittemore, A. S., Wu, A. H., Kolonel, L. N., John, E. M., Gallagher, R. P., Howe, G. R., West, D. W., Teh, C. Z., and Stamey, T. (1995). Family history and prostate cancer risk in black, white, and Asian men in the United States and Canada. *Am. J. Epidemiol.* **141**, 732–740.

Xu, J., and the International Consortium for Prostate Cancer Genetics (2000). Combined analysis of hereditary prostate cancer linkage to 1q24-25: Results from 772 families from the International Consortium for Prostate Cancer Genetics [see errata: *Am. J. Hum. Genet.* **67**, 541–542 (2000)]. *Am. J. Hum. Genet.* **66**, 945–957.

Xu, J., Zheng, S. L., Carpten, J. D., Nupponen, N. N., Robbins, C. M., Mestre, J., Moses, T. Y., Faith, D. A., Kelly, B. D., Isaacs, S. D., Wiley, K. E., Ewing, C. M., Bujnovszky, P., Chang, B., Bailey-Wilson, J., Bleecker, E. R., Walsh, P. C., Trent, J. M., Meyers, D. A., and Isaacs, W. B. (2001). Evaluation of linkage and association of HPC2/ELAC2 in patients with familial or sporadic prostate cancer. *Am. J. Hum. Genet.* **68,** 901–911.

Xue, W., Irvine, R. A., Yu, M. C., Ross, R. K., Coetzee, G. A., and Ingles, S. A. (2000). Susceptibility to prostate cancer: Interaction between genotypes at the androgen receptor and prostate-specific antigen loci. *Cancer Res.* **60,** 839–841.

Germ Cell Tumors

Jane Houldsworth
George J. Bosl
Alessia Donadio
R. S. K. Chaganti
Memorial Sloan-Kettering Cancer Center

GLOSSARY

American Joint Committee on Cancer Group responsible for determining consistent staging conventions for cancer.

differentiation Process by which an uncommitted cell develops fidelity to a particular lineage.

germ cells Cells within the seminiferous tubule destined to give rise to sperm, these include primordial germ cells, spermatocytes, and spermatids.

kit receptor Tyrosine kinase receptor, deletion of which results in testes devoid of germ cells.

meiosis Cell division of a diploid germ cell leading to the formation of haploid gametes.

pachytene Substage in meiosis after chromosome replication when homologous chromosome pairs are synapsed and genetic material is exchanged between nonsister chromatids.

Germ cell tumors (GCTs) are malignancies that arise in germ cells and retain a variable capacity to differentiate into both somatic and extraembryonic tissues. They are more common in men than in women, arise in the gonads about 10 times more frequently than at extragonadal sites, and sometimes secrete α-fetoprotein (AFP) and human chorionic gonadotropin (HCG). These two proteins represent the normal products of the embryonic yolk sac and chorion, respectively, and represent biochemical evidence for differentiation.

I. CLINICAL INTRODUCTION

Germ cell tumors are highly curable. More than 90% of patients with newly diagnosed GCTs of the testis will be cured; moreover, even after the development of regional nodal and systemic visceral metastases, multiple drug therapy, which includes cisplatin, will cure 70 to 80% of patients. Radioimmunoassays for AFP and HCG, which can detect nanogram quantities of protein, are essential to patient management. In addition, the serum level of lactate dehydrogenase (LDH) has also been shown to predict outcome. Tumor marker production (AFP, HCG, LDH) has been shown to be a predictor of outcome independent of extent of disease, histology, and primary site of disease. Because of this independent prognostic significance, the TNM staging classification of the American Joint Committee on Cancer (AJCC) was modified in 1997 to include an "S" category for serum concentrations of AFP, HCG, and LDH.

Because such a large proportion of patients with GCT will be cured with cisplatin-based chemotherapy, it has become increasingly important to stratify patients in terms of likelihood of cure. The International Germ Cell Cancer Collaborative Group developed an accepted risk classification system in which patients are assigned to good-risk, intermediate-risk, and poor-risk categories based on histology, pretreatment tumor marker levels, site of primary tumor, and site of visceral metastases.

II. PATHOLOGY OF GERM CELL TUMORS

The unique feature of GCTs lies in the differentiated and undifferentiated cell types that are identifiable on microscopic analysis. The morphological patterns mimic normal developmental differentiation patterns. Some cases demonstrate undifferentiated germ cell-like and zygote-like components (seminoma and embryonal carcinoma, respectively), some show highly developed somatic differentiation (mature teratoma), others show malignant extraembryonic differentiation (yolk sac tumor and choriocarcinoma), a few cases develop embryoid bodies, and still others show an admixture of multiple cell types. This complex differentiation occurs both *in vivo* and *in vitro*.

In clinical terms, GCTs are divided into two major subgroups: seminomatous and nonseminomatous. Seminomas retain the morphology of early spermatogonial germ cells and are exquisitely sensitive to both radiation therapy and chemotherapy. Pure seminoma

accounts for 40 to 50% of all GCTs. Nonseminomatous GCTs (NSGCTs) include all other histologies and usually appear as mixed tumors containing both undifferentiated and differentiated cell types, are relatively radioresistant (in contradistinction to seminoma), and are sensitive to chemotherapy (although probably slightly less so than seminomas). Mature teratoma constitutes the most apparent form of differentiation *in vivo*. Mature cell types, such as cartilage, neural tissue, and mucinous and nonmucinous glands, are present in an unorganized fashion. Occasionally, the mature cell types in teratomatous lesions undergo further malignant differentiation into neoplastic elements that display histological features characteristic of *de novo* tumors affecting multiple tissue types (e.g., sarcoma, carcinoma, and leukemia). The clinical phenotypes of transformed germ cells imply that GCTs are a model of deregulated differentiation and that lessons regarding the genetic control of normal differentiation can be derived from observations of altered gene expression in GCT.

In the testis, GCTs of all types are frequently, if not always, associated with intratubular germ cell neoplasia (ITGCN), the *in situ* form of GCT. ITGCN progresses to invasive GCT in nearly all cases. However, both seminomas and NSGCTs arise from cytologically identical ITGCN, implying that the genetic events responsible for germ cell transformation are different from those leading to differentiation. Because tumors limited to the primary site can contain either one histological type or admixtures of multiple cell types, the genetic events that result in differentiation are probably distinct from those that lead to invasion and metastasis. The expression of surrogate markers of differentiation including AFP and HCG secretion, cytoplasmic intermediate filaments expressed universally as cytokeratins in NSGCTs, and kit receptors make GCTs excellent models in which the genetic events that regulate transformation, differentiation, invasion, metastasis, and treatment response in normal and malignant germ cells can be studied.

III. GERM CELL TRANSFORMATION

For a GCT to develop, transformation must occur in a germ cell that normally undergoes a complex series of proliferation and differentiation programs leading ultimately to gametogenesis. The phase in the life span of a germ cell at which this occurs is unclear. In the gastrulating embryo, primordial germ cells are first recognized in the epiblast, whereupon they migrate and proliferate, finally reaching the genital ridges where the primitive gonad forms. In the human, this occurs around the seventh or eighth week of fetal life. In the male embryo, the so-called gonocytes undergo mitotic arrest until the second and third trimesters of pregnancy wherein they will differentiate into spermatogonia. After birth, proliferation of the germ cells resumes, leading to the successive development of type A, intermediate, and type B spermatogonia, retaining a population of spermatogonia with the capacity of self-renewal. It is committed type B spermatogonia that, at puberty, undergo premeiotic DNA replication and enter meiosis. Following a protracted prophase (leptotene, zygotene, pachytene, diplotene, and diakinesis), mitoses I and II occur, leading to the formation of four haploid gametes. Subsequent to spermiogenesis, the fully differentiated germ cells are recognized as spermatozoa. In the human male, the committed differentiation program of the type B spermatogonia, through the appearance of mature spermatozoa, takes approximately 60 days. Thus, in the life span of a germ cell from fetus through to the adult, there are many stages requiring strict temporal regulation, disruption of which could result in transformation.

Identification of the underlying genetic mechanisms whereby a germ cell is transformed has been aided by cytogenetic and molecular genetic studies performed on tumor specimens and derived cell lines. Initial cytogenetic studies revealed the hypertriploid chromosomal complement of these tumors, along with a number of recurrent chromosomal abnormalities. These studies revealed that virtually all GCTs exhibit multiple copies of the short arm of chromosome 12, evidenced in about 85% of cases as an isochromosome [i(12p)], and in the remaining as tandem duplications embedded in marker chromosomes. This chromosomal marker is easily identified by fluorescence *in situ* hybridization (FISH) of interphase tumor cells using a microdissected 12p painting probe, and its presence is considered diagnostic of GCTs. Because this chromosomal marker has been observed in ITGCN, the presumed precursor for all invasive GCTs, it has been suggested that this genetic lesion is among those associated with germ cell transformation per se rather than progression. Note, however, that a recent report has indicated a contrary role. Using the molecular cytogenetic technique of comparative genomic hybridization (CGH), a few GCT cases have been identified to not only exhibit extra copies of 12p, but also to show an additional amplification of DNA sequences derived from 12p11.2-12. This subregional amplification has been predominantly observed in seminomas and is thought to be involved with tumor progression.

Several studies have been initiated in order to identify the gene(s) mapped to 12p, whose presence in higher copy number and presumed increased expression play a role in the genesis of these tumors. Expression analysis of candidate genes has identified *CCND2*, mapped to 12p13, to be one such candidate. Cyclin D2 is a member of the D-type family of cyclins involved with the regulation of cell progression through the G1 phase of the mitotic cell cycle. In GCTs, cyclin D2 was aberrantly expressed in all 10 ITGCN studied, compared with normal testes where occasional spermatogonial cells exhibited detectable levels of expression. For the other histologies, patterns of cyclin D2 expression were related to the extent and type of differentiated elements present within a tumor and were similar to those reported for the comparable normal cellular counterpart. Other studies in tumors and cell lines have confirmed these findings. These results indicate perhaps that aberrant cyclin D2 expression is a necessary event early rather than later in germ cell transformation. Supportive evidence for the role of cyclin D2 in germ cell biology has come from murine knockout studies where male mice lacking cyclin D2 expression exhibit smaller, although fertile, testes. In the normal murine postnatal gonad, cyclin D2 is abundantly expressed, peaking at about 8 days after birth in spermatogonial cells undergoing mitotic division. Subsequent downregulation of cyclin D2 expression was associated with the onset of puberty and, thus, meiosis in the murine testis. Furthermore, inappropriate expression of cyclin D2 has been reported to lead to hyperplasia in mice. Thus, while evidence exists for the role of cyclin D2 in germ cell transformation, more direct evidence will come from murine transgenic studies where aberrant cyclin D2 expression can be driven by germ cell-specific promoters at various times during the life span of the germ cell.

Other studies aimed at identifying relevant genes on 12p have utilized GCTs displaying subregional amplification of 12p11.2-12 as described earlier. FISH analysis of GCT chromosome metaphase spreads of such cases has permitted a physical estimation of the commonly amplified region (750–3000 kbp). To date, genes mapped to this region and assayed for expression have not revealed good candidates. With the completion of the human genome sequence, identification of other expressed sequence tags (ESTs) within this common region will provide additional candidates for expression analysis. Recently developed high-throughput genomic and expression screening techniques are highly applicable to such studies. In this case, all ESTs and genes mapped to 12p could be spotted on a single array, which would serve for both analysis of genomic copy number within a tumor by microarray CGH and expression levels within a tumor by microarray expression analysis. Such studies should lead to the identification of cDNAs/ESTs that are present in GCTs in higher copy number and are aberrantly expressed.

Historically, ITGCN has been thought to represent the transformed counterpart of a primordial germ cell/gonocyte, based on common histological and ultrastructural features and immunohistochemical markers. It has been postulated that fetal gonocytes, which have escaped normal development into spermatogonia, may undergo abnormal cell division. Furthermore, aberrant cell cycling is thought to be affected by the kit receptor/SCF paracrine loop. Normally, kit receptor is expressed during the first trimester of pregnancy and postnatally in association with meiosis, and SCF is expressed by Sertoli cells. Thus, developmentally derailed gonocytes may aberrantly continue to express kit receptor, resulting in continued mitogenic stimulation, ultimately leading to ITGCN. Postnatal, pubertal, and postpubertal endocrinological factors are thought then to have a role in the stimulation of invasive growth of precursor ITGCN lesions. This model also has the supportive evidence of the greater incidence of GCTs in males with developmental disorders having abnormal germ cells, and the epidemiology of GCT incidence.

However, this model does not invoke a role for extra copies of 12p and presumably represents a downstream genetic lesion, despite its documented presence in virtually 100% of all adult GCTs. This striking genetic feature has been incorporated in another model, where GCTs are postulated to arise by rescue of germ cells with replicated chromosomes, in which an aberrant recombinational event has occurred during the pachytene phase of meiosis. Normally, such cells are destined to die by apoptosis, possibly affected by the relatively high levels of p53 detected at this phase of meiosis. However, if the recombinational event leads to increased copies of 12p after division and subsequent increased expression of cyclin D2, then a germ cell may aberrantly reenter a mitotic cell cycle, resulting in uncontrolled cell proliferation. This model is based primarily on genetic data, namely increased copy number of 12p, aberrant expression of cyclin D2 in ITGCN, hypertriploid chromosomal complement, and abundant expression of wild-type p53 observed in these tumors.

Both models need to be tested in a transgenic murine system, utilizing stage-specific promoters to direct expression of the implicated genes (kit receptor in the first model and cyclin D2 in the second) at the relevant phase in the germ cell life span.

In both models, the first step in germ cell transformation is the aberrant initiation of cell cycling leading to a bypass of the normal checkpoint associated with the respective differentiation programs. Such abnormal cycling would predispose genomic instability, resulting in the acquisition of additional genetic lesions culminating in neoplastic transformation. Initially, karyotypic analysis of these tumors identified a number of recurrent chromosomal abnormalities, some of which are associated with histological subtypes. In particular, breakpoints involving 1p32-36 and 7q11.2 were significantly associated with a teratomatous histology, and 1p22 with yolk sac tumors. Deletion/rearrangement at 12q, 1p32-36, and 7q and deletion at 6q13-25 comprise the most frequently observed nonrandom chromosomal aberrations.

Such studies, along with a comprehensive loss of heterozygosity (LOH) analysis by molecular genetic techniques, have revealed a number of sites with a high frequency of LOH in GCTs. These included sites of known tumor suppressor genes (TSGs) (*RB1*, *DCC*, and *NME*), of previously known chromosomal regions (1p, 3p, 5q, 9p, 10q, 11p, 11q, and 17p), and of several novel sites (1q, 2q, 3q, 5p, 9q, 12q, 18p, and

20p). Chromosome 12 harbors two sites, 12q13 and 12q22, for which the identity of the putative tumor suppressor genes is the subject of further studies. In the case of 12q22, the minimally deleted region in 12q22 has now been narrowed to 830 kbp, which is covered by a high-resolution BAC/PAC contig. Candidate genes and EST sequences identified within this region by sequencing efforts can now be tested for involvement.

Few GCTs have been reported to exhibit cytologic evidence for gene amplification in the form of double minute chromosomes and/or homogeneously staining regions, and application of CGH to GCTs has led to the identification of chromosomal regions that undergo frequent loss or gain (other than 12p). Limited studies have revealed the presence of mutations within genes that may contribute to the transformed phenotype. These include *KRAS2*, *KIT*, and *SMAD4*. Overall, these cytogenetic and molecular studies have identified lesions in chromosomal regions in common with other solid tumors, as well as unique to GCTs, and have directed further studies aimed at identifying the relevant genes and their roles in germ cell transformation.

While considering the genetic etiology of GCTs, it must be noted that a small percentage of these tumors are familial, being mostly restricted to sibpair and (more rarely) father/son family types. A recent genome-wide linkage search indicated the presence of a GCT susceptibility gene to Xq27. The identity of the relevant gene is as yet unknown, as well as its role in the etiology of sporadic GCTs.

GCTs presenting at extragonadal sites are thought to arise by the transformation of germ cells misplaced during migration early in embryogenesis. Such germ cells are presumably subject to local hormonal and growth factor influences, and thus further normal development of the germ cell is disrupted, predisposing the germ cell to transformation. However, it has been reported that in a high percentage of primary retroperitoneal GCTs, testis biopsy has revealed the presence of ITGCN. In these cases, it is likely that the retroperitoneal lesion represents a metastatic rather than a primary lesion. This is supported by the fact that metastasis to retroperitoneal lymph nodes is a common site for metastasis from a primary testicular lesion. Importantly, cytogenetic analysis of a panel of primary extragonadal GCTs has indicated comparable frequency, type, and sites of chromosomal aberrations as those observed in primary testicular GCTs. In addition, murine studies have indicated that such misplaced germ cells in embryos are eliminated by apoptosis. Nonetheless, primary mediastinal GCTs do not display ITGCN, and their origin remains controversial.

IV. EMBRYONAL-LIKE DIFFERENTIATION

Germ cell tumors exhibit an array of histologies that resemble different temporal phases of human development. Seminomas can be viewed as mitotically dividing transformed germ cells that, like normal germ cells prior to fertilization, are under inhibitory control for zygotic-like differentiation. Nonseminomas, then, have been released from this control, displaying histologies of early zygotic (embryonal carcinoma), extraembryonic (yolk sac tumor, choriocarcinoma), and embryonic (teratoma) patterns of differentiation. This implies that a transformed male germ cell has the unique potential to undergo developmental programs without a maternal contribution that would normally occur during fertilization. These tumors and derived cell lines comprise a model system in which the molecular mechanisms regulating cell proliferation/differentiation and cell fate/lineage decisions can be studied. In the case of tumors, LOH studies have indicated that a higher overall loss of genetic material is associated with highly differentiated teratomas, compared with less differentiated embryonal carcinomas. The genes at such chromosomal sites whose function is altered by loss/mutation may well act as effector genes in regulating developmentally important events. Notable among the genes deleted in teratomas were *NME1* and *NME2*, for which there is evidence of transcription factor function to negatively regulate differentiation. Further studies determined that the levels of Nm23 proteins were four- to fivefold lower in teratomas than in embryonal carcinomas. The functional consequence of this observation needs to be investigated further.

Derived human embryonal carcinoma cell lines can be maintained *in vitro* in an undifferentiated state and induced to undergo differentiation upon addition of a morphogen. Some embryonal carcinoma cell lines display the ability to differentiate along somatic and extraembryonic endodermal lineage, placing them as equivalents of cells derived from the inner cell mass in the developing embryo. One such cell line, NTera2/Clone D1 (NT2/D1), has been well studied due to its ability to differentiate along a neuronal lineage in response to all-*trans* retinoic acid, aiding in the study of neurodegenerative diseases. However, the same cell line, upon addition of other known mammalian morphogens, bone morphogenetic protein (BMP)-2, -4, and -7, is stimulated to undergo distinctly nonneuronal pathways of differentiation, whose precise lineage remains to be identified. Such cell lines can now be utilized to define the molecular mechanisms that govern the fate of these embryonic stem cell-like cells. Other GCT-derived cell lines exhibit the additional ability to differentiate into trophoblastic cells, placing them at an earlier stage in embryogenesis to trophectodermal fate decision. Embryonal (teratoma) versus extraembryonal (yolk sac tumor, choriocarcinoma) commitment mechanisms can be identified in such cell lines. In contrast, other embryonal carcinoma cell lines have little or no differentiation potential and provide an ideal system in which master regulators of differentiation induction and cell/fate decision can be identified.

The ability of some GCTs to undergo an embryonal-like developmental program without a maternal contribution has implications in genomic imprinting wherein parental imprints are erased prior to meiosis, and new patterns are laid down during gametogenesis and embryogenesis. Examination of the expression of two genes (*H19, IGF2*) that normally exhibit monoallelic expression in postfertilization somatic cells has revealed a biallelic expression pattern in GCTs. These results are consistent with a pachytene spermatocyte (imprint erased) as the cell of origin for these tumors.

V. GENETIC PATHWAYS OF RESISTANCE

Male GCTs serve as an excellent model for a curable malignancy. While over 90% of patients are cured with cisplatin-based chemotherapy, a small cohort remains that ultimately succumbs to the disease. Much effort has been spent defining the clinicopathologic features associated with a poor response. These include GCTs with hepatic, osseous, and/or brain metastases and mediastinal nonseminomatous GCTs. Patients with high serum levels of LDH, AFP, or HCG are also likely to have a poor response. Pathological examination of residual masses resected after chemotherapy often reveal the presence of teratoma, reflecting the relative resistance of this histology to therapy. In addition, GCTs displaying malignant transformation often have a poor response to cisplatin-based chemotherapy and may respond better to a therapy program tailored for the specific malignant histology.

In recent years, a few genetic lesions have been associated with clinical resistance to cisplatin-based chemotherapy. On the whole, GCTs display higher than normal levels of wild-type p53, as evidenced in immunohistochemical analysis of tumor specimens, with somewhat lower levels in more differentiated teratoma elements. Therefore, the observation of *TP53* mutations in a subset of resistant GCTs is noteworthy. While mutation of this gene is frequent in other solid tumors, it is rarely found in GCTs. Thus, functional inactivation of p53 by mutation most likely represents one genetic pathway underlying clinical resistance to cisplatin-based chemotherapeutic regimens. This was substantiated by *in vitro* studies in which a GCT-derived cell line with mutant *TP53* displayed a resistance to cisplatin treatment compared with a GCT cell line with wild-type *TP53*.

Gene amplification is another genetic mechanism whereby resistance to therapy could be achieved. A few studies have noted a gain/loss of genetic material in specimens with clinical resistance at specific loci (gain of 6q21-q24, loss of 6q15-q21), whereas one study found an association of high-level amplification of DNA sequences with a poor response to cisplatin-based chemotherapy. Amplification in 5 out of 17 resistant tumors was detected at eight chromosomal regions (other than 12p) and in none of 17 tumors resected from cured patients. Few candidate genes exist for the amplified regions, and the identity of the functionally relevant gene remains unknown. With the advent of microarray genome and expression scanning technologies, it is now possible to not only identify the amplified sequences mapped to the respective regions, but also to determine the relative expression levels. Amplified and overexpressed sequences thus identified would represent genes that might play important roles in the poor response of GCTs to therapy, as well as possibly in other tumor types.

Because GCTs are unique in their extreme sensitivity to platinum-based chemotherapeutic regimens, they represent an ideal model system in which the molecular mechanisms involved in such a response can be studied. Such studies have been performed primarily in GCT-derived cell lines and have investigated various aspects of a cell's response to DNA-damaging agents such as cisplatin. An enzyme that removes apurinic/apyrimidinic nucleotides (Ape1/ref-1) involved in the base excision repair pathway has also been shown to modulate the cellular response to chemotherapeutic agents of a GCT cell line. In this context, a poor response to chemotherapeutic agents in GCTs may derive from an increased ability to remove lesions in DNA induced by the agent. A few reports have now indicated a relatively poor ability of GCTs to remove DNA–platinum adducts. It has been suggested that this inability is rooted in reduced levels of XPA activity, a protein involved in DNA damage recognition and facilitation of the nucleotide excision repair complex. More research is needed in this area.

Generally, after exposure to genotoxic stress, cells respond either by induction of a cell cycle delay, presumably allowing DNA repair, or by cell death via an apoptotic mechanism. Clearly, the latter is invoked in GCTs, as evidenced in a number of *in vitro* studies and the *in vivo* response of most GCTs, and is thought to be primarily a p53-dependent phenomenon. Indeed, GCT cell lines exhibit a prompt induction of expression of known p53 responsive genes following exposure to a chemotherapeutic agent. The precise molecular link between this response and the induction of apoptosis is not clearly defined, and, again, application of microarray-based expression profiling analysis of cells after treatment may help identify the relevant genes. Few studies have focused on analysis of the proteins known to alter the apoptotic response of a cell to stress. These comprise the bcl2 family of proteins, and it has been found that on the whole, GCTs express low levels of antiapoptotic members of this family. One study has implicated the apoptosis antagonist bcl-X$_L$ as the regulator of apoptotic response in

GCTs rather than bcl2. Such studies are gradually elucidating the underlying molecular features that are responsible for the clinically favorable response of this tumor type to chemotherapeutic agents, with possible application to other tumor systems.

VI. CLINICAL IMPLICATIONS OF GERM CELL TUMOR BIOLOGY

A. Midline Tumors of Uncertain Histogenesis

Midline tumors of uncertain histogenesis are characterized by the presence of a midline tumor or bilateral pulmonary nodules, an undifferentiated morphology, which precluded identification of the tissue of origin, and a low but definable cure rate (approximately 15%) to cisplatin-based chemotherapy. It was suggested that the responsive subset was a group of "unrecognized" GCTs.

The presence of multiple copies of the short arm of chromosome 12 [predominantly as i(12p)] is generally considered to be diagnostic for GCTs and therefore represents a useful tool in the potential identification of such tumors. To this end, 28 tumors of uncertain histogenesis were studied using conventional and molecular cytogenetic methods to identify i(12p). Eight of the 28 tumors (28%) were found to have either i(12p) by karyotype analysis or increased 12p copy number by Southern analysis or FISH. Twenty-four patients were treated with cisplatin-based chemotherapy. Six of 7 patients (83%) whose tumor had a GCT genetic marker and only 2 of 17 patients (11%) whose tumor was without a GCT marker achieved a major response. Three of the 7 GCT patients and 3 of 24 patients (13%) overall achieved a durable, complete disappearance of disease. Thus, undifferentiated tumors with a GCT genetic marker behave clinically like GCTs in their response to therapy.

B. Malignant Transformation

In a small proportion of mature teratomas of gonadal and extragonadal origin, malignancies composed of non-germ cell histologies are found on microscopic analysis. Sarcomas predominate, but carcinomas and primitive neural tumors have also been described. In addition, acute myeloid leukemia may arise in patients with mediastinal NSGCTs (predominantly yolk sac tumors). The origin of these secondary malignancies had been postulated to be due to malignant transformation within the GCT, but the possibility of a simultaneous or metachronous development of a second unrelated malignancy could not be excluded with certainty. Using conventional cytogenetics, i(12p) has been identified in acute nonlymphocytic leukemia arising in a patient with an i(12p)-positive mediastinal NSGCT, in embryonal rhabdomyosarcoma arising in a second i(12p)-positive mediastinal NSGCT, and in a primitive neuroectodermal tumor (PNET), which arose from a testicular GCT. These findings provide conclusive evidence for the GCT clonal origin of these differentiated malignancies. Equally interesting was the cytogenetic identification of additional lesions in these tumors, which were characteristic of the differentiated malignant phenotype. The leukemia had a deletion on 5q, which is frequently seen in poor-prognosis leukemia, the rhabdomyosarcoma had a rearrangement at 2q37, a site rearranged in *de novo* rhabdomyosarcoma, and the PNET had a rearrangement at 11q24, a site rearranged in *de novo* PNET. Thus, the study of GCTs may lead not only to a better understanding of normal germ cell development and germ cell malignant transformation, but also may provide insight into the development of other tumors and provide an opportunity to identify genes involved in the development of other differentiated tumors.

C. Kit Receptor Expression in GCT

Expression of the kit receptor is predominantly associated with seminoma, consistent with its undifferentiated germ cell-like phenotype (Table I). Despite a high cure rate for testicular seminoma, a small proportion of these patients go on to a poor clinical outcome. Attempts have been made to isolate markers to predict tumors with atypically aggressive phenotypes. In one study, 105 testicular seminomas were studied to attempt to correlate morphology, immunohistochemical features, and clinical/pathological stage. Tumors were separated on the basis of atypia into "usual seminoma" and "seminomas with atypia." The presence of atypia was associated with a higher AJCC stage. Fifty-four percent of "seminomas with atypia" had AJCC stage II or III at presentation, whereas 78% of classical seminomas presented with stage I disease. Ninety percent of seminomas were found to have membrane positivity for the kit receptor. Interestingly, 43% of "seminomas with atypia" were kit receptor negative, whereas only 5% of "usual seminoma" were kit receptor negative. Based on these findings, it has been suggested that downregulation or loss of kit receptor expression may be a critical early step toward carcinomatous (i.e., nonseminomatous) differentiation.

This correlation of kit receptor expression with clinical outcome suggests that the likelihood of more aggressive growth and the development of metastases may be associated with predictable profiles of gene expression related to proliferation, differentiation, and cell death. The understanding of gene expression in GCT and how it relates to tumor stage and clinical phenotype will improve our ability to identify patients with different prognoses and design more effective, targeted therapy.

VII. COMMENT

The clinical phenotype of transformed germ cells reflects genetic events that disrupt or replace the normal cascade of coordinated gene regulation during the life span of normal germ cells. Ultimately, the accumulation of genetic events (Fig. 1) will be reflected, not only in the morphological features of the tumor,

TABLE I
KIT Receptor Expression in Human Germ Cell Tumors

Cell type	Strohmeyer (%)	Murty (%)	Total (%)
Seminoma	24/30 (80)	3/10 (30)	27/40 (68)
Nonseminomatous GCT	3/40 (8)	0/14 (0)	3/54 (66)

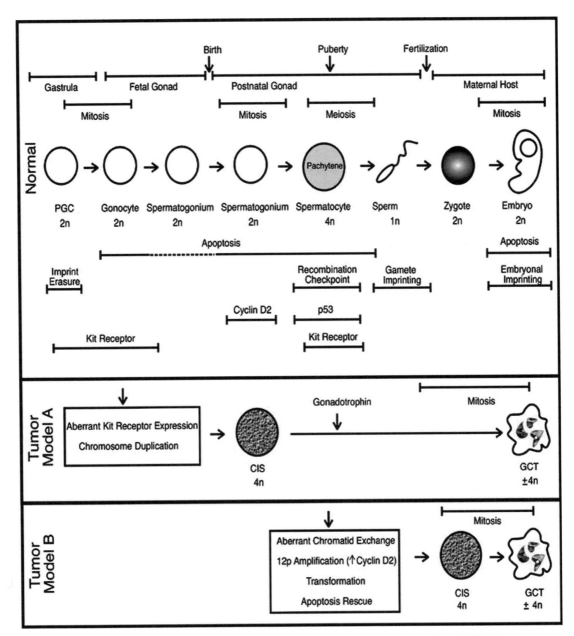

FIGURE 1 Accumulation of genetic events. Modified from Chaganti and Houldsworth (2000).

but also by its variable ability to invade, differentiate, metastasize, and respond to therapy. How these events translate into metastases and resistance is the subject of ongoing investigation.

See Also the Following Articles

CELL CYCLE CONTROL • CISPLATIN AND RELATED DRUGS • NM23 METASTASIS SUPPRESSOR GENE • RHABDOMYOSAR-COMA • TP53 TUMOR SUPPRESSOR GENE

Bibliography

Andrews, P. W. (1998). Teratocarcinomas and human embryology: Pluripotent human EC cell lines: A review. *APMIS* **106,** 158–168.

Bosl, G. J., Ilson, D. H., Rodriguez, E., Motzer, R. J., Reuter, V. E., and Chaganti, R. S. K. (1994). The clinical relevance of the i(12p) marker chromosome in germ cell tumors. *J. Natl. Cancer Inst.* **86,** 349–355.

Bosl, G. J., Sheinfeld, J., Bajorin, D., Motzer, R. J., and Chaganti, R. S. K. (2001). Cancer of the testis. *In* "Principles and Practice of Oncology" (V. T. De Vita, Jr., S. Hellman, and S. A. Rosenberg, eds.), 6th Ed., pp. 1491–1518. Lippincott Williams & Wilkins, Philadelphia.

Chaganti, R. S. K., and Houldsworth, J. (2000). Genetics and biology of adult human male germ cell tumors. *Cancer Res.* **60,** 1475–1482.

Chaganti, R. S. K., Houldsworth, J., and Bosl, G. J. (2000). Molecular biology of adult male germ cell tumors. *In* "Comprehensive Textbook of Genitourinary Oncology" (N. Z. Vogelzang, W. O. Shipley, P. T. Scardino, and D. S. Coffey, eds.), pp. 891–896. Williams & Wilkins, Baltimore.

Houldsworth, J., Reuter, V., Bosl, G. J., and Chaganti, R. S. K. (1997). Aberrant expression of cyclin D2 is an early event in human male germ cell tumorigenesis. *Cell Growth Differ.* **8,** 293–299.

Houldsworth, J., Xiao, H., Murty, V. V. V. S., Chen, W., Ray, B., Reuter, V. E., Bosl, G. J., and Chaganti, R. S. K. (1998). Human male germ cell tumor resistance to cisplatin is linked to TP53 gene mutation. *Oncogene* **16,** 2345–2349.

Koberle, B., Masters, J. R. W., Hartley, J. A., and Wood, R. D. (1999). Defective repair of cisplatin-induced DNA damage caused by reduced XPA protein in testicular germ cell tumours. *Curr. Biol.* **9,** 273–276.

Murty, V. V. V. S., and Chaganti, R. S. K. (1998). A genetic perspective of male germ cell tumors. *Semin. Oncol.* **25,** 133–144.

Nichols, C. R., Roth, B. J., Heerema, *et al.* (1990). Hematologic neoplasia associated with primary mediastinal germ cell tumors. *N. Engl. J. Med.* **322,** 1425–1429.

Rao, P. H., Houldsworth, J., Palanisamy, N., Murty, V. V. V. S., Reuter, V. E., Motzer, R., Bosl, G. J., and Chaganti, R. S. K. (1998). Chromosomal amplification is associated with cisplatin resistance of human male germ cell tumors. *Cancer Res.* **58,** 4260–4263.

Rapley, E. A., Crockford, G. P., Teare, D., *et al.* (2000). Localization to Xq27 of a susceptibility gene for testicular germ cell tumours. *Nature Genet.* **24,** 197–200.

Robertson, K. A., Bullock, H. A., Xu, Y., *et al.* (2001). Altered expression of Ape1/ref-1 in germ cell tumors and overexpression in NT2 cells confers resistance to bleomycin and radiation. *Cancer Res.* **61,** 2220–2225.

Rodriguez, E., Mathew, S., Reuter, V., *et al.* (1992). Cytogenetic analysis of 124 prospectively ascertained male germ cell tumors. *Cancer Res.* **52,** 2285–2291.

Skakkebaek, N. E., Rajpert-de Meyts, E., Jorgensen, N., *et al.* (1998). Germ cell cancer and disorders of spermatogenesis: An environmental connection? *APMIS* **106,** 3–12.

Strohmeyer, T., Peter, S., Hartmann, M., Munemitsu, S., Ackerman, R., Ulrich, A., and Slamon, D. (1991). Expression of the hst-1 and c-kit protooncogenes in human testicular germ cell tumors. *Cancer Res.* **51,** 1811–1816.

Glutathione Transferases

Shigeki Tsuchida

Hirosaki University School of Medicine, Hirosaki, Japan

GLOSSARY

aryl hydrocarbon receptor (Ah receptor) a receptor protein for 2,3,7,8-tetrachlorodibenzo-*p*-dioxin and other aromatic hydrocarbons that mediates the induction of aryl hydrocarbon hydroxylase, cytochrome P450-dependent monooxygenases, and other enzymes by these xenobiotics, possibly acting as a transcription factor.

chemoprevention the prevention of the occurrence of cancer by the administration of one or several chemical compounds.

enhancer DNA sequences that enhance transcription of a gene, located at a considerable distance, either upstream or downstream, from the start point and that can function in either orientation.

initiation a process that causes an irreversible and heritable alteration(s), resulting in a cell with the potential of developing into a clone of neoplastic cells.

monofunctional inducers agents that induce Phase II drug-metabolizing enzymes independently of the Ah receptor. Bifunctional inducers are those that bind to the Ah receptor and induce certain Phase I and Phase II drug-metabolizing enzymes.

Phase I drug-metabolizing enzymes cytochrome P450 and other enzymes that activate xenobiotics by introducing hydroxyl or epoxide groups. Phase II drug-metabolizing enzymes are those that detoxify either by conjugating these activated molecules with endogenous ligands or by destroying their reactive centers by hydrolysis, reduction, or other reactions.

promotion the stage of reversible expansion of an initiated cell population.

silencer a negative enhancer that suppresses transcription, located at a distance from the start point, and which can function in either orientation.

Glutathione transferases (GSTs) are a family of multifunctional proteins which act as enzymes and also as binding proteins in various detoxication processes. Some of these forms can function to prevent initiation of the carcinogenic processes by inactivating or detoxifying electrophilic proximate or ultimate carcinogens. During the initiation and promotion stages, specific forms of glutathione transferase are expressed in initiated and preneoplastic cells as well as in neoplastic populations. Furthermore, these forms expressed in neoplastic cells are known to participate in the mechanisms of their resistance to anticancer drugs.

I. INTRODUCTION

Glutathione transferases (EC 2.5.1.18) catalyze glutathione conjugation to electrophilic compounds, primarily produced from exogenous xenobiotics by biotransformation but which can also arise from endogenous substances. The glutathione conjugation reaction is the first step of the mercapturic acid pathway, which is one of the most important detoxication processes (Fig. 1). The second step is catalyzed by γ-

glutamyltransferase. In addition to this conjugation reaction, some forms of the enzyme exhibit isomerase activity toward ketosteroids and glutathione peroxidase activity toward lipid and nucleic acid hydroperoxides and also act as binding (carrier) proteins. With a few exceptions, GSTs exhibit conjugation activity toward 1-chloro-2,4-dinitrobenzene (CDNB). Many molecular forms of GST have been identified from various organs in a variety of species. Although microsomal and mitochondrial forms are known, most are localized in the cytosol as homodimers or heterodimers. Each form can be defined by an isoelectric point, subunit molecular weight (23,500–27,000), immunological properties, and amino acid sequence. Rat GST subunits are assigned a number that refers to the order in which they were isolated and characterized, respective forms being expressed as 1-1, 1-2, etc. After a brief description of forms and general functions of GST, the

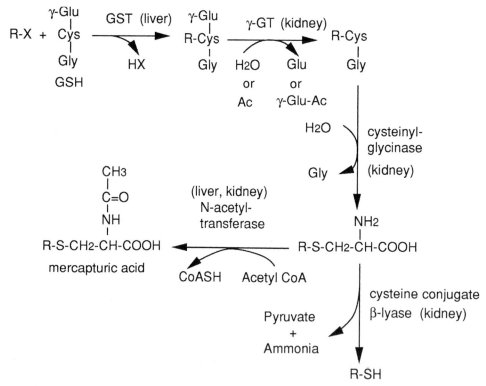

FIGURE 1 Mercapturic acid pathway of glutathione conjugates. The reaction catalyzed by cysteine conjugate β-lyase is also included. R-X, xenobiotics; GSH, glutathione; GST, glutathione transferase; γ-GT, γ-glutamyltransferase; Ac, γ-glutamyl acceptor.

involvement of these enzymes in cancers will be summarized in this article.

II. FORMS AND GENERAL FUNCTIONS

The many molecular forms of cytosolic GST are species-independently grouped into four classes, Alpha, Mu, Pi, and Theta, according to similarities in amino acid sequence, substrate specificity, sensitivity to inhibitors, and immunological cross-reactivity. So far, 13 subunits have been reported from the rat, as summarized in Table I, and homo- or heterodimers of cytosolic forms can be formed between subunits belonging to the same class. Table I also summarizes the possible correspondence of man and mouse subunits to the respective rat subunits, estimated from similarities in the properties listed earlier. Respective cDNAs encoding these subunits have been cloned and their deduced amino acid sequences reported. Within a class, even among different species, protein-coding regions are highly homologous (70–90%), while the 5'- and 3'-untranslated regions are very divergent. Between subunits belonging to different classes, sequence homology is about 30% in protein-coding regions. These subunits, even those belonging to the same class, are encoded by respective individual genes. In addition to these forms, a monomer (subunit molecular weight, 13,000) active toward 1,2-epoxy-3-(p-nitrophenoxy)propane and dichloromethane has been purified from rat liver cytosol. This form seems to be identical with the macrophage migration inhibitory factor and exhibits partial similarity to rat GST 3-3 in the N-terminal amino acid sequence. In addition, leukotriene C_4 synthase, an enzyme catalyzing the conjugation of leukotriene A_4 with glutathione to form leukotriene C_4, has been purified from microsomal fractions of human leukemia cell lines. It is a homodimer consisting of a 18-kDa subunit.

Diverse functions of GSTs are played by a whole family consisting of multiple forms. The various forms share some substrate overlap but show different activities toward a wide range of electrophiles with different chemical structures. Each subunit of GSTs seems to exhibit catalytic activity independent of other subunits, although dissociated monomers do not exhibit any activity. The reported specific functions of rat subunits are summarized in Table II. Ligandin, identified as a binding protein for steroids, bilirubin, and azodye carcinogens, corresponds to a mixture of GST 1-1 and 1-2. Other subunits also act as binding or carrier proteins for bilirubin, heme, cholic acids, and steroids. Human and mouse subunits are presumed to have activities similar to the equivalent rat subunits.

Each organ possesses a unique profile of GST forms; the liver has the highest activity and number of molecular forms. Other organs share some, but not all, forms expressed in the liver and also specifically express particular forms, e.g., GST 6-9 and 11-11 in the testis and 6-6 in the brain. Thus, the expression of GST subunits is, to a certain extent, tissue specific, as shown in Table III. In the kidney, the Alpha class (subunits 1, 2, and 8) is abundantly expressed, while the Mu class (subunits 3 and 4) occurs at a low level. In the lung, subunits 2, 8, 3, 4, and 7 are expressed, but subunit 1 is undetectable. Rat GST-P and human GST P1-1(π), both Pi class forms, are not expressed in normal adult livers except in bile ducts, while the mouse Pi class form, MII, is a major form in the adult male liver.

TABLE I
Rat Glutathione Transferase Subunits and Corresponding Human and Mouse Subunits[a]

Class	Rat	Human	Mouse
Alpha	Subunit 1 (Ya_1/Ya_2)	A1 (B_1)/ A2 (B_2)	Ya_1/Ya_2
	2 (Yc)	(2)	MI (Ya_3, Yc)
	8 (Yk)		5.7
	10 (Yfetus)		
Mu	3 (Yb_1)		MIII
	4 (Yb_2)	M1a (μ)/ M1b (ψ)	7.1
	6 (Yb_3, Yn_1)	M2 (4)	
	9 (Yn_2)		
	11 (Yo)	M3 (5.2)	
	(Yb_4)		9.3
Pi	7 (Yp, Yf)	P1 (π)	MII
Theta	5		
	12 (Yrs)	(θ, T1)	
Microsome	Microsomal	Microsomal	
Mitochondria	13		

[a]Adapted from Tsuchia and Sato (1992).

TABLE II

Specific Functions of Rat
Glutathione Transferase Subunits[a]

Subunit	Function
1	Binding steroids, bilirubin, bile acids, carcinogens, and leukotriene C_4 Isomerase activity for ketosteroids and prostaglandin H_2 ($\rightarrow$PGE$_2$ and D$_2$) Reduction of lipid peroxides and prostaglandin H_2 ($\rightarrow$PGF$_{2\alpha}$) Conjugation of benzo[a]pyrene and aflatoxin B_1-8,9-oxide
2	Reduction of lipid peroxides Conjugation of 1,2-dibromoethane
8	Conjugation of 4-hydroxyalkenals derived from lipid peroxides
10	Reduction of lipid peroxides
3	Binding bile acids Conjugation of aflatoxin B_1-8,9-oxide Release of nitrite from 4-nitroquinoline-1-oxide
4	Carrier for heme Binding steroids, thyroid hormones, and bile acids Conjugation of trans-stilbene oxide and benzo[a]pyrene Denitrosation of 1-methyl-2-nitro-1-nitrosoguanidine and 1,3-bis(2-chloroethyl)-1-nitrosourea Synthesis of hepoxilin A_3-C
6	Reduction of nucleic acid hydroperoxides Synthesis of leukotriene C_4
7	Reduction of lipid peroxides Conjugation of benzo[a]pyrene
5	Conjugation of epoxides and dichloromethane Reduction of nucleic acid hydroperoxides
12	Conjugation of arylmethyl sulfates
Microsomal	Reduction of lipid peroxides Conjugation of hexachloro-1,3-butadiene

[a]Adapted from Sato (1989).

III. PREVENTION OR STIMULATION OF CARCINOGENESIS

A. Carcinogen Metabolism

The covalent binding of electrophiles derived from carcinogens to macromolecules, especially DNA, has been considered as an initial step in chemical carcinogenesis. Such electrophilic compounds are known to be detoxified by enzymatic or, in some cases, spontaneous conjugation with glutathione. Specific GST forms are involved in the conjugation of particular carcinogens (Table II). For example, rat GST 4-4 ex-

TABLE III

Relative Organ Distribution of Rat Glutathione
Transferase Subunits[a]

Subunit	Liver	Kidney	Lung	Testis	Colon	Brain
Class Alpha						
1	+++[b]	+++	−	−	−	−
2	++	+++	++	++	−	++
8	++	++	++	−	+	−
Class Mu						
3	+++	−	+	++	+	+
4	+++	+	+	++	+	−
6	−	−	+	++	−	+
9	−	−		++		−
Class Pi						
7	−	+++	++	+	++	++

[a]Adapted from Sato (1989).

[b]Degree of expression. Negative (−), weak (+), moderate (++), and strong (+++), respectively.

hibits activity toward trans-stilbene oxide and GST 12-12 toward arylmethyl sulfates such as reactive sulfate esters produced from 7-hydroxymethyl-benz[a]anthracene by sulfotransferase. GSTs 1-1, 4-4, and 7-7 share conjugation activity toward benzo[a]pyrene-7,8-diol-9,10-oxide, but each exhibits different enantio- and regioselectivity. GSTs 1-1 and 3-3 are highly active toward aflatoxin B_1-8,9-exo epoxide, while 4-4 is preferentially active toward the endo epoxide. GST 4-4 also possesses denitrosation activity toward 1-methyl-2-nitro-1-nitrosoguanidine. Some hepatocarcinogens, including N-acetyl-2-aminofluorene, N-methyl-4-aminoazobenzene, and dimethylnitrosamine, are activated by cytochrome P450 and then conjugated spontaneously with glutathione.

B. Induction of Glutathione Transferases by Drugs

Rat GST subunits are preferentially induced by various drugs, including carcinogens and anti-carcinogenic agents such as butylated hydroxyanisole (BHA) and ethoxyquin. Although subunits 1 and 3 are inducible by almost all drugs examined, the induction of subunit 3 by 3-methylcholanthrene or β-naphthoflavone is not remarkable. Preferential induction of Alpha class GST is also reported in primary cultured human hepatocytes. Antioxidants induce mouse

TABLE IV
Induction of Mouse Liver Glutathione Transferases by Drugs[a]

	Molecular form				
	Alpha		Mu		Pi
Inducer	10.6 (MI, Ya₃Ya₃)	10.3 (Ya₁Ya₂)	8.7 (MIII)	9.3	9.0 (MII)
tert-Butylhydroxyanisole	→[b]	↑↑	↑	↑↑	→
Bisethylxanthogen	→	↑↑	↑	↑↑	→
β-Naphthoflavone	→	↑	↑	↑	→
Phenobarbital	→	↑	↑	↑	→

[a]Adapted from Stao and Tsuchida (1991).

[b]Single and double arrows pointing upward indicate slight (within fivefold) and strong (above fivefold) induction, respectively. A horizontal arrow indicates no change.

liver GST to a much higher extent than in rat liver. The major mouse forms induced by BHA are GST-9.3 in the Mu class and GST-10.3 in the Alpha class, both being undetectable in normal liver (Table IV). GST-MI, a constitutive form in normal liver, is not significantly induced.

The gene structure of rat subunit 1 provides the molecular basis for its induction by drugs. This gene possesses at least two enhancers, a xenobiotic-responsive element (XRE) and an antioxidant-responsive element (ARE), in the 5'-flanking region (Fig. 2). The former element contains the XRE core sequence found in the 5'-flanking region of the cytochrome P450 IA1 gene, while the ARE contains the 12-O-tetradecanoylphorbol-13-acetate (TPA) responsive element (TRE)-like sequence. An enhancer analogous to the rat ARE is also present in the mouse Ya (possibly identical to GST-10.3) gene and is named the electrophile-responsive element (EpRE). The oncogene products, *Jun* and *Fos* protein families, have been suggested to bind to ARE and EpRE and to be involved in the basal and inducible activities of these related elements. β-Naphthoflavone, a planar aromatic compound, activates the gene through either XRE or ARE, but the presence of *Ah* receptors and metabolism of β-naphthoflavone by cytochrome P450 IA1 are required for its transcriptional activation. On the other hand, *t*-butylhydroquinone, a phenolic antioxidant, activates the gene only through ARE, independently of *Ah* receptors or cytochrome P450 IA1. In the presence of *Ah* receptors, XRE reacts with 2,3,7,8-tetrachlorodibenzo-*p*-dioxin, but ARE does

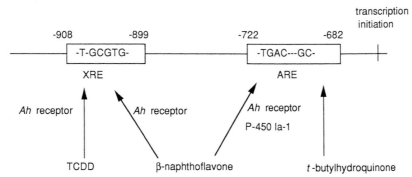

FIGURE 2 Regulatory elements of the rat subunit 1 gene. XRE, xenobiotic-responsive element-like sequence; ARE, antioxidant-responsive element; TCDD, 2,3,7,8-tetrachlorodibenzo-*p*-dioxin. The XRE core sequence is shown in the left-hand box. ARE contains a 12-O-tetradecanoylphorbol-13-acetate response element-like sequence as shown in the right-hand box. Adapted from Tsuchida and Sato (1992).

not. These results support the conclusion that Phase II drug-metabolizing enzymes, including GST, are induced by monofunctional and bifunctional inducers by different mechanisms, and that induction by monofunctional inducers such as t-butylhydroquinone is mediated by an electrophilic signal, independent of Ah receptors. Mouse EpRE is responsive to a wide variety of GST inducers, and transcriptional activation through this element seems to account for most of the enzyme elevations produced by these inducers. The element contains two repeats of the TRE-like sequence, while one base is replaced in rat ARE. This difference may be responsible for the higher extent of GST induction in mouse liver than in rat liver.

Administration of clofibrate and other peroxisome proliferators to rats results in diminished GST subunits 1 and 3 in livers. Peroxisome proliferator receptors are supposed to mediate the biological effects of these agents and act as a transcription factor. The receptors belong to the steroid hormone receptor superfamily. Ah receptors are stimulatory for induction of GST, while peroxisome proliferator receptors are inhibitory.

C. Prevention of Carcinogenesis

Chemical carcinogenesis in mouse or rat livers and other organs is known to be prevented or modulated by BHA, bisethylxanthogen, and other antioxidants. These induce GSTs and other drug-metabolizing enzymes, and their induction of GSTs closely correlates with their tumor inhibitory activity. Thus, these enzymes seem to play a central role in antioxidant-associated chemoprevention of carcinogenesis and have been used as a marker for screening potential chemopreventive agents. Microsome-mediated aflatoxin B_1 binding to DNA is reduced when mouse or rat liver GSTs are induced by BHA. The mutagenic response to aflatoxin B_1 is also reduced by BHA treatment. In mouse lung, two forms in the Mu class, preferentially induced by BHA, bind to benzo[a]pyrene (BP) metabolites, indicating antineoplastic activity of BHA against BP-induced neoplasia in this organ. Since antioxidants and other drugs have been noted to inhibit hepatocarcinogenesis induced by many different carcinogens, different GST forms are presumably responsible.

As polyaromatic hydrocarbon epoxides derived from BP and 3-methylcholanthrene are good sub-strates for GSTs composing subunits 1 or 3, which are abundant in rat liver, these carcinogens are generally not hepatocarcinogenic. GST 12-12 exhibits activity only toward arylmethyl sulfates, which are carcinogenic in rat skin, but not in the liver, where the form is abundant. Similarly, rat forms in the Mu class catalyze the glutathione-dependent liberation of nitrite from 4-nitroquinoline-1-oxide, which is tumorigenic to the lung, esophagus, and other organs where these forms are not expressed or expressed only marginally. Thus, the organ-specific distribution of GST forms involved in detoxification of carcinogens seems to be one of the factors that might play a role in suppressing carcinogenesis in particular organs.

Human GST M1-1(μ) has high activity toward trans-stilbene oxide or epoxides from BP. About half of the population is devoid of its expression due to deletion of the gene, and the GST M1-1 null phenotype is reported to be more frequent in lung cancer or urinary bladder cancer patients than in matched control smokers. Loss of this form has been also suggested as a possible marker of greater likelihood of adenocarcinoma development in the stomach or colon. Similar genetic polymorphism is also noted in the human T1 gene, about 30–40% of the population lacking the gene. However, the relationship between T1-1 phenotype and cancer susceptibility remains to be clarified.

D. Stimulation of Carcinogenesis

Although, as described earlier, GSTs are generally recognized as detoxifying enzymes, they are also involved in the activation of some carcinogens such as haloalkanes and haloalkenes. Rat GST 2-2 and 3-3 catalyze the conjugation of ethylene dibromide (1,2-dibromoethane) with glutathione to form 1-bromo-2-S-glutathionyl ethane, which reacts with DNA via an episulfonium ion, eventually resulting in the formation of S-[2-(N^7-guanyl)ethyl]glutathione. This reaction with DNA is considered to be responsible for the carcinogenesis caused by ethylene dibromide in rats, whereby pretreatment with t-butylated hydroxytoluene, an inducer of GSTs, markedly increased DNA adduct levels, while depletion of glutathione resulted in decreased levels. Dichloromethane is activated by rat GST 5-5 of the Theta class to form 5-chloromethyl glutathione, eventually resulting in formaldehyde formation. 1,2-Dichloroethane and 1,2-dibromo-3-chloropropane are also activated by GST.

Haloalkenes, including hexachloro-1,3-butadiene and trichloroethene, which induce renal tumors in the rat, are conjugated with glutathione by microsomal GST. In contrast to haloalkanes, these glutathione conjugates are not mutagenic by themselves and require further metabolism to unstable thiols via cysteinyl derivatives by the mercapturic acid pathway (Fig. 1), followed by the action of the cysteine conjugate β-lyase. Reactive thiols thus formed are considered to be involved in the induction of renal tumors.

IV. MARKERS FOR PRENEOPLASIA AND NEOPLASIA

A. Preneoplastic Foci in Rat Liver

During rat chemical hepatocarcinogenesis, GST-P (7-7) is markedly increased (30-fold or more, and above 1 mg/g wet weight of the liver) in rat liver bearing hyperplastic nodules induced by several protocols and in primary and some transplantable hepatocarcinomas. GST-P is especially low in adult rat livers, but is ubiquitous in other organs. The kidney, lung, and pancreas contain significant amounts. Immunohistochemical staining has revealed that GST-P is localized in preneoplastic foci and neoplastic tissues. Furthermore, very small GST-P-positive foci or even single cells, appearing 1 or 2 weeks after a single administration of initiators, are detectable before an increase in GST-P content becomes evident in whole liver preparations. GST-P-positive single cells are presumed to be "initiated cells," indicating a clonal origin of GST-P-positive foci and hepatomas. Unlike most drug-metabolizing enzymes, GST-P is not inducible by administration of a large variety of hepatocarcinogenic promoters or modulators, or even by hepatocarcinogens, without the appearance of preneoplastic foci and hyperplastic nodules. These advantages have established GST-P as one of the best markers for detection of early liver lesions, now widely used for analysis of hepatocarcinogenesis and in medium-term bioassay methods for carcinogens and modifiers. Exceptions are peroxisome proliferators, including clofibrate; GST-P is not expressed in hyperplastic nodules induced by these agents.

The GST-P gene is about 3000 bp long and consists of seven exons and six introns. Two enhancing elements (GPEI and GPEII) and a silencing element are present in the 5′-flanking region (Fig. 3). The GPEI contains an imperfect palindrome structure composed of two TPA response element-like sequences, each having no activity by itself, but acting synergistically. GPEI is known to be activated by the oncogene products, *Jun* and *Fos*, and other unidentified transcription factors. One *trans*-acting factor binding to the silencer seems to be very similar to the interleukin 6-dependent DNA-binding protein. The positive enhancer, GPEI, rather than the silencer has been suggested to be mainly involved in the expression of GST-P in preneoplastic foci, but the question of which transcription factors are actually responsible remains to be solved.

B. Human Cancer Tissues

GST P1-1(π), the human equivalent of rat GST-P, is also expressed in many cancer tissues, including carcinomas of the colon, stomach, esophagus, pharynx, bile duct, lung, breast, uterine cervix, and urinary bladder. In the lung tumor case, GST P1-1 is expressed in both adenocarcinomas and squamous cell carcinomas, but not in small cell lung cancers. The properties of GST P1-1 purified from several cancer tissues are not different from those of placental GST P1-1. A few bases were found to be replaced among GST P1-1 cDNAs cloned from the placenta, a breast cancer cell line, and lung but with conservation of amino acid sequences. GST P1-1 content is increased two- to sixfold in cancer tissues, as compared with the respective control tissue values. It should be noted that these organs normally express GST P1-1 as a

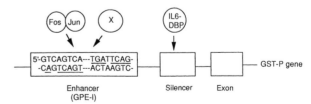

FIGURE 3 Regulatory elements of the rat GST-P gene and its transcription factors. *Fos* and *Jun*, oncogene products; X, unidentified transcription factors acting on GPEI; IL6-DBP, interleukin 6-dependent DNA-binding protein. GPEI contains dyad palindromic TRE-like sequences and TRE consensus sequences are underlined.

major form, but in lower amounts than in their cancer tissues. Alterations in expression of GST M1-1 and other forms in cancer tissues are not striking. Thus, GST P1-1 is the dominant form in cancer tissues, responsible for more than 70 to 90% of GST activity toward 1-chloro-2,4-dinitrobenzene. Cancers originating from the liver or kidney, both of which are organs normally possessing high GST activity, show less activity than the respective control tissues, mainly due to a decrease of the A1 and A2 subunits in the Alpha class, GST P1-1 being changed marginally. GST P1-1 becomes the dominant form in renal cancers. Changes in GST forms in cancer tissues are, therefore, not homogeneous. GST P1-1 is enhanced in most, but not all, cancers derived from many organs. The profiles of GST forms in cancer tissues seem to be influenced by the respective normal tissue profiles. Brain tumors (glioma), skin cancers, Wilms' tumors, malignant melanomas, seminomas, soft tissue sarcomas, and nonlymphoblastic leukemia cells also express GST P1-1. In addition, this form is also found in preneoplastic lesions, such as colon adenomas, and dysplasia of the uterine cervix and esophagus. Thus, GST P1-1 may be a useful marker not only for a wide range of cancers, but also for high-risk precancerous lesions. Elevated serum or plasma GST P1-1 contents are noted in patients with advanced cancers of the gastrointestinal tract. Despite the striking expression of GST-P in rat hepatocarcinogenesis, GST P1-1 is hardly expressed in human primary hepatocellular carcinomas. The GST P1-1 gene has an AP-1-binding site but does not have an element like GPEI observed in the rat GST-P gene, suggesting that the expression of the two genes may be regulated by different mechanisms. GST P1-1 and its mRNA levels are suggested to be negatively correlated with estrogen receptor content in breast cancer specimens.

V. ANTICANCER DRUG RESISTANCE

A. Metabolism of Anticancer Drugs

Anticancer drugs such as alkylating agents or their metabolites are conjugated with glutathione by cy-

tosolic GSTs, and some drugs by a microsomal form. These include melphalan, chlorambucil, and cyclophosphamide. Although glutathione conjugation occurs to some extent without enzymes, the mouse cytosolic GST MI in the Alpha class has significant activity toward melphalan or chlorambucil. Acrolein, a genotoxic aldehyde released in the metabolic activation of cyclophosphamide, is conjugated with glutathione by human GST P1-1. Rat GST 4-4 is known to detoxify 1,3-bis(2-chloroethyl)-1-nitrosourea (BCNU) by a glutathione-dependent denitrosation reaction. GSTs are also suggested to be involved in the conjugation of 9-deoxy-Δ^9, Δ^{12} (E)-prostaglandin D_2 (Δ^{12}-prostaglandin J_2), which exerts a cytotoxic effect on many cancer cell lines.

B. Expression of Glutathione Transferases in Drug Resistance

The relationship between intracellular glutathione levels and drug resistance has been studied extensively; glutathione is suggested as one of the major determinants of therapeutic efficacy. Among enzymes involved in glutathione metabolism, the activity of GST is most often increased in many cell lines resistant to alkylating agents, doxorubicin, mitomycin C, and cis-platinum, mainly due to Pi class forms. In cell lines which exhibit increased activities after acquisition of resistance, their sensitive precursors have generally been demonstrated to have had lower values. The activity expressed in most resistant cell lines is comparable to activities in cancer tissues. Thus, it seems likely that the increase in cell lines with low GST activity might be linked to acquisition of resistance; only a few cell lines with high activity exhibit a further increase upon becoming resistant. Several cell lines transfected with cDNAs encoding GST P1, rat subunits 1 or 3 have exhibited increased resistance to particular drugs, depending on the respective cDNAs transfected. Furthermore, treatment with inhibitors of GSTs such as ethacrynic acid and indomethacin has resulted in reduced resistance to alkylating agents in cell lines with high GST activities, suggesting the direct involvement of the enzyme in drug resistance. On the other hand, contrary to expectation, certain cell lines transfected with GST P1 cDNA were reported not to demonstrate any enhanced resistance to doxorubicin and other drugs.

In drug-resistant cell lines, particular GST forms appear to be elevated in association with the detoxication of particular anticancer drugs; rat GST 2-2 is expressed in chlorambucil-resistant cell lines and GST 4-4 in BCNU-resistant cells. The finding that the Pi-class forms are expressed in many cell lines resistant to structurally unrelated drugs is analogous to the expression of rat GST-P in hepatocarcinogenesis induced by many genotoxic carcinogens. It is not evident yet whether the Pi-class forms possess conjugation activities toward chlorambucil and other alkylating agents except for acrolein. Thus, the actual role of the Pi-class forms expressed in drug-resistant cells remains to be clarified. These forms are reversibly inactivated by active oxygen species, including hydrogen peroxide and superoxide anion. This raises the possibility that the Pi-class forms might function as scavengers to remove active oxygen metabolites escaping metabolism by superoxide dismutase, catalase, or selenium-dependent glutathione peroxidase. Since the cytotoxicity of doxorubicin or bleomycin has been suggested to be dependent on the formation of free radicals, this possible scavenger function as well as the glutathione peroxidase activity of Pi-class forms toward lipid hydroperoxides may be important as mechanisms of doxorubicin resistance.

The finding of high amounts of GST P1-1 in most established cell lines and in many cancer tissues as well as in drug-resistant cell lines suggests that GSTs may play important roles not only in acquired resistance, but also in natural resistance. A significant correlation between the expression of GST P1-1 at the time of diagnosis and the subsequent treatment results has been reported in acute nonlymphoblastic leukemia or non-small cell lung carcinomas. On the other hand, such a relation was not found for untreated ovarian tumors and the expression of GSTs did not change after the development of acquired resistance, suggesting that other mechanisms, including P-glycoprotein and topoisomerases, may be responsible in this case. The multidrug resistance-associated protein (MRP) has recently been shown to be an ATP-dependent glutathione S-conjugate transporter. Thus, glutathione conjugates of drugs formed by GSTs are possibly pumped out by this particular ATPase present on the plasma membrane. It is also reported that GST activities are not increased or are even undetectable in some resistant cell lines.

C. Sensitization of Resistant Cells by Glutathione Transferase Inhibitors

Modulation of GSTs with inhibitors has shown promise for overcoming resistance in experimental models, although the inhibition is not sufficiently specific. Thus, more specific inhibitors for GSTs, including GST P1-1, are anticipated. The three-dimensional structures of GST P1-1, rat GST 3-3, and human GST A1-1 have been reported and all exhibit very similar folding topologies, irrespective of their relatively low degree of amino acid sequence identity. The structure of these subunits is divided into two domains: domain I contains four β-strands and three α-helices, arranged in a $\beta\alpha\beta\alpha\beta\beta\alpha$ motif, while domain II is composed of five to seven α-helices (Fig. 4). The domain I of GST P1 is encoded by exons 2–4 of its gene while that of subunit 3 is due to exons 1–4. The distribution of nucleotides encoding these β-strands and α-helices in respective exons is quite similar between the two genes, except for $\alpha2$- and $\alpha8$-coding sequences in the subunit 3 gene (Fig. 5). Domain I is considered as the glutathione-binding domain and domain II seems to be primarily responsible for electrophilic substrate binding. Several amino acid residues located in proximity to the bound glutathione analog were postulated from the three-dimensional structure. Substitution mutations have revealed that these residues of GST P1, as shown in Fig. 4, in fact play an important role in the binding of glutathione. Most of these residues are located in domain I. The electrophilic substrate-binding site is suggested to be located in the C- and N-terminal regions which are in close proximity to the glutathione-binding site. Although a glutathione derivative and SH reagents were noted to modify cysteine residues of GSTs resulting in inactivation, site-directed mutagenesis revealed that none of the cysteine residues are essential for catalytic activity. The cysteine residue at the 47th position from the N terminus of the GST P1 subunit is very sensitive to these reagents and active

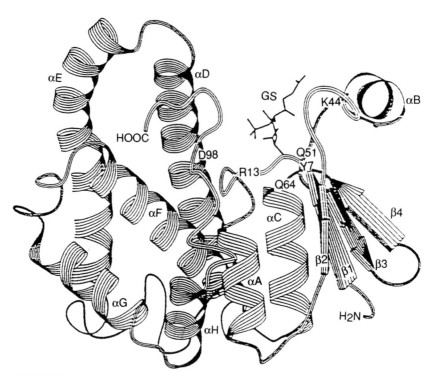

FIGURE 4 The three-dimensional structure of the pig Pi-class glutathione transferase. Amino acid residues involved in glutathione binding are imposed on the structure reported by P. Reinemer, H. D. Dirr, R. Ladenstein, J. Schäffer, O. Gallay, and R. Huber (1991). *EMBO J.* **10,** 1997. The figure is adapted with permission of Oxford University Press. The numerals denote the amino acid residues counting from the NH₂ terminus of the human GST P1 (π) subunit. Y, tyrosine; R, arginine; K, lysine; Q, glutamine; D, aspartic acid; GS, glutathione sulfonate.

oxygen metabolites such as hydrogen peroxide. The clarification of the three-dimensional structure of GST P1-1 and information on the active sites will provide the basis for the future development of specific inhibitors. Such inhibitors have promise as agents to overcome GST-mediated drug resistance.

Repression of GST P1-1 expression may also deserve consideration for sensitization of such resistant cells. Since several transcription factors acting on the positive or negative enhancers of the Pi-class forms have been identified, as already described, these factors may well become targets for repression. It is interesting in this context that GST P1-1 expression was shown to be repressed by ionizing radiation.

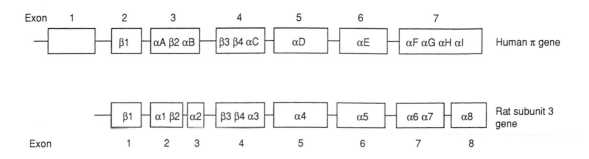

FIGURE 5 Exon structures of human GST P1 and rat subunit 3 genes and distribution of α-helix- and β-strand-coding nucleotides in respective exons. αA to αI are α-helices of the GST P1 subunit, while α1 to α8 are those of the subunit 3. β1 to β4 are β-strands of both subunits.

Acknowledgment

This article is dedicated to the late Professor Kiyomi Sato who first established the usefulness of Pi-class forms as tumor markers and guided our studies.

See Also the Following Articles

GLYCOPROTEINS AND GLYCOSYLATION CHANGES IN CANCER

Bibliography

Armstrong, R. N. (1991). Glutathione S-transferases: Reaction mechanism, structure, and function. *Chem. Res. Toxicol.* **4,** 131.

Coles, B., and Ketterer, B. (1990). The role of glutathione and glutathione transferases in chemical carcinogenesis. *Crit. Rev. Biochem. Mol. Biol.* **25,** 47.

Dirr, H., Reinemer, P., and Huber, R. (1994). X-ray crystal structures of cytosolic glutathione S-transferases: Implications for protein architecture, substrate recognition and catalytic function. *Eur. J. Biochem.* **220,** 635.

Mannervik, B., and Danielson, U. H. (1988). Glutathione transferases: Structure and catalytic activity. *CRC Crit. Rev. Biochem.* **23,** 283.

Mannervik, B., and Widersten, M. (1995). Human glutathione transferases: Classification, tissue distribution, structure and functional properties. *In* "Advances in Drug Metabolism in Man" (G. M. Pacifici and G. N. Fracchia, eds.), p. 407. European Commision, Luxembourg.

Rushmore, T. H., and Pickett, C. B. (1993). Glutathione S-transferases, structure, regulation, and therapeutic implications. *J. Biol. Chem.* **268,** 11475.

Sato, K. (1989). Glutathione transferases as markers of preneoplasia and neoplasia. *Adv. Cancer Res.* **52,** 205.

Sato, K., and Tsuchida, S. (1991). Glutathione transferases in normal, preneoplastic, and neoplastic tissues: Forms and functions. *In* "Biochemical and Molecular Aspects of Selected Cancers" (T. G. Pretlow, II and T. P. Pretlow, eds.), Vol. 1, p. 177. Academic Press, San Diego.

Tew, K. D., Pickett, C. B., Mantle, T. J., Mannervik, B., and Hayes, J. D. (eds.) (1993). "Structure and Function of Glutathione Transferases." CRC Press, Boca Raton, FL.

Tsuchida, S., and Sato, K. (1992). Glutathione transferases and cancer. *Crit. Rev. Biochem. Mol. Biol.* **27,** 337.

van Bladeren, P. J., and van Ommen, B. (1991). The inhibition of glutathione S-transferases: Mechanisms, toxic consequences and their therapeutic benefits. *Pharmacol. Ther.* **51,** 35.

Glycoproteins and Glycosylation Changes in Cancer

Samuel B. Ho
University of Minnesota Medical School, Minneapolis

Young S. Kim
University of California, San Francisco

GLOSSARY

carbohydrate antigens sugar molecules that are covalently linked to proteins or lipids. Individual or groups of sugar molecules can be recognized by polyclonal or monoclonal antibodies.

expression cloning a technique used to isolate cDNA clones of a particular protein. Antibodies that recognize a specific protein are used to screen a cDNA library made from RNA isolated from a tissue that highly expresses the protein of interest. Immunoreactive clones are isolated and cDNA inserts sequenced.

glycoprotein a protein with carbohydrate sugars covalently attached. Glycoproteins can be categorized as O-linked (carbohydrates linked to the hydroxyl group of serine or threonine) or N-linked (carbohydrates linked to the amide nitrogen of asparagine).

glycosyltransferase enzymes that catalyze the transfer of carbohydrate molecules to a glycoprotein or glycolipid.

mucins large, heavily glycosylated O-linked glycoproteins characterized by a domain of tandem repeats rich in serine and/or threonine amino acid glycosylation sites.

Alterations of glycoproteins have long been described in carcinomas. These changes produce tumor-associated antigens which can be exploited for both the diagnosis and the treatment of cancer. Tumor-associated antigens are commonly found on large, heavily glycosylated proteins known as mucins. Mucins are produced in large amounts by epithelial tissues, especially by gastrointestinal tissues. Recent research using monoclonal antibodies and molecular cloning techniques has greatly advanced our knowledge of the structure and function of mucin-type glycoproteins in both normal tissues and cancer.

I. INTRODUCTION

Glycosylation is one of the most common posttranslational modifications of proteins. The pattern of glycosylation is determined by the type of protein substrate and the complement of carbohydrate donors and glycosyltransferase enzymes present within a cell. The addition of carbohydrates to proteins confers important physical properties to the proteins. For example, carbohydrates alter the tertiary structure of the protein and limit the approach of other macromolecules resulting in resistance to protease digestion and increased water-binding capacity. In addition, the diversity of terminal carbohydrates on glycoproteins serve as biological signals for protein targeting and cell–cell interactions. Alterations of glycosylation patterns in malignant cells may influence the biological behavior of these cells. These changes also result in cancer-specific antigens that can be exploited for cancer diagnosis and therapy. O-linked glycoproteins of normal and neoplastic gastrointestinal tissues have been extensively studied and will be reviewed here.

II. GLYCOPROTEIN STRUCTURE

Glycoproteins can be divided into two categories, N-linked and O-linked. Carbohydrates added to the amide nitrogen of asparagine are considered to be N-linked, and carbohydrates added to the OH group of serine or threonine are considered O-linked. N-linked glycoproteins are the most common. The functional roles of N-lined glycosylation include targeting of lysosomal enzymes, determination of polypeptide folding patterns, and providing specific cellular recognition targets. O-linked glycoproteins are usually found in cell surface and secreted products. O-linked glycoproteins are typically heavily glycosylated, containing 65–85% carbohydrate by weight and possessing regions with a high content of serine and threonine.

Large heavily glycosylated O-linked glycoproteins include proteoglycans and mucins. Proteoglycans are characterized by uronic acid-containing glycosaminoglycan carbohydrates. Proteoglycans are secreted as components of the extracellular matrix or are anchored in the plasma membrane as integral membrane proteins. Mucins are the largest of the O-linked glycoproteins, containing heavily glycosylated regions of 600–1200 amino acids in length and 65–85% carbohydrate by weight. Secreted mucins form polymers by binding end to end through disulfide linkages, resulting in apparent molecular weights of 10^7 and high levels of viscoelasticity. Mucin proteins are the major structural protein of mucous gels which are essential to epithelial protection against abrasion, pH extremes, proteases, bile acids, foreign ligands, and infectious agents. Large quantities of mucins are synthesized by gastrointestinal epithelia and respiratory and reproductive epithelia; alterations of mucin proteins are a characteristic feature of adenocarcinoma.

III. PROTEIN STRUCTURE OF O-LINKED MUCIN GLYCOPROTEINS

Biochemical analysis and characterization of mucin proteins have been limited because of their large size and abundant glycosylation. Recently, much has been learned about the structure and possible functions of mucins from molecular sequence data derived from the cloning of several human and animal mucins. These data have demonstrated that all mucins share certain structural features. For example, all the mucin proteins sequenced to date contain regions with a high proportion of threonine and/or serine glycosylation sites. These threonine- and serine-rich sequences are repeated in tandem along the length of the molecule, and thus are called tandem repeats. Nonrepetitive sequences are found beyond the tandem repeat regions. Each mucin can be distinguished by the specific amino acid sequences and the lengths of these tandem repeats (Table I). Contrary to previous definitions, mucins do contain a small number of N-linked oligosaccharide attachment sites in both the tandem repeat and the nonreptitive domains. The high density of carbohydrates enables the molecule to bind high volumes of water, which contributes to

TABLE I

Human Mucin Genes

Designation	Source	Type[a]	No. of amino acids in tandem repeat	Chromosomal location	Tandem repeat amino acid sequence	Reference[b]
MUC1	Mammary Pancreatic	mem	20	1q21q24	GSTAPPAHGVTSAPDTRPAP	1,2,3
MUC2	Intestinal	sec	23	11p15	PTTPITTTTTVTPTPTPTGTQT	4
	Trachea	sec	23		PYPYPITTTTVTPTPTPT(G/S)TQT	5
MUC3	Intestinal	sec	17	7	HSTPSFTSSITTTETTS	6
MUC4	Tracheobronchial	sec	16	3	(T)SS(A)ST(GHA)T(P)L(P)VT(D)[c]	7
MUC5	Tracheobronchial	sec	8	11p15	TTSTTSAP	8
MUC6	Gastric	sec	169	11p15	SPFSSTGPMTATSFQTTTTYPTTSHPQTTLPTHVPPFSTSLVTP STGTVITPTHAQMATSASIHSTPTGTIPPPTTLKATGSTHT APPMTPTTSGTSQAHSSFSTAKTSTSLHSHTSSTHHPEVTP TSTTTITPNPTSTGTSTPVAHTTSATSSRLPTPFTTHSPPTGS	9
MUC7	Salivary	sec	23	4	TTAAPPTPSATTPAPPSSSAPPG	10

[a] mem, membrane bound; sec, secreted.

[b] Key to references: (1) Gendler et al. (1990). JBC **265**, 15286; (2) Ligtenberg et al. (1990). JBC **265**, 5573; (3) Lan et al. (1990). JBC **265**, 15294; (4) Gum et al. (1989). JBC **264**, 6480; (5) Jany (1991). J. Clin. Invest. **87**, 77; (6) Gum et al. (1990). BBRC **171**, 407; (7) Porchet et al. (1991). BBRC **175**, 414; (8) Aubert et al. (1991). Am. J. Res. Cell. Mol. Biol. **5**, 178; (9) Toribara et al. (1993). JBC **268**, 5879; (10) Bobek et al. (1993). JBC **268**, 20563.

[c] Imperfectly conserved.

their high viscosity in solution. In addition, the carbohydrates protect the mucin peptide from hydrolysis when exposed to luminal proteases or pH extremes.

Two families of mucins have been characterized to date. The first is a *membrane-bound* glycoprotein which is synthesized by most, if not all, epithelial tissues. Characterization of this mucin resulted from studies of the high molecular weight glycoproteins [previously labeled as PUM, PEM (polymorphic epithelial mucin), MAM-6, PAS-O, EMA, NPG, and DF-3] that occur in human breast milk and are highly expressed in breast and other adenocarcinomas. Data from full-length cDNA sequencing indicate that two-thirds of this protein consist of 20-amino-acid tandem repeats, which contain 25% serum or threonine glycosylation sites (Table I). The carboxyl terminus contains a putative transmembrane sequence and a 69-amino-acid cytoplasmic tail (Fig. 1). Interaction of the cytoplasmic tail with the actin cytoskeleton has been demonstrated, suggesting that this segment may represent a cytoplasmic "anchor" for the protein. Cysteine residues are located in the transmembrane-spanning region and may be modified by lipids to aid in insertion of the protein into the membrane. The corresponding gene was designated MUC1 and contains 7 exons and 6 introns, and is located on chromosome 1q21-24. This gene is highly polymorphic due to variable numbers of tandem repeats in each al-lele. By convention, mucin genes are designated MUC and are numbered in order of their publication.

These large membrane-bound molecules are thought to play an important role in epithelial cell surface protection. The MUC1 polypeptide is a polymorphic protein ranging from 120 to 300 kDa in size, and forms a single rod-like molecule extending above a short transmembrane sequence. Unlike the secreted mucins, MUC1 mucins do not form multimers by disulfide bonding. They are typically localized to the apical membrane of epithelial cells, with the tandem-repeat domain extending approximately 150 nm above the cell surface. This structure is thought to physically shield epithelial surface antigens or receptors from luminal agents. Several investigators have shown that transfection of a cancer cell line with a full-length cDNA encoding a MUC1 protein resulted in a high level expression of MUC1 protein at the cell surface. This resulted, in turn, in diminished cell–cell aggregation, which was not altered after the removal of sialic acid residues by neuraminidase. These results indicate that overexpression of MUC1 protein may result in steric interference with extracellular matrix or cellular adhesion molecules. It was also speculated that insertion of MUC1 mucin molecules in normal ductular structures would inhibit adhesive interactions of opposing apical membranes and facilitate duct patency.

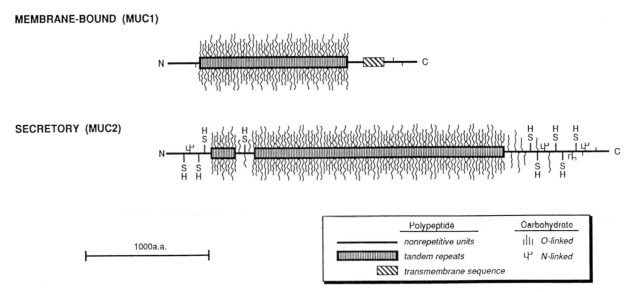

FIGURE 1   Structures of membrane-bound and secreted mucin glycoproteins based on cDNA sequence data.

Several other cell surface proteins with mucin-like regions have been described. These include complement recognition factor, platelet glycoprotein Ib, sucrase-isomaltase, GLYCAM 1, MAdCAM-1, glycophorin, and leukocyte leukosialin (CD34) molecules. These proteins have small regions containing a high proportion of serine and threonine glycosylation sites, but lack a regular tandem repeat structure. The short segments of O-linked carbohydrate within these proteins confer a rigid rod-shaped conformation to this portion of the molecule. Many of these proteins are thought to function as cell adhesion molecules.

The second family of mucins consists of the *secreted* or soluble mucins. These mucins constitute the major structural component of mucous gels that cover the respiratory, gastrointestinal, and reproductive tracts. Biochemical and expression cloning experiments have demonstrated considerable heterogeneity in mucins purified from both the respiratory tract and various regions of the intestine (Table I). Sequence analysis of cDNA clones corresponding to the MUC2 mucin gene indicates that the majority of the mucin molecule consists of an extended array of tandem repeats of 23 amino acids that are rich in threonine and proline. A second intestinal mucin cDNA was isolated and encoded 17-amino-acid tandem repeats rich in threonine and serine. The corresponding gene was localized to chromosome 7 and was termed MUC3. Several laboratories have isolated a number of tracheobronchial mucins, which include MUC4 and MUC5. Expression cloning indicates that human gastric mucosa expresses high levels of MUC5 and MUC6 mucin, the latter characterized by the longest tandem repeat sequence yet published (169 amino acids). Recently, a low molecular weight mucin has been cloned from a human salivary gene library (MUC7).

Studies using mucin-specific cDNA probes and antibodies indicate that the expression of secretory mucin genes is organ- and cell-type specific. MUC2 mRNA and protein are highly expressed in goblet cells of normal jejunum, ileum, and colon. MUC3 mRNA and protein are highly expressed in columnar and goblet cells of normal jejunum, ileum, colon, and gallbladder. These levels are contrasted with very low to undetectable levels in other epithelia (bronchus,

breast, stomach, esophagus). Conversely, MUC6 mRNA and protein are primarily found in gastric epithelium, and MUC5 is expressed in both bronchial and gastric tissues. The functional importance of different secretory mucin gene products found in different organs is unknown.

In addition, a variety of mucins from animal species have also been sequenced. Numerous unique tandem repeat sequences have been identified in these mucins which do not share homology with tandem repeats of human mucins. In contrast, the carboxyl-terminal sequence of animal and human mucins demonstrates extensive sequence similarity. Unique regions upstream and downstream of the tandem repeat array of the human MUC2 molecule have been sequenced. The carboxyl-terminal domain contains 984 residues and is divided into mucin-like repetitive units (139 residues) and cysteine-rich (845 residues) subdomains (Fig. 1). The cysteine-rich subdomain exhibits varying degrees of sequence similarity to a wide range of mucins. The degree of similarity is greatest with rat intestinal mucin protein. Lesser similarity was present with porcine submaxillary mucin, bovine submaxillary mucin-like protein, frog integumentary mucin B.1, and canine tracheobronchial mucin. Most of the cysteine residues within these regions are conserved, indicating their functional importance. The MUC2 protein demonstrates both amino- and carboxyl-terminal sequence similarity with the amino- and carboxyl-terminal domains of the von Willebrand factor. The von Willebrand factor is characterized by the formation of large oligomers (> 12,000,000 Da) via disulfide linkages between the amino- and carboxyl-terminal domains. In addition, both rat intestinal mucin and frog integumentary mucin have also been shown to contain carboxyl-terminal sequence similarity with the von Willebrand factor. These data indicate that these structural regions are necessary for the formation of protein polymers and may also play a role in the regulation of polymer formation. Electron microscopic studies have demonstrated that secreted mucins form long polymers, with molecules linked end to end. Thus, mucin monomers are thought to be linked together by terminal disulfide bonds via cysteine residues in the terminal nonrepetitive domains, and reduction of disulfide bonds has been shown to result in loss of viscosity in mucous gels.

GLYCOPROTEINS AND GLYCOSYLATION CHANGES

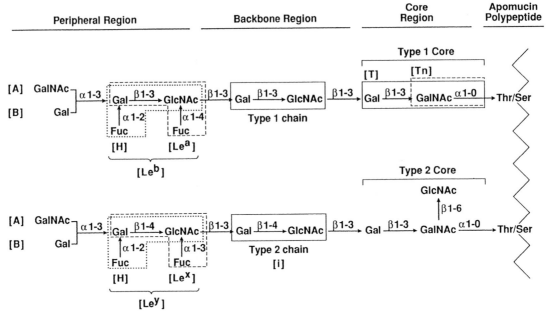

FIGURE 2 Carbohydrate side chain structures of O-linked glycoproteins.

IV. CARBOHYDRATE STRUCTURE OF O-LINKED GLYCOPROTEINS

Mucin glycoproteins contain five different sugars: N-acetylgalactosamine (GalNAc), N-acetylglucosamine (GlcNAc), N-acetylneuraminic acid (NeuAc or sialic acid) galactose (Gal), and fucose (Fuc). Mucin glycoproteins do not contain uronic acids found in proteoglycans nor mannose found in N-linked glycoproteins. These sugars form chains on the mucin peptide which can be divided into three regions: inner core, backbone, and peripheral (Fig. 2). Core oligosaccharides are first formed by the addition of GalNAc to the mucin peptide. This antigen is known as the Tn antigen. Further glycosylation of this GalNAc can be terminated by the addition of a sialic acid residue, which creates the sialosyl-Tn antigen. However, in normal tissues sialosyl-Tn usually does not occur, instead the Tn antigen is glycosylated to form core structures such as core 1, Galβ1-3GalNAc-R; the branched structure core 2, Galβ1-3(GlcNAcβ1-6)GalNAc-R; or core 3, GlcNAcβ1-3GalNAc-R. At least six types of core oligosaccharide arrangements

have been described in mucins and are listed in Fig. 3. Core type 3 predominates in normal colonic mucins and core types 1 and 2 are found in normal gastric mucins.

The core regions are elongated by two major types of backbone chains. The type 1 chain consists of Galβ1-3GlcNAc (also named "lacto") and the type 2 chain (named "neolacto") consists of Galβ1-4Glc-NAc (Fig. 2). Neolacto chains are also known as the "i" antigen. The backbone oligosaccharides may also branch via a β1-6 linkage of the GlcNAc of one type

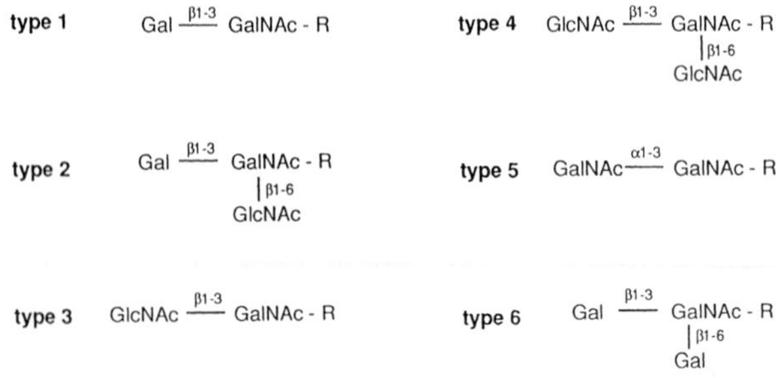

type 1	Gal $\xrightarrow{\beta 1\text{-}3}$ GalNAc - R	type 4	GlcNAc $\xrightarrow{\beta 1\text{-}3}$ GalNAc - R $\mid \beta 1\text{-}6$ GlcNAc
type 2	Gal $\xrightarrow{\beta 1\text{-}3}$ GalNAc - R $\mid \beta 1\text{-}6$ GlcNAc	type 5	GalNAc $\xrightarrow{\alpha 1\text{-}3}$ GalNAc - R
type 3	GlcNAc $\xrightarrow{\beta 1\text{-}3}$ GalNAc - R	type 6	Gal $\xrightarrow{\beta 1\text{-}3}$ GalNAc - R $\mid \beta 1\text{-}6$ Gal

FIGURE 3 Core carbohydrate structures found in O-linked glycoproteins.

2 chain onto the Gal of another type 2 chain, which forms the "I" antigen. Backbone chains may also be branched by a mixture of type 1 and type 2 chain linkages.

The nonreducing ends of backbone sequences are often terminated with carbohydrates which create ABH and Lewis type blood group antigens. The antigen formed is dependent on the presence of specific glycosyltransferases, such as the protein products of secretor gene (Se) and Lewis (Le) genes. The secretor gene encodes for an α1-2 fucosyltransferase which transfers a fucose to terminal Gal residues of type 1 or type 2 chains to form the blood group H determinant. This in turn becomes the substrate for blood group A and B α1-3 glycosyltransferases, resulting in chain termination. The Lewis gene encodes for an α1-4 fucosyltransferase which adds a fucose to penultimate GlcNAc residues, resulting in the Le^a antigen on type 1 chains and the Le^x antigen on type 2 chains. Activation of both the secretor gene and the Lewis gene products results in the formation of difucosylated antigens: Le^b on type 1 chains and Le^y on type 2 chains (see Fig. 2). Approximately 20–25% of the population lack blood group H fucosyltransferase and are termed "nonsecretors." These individuals normally express little or no ABH, Le^b, and Le^y antigens.

Up to half the oligosaccharides in mucins carry acidic groups, which are responsible for the polyanionic nature of mucins. Sialic acid residues can be found attached to core or peripheral carbohydrates. Sialic acid and sulfate are usually present on different oligosaccharide units, and sulfation predominantly occurs on longer oligosaccharide chains. Sulfates may also be attached via Gal or GlcNAc sugars.

V. GLYCOSYLTRANSFERASE ENZYMES

The addition of each oligosaccharide is controlled by specific glycosyltransferases located in the Golgi apparatus of the cell. Control of carbohydrate antigen synthesis depends on substrate availability and the types and activities of glycosyltransferase enzymes. It is estimated that approximately 100 different glycosyltransferase enzymes are required to synthesize the diverse types of carbohydrate patterns found on glycoproteins and glycolipids. To date, a number of glycosyltransferase enzymes have been characterized by molecular sequencing (Table II).

Sequence data indicate that these enzymes share a common domain structure, consisting of an amino-terminal cytoplasmic domain, a signal-anchor domain,

TABLE II
Cloned Glycosyltransferase Enzymes

Family	Glycosyltransferase	Reference[a]
Sialyltransferases	Galα2,6-ST	1
	Galβ1,3(4)GlcNAcα2,3-ST	2
	Galβ1,3GalNAcα2,3-ST	3
Galactosyltransferases	GlcNAcβ1,4-GT	4,5
	Galα1,3-GT	6,7
Fucosyltransferases	GlcNAcα1,3-FT	8
	Galα1,2-FT	9
N-Acetylgalactosaminyltransferase	Galα,2-GALNAcT	10

[a]Key to references: *(1)* Weinstein *et al.* (1987), JBC **263,** 17735; *(2)* Wen *et al.* (1992). JBC **267,** 21011; *(3)* Gillespie *et al.* (1992). JBC **267,** 21004; *(4)* Shaper *et al.* (1986). *Proc. Natl. Acad. Sci. USA* **83,** 1573; *(5)* Narimatsu *et al.* (1986). *Proc. Natl. Acad. Sci. USA* **83,** 4720; *(6)* Joziasse *et al.* (1989). JBC **264,** 14290; *(7)* Larsen *et al.* (1989). *Proc. Natl. Acad. Sci. USA* **87,** 6674; *(8)* Goelz *et al.* (1990). *Cell* **63,** 1349; *(9)* Yamamoto *et al.* (1990). *Nature* **345,** 229; *(10)* Yamamoto *et al.* (1990). JBC **265,** 1146.

and a large luminal carboxyl-terminal catalytic domain. Variable homology exists between different types of glycosyltransferase enzymes. Members of the sialyltransferase family contain a 55-amino-acid region in the center of the molecule with 45–56% homology, which may represent the acceptor- or donor-binding site. Outside this region these molecules share no homology. Marked homology was demonstrated for blood group A enzyme (Fucα1,2Galα1,3GalNAc-transferase) and the blood group B enzyme (Fucα1, 2Galα1,3Gal-transferase), which differ in only 4 amino acids. In contrast, cDNAs of two galactosyltransferases (Galβ1,4Glc-NAcα1,3-galactosyltransferase and GlcNAcβ1,4-galactosyltransferase) dem-onstrate no homology.

The regulation of glycosyltransferase enzymes is poorly understood. J. C. Paulson and other investigators have demonstrated that expression of glycosyltransferase genes demonstrates tissue- and cell-specific differences, which is determined at the level of transcription. Galα2,6-sialyltransferase mRNA varies up to 100-fold in various rat tissues as does its enzyme activity. Genomic sequencing of Galα2,6-sialyltransferase indicates that multiple transcripts are produced via a combination of alternative splicing and alternate promoter use which is regulated in a tissue-specific fashion. Whether other glycosyltransferase enzymes have similar organizational and regulatory construction remains unknown.

Few examples exist of the regulation of glycosyltransferases by polypeptide sequences. Glycosyltransferases responsible for specific N-linked carbohydrate addition to lysozomal enzymes, luteinizing hormone and thyroid-stimulating hormone pituitary hormones, and neural cell adhesion molecule N-CAM all appear to contain polypeptide recognition sites. More commonly, polypeptide chains may regulate glycosyltransferase activity by conformational restraints surrounding glycosylation sites. For example, the presence of adjacent proline or GalNAc residues to serine or threonine glycosylation sites can influence the activities of polypeptide:GalNAc transferase enzymes (responsible for the initial glycosylation of mucin core peptides). These data indicate that the glycosyltransferase enzymes, the carbohydrate donors, and the polypeptide sequence acceptors present within a cell

all may contribute to determining peripheral carbohydrate structures.

VI. ALTERATIONS OF MUCIN-ASSOCIATED CARBOHYDRATES IN CANCER

A. Peripheral and Backbone Carbohydrates

Peripheral carbohydrate antigens are commonly altered on glycoproteins and glycolipids synthesized by adenocarcinomas. The overall carbohydrate content of cancers is generally reduced compared with normal tissues. For example, biochemical analysis reveals that all five sugars are reduced in colon cancer mucin, and the overall carbohydrate content of colon cancers is approximately 50% that of normal colon. This results from a decrease in both the number and the length of oligosaccharide chains. Qualitative alterations of carbohydrate antigens have been extensively catalogued using immunohistochemical studies with monoclonal antibodies. In general, these alterations may be grouped into five categories (Table III).

1. *Increased* quantities of antigen compared with normal tissues.
2. *Reappearance* of normal antigens that are usually present in fetal tissue ("oncofetal antigens").
3. Expression of antigens *incompatible* with the patients blood type.
4. *Deletion* of antigens normally expressed in normal tissues, which may result in exposure of precursor or inner core antigenic structures.
5. *Neosynthesis* of new and unique antigens.

Alterations of blood group-related antigens in colorectal cancers exemplify these changes. In the fetus, A, B, H, Le[a], and Le[b] antigens are expressed throughout the colon; however, all but Le[a] disappear in the distal colon after birth. These antigens commonly reappear in premalignant adenomas and carcinomas arising in the distal colon. Conversely, deletion of normally appearing A, B, H, and Le[b] antigen frequently occurs in cancers arising in the proximal colon, and deletion of Le[a] antigens occurs in distal colonic cancers. Blood group H antigen is a structural

TABLE III
Mucin Glycoprotein Antigens in Normal and Neoplastic Gastrointestinal Tissues[a]

Antigenic alteration	Normal colon	Colon adenoma	Colon cancer	Normal pancreas	Chronic pancreatitis	Pancreatic cancer	Normal stomach	Gastric cancer
Reappearance								
A, B, H (distal colon)	1	73	70–100					
Le^b (distal colon)	5	90	95					
Incompatibility								
A, B, H, Le^b	0	38	61	0		13	Le^a 0	Le^a 73
Deletion								
A, B, Le^b (proximal colon)	0	18	43	0		33 (B antigen)	Le^{ab} 0	Le^{ab} 22
Le^a	0	21	0					
Core carbohydrate exposure								
Tn	14	100	72–81	0		100	92	87
T	0	100	71	53–70		44–100	0	
Sialosyl-Tn	0	60–100	93–96	0		97–100	0	92–100
Core mucin peptide exposure								
MUC1	10	57	71	100		100	100	91
MUC2	92	100	91	0		18	0	42
MUC3	47	53	60	0		45	0	45
Neosynthesis								
Sialosyl-Le^a	0–45	51–81	59–82	100		80–84	16	48
Le^x (SSEA-1)	89 p[b], 46 p	73 p, 90 d	92 p, 92 d	0	0	71	100	66
Extended Le^x (FH1)	0–8	50	82–86					
Sialosyl-extended Le^x (1B9)	8–15	45–56	60–67	0	20	57		
Difucosyl-Le^x (FH4)	0–8	46	96	0	20	54		
Sialosyl-difucosyl Le^x (FH6)	0	60–65	72–82	0	20	63		
Extended Le^y (CC1, CC2)	21–38 p, 0–6 d	33–60 p, 39–50 d	83 p, 58–79 d	55–73	30–50	37–49	0	67
Trifucosyl Le^y (KH-1)	27 p, 0 d	67 p, 43 d	70 p, 53 d	32	40	31		

[a]Expressed as the percentage of specimens with positive immunoreactivity.
[b]p, proximal colon; d, distal colon.

precursor to A and B antigens, is found in 90% of colon cancers, and is generally present when appropriate A and B antigens are not expressed. In addition, expression of A, B, H, and Le^b antigens that are incompatible with the patients blood type may occur in 38 and 61% of colonic adenomas and carcinomas, respectively. This alteration is more specific for neoplasia since it was not observed in hyperplastic polyps or fetal colonic mucosa. Incompatible blood group antigen expression has also been described in gastric, pancreatic, and hepatocellular adenocarcinomas. Individuals who have the "secretor" gene express gastric mucins with the Le^{a-b+} phenotype. Gastric dysplasia and cancer occurring in these individuals frequently express incompatible Le^a antigen.

"Neosynthesis" of novel oligosaccharides in adenocarcinomas also results in more cancer-specific markers. Sialosylation of simple or fucosylated type 1 backbone chains produces the CA-50 antigen ($NeuAc\alpha1,3Gal\beta1,3GlcNAc$) and sialosyl-$Le^a$ antigen [$NeuAc\alpha1,3Gal\beta1,3(Fuc\alpha1,4)GlcNAc$, also known as CA19-9 and GICA]. These antigens are found on glycolipids and glycoproteins of a variety of adenocarcinomas; however, they are released into the circulation or secreted into pancreatic secretions on mucin-like glycoproteins. In contrast with normal colon, sialosyl-Le^a expression is increased in fetal colon, in hyperplastic and adenomatous polyps, and in most colorectal cancers regardless of location or differentiation. However, sialosyl-Le^a expression does not correlate with stage, DNA aneuploidy, or prognosis in colorectal carcinoma patients. Most endometrial, gastric, and pancreatic carcinomas express focal sialosyl-Le^a immunoreactivity, whereas this is rarely found in breast adenocarcinomas.

"Neosynthetic" alterations of the type 2 backbone chains have been described in adenocarcinomas of the gastrointestinal tract, breast, and lung. Type 2 chains synthesized as simple, repeating, unbranched structures are highly expressed in colon, liver, and lung carcinomas, and are absent or weakly expressed in corresponding normal tissues. S. Hakomori and coworkers have shown that fucosylated and/or sialosylated type 2 chains are also preferentially expressed by carcinomas compared with normal epithelium. Distribution of these antigens in colon and pancreatic disease has been described in detail (Table III). Short chain Le^x determinants are expressed in the normal colon with a decreasing proximal to distal gradient and are absent in normal pancreas. Expression of this antigen is enhanced in colorectal and particularly in pancreatic cancer. Extended difucosyl and extended-sialylated Le^x-type antigens are rarely expressed in normal colon and pancreas or chronic pancreatitis specimens. In contrast, these antigens are expressed in the majority of adenomatous polyps and colon and pancreatic cancers. The difucosyl-Le^x structure was the most colon cancer-specific epitope in one study. Expression of these antigens in adenomatous polyps correlates with criteria indicative of greater potential for malignant transformation (increasing size, villous histology, and dysplasia). The finding of difucosyl-Le^x immunoreactivity in the majority of hyperplastic colonic polyps indicates that this antigen may also become expressed in mucosa abnormal growth characteristics which are not considered to be premalignant.

The extended and trifucosylated type 2 chain (Le^y-type) antigens are weakly expressed in normal colon (proximal sites only) but are highly expressed in the majority of adenomas with an increased risk for malignant transformation and in colon cancers. These epitopes are absent in hyperplastic polyps. In contrast, these extended or polyfucosylated Le^y antigens do not discriminate among normal, benign, or malignant disease in the pancreas.

B. Core Carbohydrates

Core carbohydrate structures frequently are expressed in O-linked glycoproteins derived from adenocarcinomas, which correlates with the overall diminished amount of carbohydrates and the resultant "unmasking" of these structures (Fig. 4). Tn and T antigens have been shown to be present on greater than 90% of primary adenocarcinomas and their metastases. In contrast, they are hidden in normal tissues as evidenced by their appearance if the tissue is treated with neuraminidase. Exposure of these epitopes in cancer patients results in the stimulation of an immune response, resulting in circulating antibodies directed against these antigens. Sialosyl-Tn is also a "pan-carcinoma" epitope. This antigen is detected by immunohistochemical techniques in adenocarcinomas of the colon (94%), breast (84%), lung (non-small cell, 96%), and ovary

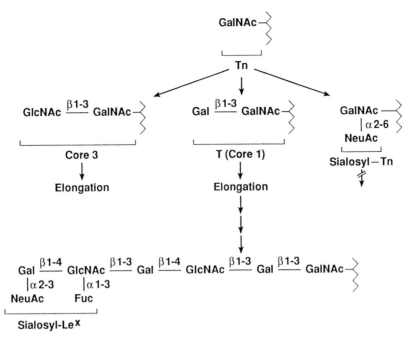

FIGURE 4 Possible glycosylation pathways of core Tn antigen of O-linked glycoproteins. In normal tissues the Tn antigen is glycosylated to form one of the core carbohydrate structures, which is elongated by type 1 or type 2 chains and terminated by a blood group carbohydrate antigen. In cancer tissues the Tn antigen can be sialosylated, which terminates glycosylation, or it can be elongated to form an antigen normally found in lesser amounts in normal tissues, such as the sialosyl-Le[x] antigen pictured.

(100%) and in most pancreatic, gastric, and esophageal cancers evaluated. Tn, T, and sialosyl-Tn epitopes also are frequently identified in the normal appearing "transitional" mucosa adjacent to colorectal cancers, indicating that other factors besides malignancy may affect expression of these epitopes.

Conversion of core carbohydrate structures also occurs in adenocarcinoma mucins. Detailed analyses of core carbohydrate structures isolated from a human rectal cancer indicate that carbohydrates occur on a variety of core types, namely core types 1, 3, and 5. Similarly, core carbohydrates isolated from a human colon cancer cell line included core types 1, 2, and 4. This markedly contrasts with normal colonic mucins which contain primarily core 3 structures.

C. Mucin-Related Antigens with Undetermined Epitopes

Several of these mucin-associated antigens are not fully characterized chemically. These include crypt cell antigen, M1, SIMA, LIMA, Cora antigen, NCC-CO-450 antigen, DuPan-2, SPan-1, YPan-1, and CA-125. These antigens are generally strongly expressed by a variety of adenocarcinomas relative to corresponding normal tissues and are frequently secreted into the circulation (Table IV).

D. Biochemical Mechanisms of Altered Carbohydrate Antigens

The biochemical mechanisms responsible for these blood group antigen alterations in colon cancers compared with normal colon remain unclear. Possibilities include decreased activities of glycosyltransferase enzymes, lack of appropriate enzymatic substrates, loss of glycosyltransferase specificity for specific substrates, *de novo* expression of a novel glycosyltransferase, increased glycosidase activities, or masking of antigen by synthesis of neoantigens. Changes in carbohydrate structures demonstrated in cancers have been related to changes in the relevant glycosyltransferase, and the aberrant expression of a glycosyltransferase in cancer tissue has been demonstrated. In colorectal cancers most studies have reported decreased activities of a variety of glycosyltransferases in colon cancers compared with adjacent normal colon. More specifically, Itzkowitz and coworkers compared the presence of immunoreactive blood group antigens with the activities of glycosyltransferase and glycosidase enzymes in normal colon and colon cancers. Despite the fact that blood group A, B, H, and Le[b] antigens are not found in distal colon, the activities of their corresponding glycosyltransferase enzymes were the same in proximal and distal normal colonic specimens. Cancers demonstrated lower A transferase activities compared with normal mucosa; however, blood group A immunoreactivity was present in 9 of 10 of these cancers. Two cancers lacked blood group B immunoreactivity, and B transferase activity was decreased. The H antigen was expressed in the cancers of all blood type O patients and also in the cancers of one blood type B patient and one blood type A patient. Blood group H (α1,2 fucosyl) transferase activities in these cancers did not differ from normal colon in both proximal and distal locations. Blood group A and B glycosidase activities were also similar in cancer and normal tissue. These studies indicate that the presence of a specific glycosyltransferase enzyme is a necessary but not sufficient factor to account for blood group antigen expression and that lack of precursor substance (via diversion of precursors into alternate synthetic pathways) was the most likely explanation of the absence of A, B, or H antigens in the distal colon. The availability of molecular probes for various glycosyltransferase enzymes may help clarify the mechanisms of altered carbohydrates in cancer glycoproteins.

VII. ALTERED MUCIN GENE EXPRESSION IN CANCER

A. Mucin Gene-Related Alterations

Less is known concerning alterations of specific mucin peptides in adenocarcinomas. Biochemical and mo-

lecular experiments have demonstrated that mucin protein and mRNA levels are frequently altered in adenocarcinomas compared to corresponding normal tissues. Alterations include increased expression, loss of expression, and aberrant expression. Antibodies that recognize the core tandem repeat sequences of mucins often demonstrate increased immunoreactive mucin proteins in cancers compared with normal tissues, most likely due to incomplete glycosylation and unmasking of peptide epitopes (Table III). Increased core peptide immunoreactivity correlates with increased mucin mRNA in breast and well-differentiated lung adenocarcinomas compared with normal tissue. MUC2 and MUC3 mRNA levels are increased in colloid colon cancer compared with normal colon; however, in well- and moderately well-differentiated colon cancers, MUC1, MUC2, and MUC3 mRNA levels are decreased. Gastric cancers of all histologic subtypes demonstrate decreased MUC5 and MUC6 gene expression. In addition, focal aberrant expression of MUC2, MUC3, and MUC4 genes can occur in breast, lung, gastric, and pancreatic cancers. Coexpression of multiple mucin genes is more frequently observed in advanced gastric cancers compared with early Stage I and II gastric cancers. These data demonstrate that neoplastic transformation is associated with dysregulated expression of both membrane-found and secreted mucin core protein epitopes, presumably due to both altered mucin mRNA levels and altered mucin glycosylation.

Little information exists concerning structural alterations of mucin genes in cancers. G. R. Merlo, D. W. Kufe, and co-workers examined 110 breast adenocarcinomas for MUC1 restriction fragment-length polymorphisms. Seventy of 110 breast cancer specimens were constitutionally heterozygous (informative). Twenty (29%) of the tumor DNAs demonstrated loss of one MUC1 allele. Eight (11%) of the tumor DNAs demonstrated increased MUC1 gene copy number in one allele. Of these, one case with increased copy number resulted from trisomy of chromosome 1. These data indicate that the MUC1 locus is frequently altered in these adenocarcinomas. Further studies of the relationship of MUC1 and secreted mucin gene abnormalities with alterations of mucin transcription and translation will clarify this issue.

VIII. CLINICAL APPLICATIONS OF CANCER-ASSOCIATED GLYCOPROTEIN ANTIGENS

A. Serologic Markers of Cancer

Glycoprotein antigens listed in Table IV show potential for their use in specific clinical circumstances, such as evaluating response to therapy or for prediction of relapse in patients with initially elevated serum levels. In the circulation these antigens are generally found on high molecular weight mucin-type glycoproteins. Most clinically useful markers are peripheral or core carbohydrate antigens which are highly expressed in cancers and rarely expressed in normal tissues. However, to date, no serologic marker has been shown to be sensitive or specific enough in early stage disease to be reliable as a tool for screening or diagnosing of adenocarcinomas.

Immunohistochemical studies indicate that different mucin-related carbohydrate antigens are frequently coexpressed by individual adenocarcinomas; however, certain adenocarcinomas may preferentially release one type of antigen into the circulation. As illustrated in Table IV, sialosylated type 1 backbone chain epitopes recognized by 19-9 and Ca-50 and the indeterminate epitopes SPan-1 and DuPan-2 are more commonly detected in serum of patients with pancreatic adenocarcinoma compared with colonic, gastric, lung, or breast adenocarcinomas. SPan-1 (which is a sialosylated epitope similar but not identical to sialosyl Le[a]) provides greater sensitivity and predictive value than 19-9 and DuPan-2 in patients with pancreatic carcinoma, and all three are much more sensitive and specific compared with carcinoembryonic antigen (CEA) assays in these patients. Similarly, TAG-72 and CA 19-9 have demonstrated comparable sensitivity and improved specificity in serologic assays of patients with colorectal cancer when compared with CEA. Numerous mucin-related epitopes are detectable in ovarian cancers; however, CA-125 remains the most frequently detected epitope in the circulation of these patients. CA-125 has been shown to be superior to 15-3, CA19-9, TAG-72, and CA-50 in predicting the clinical course of these patients.

MUC1-related mucin polypeptide antigens are also detectable in the serum of patients with adenocarcinomas of the breast, gastrointestinal tract, lung, and ovary. The antigen 15-3 is detected using a bideterminant radioimmunoassay using antibodies DF3 and 115D8. Hayes and co-workers have shown this assay to be more sensitive than CEA assays in patients with primary and metastatic breast cancer, and also to correlate with clinical disease course in the majority of these patients. The specificity of this test is limited due to the high frequency of elevated levels in patients with chronic hepatitis or cirrhosis. Serologic assays for MUC2- or MUC3-related polypeptide epitopes are currently being developed.

Mucins with Le[x]- or Le[y]-related type 2 chain antigens are secreted into the circulation in many adenocarcinoma patients (Table IV). Studies from Hakomori's laboratory indicate that mono and dimeric Lex antigens are found in the serum of 85% of adenocarcinoma patients compared to lower levels detected in 33% of normal sera. This glycoprotein is distinct from glycoproteins carrying CEA or sialosyl-Lea epitopes. The presence of this antigen in the serum of colon cancer patients correlates with the more invasive disease: Dukes A, 20%; Dukes B, 45%; Dukes C, 67%; and Dukes D, 74%.

B. Glycoprotein Carbohydrate Antigens and Cancer Prognosis

Qualitative changes in glycoprotein oligosaccharides may also play an important role in determining the biological behavior of adenocarcinoma cells. For example, histochemical studies have suggested that sialomucin content is higher in colorectal cancers which are more aggressive and associated with a poor prognosis. The core glycosidic sialosyl-Tn glycoprotein epitope was examined by immunohistochemical techniques in 128 primary colorectal carcinoma specimens. Sialosyl-Tn expression was observed in 87.5% of specimens and did not correlate with tumor location, Dukes stage, differentiation, or ploidy status. However, sialosyl-Tn positivity was associated with diminished 5-year survival compared with sialosyl-Tn negative patients (73% vs 100%, $P < 0.05$). Multivariate regression analysis indicated that DNA ploidy ($P < 0.001$) and sialosyl-Tn expression ($P < 0.05$) were the two most important variables for prediction of disease free and overall survival. Increased expression of the

TABLE IV

Serologic Detection of Carbohydrate and Mucin-Type Glycoprotein Antigens[a]

Name	Antigen	Normal	Benign[b] disease	Carcinoma Colorectal	Pancreas	Stomach	Liver	Breast	Lung	Ovary
49H.8 (T-F antigen)	T	9	—	61	—	—	—	52	54	55
TAG-72	Sialosyl-Tn	1	4–8	19–25 early[c] 35–79 late	46–74	44–48	—	7–39	27	52–66
JT10e	Sialosyl-Tn	6	10	38	42	31	38	32	28	15
AH-6	Le^y	3	4–7	7	41	18	34	5	16	15
FH2	Le^x	2	5–8	10	22	9	15	2	7	14
SH1/SH2	Mono and dimeric Le^x	1	13	39 early 68 late	—	—	—	60	60	—
CSLEX1	Sialosyl-Le^x	0.7–4	0.9–14	25–44	33–37	19–26	—	19–52	29–52	—
FH6	Sialosyl-difucosyl Le^x	0–3	2–13	25	32–66	16 early 33 late	24	14–20	42–71	23
CA19-9	Sialosyl-Le^a	0.6	1.5–22 (pancreatitis)	4–25 early 47–67 late	79–87	36–50	51	18	25 early 40–50 late (all types)	26
SPan-1	Sialosyl-Le^a-type epitope	0–2	5–54 (liver disease)	13–41	81–93	23	59	—	—	—
CA-50	Sialosyl-type 1 backbone chain	0.7	8–34 (liver disease)	50 early 75 late	71	43	—	48	52	29–40
DU-PAN-2	Neuraminidase/alkaline sensitive epitope	0–4	5–20	6–11	68–87	19–40	44–85	0	14	0
MAM-6 (115D8)	MUC1 mucin epitope	4.5	3–80 (liver disease)	21	—	—	—	23 early 62 late	33	78
15-3	MUC1 peptide	1–9	8–44 (liver disease)	61	80	14	36	29 early 73 late	71	66
CSAp	Heat/thiol-sensitive epitope	3	18	61	20	20	—	5	—	—
CA-125	Mucin peptide epitope	1	6–10	22	59	11	40	12	19 early 23 late	68–87
NCC-CO-450	Nonsialic acid carbohydrate epitope	3	—	56	50	40	25	42	—	—

[a]Expressed as the percentage of patients with serum levels above normal limits.
[b]Condition in parentheses is associated with highest percentage of positive tests.
[c]Early, stage 1–2 disease; late, stage 3–4 disease.

sialosyl-Le^x antigen in colon cancers has also been shown to correlate with poor survival.

Recent studies from Lee *et al.* and Miyake *et al.* indicate that alterations of blood group-related oligosaccharides may also predict the biological behavior of primary lung cancers. In the first study, deletion of blood group A antigen was associated with diminished survival compared with blood group A antigen-positive cases. In this series the expression of blood group B or H antigens did not correlate with survival. Deletion of the A and B blood group results in the exposure of H, Le^y, and Le^b antigens. This deletion is identified by monoclonal antibody MIA-15-5, which recognizes Fucα1-2Galβ1-R on type 1 or type 2 backbone chains. In the second study, adenocarcinomas and squamous cell carcinomas of the lung with positive MIA-15-5 reactivity demonstrated decreased survival in patients with blood groups A and AB. The mechanism responsible for this observation is unknown; however, blood group H antigens may play a role as recognition sites for cell motility factors or adhesion molecules.

C. Glycoprotein Carbohydrate Antigens and Cancer Metastases

Increased metastatic potential may be one mechanism whereby altered cell surface glycoproteins influence cancer survival. Sialosylated cell surface glycoproteins have been associated with enhanced metastatic potential in a variety of malignant cell types in experimental systems. Furthermore, inhibition of glycoprotein glycosylation by the use of competitive inhibitors of sialyltransferase or polypeptidyl-GalNAc transferase or the enzyme tunicamycin results in diminished metastatic abilities of cancer cell lines.

Metastatic colon cancers have been reported to express altered lectin reactivities and increased expression of sialosyl-Tn and sialosyl-extended Le^x glycoconjugates. Levels of these sialosylated mucin antigen levels are higher in metastases compared with primary tumors and lower in early stage primary tumors compared with more invasive or later stage primary tumors. Accordingly, the levels of sialosyl-extended Le^x in colorectal cancers have been shown to correlate with early recurrence and metastasis.

The mechanism by which sialosylation alters metastatic abilities of cells may be multifactorial. Sialosylation of mucin and other glycoconjugate epitopes may affect growth regulation, cellular adhesion, and/or cell-substratum invasion. Sialylated tumor-associated antigens have recently been shown to be the ligands for binding to selectin-type molecules. Selectins are a family of cell adhesion molecules that share a common structural motif consisting of an NH$_2$ terminal lectin-like domain, an epidermal growth factor repeat, and a variable number of complement regulatory-like modules. These molecules are expressed on the cell surfaces of white blood cells, platelets, and endothelial cells. The ligands for the lectin-like domain of selectins have been shown to include Le^x, sialylated Le^x, and sialylated Le^a carbohydrates. Since these structures are commonly expressed on malignant cells, they may play a role in selectin-mediated adhesion to endothelial cells and platelets with resultant initiation of metastasis.

In addition, mucin glycoproteins demonstrate inhibitory effects on certain immune effector cells. For example, MUC1-type mucin (DF3 antigen) purified from a breast carcinoma cell line and human breast milk has been shown to prevent the adherence of eosinophils to human immunoglobulin-conjugated targets. These data raise the possibility that MUC1 mucin may protect epithelial cells from the cytotoxic effects of activated inflammatory cells. This may promote metastases by serving as one mechanism by which mucin-producing cancer cells avoid immune destruction.

D. Altering Cancer Progression: Glycoprotein-Related Antigens as Targets for Immunotherapy

Altered mucin glycoprotein-related antigens may serve as targets for an anti-tumor immune response in cancer patients. O. J. Finn and co-workers have shown that cytotoxic T cells derived from patients with breast, pancreatic, or ovarian cancer recognize cell surface MUC1-type core tandem repeat sequences. Mucin-specific T cells preferentially recognize mucins made by malignant cells rather than normal cells. This recognition is not major histocompatability complex restricted, presumably because the extensive tandem repeats facilitate cross-linking of T-cell receptors on mucin-specific T cells. Transfection of autologous or allogenic B cells with MUC1 mucin cDNA results in cells that are able to present this antigen and become susceptible to lysis by specific cytotoxic T cells. Treatment of the cells with inhibitors of O-glycosylation increased their susceptibility to lysis. Target cells transfected with the same mucin construct exhibited a variety of tumor-associated epitopes, which were also increased when the cells were incubated with inhibitors of O-glycosylation. In addition, cytotoxic T cells readily recognize target cells that are transfected with cDNA encoding only two 20-amino-acid tandem repeat sequences. These data indicate that differences in glycosylation are responsible for tumor-associated mucin antigen expression and T-cell recognition rather than differences in the mucin protein itself. Stimulation of cytotoxic T cells by core sequences of other mucins such as MUC2 and MUC3 have not been examined to date.

Stimulation of an anti-tumor immune response can also be accomplished by immunization with specific carbohydrate antigens. Fung and co-workers found that immunization of mice with a synthetic T antigen linked to the carrier protein keyhole limpet hemocyanin resulted in IgG antibody and T-cell-mediated delayed hypersensitivity responses. This resulted in suppression of T antigen expressing TA3-HA tumor cells. In addition, Singhal, Fohn, and Hakomori found that mice immunized with asialo-ovine submaxillary mucin demonstrated a T-cell response against Tn antigen and resistance to the growth of syngeneic TA3-HA tumor cells.

Monoclonal antibodies against mucin-related antigens may also be used for targeting radioisotopes (^{131}I, ^{111}In, [131]Tc) or cytotoxic drugs. Heterogeneity of antigen expression in tissues may be overcome with the use of relatively tumor-specific monoclonal antibodies which recognize different epitopes. Producing "humanized" murine monoclonal antibodies is necessary to avoid immunologic destruction of these antibodies. Future research will continue to focus on aberrantly glycosylated antigens on cell surface and secreted glycoproteins for immunotherapy and anti-tumor vaccines.

See Also the Following Articles

CELL–MATRIX INTERACTIONS • GLUTATHIONE TRANSFERASES • P-GLYCOPROTEIN AS A GENERAL ANTIAPOPTOTIC PROTEIN

Bibliography

Bresalier, R. S., Niu, Y., Byrd, J. C., Duh, Q. Y., Toribara, N. W., Dahiya, R., and Kim, Y. S. (1991). Mucin production by human colonic carcinoma cells correlates with their metastatic potential in animal models of human colon cancer metastasis. *J. Clin. Invest.* **87,** 1037–1045.

Carraway, K. L., Fregien, N., Carraway, K. L., III, and Carraway, C. A. C. (1992). Tumor sialomucin complexes as tumor antigens and modulators of cellular interactions and proliferation. *J. Cell. Sci.* **103,** 299–307.

Fung, P. Y. S., Madej, M., Koganty, R. R., and Longenecker, B. M. (1990). Specific immunotherapy of a murine mammary adenocarcinoma using a synthetic tumor-associated glycoconjugate. *Cancer Res.* **50,** 4308–4314.

Hakomori, S. I. (1989). Aberrant glycosylation in tumors and tumor-associated carbohydrate antigens. *Adv. Cancer Res.* **52,** 257–331.

Ho, S. B., Shekels, L. L., Toribara, N. W., Kim, Y. S., Lyftogt, C., Cherwitz, D. L., and Niehans, G. A. (1995). Mucin gene expression in normal, preneoplastic, and neoplastic human gastric epithelium. *Cancer Res.* **55,** 2681–2690.

Irimura, T., Nakamori, S., Matsushita, Y., Taniuchi, Y., Todoroki, N., Tsuji, T., Izumi, Y., Kawamura, Y., Hoff, S. D., Cleary, K. R., and Ota, D. M. (1993). Colorectal cancer metastasis determined by carbohydrate-mediated cell adhesion: Role of sialyl-LeX antigens. *Semin. Cancer Biol.* **4,** 319–324.

Jerome, K. R., Domenech, N., and Finn, O. J. (1993). Tumor-specific cytotoxic T cell clones from patients with breast and pancreatic adenocarcinoma recognize EBV-immortalized B cells transfected with polymorphic epithelial mucin complementary DNA. *J. Immunol.* **151,** 1654–1662.

Miyake, M., Taki, T., Hitomi, S., and Hakomori, S.-I. (1992). Correlation of expression of H/LeY/LeB antigens with survival in patients with carcinoma of the lung. *N. Engl. J. Med.* **327,** 14–18.

Paulson, J. C. (1989). Glycosyltransferases: Structure, localization, and control of cell type-specific glycosylation. *J. Biol. Chem.* **264,** 17615–17618.

Strous, G. J., and Dekker, J. (1992). Mucin-type glycoproteins. *Crit. Rev. Biochem. Mol. Biol.* **27,** 57–92.

Graft versus Leukemia and Graft versus Tumor Activity

Cornelius Schmaltz
Marcel R. M. van den Brink
Memorial Sloan-Kettering Cancer Center

I. Introduction
II. Experimental and Clinical Evidence
III. Mechanisms of the Graft versus Leukemia/Graft versus Tumor (GvL/GvT) Effect
IV. Attempts to Separate Graft-versus-Host Disease and GvL/GvT
V. Clinical Application and Future Direction

GLOSSARY

donor leukocyte infusion Infusion of donor leukocytes (or mononuclear cells) into patients with malignancies, usually after HCT. The intent is to induce a (→) graft-versus-leukemia or (→) graft-versus-tumor effect in order to treat or prevent relapse of the malignant disease.

graft-versus-host disease (GvHD) Condition that is caused by the attack of alloreactive donor cells against host tissues. Bowel, liver, and skin are classic target organs, but other tissues (lungs, thymus) might also be affected. GvHD is a major complication of (→) hematopoetic cell tranplantation or (→) donor leukocyte infusion and contributes significantly to transplant-related mortality.

graft-versus-leukemia and graft-versus-tumor effect Killing (or growth inhibition) of leukemia/tumor cells by allogeneic donor cells after (→) hematopoetic cell transplantation or (→) donor leukocyte infusion. Therapeutic use of this effect for the treatment of leukemia/solid tumors contributes to leukemic/tumor control and eventually to a decrease in death from leukemia/tumor and/or prolonged survival.

hematopoetic cell transplantation (HCT) Transfer of autologous or allogeneic lymphohematopoetic cells. Originally conceived as bone marrow transplantation, alternative sources of stem cells, such as umbilical cord blood cells or peripheral blood stem cells, are increasingly being used. While autologous HCT is used as a rescue after myeloablative chemo- or radiation therapy, allogeneic HCT provides the additional therapeutic advantage of a (→) graft-versus-leukemia or (→) graft-versus-tumor effect when used in patients with malignancies. Preparative regimens prior to HCT have traditionally consisted of myeloablative radio- and/or chemotherapy, but (→) nonmyeloablative regimens for use with allogeneic HCT have been developed.

nonmyeloablative stem cell tranplantation (NST) Also called "minitransplants," NST is a term used for recently developed less intensive preparative regimens prior to (→)

hematopoetic cell transplantation. NST uses the (→) graft-versus-leukemia or (→) graft-versus-tumor effect as its primary therapeutic modality. While NST has the advantage of decreased toxicity from the preparative regimen, it still carries the risks of (→) graft-versus-host disease and prolonged immunosuppression.

Since the 1950s there has been experimental and subsequently clinical evidence for an effect of allogeneic hematopoetic cells against leukemias (graft versus leukemia, GvL) and, more recently, solid tumors (graft versus tumor, GvT). The success of donor leukocyte infusions (DLI) as a therapy for relapsed chronic myelogenous leukemia (CML) after bone marrow transplant (BMT) is the ultimate proof of the antitumor activity of allogeneic cells. The mechanisms responsible for this effect, in particular the specific effector cell(s), the target antigens, and the cytotolytic pathways, remain under investigation. These mechanisms and other strategies (timing of lymphocyte infusion, suicide vectors, cytokines) are being studied by many investigators in an effort to separate GvL/GvT from its main side effect, graft-versus-host disease (GvHD). Evidence that GvL/GvT activity is an essential component of conventional hematopoetic cell transplants (HCT) and the success of DLI have resulted in the development of nonmyeloablative stem cell transplantation (NST), which depends largely on the induction of GvL/GvT to mediate antitumor activity. Future developments are likely to include a broadening of clinical indications, mainly in the field of solid tumors, as well as more refined *ex vivo* manipulation of graft and vaccinations strategies. In summary, GvL/GvT has evolved from a useful side effect of allogeneic stem cell transplantation into the primary focus of novel approaches in stem cell and adoptive therapies.

I. INTRODUCTION

The terms graft versus leukemia and graft versus tumor describe the therapeutic effects of allogeneic cells against malignancies after hematopoetic cell trans-

plantation or donor leukocyte infusion. In its simplest form, this effect is observed with the transplantation of unmanipulated grafts, but manipulation of these cells *ex vivo* before reinfusion is an increasingly important therapeutical modality and links this effect to strategies described elsewhere in this encyclopedia.

The earliest description of a GvL effect dates back to murine BMT experiments in the 1950s, when it was found that mice reconstituted with "homologous" (allogeneic) bone marrow after leukemia inoculation and irradiation had prolonged survival when compared to mice reconstituted with "isologous" (syngeneic) marrow. With the introduction of allogeneic HCT as a treatment option for human hematologic malignancies starting in the 1970s, GvL entered the realm of clinical medicine. It has since been increasingly recognized as an important mechanism by which HCT eliminates leukemia cells in addition to the effects of the high-dose chemotherapy or radiation therapy used in the conditioning regimen. Two important developments of the 1990s have focused even more attention on GvL: The discovery that DLI can induce remissions in patients with relapsed leukemias after HCT and the development of stem cell transplantation with nonmyeloablative conditioning regimens.

Today, GvL/GvT has moved to the forefront of clinical strategies as well as immunological and oncological research: DLI has come into routine clinical practice and is currently the standard of care for relapsed CML post-HCT. The most firm and compelling evidence to date of a clinically relevant graft-versus-solid tumor effect has been established in patients with metastatic renal cell carcinoma who were treated with nonmyeloablative HCT. Multiple strategies to characterize target antigens of GvL/GvT, to enhance GvL/GvT, and to separate it from harmful GvHD are being pursued.

II. EXPERIMENTAL AND CLINICAL EVIDENCE

Since the original mouse experiments by Barnes and Loutit, it has been firmly established in many murine models that donor T cells [and natural killer (NK) cells] prolong survival or contribute to the eradication of hematopoetic malignances. A smaller number of animal studies has addressed the effect of grafts against solid tumors, but several published studies demonstrate this effect.

A. Graft versus Leukemia

In the clinical setting, evidence for graft versus leukemia was initally difficult to separate from the effect of high-dose chemotherapy or radiation in the conditioning regimen and was derived from indirect observations.

1. A number of case reports indicate a temporal association between withdrawal of immunosuppression and/or a flare of graft-versus-host disease and the induction of complete remission in relapsed patients after HCT.

2. The incidence of leukemic relapse is lower after matched sibling BMT than after grafts from identical twins. Similarly, several studies have shown increased relapse rates after autologous compared to allogeneic transplant, but these data may be compromised by the possibility of tumor cell contamination in the autograft.

3. Large retrospective studies confirm that both acute and chronic GvHD are protective against relapse after GvHD.

4. The incidence of leukemic relapse is higher in recipients of T-cell-depleted (TCD) allogeneic marrow than in recipients of unmodified allogeneic marrow. This difference holds up even if adjusted for the presence or absence of GvHD. In fact, one large retrospective study by the International Bone Marrow Transplant Registry (IBMTR) found that the risk of relapse was still higher for recipients of TCD marrow with GvHD than for recipients of non-TCD marrow without GvHD. In addition to providing evidence for the existence of a GvL effect, these observations also underline the pivotal role of T cells as mediators of this effect. However, widely varying methods for T-cell depletion and more recent developments in this field necessitate a more specific analysis of different methods of T cell depletion (see Section IV).

5. The most direct and relatively recently discovered evidence for GvL in the clinical setting is the effec-

tiveness of donor leukocyte infusion. In 1990, Kolb and co-workers reported complete remissions in three patients who received a transfusion of donor lymphocytes ("buffy coat") for hematological relapse of CML after BMT. Interferon-α had failed in these patients and they did not receive any further chemotherapy. The effect of DLI was durable and was associated with only mild and treatment responsive GvHD in two of the three patients. DLI has since become standard therapy for CML and induces complete (molecular) remissions in the majority of patients with cytogenetic (88%) or hematological (72%) relapse and in 22% of patients with relapse in accelerated or blast phase. Although the numbers are smaller, DLI seems to be considerably less effective for other hematological malignancies in the order of CML>acute myeloid leukemia (AML)>acute lymphoid leukemia (ALL). The relative ineffectiveness of DLI in ALL is in contrast to the close correlation between GvHD and protection from relapse, as well as the superiority of allogeneic over syngeneic HCT in this disease. Small series and anecdotal reports of responses in juvenile myelomonocytic leukemia (JMML), multiple myeloma (MM), polycythemia vera, and myelodysplastic syndrome (MDS) exist.

B. Graft versus Solid Tumor

Until very recently, clinical evidence for a graft-versus-solid tumor effect was anecdotal at best. A limited number of case reports describe remissions after allogeneic bone marrow transplantation for adult nephroblastoma, metastatic ovarian cancer, metastatic renal cell cancer, and metastatic and locally recurrent breast cancer. One study of allogeneic HCT in 10 patients with metastatic breast cancer showed a modest benefit with one patient in complete remission, four in partial remission, and four with stable disease. Because all these transplants were performed with high-dose chemotherapy and/or radiation as myeloablative regimen, it is impossible to separately evaluate the efficacy of a potential graft-versus-tumor effect. Such a comparison is feasible, however, in pediatric high-risk neuroblastoma, for which a large number of autotransplants and a smaller number of allograft procedure have been performed.

Several matched pair analyses and case control studies have demonstrated no benefit or even a worse outcome for allogeneic compared to autologous transplantation, thereby negating a GvT effect for this malignancy.

Nonmyeloablative stem cell transplant is a recently developed strategy that relies to a larger extent than conventional HCT on a GvL effect. It attempts to achieve complete chimerism with a less intensive, mostly immunosuppressive, fludarabine-based conditioning regimen. This regimen is designed not to eradicate the malignancy, but to provide sufficient immunosuppression to achieve engraftment of an allogeneic graft, which in turn attacks the disease via GvL. Posttransplant DLI can augment this effect if needed. The most experience with this approach has so far been generated in low-grade lymphomas, for which the GvL benefit of an allogeneic transplant had previously been offset (particularly in the elderly patient population) by a high transplant-related mortality. This relatively new strategy is currently being tested at many centers and it remains to be seen if the promise of less side effects (especially GvHD) with this concept holds true.

The most convincing evidence to date for a clinically relevant GvT effect has been published by Childs and co-workers in patients with metastatic renal cell carcinoma. Metastatic renal cell tumor has an extremely poor prognosis and is usually resistant to systemic chemotherapy. In their study, Childs and colleagues treated 19 consecutive patients with a nonmyeloablative regimen of cyclophosphamide and fludarabine, followed by a matched (or one antigen mismatched) sibling peripheral blood stem cell allograft. Cyclosporine was used as GvHD prophylaxis. Patients were eligible to receive additional DLI depending on their degree of chimerism, the absence of GvHD, and their disease status. They found that 3 of 19 patients remained in full remission and 9 additional patients with partial response were alive 3–18 months posttransplant. A response was significantly associated with the development of GvHD and/or the withdrawal of immunosuppression. GvHD was the major side effect (2 patients with grade IV, 1 with grade III, and 7 with grade II) and there were two transplant-related deaths (1 from steroid-resistant GvHD, 1 from bacterial sepsis).

III. MECHANISMS OF THE GRAFT VERSUS LEUKEMIA/GRAFT VERSUS TUMOR (GvL/GvT) EFFECT

The mechanisms that underlie the GvL/GvT effect are of great interest not only with regard to their basic immunological mechanisms, but also with regard to the clinical goal of enhancing GvL/GvT, while at the same time trying to prevent GvHD. This section concentrates on three central questions in the study of the mechanisms of the GvL/GvT effect that are relevant in different attempts to separate GvL/GvT from GvHD.

1. Which subset of cells exerts the GvL/GvT effect?
2. How do these cells make the distinction between malignant cells and normal host tissue?
3. How do these cells kill or inhibit or inactivate the malignant cells?

Unfortunately, several decades of extensive investigations have not yielded a simple answer to any of these questions. There is, however, growing evidence for a multifactorial network of several effector populations, host targets, and effector mechanisms whose importance might vary significantly in different species, strains, tumor models, and MHC or minor histocompatibility antigen (miHA) mismatches.

A. The Effector Cell

T cells are critical in the GvL/GvT response. This is true in virtually all animal models tested as well as in humans and evidence for this is very convincing. The depletion of T cells from the graft in animal models or in human HCT increases the risk of relapse or (depending on the stringency of T-cell depletion) in fact abrogates any GvL/GvT effect. In mouse models, a dose–response curve according to the number of transplanted T cells can be established.

Significant controversy exists regarding the relative role of different T-cell subsets. CD8$^+$ as well as CD4$^+$ cells have been shown to contribute to GvL in mouse models. The effect seems to be very model dependent. O'Kunewick and colleagues, for example, reported that CD8 depletion lowered GvL in an MHC-matched model, whereas in a MHC-mismatched model, only CD4 but not CD8 depletion had an effect on GvL. Human *in vitro* studies have demonstrated an increased frequency of leukemia-specific CTL predominantly of the CD4$^+$ subtype. While a majority of clinical trials using selective T-cell depletion of the graft (in HCT or posttransplant DLI) focus on CD8 depletion, at least one study reports good results with CD4$^+$ depletion and a fixed number of marrow CD8$^+$ cells in the graft.

NK cells are another lymphocyte population that has been shown to have a potent antitumor effect and play a role in post-HCT GvL in murine studies. In humans, an early rise in lymphokine-activated killer cells of NK and of T-cell phenotype has been observed after allogeneic BMT and DLI.

Several murine studies are beginning to address the role of NKT cells, a recently described lymphocyte subset that expresses the αβ T-cell receptor as well as the murine NK marker NK1.1 and is characterized by heavily biased TCR gene usage and high levels of cytokine production. Interestingly, they occur at a much higher frequency in the marrow than in the peripheral blood and play a role in downregulating GvHD. NKT cells *in vivo* reject chemically induced tumors in mice; however, their importance in the role of post-HCT GvL/GvT has not been studied.

B. Target Antigens

Target antigens for a GvL/GvT effect can be divided into ubiquitous, tissue-restricted, and leukemia or tumor-specific antigens (Table I).

1. Ubiquitous antigens include the major histocompatibility antigens (MHC), which are irrelevant in so-called "matched" sibling or matched unrelated donor transplants. In partially mismatched transplants they contribute to GvL/GvT in experimental models as well as in human clinical studies, but have the major disadvantage of also being targets for GvHD activity. Ubiquitously expressed minor histocompatibility antigens (miHA) have been identified and can be recognized by cytotoxic T cells. These T-cell clones are also capable of antigen-specific *in vitro* growth inhibition of leukemic precursors. While these antigens are potentially relevant in matched transplants, their use in exploiting a GvL

TABLE I

Candidate Leukemia/Tumor Antigens with Potential GvL/GvT Reactivity

Ubiquitous
  Major histocompatibility antigens (irrelevant in "matched" transplants)
  Minor histocompatibility antigens: HA-3, H-Y
Tissue restricted
  Minor histocompatibility antigens
    HA-1 (lymphohematopoetic system)
    HA-2 (lymphohematopoetic system)
Overexpressed on leukemia/tumor cells
  Proteinase-3
  Myeloperoxidase
  WT-1
Leukemia/tumor specific
  Bcr-abl fusion proteins
    p210 (CML)
    p190 (ALL)
  Other translocations
    PML-RAR α (APML)
    ETV6-AML1 (AML)
    MLL-AF4 (infant ALL, secondary AML)
  G250 (renal cell carcinoma)
  RAGE-1 (renal cell carcinoma)

effect is limited again by the fact that they are also target antigens for GvHD.

2. Of greater therapeutic interest are tissue-restricted miHA, which are only expressed on hematopoetic cells. This group includes HA-1 and HA-2, and these antigens are of considerable interest as a target for GvL. A protocol using *in vitro*-generated donor CTL specific for host HA-1 or HA-2 is currently being developed by Goulmy and co-workers. The limitation of this protocol is that it is restricted to donor/recipient pairs that (a) are both HLA-A2 positive and (b) are discordant for HA-1 or HA-2, both of which are not highly polymorphic (HA-1 is present in 69% of HLA-A2-positive individuals, HA-2 in 95%). Another note of caution in this attempt is the somewhat surprising finding that despite its restriction to hematopoetic tissue, HA1 mismatches have been correlated with higher frequencies of GvHD.

3. A third group of GvL target antigens consists of leukemia- or tumor-specific antigens. These are attractive therapeutic targets because of their absence on normal tissues and therefore the selective toxicity of a potential GvL effect. While their importance as

targets for allogeneic cells in an unmodified BMT is unclear, several groups have tried to engineer an immune response to peptides derived from leukemia-specific fusion proteins, the most prominent arguably being the different versions of BCR/ABL, which define CML and certain high-risk ALL. There is some limited evidence of success with vaccination strategies derived from these proteins, and further clinical studies are being carried out. In renal cell carcinoma, studies have defined several apparently tumor-specific antigens, with potential relevance for T-cell-based therapy, among them RAGE-1 and G250. Other examples from this class of GvL/GvT target antigens are tissue-restricted proteins that are strongly overexpressed on tumor cells and therefore become tumor specific for practical purposes. These include tyrosinase in melanoma, Her2/neu in breast cancer, and wt1 in acute leukemias. Proteinase 3, a myeloid tissue-restricted protein overexpressed on CML cells, has been demonstrated to play an important role in the *in vivo* immune response of patients with CML post-BMT. All of these antigens are actively being investigated in preclinical or clinical studies as targets for an allo- or autoimmune response, enhanced through different vaccination strategies. While many of these engineered immune responses surpass the definition of a GvL/GvT effect per se and are described in more detail elsewhere, attempts to enhance GvL by immunizing the donor are bringing these two approaches together.

The difficulties encountered in targeting leukemia- or tumor-specific antigens are closely related to known immune evasion mechanisms of the leukemias/ tumors. These include problems with (a) the processing of the antigen and the presentation on a professional antigen-presenting cell (APC) needed to elicit a primary T-cell response, (b) the continued expression of sufficient amounts of antigen on the leukemia/tumor cell in the context of MHC molecules, and (c) induction of anergy. While there is some evidence that leukemic cells might be able to act as (though not very efficient) antigen-presenting cells (with costimulatory molecules and adhesion molecules), they might also induce anergy if they express the antigen in the absence of costimulatory molecules. The uptake of apoptotic tumor cells by professional APCs is probably required in most cases in or-

der to elicit a primary T-cell response. Finally, in the course of malignant progression, tumor cells frequently downregulate the surface expression of the antigen and/or the expression of MHC class I, thereby evading the recognition of potential tumor-specific T cells.

C. Cytotoxic Pathways

More recent studies have focused on the cytolytic pathways used by T cells (and other effector cells) to kill tumor cells. FasL- and perforin-deficient donor T cells have been compared with wild-type T cells in their ability to induce GvHD and GvL responses in several murine models. While the FasL-Fas pathway does not seem to contribute significantly to a GvL response, perforin-deficient donor T cells are not able to induce a GvL effect, pointing to a crucial importance of this pathway in the GvL activity. Similar studies with blocking antibodies against tumor necrosis factor (TNF)-deficient T cells demonstrated a role for TNF as a killing mechanism for GvL. A number of recently described additional members of the TNF receptor superfamily, such as tumor necrosis factor-related apoptosis-inducing ligand (TRAIL), tumor necrosis factor-related activation-induced cytokine (TRANCE), and tumor necrosis factor-like weak inducer of apoptosis (TWEAK), have not been studied with regards to their relevance in GvL. Especially TRAIL deserves further examination in this regard because it possesses very impressive selective antitumor activity in its soluble form. These data suggest that GvL/GvT activity could potentially be differentiated from GvHD activity through the differential use of cytolytic pathways by donor effector cells.

IV. ATTEMPTS TO SEPARATE GRAFT-VERSUS-HOST DISEASE AND GvL/GvT

Although GvHD and GvL/GvT are clearly linked, as discussed in Section II.A.3, large clinical studies also provide evidence that it is possible to achieve a GvL/GvT effect without overt GvHD. The incidence of relapse is higher in recipients of a syngeneic transplant than in recipients of an allogeneic transplant without GvHD. Similarly, the study by Horowitz and co-workers found a higher relapse rate for recipients of TCD grafts with GvHD than for recipients of unmodified allogeneic grafts without GvHD. A number of strategies to achieve a GvL/GvT effect in the absence of GvHD have been employed and are under investigation.

1. Delayed T-cell add-back. Murine studies have clearly shown that separating the timing of T-cell infusion from the "cytokine storm" caused by the conditioning regimen significantly reduces the incidence of GvHD while conserving the GvL effect. Clinical studies with delayed prophylactic T-cell infusion after a T-cell-depleted graft have yielded encouraging results. In CML a TCD BMT can be followed by titrated T-cell infusion only in the case of relapse and still efficiently induce remission.

2. T-cell suicide vectors. An inducible suicide vector, transfected into T cells, gives the option of deleting T cells *in vivo* in the case of significant GvHD. This strategy would leave recipients who do not develop GvHD with the full T-cell-mediated GvL effect, while recipients who do develop GvHD have at least had an initial GvL effect and can be rescued from their GvHD.

3. T-cell (subset) depletion. The plethora of strategies employed for T-cell depletion necessitates a detailed investigation of the effects of different techniques. Earlier observations that T-cell depletion does not alter overall survival because the decrease in GvHD mortality is accompanied by an increase in relapse and graft failure (see Section II.A.3) need to be reevaluated. Our institution and others have reported single institution studies with excellent results for T-cell-depleted grafts. A recent comparison of different techniques of T-cell depletion showed an advantage in overall survival for recipients of marrows depleted with T-cell antibodies with narrow specificity. Even more specific methods of negatively selecting alloreactive T cells or positively selecting leukemia-reactive lymphocytes are under development.

4. Identification of specific tumor or GvHD antigens. As outlined in Section III.B, vaccination or *in vitro* activation and amplification of donor lymphocytes against tumor antigens could lead to enhanced GvL effect, whereas matching patients for miHC antigens could potentially further reduce GvHD.

5. Cytokine administration. Cytokines that can selectively upregulate GvL or downregulate GvHD activity of donor lymphocytes (sometimes by polarizing them to a Th-2 phenotype, which is presumed to dampen the development of GvHD) have been tested and are continously being sought. A number of agents have been used in animal models (including interleukin (IL)-11, IL-10, IL-12, interferon-γ) or patients (including IL-2, anti-TNF antibodies, G-CSF), none with overwhelming success or only at the price of significant side effects. Two of the most recent cytokines under investigation that have shown promise in murine studies are keratinocyte growth factor and IL-7.

V. CLINICAL APPLICATION AND FUTURE DIRECTIONS

The GvL effect has been used clinically since the 1970s when the allogeneic bone marrow transplant was introduced as a therapy for hematological malignancies. Initially it was difficult to differentiate its antitumor effect from that of the myeloablative conditioning regimen. With the introduction of DLI in the early 1990s and the introduction of nonmyeloablative stem cell transplants in the late 1990s, the GvL/GvT effect has moved to the center of HCT approaches. An increasing number of malignancies has been recognized as susceptible to GvL/GvT effects (Table II).

However, susceptibility to GvL does not automatically translate into effective and proven therapy of these diseases with one of the three treatment categories that make use of the GvL/GvT effect clinically: conventional HCT, DLI, and NST.

Allogeneic myeloablative HCT continues to be standard therapy (in the presence of a suitable donor) for certain high-risk ALL in first complete reunion (CR1), for almost all ALL in CR2, for AML in CR1, for CML, for JMML, for MDS, and for a subset of patients with MM. It is being evaluated for a number of other diseases.

DLI is an established therapy for relapsed CML post-HCT. Its efficacy in other relapsed hematologic malignancies (AML, ALL, MDS) is small or minimal. A recent phase I protocol studied its feasibility as a primary therapy for patients with different malignancies and reported some evidence of a GvT effect in this setting.

TABLE II
Susceptibility of Different Malignancies to GvL/GvT Effect

	(Post-HCT) DLI alone effective		Other clinical evidence[a]		References
Chronic myeloid leukemia	++	Standard therapy for relapse post-BMT, effective in >70%	++	GvHD TCD	Horowitz et al. (1990); Kolb et al. (1990, 1995)
Acute myeloid leukemia	+	Remission induction in 15–30% of patients	++	GvHD	Collins et al. (1997); Horowitz et al. (1990); Kolb et al. (1995)
Acute lymphoid leukemia	(+)	Remission induction in 0–18% of patients	++	GvHD	Collins et al. (1997); Horowitz et al. (1990); Passweg et al. (1998)
Chronic lymphoid leukemia			+	NST	deMagalhaes-Silverman et al. (1997); Khouri et al. (1998)
Juvenile mylelomonocytic leukemia			(+)	Case report of remission induction with discontinuation of immunosuppression and flare-up of GvHD, one report of NST	Orchard et al. (1998); Slavin et al. (1998)
Multiple myeloma	+	Effective in small series	(+)	Case reports of NST	Collins et al. (1997); Porter et al. (1999); Slavin et al. (1998)
Myelodysplastic syndrome	+	Effective in small series			Collins et al. (1997); Kolb et al. (1995); Porter et al. (1996)
Polycythemia vera	(+)	Effective in single case			Kolb et al. (1995)
Non-Hodgkin's lymphoma	?	No remission in seven reported cases	(+)	NST?	Carella et al. (2000); Collins et al. (1997); Slavin et al. (1998)
Hodgkin's disease	(+)	Only one remission in five reported cases	(+)	NST?	Carella et al. (2000); Porter et al. (1999)
Renal cell carcinoma			+	NST	Childs et al. (2000)
Breast cancer			(+)	Case report of regression of liver metastases in association with GvHD	Ben-Yosef et al. (1996); Ueno et al. (1998)
Ovarian center			(+)	Case report of remission induction with flare-up of GvHD	Bay et al. (2000)
Melanoma	?	No remission in three reported cases, but model system for other T-cell-mediated therapies			Porter et al. (1999)
Neuroblastoma			−	Allo-BMT inferior to auto-BMT in multiple studies	Ladenstein et al. (1994); Matthay et al. (1995); Matthay et al. (1994); Philip et al. (1997)

[a]GvHD, increased relative risk of relapse for patients without GvHD; TCD, increased relative risk of relapse for recipients of T-cell-depleted grafts; NST, nonmyeloablative stem cell transplants effective.

NSTs are still a new concept with limited follow-up, and some controversy still exists as to the morbidity of this approach. It remains to be seen if terms like "minitransplants" or "transplant lite" hold true to their promise. It is not yet state-of-the art therapy for any particular disease, although considerable experience exists in the field of low-grade lymphoma and it is proposed as a valid treatment option for this indication. Other hematologic malignancies and renal cell carcinoma are being evaluated as targets for this promising application of the GvL effect.

Future developments are certain to happen at a fast pace in the field of GvL/GvT. It is already arguably the only form of cancer immunotherapy that has made a significant clinical impact and has earned itself a place in the therapeutic repertoire for a number of malignancies. Recent progress in the field (especially the development of nonmyeloablative HCT) suggests that its scope is still expanding. Basic research and animal studies are going to further dissect the mechanisms of GvL/GvT, focusing on, but not limited to, the issues that were highlighted in Section III. The potential separation of GvL/GvT from GvHD will continue to be a major area of concern for researchers and clinicans alike; despite a vast array of studies, progress on this front has been slow over the last decades. Clinically, major areas of development are likely to be the optimization and more detailed indications for NST in hematological malignancies and solid tumors, as well as vaccination and adoptive immunotherapy strategies in the context of HCT that go beyond the scope of the GvL/GvT effect as discussed in this article.

See Also the Following Articles

ACUTE LYMPHOBLASTIC LEUKEMIA • ACUTE MYELOCYTIC LEUKEMIA • CANCER VACCINES: GENE THERAPY AND DENDRITIC CELL-BASED VACCINES • CELL-MEDIATED IMMUNITY TO CANCER • CHRONIC MYELOGENOUS LEUKEMIA • MONOCLONAL ANTIBODIES: LEUKEMIA AND LYMPHOMA • STEM CELL TRANSPLANTATION • TUMOR ANTIGENS

Bibliography

Alyea, E. P., Soiffer, R. J., Canning, C., Neuberg, D., Schlossman, R., Pickett, C., Collins, H., Wang, Y., Anderson, K. C., and Ritz, J. (1998). Toxicity and efficacy of defined doses of CD4(+) donor lymphocytes for treatment of relapse after allogeneic bone marrow transplant, *Blood* **91**, 3671–3680.

Apperley, J. F., Mauro, F. R., Goldman, J. M., Gregory, W., Arthur, C. K., Hows, J., Arcese, W., Papa, G., Mandelli, F., Wardle, D., *et al.* (1988). Bone marrow transplantation for chronic myeloid leukaemia in first chronic phase: Importance of a graft-versus-leukaemia effect [published erratum appears in *Br. J. Haematol.* 70(2), 261 (1988)]. *Br. J. Haematol.* **69**, 239–245.

Ashkenazi, A., Pai, R. C., Fong, S., Leung, S., Lawrence, D. A., Marsters, S. A., Blackie, C., Chang, L., McMurtrey, A. E., Hebert, A., *et al.* (1999). Safety and antitumor activity of recombinant soluble Apo2 ligand. *J. Clin. Invest.* **104**, 155–162.

Attal, M., Socie, G., Molina, L., Jouet, J. P., Pico, J., Kuentz, M., Blaise, D., Milpied, N., Ifrah, N., Payen, C., and Tanguy, M. L. (1997). Allogeneic bone marrow transplantation for refractory and recurrent follicular lymphoma: A case-matched analysis with autologous and recurrent follicular lymphoma: A case-matched analysis with autologous transplantation from the French bone marrow transplant group registry data. *Blood* **90**(Suppl.1), 255a.

Barnes, D. W. H., and Loutit, J. F. (1956). Treatment of murine leukemia with x-rays and homologous bone marrow. *Br. Med. J.* **2**, 626–627.

Barnes, D. W. H., and Loutit, J. F. (1957). Treatment of murine leukaemia with X-rays and homologous bone marrow. *Br. J. Haematol.* **3**, 241–252.

Barrett, A. J., Mavroudis, D., Tisdale, J., Molldrem, J., Clave, E., Dunbar, C., Cottler-Fox, M., Phang, S., Carter, C., Okunnieff, P., *et al.* (1998). T cell-depleted bone marrow transplantation and delayed T cell add-back to control acute GVHD and conserve a graft-versus-leukemia effect. *Bone Marrow Transplant.* **21**, 543–551.

Bartels, C. J., Rosenberg, S. A., and Yang, J. C. (1996). Adoptive cellular immunotherapy of cancer in mice using allogeneic T cells. *Ann. Surg. Oncol.* **3**, 67–73.

Bay, J. O., Choufi, B., Pomel, C., Dauplat, J., Durando, X., Tournilhac, O., Travade, P., Plagne, R., and Blaise, D. (2000). Potential allogeneic graft-versus-tumor effect in a patient with ovarian cancer. *Bone Marrow Transplant.* **25**, 681–682.

Ben-Yosef, R., Or, R., Nagler, A., and Slavin, S. (1996). Graft-versus-tumour and graft-versus-leukaemia effect in patient with concurrent breast cancer and acute myelocytic leukaemia. *Lancet* **348**, 1242–1243.

Carella, A. M., Cavaliere, M., Lerma, E., Ferrara, R., Tedeschi, L., Romanelli, A., Vinci, M., Pinotti, G., Lambelet, P., Loni, C., *et al.* (2000). Autografting followed by nonmyeloablative immunosuppressive chemotherapy and allogeneic peripheral-blood hematopoietic stem-cell transplantation as treatment of resistant Hodgkin's disease and non-Hodgkin's lymphoma. *J. Clin. Oncol.* **18**, 3918–3924.

Champlin, R. E., Passweg, J. R., Zhang, M. J., Rowlings, P. A.,

Pelz, C. J., Atkinson, K. A., Barrett, A. J., Cahn, J. Y., Drobyski, W. R., Gale, R. P., et al. (2000). T-cell depletion of bone marrow transplants for leukemia from donors other than HLA-identical siblings: Advantage of T-cell antibodies with narrow specificities. Blood **95**, 3996–4003.

Childs, R., Chernoff, A., Contentin, N., Bahceci, E., Schrump, D., Leitman, S., Read, E. J., Tisdale, J., Dunbar, C., Linehan, W. M., et al. (2000). Regression of metastatic renal-cell carcinoma after nonmyeloablative allogeneic peripheral-blood stem-cell transplantation. N. Engl. J. Med. **343**, 750–758.

Childs, R. W., Clave, E., Tisdale, J., Plante, M., Hensel, N., and Barrett, J. (1999). Successful treatment of metastatic renal cell carcinoma with a nonmyeloablative allogeneic peripheral-blood progenitor-cell transplant: Evidence for a graft-versus-tumor effect. J. Clin. Oncol. **17**, 2044–2049.

Collins, R. H., Jr., Rogers, Z. R., Bennett, M., Kumar, V., Nikein, A., and Fay, J. W. (1992). Hematologic relapse of chronic myelogenous leukemia following allogeneic bone marrow transplantation: Apparent graft-versus-leukemia effect following abrupt discontinuation of immunosuppression. Bone Marrow Transplant. **10**, 391–395.

Collins, R. H., Jr., Shpilberg, O., Drobyski, W. R., Porter, D. L., Giralt, S., Champlin, R., Goodman, S. A., Wolff, S. N., Hu, W., Verfaillie, C., et al. (1997). Donor leukocyte infusions in 140 patients with relapsed malignancy after allogeneic bone marrow transplantation. J. Clin. Oncol. **15**, 433–444.

de Bueger, M., Bakker, A., Van Rood, J. J., Van der Woude, F., and Goulmy, E. (1992). Tissue distribution of human minor histocompatibility antigens: Ubiquitous versus restricted tissue distribution indicates heterogeneity among human cytotoxic T lymphocyte-defined non-MHC antigens. J. Immunol. **149**, 1788–1794.

Deichman, G. I., Kashkina, L. M., Kluchareva, T. E., Vendrov, E. L., and Matveeva, V. A. (1983). Inhibition of experimental and spontaneous lung metastases of highly metastatic Syrian hamster sarcoma cells by non-activated bone marrow and peritoneal exudate cells. Int. J. Cancer **31**, 609–615.

deMagalhaes-Silverman, M., Donnenberg, A., Hammert, L., Lister, J., Myers, D., Simpson, J., and Ball, E. (1997). Induction of graft-versus-leukemia effect in a patient with chronic lymphocytic leukemia. Bone Marrow Transplant. **20**, 175–177.

den Haan, J. M., Sherman, N. E., Blokland, E., Huczko, E., Koning, F., Drijfhout, J. W., Skipper, J., Shabanowitz, J., Hunt, D. F., Engelhard, V. H., et al. (1995). Identification of a graft versus host disease-associated human minor histocompatibility antigen. Science **268**, 1476–1480.

Doney, K., Fisher, L. D., Appelbaum, F. R., Buckner, C. D., Storb, R., Singer, J., Fefer, A., Anasetti, C., Beatty, P., Bensinger, W., et al. (1991). Treatment of adult acute lymphoblastic leukemia with allogeneic bone marrow transplantation: Multivariate analysis of factors affecting acute

graft-versus-host disease, relapse, and relapse-free survival. Bone Marrow Transplant. **7**, 453–459.

Eibl, B., Schwaighofer, H., Nachbaur, D., Marth, C., Gachter, A., Knapp, R., Bock, G., Gassner, C., Schiller, L., Petersen, F., and Niederwieser, D. (1996). Evidence for a graft-versus-tumor effect in a patient treated with marrow ablative chemotherapy and allogeneic bone marrow transplantation for breast cancer. Blood **88**, 1501–1508.

Falkenburg, J. H., Goselink, H. M., van der Harst, D., van Luxemburg-Heijs, S. A., Kooy-Winkelaar, Y. M., Faber, L. M., de Kroon, J., Brand, A., Fibbe, W. E., Willemze, R., et al. (1991). Growth inhibition of clonogenic leukemic precursor cells by minor histocompatibility antigen-specific cytotoxic T lymphocytes. J. Exp. Med. **174**, 27–33.

Fefer, A., Sullivan, K., Weiden, P., et al. (1987). Graft versus leukemia effect in man: The relapse rate of acute leukemia is lower after allogeneic than after syngeneic marrow transplantation. In "Cellular Immunotherapy of Cancer" (R. Truitt, R. P. Gale, and M. M. Bortin, eds.), pp. 401–408. A. R. Liss, New York.

Gale, R. P., and Champlin, R. E. (1984). How does bone-marrow transplantation cure leukaemia? Lancet **2**, 28–30.

Gale, R. P., Horowitz, M. M., Ash, R. C., Champlin, R. E., Goldman, J. M., Rimm, A. A., Ringden, O., Stone, J. A., and Bortin, M. M. (1994). Identical-twin bone marrow transplants for leukemia. Ann. Intern. Med. **120**, 646–652.

Giralt, S., Hester, J., Huh, Y., Hirsch-Ginsberg, C., Rondon, G., Seong, D., Lee, M., Gajewski, J., Van Besien, K., Khouri, I., et al. (1995). CD8-depleted donor lymphocyte infusion as treatment for relapsed chronic myelogenous leukemia after allogeneic bone marrow transplantation. Blood **86**, 4337–4343.

Glass, B., Uharek, L., Zeis, M., Loeffler, H., Mueller-Ruchholtz, W., and Gassmann, W. (1996). Graft-versus-leukaemia activity can be predicted by natural cytotoxicity against leukaemia cells. Br. J. Haematol. **93**, 412–420.

Goldman, J. M., Gale, R. P., Horowitz, M. M., Biggs, J. C., Champlin, R. E., Gluckman, E., Hoffmann, R. G., Jacobsen, S. J., Marmont, A. M., McGlave, P. B., et al. (1988). Bone marrow transplantation for chronic myelogenous leukemia in chronic phase: Increased risk for relapse associated with T-cell depletion. Ann. Intern. Med. **108**, 806–814.

Goulmy, E. (2000). Alloimmune T cells for adoptive therapy of hematological malignancies. In "Hematology 2000" (G. P. Schechter, N. Berliner, and M. J. Telen, eds.), pp. 366–370. The American Society of Hematology, Washington, DC.

Goulmy, E., Schipper, R., Pool, J., Blokland, E., Falkenburg, J. H., Vossen, J., Grathwohl, A., Vogelsang, G. B., van Houwelingen, H. C., and van Rood, J. J. (1996). Mismatches of minor histocompatibility antigens between HLA-identical donors and recipients and the development of graft-versus-host disease after bone marrow transplantation. N. Engl. J. Med. **334**, 281–285.

Herrera, C., Martin, C., Garcia-Castellano, J. M., et al. (1995).

Prevention of GvHD by selective CD4 + T cell depletion plus adjustment of the CD8 cell content in donor bone marrow. *Blood* **86**(Suppl. 1), 571a.

Higano, C. S., Brixey, M., Bryant, E. M., Durnam, D. M., Doney, K., Sullivan, K. M., and Singer, J. W. (1990). Durable complete remission of acute nonlymphocytic leukemia associated with discontinuation of immunosuppression following relapse after allogeneic bone marrow transplantation: A case report of a probable graft-versus-leukemia effect, *Transplantation* **50**, 175–177.

Hoffmann, T., Theobald, M., Bunjes, D., Weiss, M., Heimpel, H., and Heit, W. (1993). Frequency of bone marrow T cells responding to HLA-identical non- leukemic and leukemic stimulator cells. *Bone Marrow Transplant.* **12**, 1–8.

Horowitz, M. M., Gale, R. P., Sondel, P. M., Goldman, J. M., Kersey, J., Kolb, H. J., Rimm, A. A., Ringden, O., Rozman, C., Speck, B., *et al.* (1990). Graft-versus-leukemia reactions after bone marrow transplantation. *Blood* **75**, 555.

Hupperets, P. S., Havenith, M. G., and Blijham, G. H. (1992). Recurrent adult nephroblastoma: Long-term remission after surgery plus adjuvant high-dose chemotherapy, radiation therapy, and allogeneic bone marrow transplantation. *Cancer* **69**, 2990–2992.

Jiang, Y. Z., Kanfer, E. J., Macdonald, D., Cullis, J. O., Goldman, J. M., and Barrett, A. J. (1991). Graft-versus-leukaemia following allogeneic bone marrow transplantation: Emergence of cytotoxic T lymphocytes reacting to host leukaemia cells. *Bone Marrow Transplant.* **8**, 253–258.

Jiang, Y. Z., Mavroudis, D. A., Dermime, S., Molldrem, J., Hensel, N. F., and Barrett, A. J. (1997). Preferential usage of T cell receptor (TCR) V beta by allogeneic T cells recognizing myeloid leukemia cells: Implications for separating graft-versus-leukemia effect from graft-versus-host disease. *Bone Marrow Transplant.* **19**, 899–903.

Kersey, J. H., Weisdorf, D., Nesbit, M. E., LeBien, T. W., Woods, W. G., McGlave, P. B., Kim, T., Vallera, D. A., Goldman, A. I., Bostrom, B., *et al.* (1987). Comparison of autologous and allogeneic bone marrow transplantation for treatment of high-risk refractory acute lymphoblastic leukemia. *N. Engl. J. Med.* **317**, 461–467.

Khouri, I. F., Keating, M., Korbling, M., Przepiorka, D., Anderlini, P., O'Brien, S., Giralt, S., Ippoliti, C., von Wolff, B., Gajewski, J., *et al.* (1998). Transplant-lite: Induction of graft-versus-malignancy using fludarabine- based nonablative chemotherapy and allogeneic blood progenitor-cell transplantation as treatment for lymphoid malignancies. *J. Clin. Oncol.* **16**, 2817–2824.

Kolb, H. J., Mittermuller, J., Clemm, C., Holler, E., Ledderose, G., Brehm, G., Heim, M., and Wilmanns, W. (1990). Donor leukocyte transfusions for treatment of recurrent chronic myelogenous leukemia in marrow transplant patients. *Blood* **76**, 2462–2465.

Kolb, H. J., Schattenberg, A., Goldman, J. M., Hertenstein, B., Jacobsen, N., Arcese, W., Ljungman, P., Ferrant, A., Verdonck, L., Niederwieser, D., *et al.* (1995). Graft-versus-leukemia effect of donor lymphocyte transfusions in marrow grafted patients: European Group for Blood and Marrow Transplantation Working Party Chronic Leukemia. *Blood* **86**, 2041–2050.

Krijanovski, O. I., Hill, G. R., Cooke, K. R., Teshima, T., Crawford, J. M., Brinson, Y. S., and Ferrara, J. L. (1999). Keratinocyte growth factor separates graft-versus-leukemia effects from graft-versus-host disease. *Blood* **94**, 825–831.

Kwak, L. W., Taub, D. D., Duffey, P. L., Bensinger, W. I., Bryant, E. M., Reynolds, C. W., and Longo, D. L. (1995). Transfer of myeloma idiotype-specific immunity from an actively immunised marrow donor. *Lancet* **345**, 1016–1020.

Ladenstein, R., Lasset, C., Hartmann, O., Klingebiel, T., Bouffet, E., Gadner, H., Paolucci, P., Burdach, S., Chauvin, F., Pinkerton, R., *et al.* (1994). Comparison of auto versus allografting as consolidation of primary treatments in advanced neuroblastoma over one year of age at diagnosis: Report from the European Group for Bone Marrow Transplantation. *Bone Marrow Transplant.* **14**, 37–46.

Lee, C. K., Gingrich, R. D., deMagalhaes-Silverman, M., Hohl, R. J., Joyce, J. K., Scott, S. D., Wen, B. C., and Schlueter, A. (1999). Prophylactic reinfusion of T cells for T cell-depleted allogeneic bone marrow transplantation. *Biol. Blood Marrow Transplant.* **5**, 15–27.

Mackinnon, S., Papadopoulos, E. B., Carabasi, M. H., Reich, L., Collins, N. H., Boulad, F., Castro-Malaspina, H., Childs, B. H., Gillio, A. P., Kernan, N. A., *et al.* (1995). Adoptive immunotherapy evaluating escalating doses of donor leukocytes for relapse of chronic myeloid leukemia after bone marrow transplantation: Separation of graft-versus-leukemia responses from graft-versus-host disease. *Blood* **86**, 1261–1268.

Martin, P. J., Clift, R. A., Fisher, L. D., Buckner, C. D., Hansen, J. A., Appelbaum, F. R., Doney, K. C., Sullivan, K. M., Witherspoon, R. P., Storb, R., *et al.* (1988). HLA-identical marrow transplantation during accelerated-phase chronic myelogenous leukemia: Analysis of survival and remission duration. *Blood* **72**, 1978–1984.

Matthay, K. K., O'Leary, M. C., Ramsay, N. K., Villablanca, J., Reynolds, C. P., Atkinson, J. B., Haase, G. M., Stram, D. O., and Seeger, R. C. (1995). Role of myeloablative therapy in improved outcome for high risk neuroblastoma: Review of recent Children's Cancer Group results. *Eur. J. Cancer* **4**, 572–575.

Matthay, K. K., Seeger, R. C., Reynolds, C. P., Stram, D. O., O'Leary, M., Harris, R. E., Selch, M., Atkinson, J. B., Haase, G., Hammond, G. D., *et al.* (1994). Comparison of autologous and allogeneic bone marrow transplantation for neuroblastoma. *Prog. Clin. Biol. Res.* **385**, 301–307.

Mavroudis, D. A., Dermime, S., Molldrem, J., Jiang, Y. Z., Raptis, A., van Rhee, F., Hensel, N., Fellowes, V., Eliopoulos, G., and Barrett, A. J. (1998). Specific depletion of alloreactive T cells in HLA-identical siblings: A method for separating graft-versus-host and graft-versus-leukaemia reactions. *Br. J. Haematol.* **101**, 565–570.

Molldrem, J. J., Lee, P. P., Wang, C., Felio, K., Kantarjian, H. M., Champlin, R. E., and Davis, M. M. (2000). Evidence that specific T lymphocytes may participate in the elimination of chronic myelogenous leukemia. *Nature Med.* **6,** 1018–1023.

Morecki, S., Moshel, Y., Gelfend, Y., Pugatsch, T., and Slavin, S. (1997). Induction of graft vs. tumor effect in a murine model of mammary adenocarcinoma. *Int. J. Cancer* **71,** 59–63.

Morecki, S., Yacovlev, E., Diab, A., and Slavin, S. (1998). Allogeneic cell therapy for a murine mammary carcinoma. *Cancer Res.* **58,** 3891–3895.

Moscovitch, M., and Slavin, S. (1984). Anti-tumor effects of allogeneic bone marrow transplantation in (NZB X NZW)F1 hybrids with spontaneous lymphosarcoma. *J. Immunol.* **132,** 997–1000.

Naparstek, E., Or, R., Nagler, A., Cividalli, G., Engelhard, D., Aker, M., Gimon, Z., Manny, N., Sacks, T., Tochner, Z., *et al.* (1995). T-cell-depleted allogeneic bone marrow transplantation for acute leukaemia using Campath-1 antibodies and posttransplant administration of donor's peripheral blood lymphocytes for prevention of relapse. *Br. J. Haematol.* **89,** 506–515.

Neumann, E., Engelsberg, A., Decker, J., Storkel, S., Jaeger, E., Huber, C., and Seliger, B. (1998). Heterogeneous expression of the tumor-associated antigens RAGE-1, PRAME, and glycoprotein 75 in human renal cell carcinoma: Candidates for T-cell-based immunotherapies? *Cancer Res.* **58,** 4090–4095.

Nimer, S. D., Giorgi, J., Gajewski, J. L., Ku, N., Schiller, G. J., Lee, K., Territo, M., Ho, W., Feig, S., Selch, M., *et al.* (1994). Selective depletion of CD8+ cells for prevention of graft-versus-host disease after bone marrow transplantation: A randomized controlled trial. *Transplantation* **57,** 82–87.

O'Kunewick, J. P., Kociban, D., Machen, L., and Buffo, M. (1992). Effect of selective donor T-cell depletion on the graft-versus-leukemia reaction in allogeneic marrow transplantation. *Transplant. Proc.* **24,** 2998–2999.

O'Kunewick, J. P., Kociban, D. L., Machen, L. L., and Buffo, M. J. (1995). Evidence for a possible role of Asialo-GM1-positive cells in the graft- versus-leukemia repression of a murine type-C retroviral leukemia. *Bone Marrow Transplant.* **16,** 451–456.

Odom, L. F., August, C. S., Githens, J. H., *et al.* (1981). "Graft-versus-leukemia" reaction following bone marrow transplantation for acute lymphoblastic leukemia. *In* "Graft-versus-Leukemia in Man and Animal Models" (J. P. O'Kunewick and R. F. Meredith, eds.), pp. 25–43. CRC Press, Boca Raton, FL.

Odom, L. F., August, C. S., Githens, J. H., Humbert, J. R., Morse, H., Peakman, D., Sharma, B., Rusnak, S. L., and Johnson, F. B. (1978). Remission of relapsed leukaemia during a graft-versus-host reaction: A "graft-versus-leukaemia reaction" in man? *Lancet* **2,** 537–540.

Orchard, P. J., Miller, J. S., McGlennen, R., Davies, S. M., and Ramsay, N. K. (1998). Graft-versus-leukemia is sufficient to induce remission in juvenile myelomonocytic leukemia. *Bone Marrow Transplant.* **22,** 201–203.

Papadopoulos, E. B., Carabasi, M. H., Castro-Malaspina, H., Childs, B. H., Mackinnon, S., Boulad, F., Gillio, A. P., Kernan, N. A., Small, T. N., Szabolcs, P., *et al.* (1998). T-cell-depleted allogeneic bone marrow transplantation as postremission therapy for acute myelogenous leukemia: Freedom from relapse in the absence of graft-versus-host disease. *Blood* **91,** 1083–1090.

Passweg, J. R., Tiberghien, P., Cahn, J. Y., Vowels, M. R., Camitta, B. M., Gale, R. P., Herzig, R. H., Hoelzer, D., Horowitz, M. M., Ifrah, N., *et al.* (1998). Graft-versus-leukemia effects in T lineage and B lineage acute lymphoblastic leukemia. *Bone Marrow Transplant.* **21,** 153–158.

Peniket, A. J., Ruiz de Elvira, M. C., Taghipour, G., de Witte, T., Tazelaar, P. J., Carella, A., Vernant, J. P., Schaefer, U. W., Cleeven, M., Boogaerts, M. A., *et al.* (1990). Allogeneic transplantation for lymphoma produces a lower relapse rate than autologous transplantation but survival is worse because of higher treatment related mortality: A report of 764 cases from the EBMT lymphoma registry. *Blood* **90**(Suppl.1), 255a.

Philip, T., Ladenstein, R., Lasset, C., Hartmann, O., Zucker, J. M., Pinkerton, R., Pearson, A. D., Klingebiel, T., Garaventa, A., Kremens, B., *et al.* (1997). 1070 myeloablative megatherapy procedures followed by stem cell rescue for neuroblastoma: 17 years of European experience and conclusions: European Group for Blood and Marrow Transplant Registry Solid Tumour Working Party. *Eur. J. Cancer* **33,** 2130–2135.

Pinilla-Ibarz, J., Cathcart, K., and Scheinberg, D. A. (2000). CML vaccines as a paradigm of the specific immunotherapy of cancer. *Blood Rev.* **14,** 111–120.

Porter, D. L., Connors, J. M., Van Deerlin, V. M., Duffy, K. M., McGarigle, C., Saidman, S. L., Leonard, D. G., and Antin, J. H. (1999). Graft-versus-tumor induction with donor leukocyte infusions as primary therapy for patients with malignancies. *J. Clin. Oncol.* **17,** 1234.

Porter, D. L., Roth, M. S., Lee, S. J., McGarigle, C., Ferrara, J. L., and Antin, J. H. (1996). Adoptive immunotherapy with donor mononuclear cell infusions to treat relapse of acute leukemia or myelodysplasia after allogeneic bone marrow transplantation. *Bone Marrow Transplant.* **18,** 975–980.

Reittie, J. E., Gottlieb, D., Heslop, H. E., Leger, O., Drexler, H. G., Hazlehurst, G., Hoffbrand, A. V., Prentice, H. G., and Brenner, M. K. (1989). Endogenously generated activated killer cells circulate after autologous and allogeneic marrow transplantation but not after chemotherapy. *Blood* **73,** 1351–1358.

Ringden, O., and Horowitz, M. M. (1989). Graft-versus-leukemia reactions in humans: The Advisory Committee of the International Bone Marrow Transplant Registry. *Transplant. Proc.* **21**, 2989–2992.

Rondon, G., Giralt, S., Huh, Y., Khouri, I., Andersson, B., Andreeff, M., and Champlin, R. (1996). Graft-versus-leukemia effect after allogeneic bone marrow transplantation for chronic lymphocytic leukemia. *Bone Marrow Transplant.* **18**, 669–672.

Sanders, J. E., Flournoy, N., Thomas, E. D., Buckner, C. D., Lum, L. G., Clift, R. A., Appelbaum, F. R., Sullivan, K. M., Stewart, P., Deeg, H. J., *et al.* (1985). Marrow transplant experience in children with acute lymphoblastic leukemia: An analysis of factors associated with survival, relapse, and graft-versus-host disease. *Med. Pediatr. Oncol.* **13**, 165–172.

Sehn, L. H., Alyea, E. P., Weller, E., Canning, C., Lee, S., Ritz, J., Antin, J. H., and Soiffer, R. J. (1999). Comparative outcomes of T-cell-depleted and non-T-cell-depleted allogeneic bone marrow transplantation for chronic myelogenous leukemia: Impact of donor lymphocyte infusion. *J. Clin. Oncol.* **17**, 561–568.

Slavin, S., Nagler, A., Naparstek, E., Kapelushnik, Y., Aker, M., Cividalli, G., Varadi, G., Kirschbaum, M., Ackerstein, A., Samuel, S., *et al.* (1998). Nonmyeloablative stem cell transplantation and cell therapy as an alternative to conventional bone marrow transplantation with lethal cytoreduction for the treatment of malignant and nonmalignant hematologic diseases. *Blood* **91**, 756–763.

Smyth, M. J., Thia, K. Y., Street, S. E., Cretney, E., Trapani, J. A., Taniguchi, M., Kawano, T., Pelikan, S. B., Crowe, N. Y., and Godfrey, D. I. (2000). Differential tumor surveillance by natural killer (NK) and NKT cells. *J. Exp. Med.* **191**, 661–668.

Sullivan, K. M., and Shulman, H. M. (1989). Chronic graft-versus-host disease, obliterative bronchiolitis, and graft-versus-leukemia effect: Case histories. *Transplant. Proc.* **21**, 51–62.

Sullivan, K. M., Weiden, P. L., Storb, R., Witherspoon, R. P., Fefer, A., Fisher, L., Buckner, C. D., Anasetti, C., Appelbaum, F. R., Badger, C., *et al.* (1989). Influence of acute and chronic graft-versus-host disease on relapse and survival after bone marrow transplantation from HLA-identical siblings as treatment of acute and chronic leukemia [published erratum appears in *Blood* **74**(3), 1180 (1989)]. *Blood* **73**, 1720–1728.

Sykes, M., Abraham, V. S., Harty, M. W., and Pearson, D. A. (1993). IL-2 reduces graft-versus-host disease and preserves a graft-versus-leukemia effect by selectively inhibiting CD4+ T cell activity. *J. Immunol.* **150**, 197–205.

Townsend, R. M., Paterson, A., Hsieh, M. H., and Korngold, R. (1996). Studies of the graft-versus-myeloid leukemia responses following murine bone marrow transplantation. *Blood* **88**(Suppl. 1), 244a.

Tricot, G., Vesole, D. H., Jagannath, S., Hilton, J., Munshi, N., and Barlogie, B. (1996). Graft-versus-myeloma effect: Proof of principle. *Blood* **87**, 1196–1198.

Truitt, R. L., and Atasoylu, A. A. (1991). Contribution of CD4+ and CD8+ T cells to graft-versus-host disease and graft-versus-leukemia reactivity after transplantation of MHC- compatible bone marrow. *Bone Marrow Transplant.* **8**, 51–58.

Tsukada, N., Kobata, T., Aizawa, Y., Yagita, H., and Okumura, K. (1999). Graft-versus-leukemia effect and graft-versus-host disease can be differentiated by cytotoxic mechanisms in a murine model of allogeneic bone marrow transplantation. *Blood* **93**, 2738–2747.

Ueno, N. T., Rondon, G., Mirza, N. Q., Geisler, D. K., Anderlini, P., Giralt, S. A., Andersson, B. S., Claxton, D. F., Gajewski, J. L., Khouri, I. F., *et al.* (1998). Allogeneic peripheral-blood progenitor-cell transplantation for poor-risk patients with metastatic breast cancer. *J. Clin. Oncol.* **16**, 986–993.

van Besien, K., Sobocinski, K. A., Rowlings, P. A., Murphy, S. C., Armitage, J. O., Bishop, M. R., Chaekal, O. K., Gale, R. P., Klein, J. P., Lazarus, H. M., *et al.* (1998). Allogeneic bone marrow transplantation for low-grade lymphoma. *Blood* **92**, 1832–1836.

van der Harst, D., Goulmy, E., Falkenburg, J. H., Kooij-Winkelaar, Y. M., van Luxemburg-Heijs, S. A., Goselink, H. M., and Brand, A. (1994). Recognition of minor histocompatibility antigens on lymphocytic and myeloid leukemic cells by cytotoxic T-cell clones. *Blood* **83**, 1060–1066.

Verdonck, L. F., Lokhorst, H. M., Dekker, A. W., Nieuwenhuis, H. K., and Petersen, E. J. (1996). Graft-versus-myeloma effect in two cases. *Lancet* **347**, 800–801.

Vissers, J. L., De Vries, I. J., Schreurs, M. W., Engelen, L. P., Oosterwijk, E., Figdor, C. G., and Adema, G. J. (1999). The renal cell carcinoma-associated antigen G250 encodes a human leukocyte antigen (HLA)-A2.1-restricted epitope recognized by cytotoxic T lymphocytes. *Cancer Res.* **59**, 5554–5559.

Walczak, H., Miller, R. E., Ariail, K., Gliniak, B., Griffith, T. S., Kubin, M., Chin, W., Jones, J., Woodward, A., Le, T., *et al.* (1999). Tumoricidal activity of tumor necrosis factor-related apoptosis- inducing ligand in vivo. *Nature Med.* **5**, 157–163.

Weiden, P. L., Flournoy, N., Thomas, E. D., Prentice, R., Fefer, A., Buckner, C. D., and Storb, R. (1979). Antileukemic effect of graft-versus-host disease in human recipients of allogeneic-marrow grafts. *N. Engl. J. Med.* **300**, 1068–1073.

Weiden, P. L., Sullivan, K. M., Flournoy, N., Storb, R., and Thomas, E. D. (1981). Antileukemic effect of chronic graft-versus-host disease: Contribution to improved survival after allogeneic marrow transplantation. *N. Engl. J. Med.* **304**, 1529–1533.

Weisdorf, D. J., Nesbit, M. E., Ramsay, N. K., Woods, W. G., Goldman, A. I., Kim, T. H., Hurd, D. D., McGlave, P. B., and Kersey, J. H. (1987). Allogeneic bone marrow transplantation for acute lymphoblastic leukemia in remission:

Prolonged survival associated with acute graft-versus- host disease. *J. Clin. Oncol.* **5,** 1348–1355.

Weiss, L., Reich, S., and Slavin, S. (1995). The role of antibodies to IL-2 receptor and Asialo GM1 on graft-versus-leukemia effects induced by bone marrow allografts in murine B cell leukemia. *Bone Marrow Transplant.* **16,** 457–461.

Zeis, M., Uharek, L., Glass, B., Gaska, T., Steinmann, J., Gassmann, W., Loffler, H., and Muller-Ruchholtz, W. (1995). Allogeneic NK cells as potent antileukemic effector cells after allogeneic bone marrow transplantation in mice. *Transplantation* **59,** 1734–1736.

Zeng, D., Lewis, D., Dejbakhsh-Jones, S., Lan, F., Garcia-Ojeda, M., Sibley, R., and Strober, S. (1999). Bone marrow NK1.1(−) and NK1.1(+) T cells reciprocally regulate acute graft versus host disease. *J. Exp. Med.* **189,** 1073–1081.

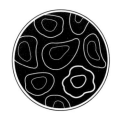

Head and Neck Cancer

Barbara Burtness
Yale University School of Medicine

GLOSSARY

field cancerization The coexistence of many areas of premalignant change in an organ or region of the body after a carcinogenic exposure.

larynx preservation The use of conservative surgery, or the substitution of chemotherapy and radiation for surgery, to preserve the larynx in patients with cancer of the larynx or hypopharynx.

nasopharynx cancer Tumors arising within the nasopharyngeal space. These are not readily amenable to surgical removal, but are sensitive to combined chemotherapy and radiation, which is the current standard of care.

retinoid Vitamin A and its analogs and derivatives, some of which suppress the progression of premalignant epithelial lesions to squamous cell cancer.

salivary gland Gland located in the head and neck that secretes saliva.

second primary A second cancer arising in a cancer survivor. In patients with head and neck cancer, these are often located in the upper aerodigestive tract and arise because of the same carcinogenic exposures as the first cancer.

squamous cell carcinoma Malignant neoplasm arising from the mucosal epithelium.

xerostomia Dry mouth. This is caused by decreased saliva production after radiation or surgical removal of the salivary glands.

T he majority of invasive cancers arising in the head and neck are squamous cell cancers. Tumors arise in epithelial tissue that is constantly exposed to the environment and are generally diseases of geno-toxic exposure and/or infection rather than of inherited high penetrance ongogenic mutations. Although the rate of cure for these cancers exceeds 60%, the morbidity of the cancers persists long after treatment in many cases because both tumor and treatment damage organs required for speech and swallowing. Premalignant lesions are often scattered throughout the mucosa of the aerodigestive tract, either because transformed cells migrate through the mucosal layer or because the sequence of genetic events leading to transformation occurs independently in many loci in the exposed epithelium. Because of this "field cancerization," second cancers commonly arise in this region among patients cured of a primary tumor of the upper aerodigestive tract.

I. EPIDEMIOLOGY

Approximately 40,300 new cases of head and neck cancer were expected in the United States in the year 2000; the majority of these arise in the oral cavity or larynx (Fig. 1).

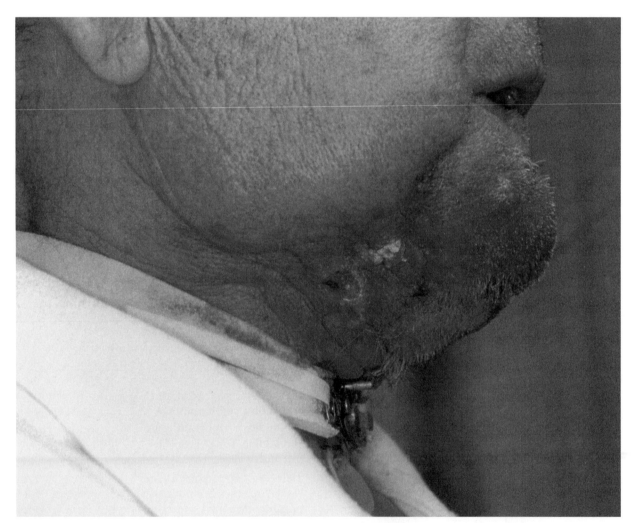

FIGURE 1 Locally advanced squamous cell carcinoma arising from base of tongue, with extension into skin. The patient has undergone tracheostomy. Photo by E. Knill-Selby.

A. Nasopharynx

The incidence of nasopharynx cancer varies dramatically among geographic regions. The disease is endemic in southern China and North Africa. Epstein–Barr virus is the likely etiologic agent, although major histocompatibility complex types H2, BW46, and B17 and diets rich in salt-cured fish and meat also play a role. Nasopharynx cancer occurs in a younger age group than is common with other sites of head and neck cancer, and the association with tobacco and alcohol use is weaker.

B. Nasal Cavity and Paranasal Sinuses

These are the least frequent sites of origin for head and neck cancers in the United States. In Asia and South Africa, tumors of these sites occur more commonly than they do in the United States. Especially for nasal cavity tumors, occupational exposure to agents such as nickel, chromium, and radium appears to be a significant risk factor.

C. Oral Cavity, Oropharynx, Larynx, and Hypopharynx

These cancers occur most commonly in users of tobacco and alcohol. The risk is related to the amount of tobacco used and the duration of use and is dramatically increased by the topical coagent ethanol. Genetic susceptibility, vitamin A deficiency, and papillomavirus infection, especially with papillomavirus type 16, are important contributing factors to risk. In addition, for cancers of the lip, pipe smoking, sun exposure, and immunosuppression have been related to risk. The median age is approximately 60 years for most sites, and the male to female ratio is 3 to 4:1 for most sites. The incidence in women may be increasing for certain sites. The risk of developing a laryngeal cancer is also increased by exposure to paint fumes, plastic by-products, wood dust, and asbestos and by long-standing gastroesophageal reflux disease.

II. MOLECULAR BIOLOGY

The epidermal growth factor receptor (EGF-R) is a transmembrane tyrosine kinase growth factor receptor that dimerizes and is activated by the binding of a number of ligands, including the epidermal growth factor. Upon activation, a signal transduction cascade is initiated, which is mitogenic. The receptor is overexpressed in >90% of squamous cell cancers of the head and neck. Receptor overexpression is associated in other tumor types with relative chemotherapy insensitivity and poor prognosis.

The most common molecular abnormality in squamous cancers arising in the head and neck is deletion or an inactivating mutation of the cell cycle regulatory gene p16 (CDK2), which is a negative regulator of cyclin D1. Cyclin D1 is itself overexpressed in approximately 30% of squamous cell cancers of the head and neck.

III. PATHOLOGY

A. Nasopharynx

The three histologic subtypes of nasopharyngeal carcinoma are keratinizing or nonkeratinizing squamous cell carcinomas and undifferentiated carcinomas, also known as lymphoepitheliomas. Keratinizing squamous cancers at this site are uncommon except in the United States, and undifferentiated cancers are the most common nasopharyngeal cancers.

B. Nasal Cavity and Paranasal Sinuses

Tumors arising in the nasal cavity and paranasal sinuses are most commonly squamous cell cancers, but adenocarcinomas and esthesioneuroblastomas may be seen. Tumors of the salivary glands, which are generally adenocarcinomas, adenoid cystic carcinomas, or mucoepidermoid cancers, may arise in the sinuses. Lymphomas and sarcomas very rarely arise in the sinuses.

C. Salivary Gland

Most tumors of the salivary glands are benign. Benign mixed tumor, previously called pleomorphic adenoma, usually arises from the parotid gland, but may arise from other salivary tissue as well. Such neoplasms contain proliferations of mucoid, cartilagenous, and other tissues, but without a high mitotic rate or perivascular or perineural invasion. They grow slowly, sometimes to large size, but except for rare cases in which the facial nerve is entrapped, remain asymptomatic.

Malignant tumors of the salivary glands are classified as mucoepidermoid carcinomas, adenocarcinomas and squamous cell carcinomas, malignant mixed tumors, and adenoid cystic carcinomas. Mucoepidermoid and adenocarcinomas spread to regional nodes early in the course, and high-grade adenocarcinomas of the salivary gland are likely to ultimately metastasize to distant organs. Adenoid cystic cancers also metastasize distantly more commonly than most tumors of this region, but are often characterized by an indolent natural history.

D. Oral Cavity, Oropharynx, Larynx and Hypopharynx

The most common histology in these sites is squamous cell cancer.

IV. ANATOMY

Each site within the aerodigestive tract has its own pattern of drainage to the regional lymph nodes, of which there are nearly 200. Initial drainage is into lymph nodes on the same side as the primary tumor. As the cancer progresses, lymph nodes on the opposite side of the neck are likely to become involved—this pattern of progression is much more common than growth of metastases in distant organs such as the lungs.

A. Nasopharynx

Lymphatic drainage from this area is to retropharyngeal nodes and along the jugular vein and spinal accessory nerve.

B. Nasal Cavity and Paranasal Sinuses

The lymphatic drainage of these areas is to the retropharyngeal and submandibular lymph nodes.

C. Oral Cavity and Oropharynx

Tumors of the lip, alveolar ridge, and retromolar area drain to the superior cervical nodes; those of the tongue drain preferentially to midlevel neck nodes and of the oropharynx to the lower neck nodes.

D. Larynx

The larynx is conventionally divided into subsites with different lymphatic drainage and natural history. The supraglottic and subglottic larynx drain independently to ipsilateral nodes and ultimately into the deep cervical chain. There is little lymphatic drainage from the true vocal cords.

E. Hypopharynx

The hypopharynx includes the posterior wall of the pharynx, the postcricoid, and the pyriform sinuses formed in the anterolateral aspects of the hypopharynx by the larynx. Tumors arising in this area are usually asymptomatic early in the course and spread rapidly through the abundant lymphatics of this region. Metastases are generally to the retropharyngeal nodes and deep cervical nodes.

F. Salivary Gland

The parotid gland is enclosed by a capsule and is located anterior to and below the external ear; its deepest aspect is in the parapharyngeal space. The facial nerve travels through the gland. Lymphatic drainage is to intraparotid nodes and the superficial and deep jugular chains.

V. CLINICAL PRESENTATION

A. Nasopharynx

Otitis media is a rare occurrence in the healthy adult. Its occurrence should always raise a suspicion of nasopharyngeal pathology, and nasopharynx cancer and Wegener's granulomatosis both should be excluded. Tumor may extend to the base of skull, causing cranial nerve abnormalities, into muscle causing trismus and along vascular bundles. A neck mass is a common presentation and rarely proptosis or cerebrospinal fluid rhinorrhea may be the presenting sign.

B. Oral Cavity

Oral cavity tumors present with ulceration or pain. These cancers are amenable to early detection by inspection of the oral cavity. Dental personnel are ideally placed to perform such screening; however, use of dental services is lower among persons of low socio-economic status.

Cancers of the tongue present with pain, impaired speech, or impaired swallowing. Those of the buccal mucosa often go undetected until they are painful or bleeding. If there has been invasion of muscle, trismus may be the presenting symptom.

C. Larynx

Larynx cancer arising on the vocal folds often presents with hoarseness relatively early in the course. In contrast, tumors arising in the supraglottic larynx are initially asymptomatic, and by the time throat or ear pain is noted by the patient, there may be clinical or subclinical involvement of the cervical lymph nodes.

D. Squamous Cell Carcinoma of the Cervical Nodes

The most likely cause of this syndrome is metastasis of cancer cells from a primary tumor of the head and neck. Thorough evaluation of the area with laryngoscopy and CT scanning, or the subsequent clinical course, will reveal a head and neck tumor in up to 40% of these cases, and standard management includes treatment of the presumed primary site if it cannot be located initially.

VI. DIAGNOSIS AND STAGING

Diagnosis of cancers of the head and neck is generally made by laryngoscopy and biopsy.

Appropriate staging requires knowledge of the local extent of the primary tumor, as well as the location and size of regional lymph nodes to which malignant cells have metastasized. Metastasis to distant sites such as the lung or bones may occur, but is infrequent at the time of presentation.

The stage of disease is assigned according to American Joint Committee on Cancer criteria. Guidelines for assigning tumor stage (T) vary according to the anatomic site of tumor origin. Nodal (N) and metastatic (M) stage are as follows:

Regional Nodes

NX: Regional nodes cannot be assessed

N0: No regional lymph nodes

N1: Metastasis in a single ipsilateral lymph node of 3 cm or less in greatest dimension

N2a: Metastasis in a single ipsilateral lymph node, more than 3 but less than 6 cm

N2b: Metastasis in multiple ipsilateral lymph nodes, none more than 6 cm in greatest dimension

N2c: Metastasis in bilateral or contralateral lymph nodes, none more than 6 cm in greatest dimension

N3: Metastasis in a lymph node more than 6 cm in greatest dimension

Stage	Tumor (T)$_{\text{site specific}}$	Nodes (N)	Metastases (M)
0	Tis (*in situ* cancer)	N0	M0
I	T1	N0	M0
II	T2	N0	M0
III	T3	N0	M0
	T1–T2	N1	M0
	T3	N0	M0
IVA	T4	N0–N2	M0
IVB	T4	N3	M0
IVC	T0–4	N0–3	M1

Cross-sectional images of the pharynx and neck are obtained with CT scanning to assess the local extent of the primary tumor, detect bony erosion, and evaluate regional lymph nodes for involvement using criteria that incorporate nodal size, shape, and number.

VII. LARYNX PRESERVATION

Management of larynx cancer is dictated by the location of the primary, the stage of the cancer, and the medical condition of the patient. Treatment decisions should be made with input from a multidisciplinary team, including a head and neck surgeon, radiotherapist, and medical oncologist. Lesions of the supraglottic larynx and early lesions of the true cords can be managed by partial laryngectomy or by radiotherapy alone. In some circumstances, radiotherapy will result in less impairment of speech than partial laryngectomy, with cure rates after primary radiotherapy, with surgical salvage in those patients who relapse in the same site, comparable to those after partial laryngectomy. The radiation tolerance of the upper aerodigestive tract is relatively high, although xerostomia and swallowing deficits may result. Some studies have suggested that twice daily administration of radiation treatments achieves somewhat better results in individual anatomic sites. Further research is ongoing into this question, as well as the role of concurrent chemotherapy administration of the use of systemic modulators of hypoxia within the treated area.

For more advanced tumors of the true cords and for most subglottic tumors, complete resection of the larynx is recommended. This results in loss of normal speech, and thus alternatives to the primary surgical approach have been sought. A number of investigators have demonstrated that initial chemotherapy and radiation, with surgery reserved for patients with a poor response to therapy or recurrence of disease, results in preservation of the larynx in about two-thirds of patients, with equivalent survival rates to immediate surgery. Patients with T4 tumors are most likely to suffer local recurrence.

VIII. MANAGEMENT OF NASOPHARYNX CANCER

The anatomic location generally precludes a curative resection of nasopharyngeal tumors. Standard therapy is combined modality radiation therapy and cisplatin chemotherapy. This approach has been demonstrated by randomized trial to lead to significant improvements in the response rate, a fourfold increase in time to progression, and an increase in 2-year survival from 55 to 80%.

IX. SURGERY

Recurrence of head and neck cancers at the primary site or in regional lymph nodes is a more common event than distant metastasis. For this reason, the margins of the tissue removed surgically are always carefully assessed because the presence of cancer cells at the edge of the resection predicts for recurrence. There has been interest in increasing the sensitivity of detection of malignant cells at the margin with the use of techniques that recognize cells carrying the same genetic abnormality as the tumor. Pilot trials suggest that molecular detection of abnormal cells at the margin, even if the margin appears free from cancer cells by conventional microscopy, predicts for a higher rate of local recurrence.

Selective to radical surgical dissection of the regional lymph node-bearing areas is performed to improve the accuracy of staging and increase the likelihood of curing the patient by surgery. The use of radical surgery if there is no clinical lymphadenopathy has decreased as the use of radiotherapy to treat microscopic residua of the tumor has become standard whenever metastases to the neck are detected.

Advances in surgical reconstruction, such as the use of free vacular flaps, have contributed to improved functional outcomes, as well as decreased postoperative complications.

X. ADJUVANT THERAPY

Postoperative radiation therapy is given when the extent of metastatic disease in the cervical lymph nodes points to a high likelihood of relapse within the regional node-bearing area. Compared with historical controls or patients offered preoperative therapy, postoperative radiation results in a lower locoregional relapse rate.

XI. MANAGEMENT OF UNRESECTABLE DISEASE

When a newly diagnosed cancer is found to be too extensive for curative treatment with surgery or radiation, systemic therapy is generally offered first. If the tumor is locally advanced without evidence of distant metastases, a good response to initial chemotherapy may make it possible to offer the patient definitive radiotherapy or surgery. In patients who have relapsed after surgery and radiotherapy, systemic therapy is not curative, but may result in a sufficient response for relief of symptoms and prolongation of survival.

XII. MANAGEMENT OF METASTATIC DISEASE

Systemic chemotherapy with cisplatin–based combination therapy is standard for the relatively well patient. The likelihood of a response to chemotherapy is 25% and the 1 year survival for patients treated in this manner is 30–40%. Patients with poor nutrition, poor performance status, or hypercalcemia have a worse prognosis and generally fare poorly with this treatment. Such patients are treated either with single agent methotrexate or with best supportive care.

XIII. SYMPTOM MANAGEMENT

The quality of life for the survivor of a carcinoma of the head and neck will depend to a great extent on the degree of impairment of swallowing, olfaction and speech. Evaluation of new therapies should always include assessments of these end points, and the post-treatment management of these patients should include assessment of swallowing with rehabilitation and nutritional support as needed.

Loss of speech, with the loss of the ability to communicate during a period of emotional and physical stress, is one of the most important complications faced by many survivors of head and neck cancer. Options for voice rehabilitation include learning to inhale air into the upper esophagus and then expel it in such as way that short sentences are audible; use of a handheld—usually electric—artificial larynx; or occlusion of the surgical tracheostomy with the thumb or with a valved prosthesis.

Late effects of treatment for head and neck cancer include necrosis of bone (osteonecrosis) or soft tissue,

chronic fibrosis, trismus, dry mouth, and chronic fibrosis, all of which may follow radiation; inner ear toxicity, nerve injury, and kidney dysfunction following cisplatin chemotherapy; and breakdown of tissue flaps used in surgical reconstruction or chronic scarring after surgery.

XIV. EXPERIMENTAL THERAPY

A. Targeting EGF-R

A chimeric monoclonal antibody that competitively inhibits the activation of EGF-R has been developed. This can safely be given in combination with standard chemotherapy agents, and a cooperative group trial is currently comparing a standard cisplatin chemotherapy regimen with the combination of cisplatin with the antibody to EGF-R. The results of this trial are expected in 2002. Likewise, small molecular kinase inhibitors that target EGF-R function have also been developed and are in the early stages of clinical testing.

B. Hypoxic Cell Sensitizers

Hypoxic cells are known to be relatively radioresistant, and tumors with larger proportions of hypoxic cells may be radioresistant. Novel pharmaceutical agents that sensitize hypoxic cells to radiation injury are currently in clinical trial.

XV. CHEMOPREVENTION

Trials of chemoprevention have been conducted in patients with the oral premalignant condition oral leukoplakia and in patients with prior cancers of the head and neck region. A reduction in the extent of oral leukoplakia and the degree of dysplasia in leukoplakia lesions were observed in randomized trials of isotretinoin, vitamin A, retinamide, and fenretinide. The regimens were associated with a number of unpleasant side effects; low-dose isotretinoin has been the regimen with the best balance of efficacy and tolerability. Premalignant lesions with decreased expression of the retinoic acid receptor β do not respond well to retinoid therapy.

See Also the Following Articles

EPSTEIN-BARR VIRUS • ESOPHAGEAL CANCER • GASTRIC CANCER • HEPATOCELLULAR CARCINOMA

Bibliography

Baselga, J., Pfister, D., Cooper, M. R. *et al.* (2000). Phase I studies of anti-epidermal growth factor receptor chimeric monoclonal antibody C225 alone and in combination with cisplatin. *J. Clin. Oncol.* **18,** 904.

Brennan, J. A., Mao, L., Hruban, R. H. *et al.* (1995). Molecular assessment of histopathologic staging. *N. Eng. J. Med.* **332,** 429–435.

Califano, J., van der Riet, P., Westra, W. *et al.* (1996). A genetic progression model for head and neck cancer: Implications for field cancerization. *Cancer Res.* **56,** 2488–2492.

Fremgen, A. M., Bland, K. I., McGinnis, L. S. *et al.* (1999). Clinical highlights from the National Cancer Data Base, 1999. *Ca. Cancer J. Clin.* **49,** 145–158.

Gillison, M. L., Koch, W. M., and Shah, K. V. (1999). Human papillovirus in head and neck squamous cell carcinoma: Are some head and neck cancers a sexually transmitted disease? *Curr. Opin. Oncol.* **11,** 191–199.

Hong, W. K., and Lotan, R. (1993). "Retinoids in Oncology." Dekker, New York.

Sidransky, D., Schantz, S. P., Harrison, L. B., Forastiere, A. A., and Sessions, R. B. (1997). Cancer of the head and neck. *In* "Cancer: Principles and Practice of Oncology" (V. T. De-Vita, Jr., S. Hellman, and S. A. Rosenberg, eds.), 5th Ed. Lippincott-Raven, Philadelphia.

Urba, S. (ed.) (1999). Head and neck cancer. *Hematol. Oncol. Clin. North Am.* **13,** 679–687.

Hepatitis B Viruses

Charles E. Rogler

Albert Einstein College of Medicine, Bronx, New York

I. Introduction
II. Characteristics of Transient and Persistent Infections
III. Persistent Infections: A Triple Threat for the
   Malignant Transformation of Hepatocytes

GLOSSARY

hepadnavirus A DNA virus with a partially single-stranded circular DNA genome that replicates by a novel reverse transcription mechanism, primarily in the liver of the host. Hepadnaviruses produce acute and persistent infections and promote hepatocarcinogenesis in the host liver.

heptocellular carcinoma A primary malignant tumor that originates from transformed hepatocytes in the liver.

hit and run mechanism Process by which hepadnavirus DNA integrates into host chromosomal DNA and then is excised along with some host DNA.

N-myc 2 A functional retroposon in the woodchuck genome that is a highly preferred target for activation by integration of enhancer elements from woodchuck hepatitis virus DNA.

persistent infection Infections of the liver that are not cleared after 6 months and generally persist for years.

triple threat The combination of (1) a hepatocyte injury,

death, and regeneration cycle in infected livers, (2) viral DNA integration and its consequences, and (3) action of the hepadnavirus X gene to deregulate cellular controls.

The aim of this article is to provide a succinct and integrated view of hepadnavirus infections and the broad roles of these viruses in malignant transformation in the liver. Hepadnaviruses (hepadnaviridae) are DNA viruses with small DNA genomes of about 3 kbp. Following the identification of human hepatitis B virus (HBV) by Blumberg and colleagues in 1967, related viruses were subsequently found in woodchucks, ground squirrels, ducks, geese, and herons. A major feature of hepadnaviruses is their very narrow host range and marked tissue specificity. While the liver is the major site of virus replication, low levels of virus production have been reported in the pancreas, spleen, and peripheral blood leukocytes. The woodchuck hepatitis virus (WHV) is the mammalian virus that most closely resembles HBV in its ability to cause liver disease and, in particular, hepatocellular carcinoma.

I. INTRODUCTION

I. General Description of the Viral Replication Cycle

Hepadnaviruses have partially double-stranded DNA genomes of approximately 3.3 kbp nucleotides in length that are held in a relaxed circular (RC) conformation by cohesive overlaps at their 5′ ends. Following infection, the genome is converted into a covalently closed circular DNA molecule, which is transported into the cell nucleus where it acts as a template for the transcription of three major viral RNA species. Pregenomic RNA, which spans the entire genome and is terminally redundant, is packaged together with the viral reverse transcriptase into subviral particles composed of 180 or 240 core subunits. Following the packaging reaction, pregenomic RNA is reverse transcribed into DNA by the viral reverse transcriptase. DNA-containing cores then interact with the viral envelope components in the endoplasmic reticulum and, following their transport through the secretory pathway, exit the cell as enveloped virions.

While over 90–95% of infectious "Dane" particles contain RC DNA genomes, approximately 5% of the infectious particles contain double strand linear (DSL) viral DNA molecules. These molecules can be circularized in hepatocytes and they replicate by a mechanism that Summers has designated "illegitimate replication" because their replication leads to the formation of a spectrum of mutant viruses. The existence of these DSL viral DNA molecules in hepatocytes may be important in hepatocarcinogenesis associated with persistent infections. Studies from the Rogler laboratory have shown that viruses containing only DSL DNA genomes integrate into host chromosomal DNA with a fourfold increased frequency compared with wild-type RC DNA molecules. Newly acquired viral DNA integrations closely resemble these linear molecules in structure, whereas integrations present in HCCs from long-term carriers are generally highly rearranged, suggesting that rearrangement of integrations occurs during long-term infections. Possible carcinogenic consequences of such rearrangements are discussed later.

II. CHARACTERISTICS OF TRANSIENT AND PERSISTENT INFECTIONS

A. Establishment and Clearance of Transient Infections

HBV generally causes transient infections in adults and chronic infections due to perinatal exposure. Transient infections are characterized by an asymptomatic incubation period that can be followed by a viremic phase typically running a course of 1–6 months. Although the entire hepatocyte population of the liver can be infected, the virus is rapidly cleared from the serum with either coincident or delayed clearance of infected hepatocytes from the liver. One scenario is that infected hepatocytes are killed by cytotoxic T lymphocytes and that regenerated hepatocytes are protected from reinfection by antibodies against the virus or by a cellular antiviral response induced by cytokines secreted by infiltrating lymphocytes. An alternative possibility supported by data from the Chisari and other laboratories is that cytokines induce an antiviral response in hepatocytes that leads to the elimination of virus and cure of the infected hepatocytes in the absence of hepatocyte killing. These hypotheses are not necessarily mutually exclusive and may both be active at different phases of infection, as is described later.

This second hypothesis is supported by a growing body of evidence that includes elegant studies with HBV transgenic mice that demonstrate rapid clearance of viral RNA and DNA replication forms that is dependent on the secretion of interferon (INF) γ and tumor necrosis factor (TNF) α by lymphocytes that migrate to the liver. Furthermore, infection studies with chimpanzees have shown that there is a period of viral clearance during acute infection when INF-γ and TNF-α are produced and hepatocyte death is not apparent. This is followed by a later phase of hepatocyte death when neutralizing antibodies are produced. These data suggest that viral clearance in chimpanzees may have a previously unappreciated biphasic nature. During the first phase, virus titer is dramatically reduced via a noncytopathic cytokine-mediated mechanism, followed by a second phase in which the immune system may clear the remaining infected hepatocytes via cytopathic CTL-mediated clearance mechanisms.

B. Establishment of Persistent Infections

When HBsAg persists in the serum of an individual for 6 months or longer, the infection is considered chronic. The basis for chronic infection lies in the failure of the immune response to clear the infection. As a consequence, infections are almost always chronic following exposure of newborn children or of immunocompromised individuals. Chronic infections in adults are often associated with severe and progressive liver disease, leading to cirrhosis and liver cancer. Interferon α and lamivudine are currently approved therapeutic agents for chronic HBV infection. The mechanism by which INF-α suppresses virus replication is not yet known. One possibility is that it suppresses virus replication in hepatocytes and the other is that it indirectly stimulates the immune system. The latter possibility is supported by evidence indicating that patients with liver disease due to a strong immune response to infected hepatocytes have the highest chances for recovery during therapy with the drug.

The mechanism by which lamivudine inhibits virus replication is inhibition of viral DNA synthesis by the HBV reverse transcriptase. As a consequence of monotherapy, lamivudine-resistant variants replace wild-type virus after about a year of therapy. However, lamivudine-resistant variants appear to replicate at an attenuated level compared with wild-type virus and, perhaps as a consequence, lamivudine therapy is generally associated with noticeable amelioration of liver disease.

III. PERSISTENT INFECTIONS: A TRIPLE THREAT FOR THE MALIGNANT TRANSFORMATION OF HEPATOCYTES

A. First Threat: A Cycle of Cell Death and Regeneration

Persistent infections are established in the liver when the host mounts an incomplete immune response to viral infection of the liver as discussed earlier. The limited immune responses are generally responsible for a spectrum of pathophysiological reactions in the liver that vary from mild portal hepatitis to chronic active hepatitis. In humans, cirrhosis is a common sequelae of persistent HBV infection, whereas cirrhosis does not occur in WHV carrier woodchucks. However, in both humans and woodchucks, a central ingredient provided by the immune response is the initiation and maintenance of a continuous cycle of cell death and regeneration in the liver. This cycle ensures that mutations that occur in regenerating hepatocytes will be fixed into cells of the next generation, and the cycle also provides an environment in which cells with a selective advantage will have the opportunity to be selectively amplified due to the need for hepatocyte replacement.

During long-term persistent infections, stress is placed on the regenerative capacity of the liver, and the liver begins to call upon its stem cell compartment for replacement of lost hepatocytes. The growth and accumulation of liver stem cells, called "oval cells," during chronic infection were first observed in WHV carrier woodchucks. A monoclonal antibody marker provided evidence that woodchuck oval cells proliferate near the portal tracts and then differentiate into hepatocytes as they expand out into the liver parenchyma. Interestingly, the monoclonal antibody identified some of these hepatocytes in precancerous lesions, called altered hepatic foci (AHF). Because HCCs develop from the progression of cells in AHFs, these data, plus a large literature from rat hepatocarcinogenesis, support the notion that woodchuck oval cells are precursors of a subset of HCCs. The amplification of oval cells has broad significance, as it has also been confirmed to occur in HBV carrier livers.

Under certain circumstances, HBV replication causes the production of ground glass hepatocytes that accumulate large amounts of HBV envelope protein. A transgenic mouse model in which the large HBV envelope protein was highly overexpressed led to the production of hepatocytes in the mouse liver that resemble ground glass cells. This pattern of large envelope overexpression caused hepatocyte injury and death and induced liver regeneration and eventually HCC in virtually all the mice. Interestingly, only those hepatocytes that deleted or inactivated the transgene and eliminated envelope protein expression survived to progress to malignancy. Within this chronic nonimmune-mediated liver damage environment in which toxic oxygen radicals are overproduced and random mutagenesis is highly increased, hepatocarcinogenesis ensues via a typical multistage mechanism. HBV DNA integration does not occur in this model, as only the HBV envelope gene is present in the mice. These data demonstrate that overexpression of viral protein can act as a carcinogenic agent but that the agent can be eliminated from the cells and the cells can continue to progress toward cancer.

As shown later, a similar situation may exist with the HBV X protein that is expressed during persistent infection but is absent from many HCCs. The multistage nature of hepatocarcinogenesis in mice with the production of precancerous foci that are negative for HBV envelope proteins clearly demonstrates the need for additional mutagenic events for carcinogenesis to proceed. In WHV and HBV carriers, these may be mediated by viral DNA integrations.

B. Second Threat: Oncogene Activation and "Hit and Run" Mutagenesis via Viral DNA Integration

1. Oncogene and Growth Factor Activation

Hepadnavirus DNA integrations into host chromosomes were first implicated in hepatocarcinogenesis when they were observed to occur in all of the cells in HCCs from HBV carriers and soon after in HCCs from WHV carrier woodchucks. Because clonal integrations of other retroviruses had been shown to activate a cellular protooncogene, c-myc, hepadnavirus integrations were cloned and sequenced with the aim of identifying a commonly activated cellular protooncogene. In the case of WHV, this search led the Buendia laboratory to the identification of a myc gene family member, N-myc 2, that was commonly activated in HCCs that arise in chronic carrier woodchucks.

Interestingly, WHV DNA integrations were observed in two cellular N-myc genes located at two separate locations in the woodchuck genome. These included the normal N-myc protooncogene and a second N-myc 2 gene, which is a functional retroposon. The N-myc 2 retroposon is not expressed in normal liver and is the most frequent WHV integration target. The predominant mechanism of activation is through integration of a fragment of the WHV genome that contains either of the two strong WHV liver-specific enhancer elements. This "enhancer insertion" mechanism is characteristic in that integration of the enhancer element can occur immediately upstream of N-myc 2 or in the 3′-untranslated region of the gene.

In an unexpected finding, a second common long distance integration site was identified approximately 200 kb upstream from the N-myc 2 gene. This site does not contain an expressed gene, and WHV DNA integration at this site is believed to mediate N-myc 2 expression also via a long distance enhancer insertion mechanism that may utilize a chromatin matrix attachment site that is near the integration site. A direct role of N-myc in the tumorigeneic phenotype has been confirmed in N-myc transgenic mice and in cell cultures that lose oncogenic properties when N-myc 2 is inactivated using antisense technology.

2. Coexpression of Insulin-like Growth Factor 2

One general finding has been that myc protooncogene activation is a double-edged sword in that it can either lead to cell proliferation or it promotes apoptosis of the cells. Many studies have shown that coexpression of a growth factor along with c-Myc drives cells into growth as opposed to apoptosis. In this regard, a key observation in woodchucks was the coordinate activation of the fetal liver growth factor, IGF-2, along with N-myc 2 activation in precancerous lesions. The coexpression of N-myc 2 and IGF-2 in early precancerous lesions, called altered hepatic foci, suggested a role for these genes early in carcinogenic progression, and their continued use in HCCs confirmed a selection for their high-level expression during carcinogenesis. Furthermore, IGF-2 was directly shown to block N-myc 2-induced apoptosis of cultured liver epithelial cells and it promotes the growth of cultured hepatocytes by an autocrine mechanism. Activation of IGF-2 has been found to be a common event in human HCC also.

3. Hit and Run Mutagenesis

While studies with WHV DNA integrations have been successful in linking viral DNA integration with a commonly activated oncogene, parallel studies with HBV DNA integrations have not successfully identified a commonly activated oncogene. HBV DNA integrations into some very provocative and potentially oncogenic genes have been identified, including integration and alteration of a steroid hormone receptor gene and the human cyclin A gene. In fact, altered cyclin A proteins have been shown to have growth regulatory properties.

HBV DNA integrations in HCCs from young children are generally colinear with an intact HBV DNA DSL integration precursor molecule. In contrast, integrations present in tumors from older adults are almost exclusively highly rearranged, with inverted repeats and deletions of HBV DNA. Another key feature of these integrations is that they are often associated with alteration of the host DNA at the site of integration. Chromosomal abnormalities linked to integrations include translocations, deletions, and direct or inverted duplications. These mechanisms can function to inactivate tumor suppressor genes as well as activate protooncogenes.

A predicted feature of the observations just mentioned is that newly acquired hepadnavirus integrations may be unstable in the genome and may function as "hit and run" mutagens that mediate the rearrangement of chromosomal DNA. Studies of the natural history of hepadnavirus integrations in cell cultures have directly demonstrated the "hit and run" mechanism and suggested that the loss of newly acquired integrations may be an important mutagenic mechanism during hepatocarcinogenesis. For example, in cell culture, host chomosomal DNA adjacent to integrated viral DNA was deleted when a viral DNA integration was lost from the cells.

Additional studies have shown that duck hepatitis B virus (DHBV) integrates frequently during acute infections. Furthermore, DHBV DNA integration in cell cultures is dramatically increased by treatments that promote DNA nicking or that block DNA repair in hepatocytes. These data support the hypothesis that sites of DNA damage may serve as integration sites. Viral DNA integrations can also accumulate in sequential cell generations. However, linear accumu-lation appears to be counterbalanced by the loss of new integrations that occur when the genome is destabilized by agents that prevent DNA repair.

4. Integration Precursor Molecules and Topoisomerase I

Cell culture studies have also demonstrated that DSL DHBV DNA molecules integrate at a much higher frequency than circular DHBV DNA molecules. Linearization of viral DNA at specific sites at the 5' ends of minus and plus strands must occur in order for integration to preferably occur at these sites. One cellular enzyme that may participate in the integration mechanism is topoisomerase I because it cleaves viral and cellular DNA at or near preferred sites of integration, and this enzyme can mediate nonhomologous recombination events of foreign DNA with host chromosomes. In fact, WHV DNA integration events can be duplicated *in vitro* with purified topoisomerase I, and sequence analysis of naturally occurring HBV DNA integration junctions shows an overwhelming association with preferred topoisomerase I cleavage sites in both viral and cellular DNAs at the junctions.

C. Third Threat: Hepadnavirus X Protein

A role for the mammalian hepadnavirus X protein in hepatocarcinogenesis has been proposed from the time it was first identified in a position in the HBV genome that is analogous to the position of other oncogenes in oncogenic retroviruses. However, several lines of evidence have been obtained to link X gene expression with the malignant transformation of hepatocytes. The current challenge in the field is to begin to link together the disparate lines of evidence from many variable experimental systems into coherent testable models and to test the models in liver relevant animal and cell culture systems.

1. Expression of X in Chronically Infected Liver and HCCs

The X gene promoter is weak, and a chronic problem in the field has been the determination of when and where the X protein is actually expressed in chronic infections. The clearest demonstration of X protein presence and quantitation comes from studies of chronically infected woodchuck liver using an excellent rabbit polyclonal antibody against the complete WHV X (WHx) protein. These studies clearly detected WHx in persistently infected hepatocytes and estimated the steady-state level to be approximately 40,000 molecules per hepatocyte. Metabolic labeling demonstrated that 80% of the rapidly labeled X was cytoplasmic with 20% located in the nucleus.

An important finding of the woodchuck studies was that WHx was only present in tissues that carried out productive WHV replication. This included a subset of woodchuck HCCs that continued to replicate WHV. Importantly, WHx was *not observed* in any poorly differentiated woodchuck HCCs that were nonpermissive for WHV replication. This has important implications for hepatocarcinogenesis in woodchucks because the WHx protein associates most closely with viral replication and is not required for malignancy in poorly differentiated HCCs that are nonpermissive for viral replication.

The expression of HBx from integrated hepadnavirus DNAs has been a controversial topic. However, elegant studies from the Brechot laboratory have identified HBV DNA integrations that contain mutant HBx genes that have important antiapoptotic activities. These studies have directly demonstrated that mutant HBx proteins can be expressed from HBV integrations and that their antiapoptotic activities can function to promote carcinogenic progression in the liver. Both HBV and WHV transgenic mouse data support a weak tumor promoter role for their respective X proteins. A tumor promoter role has been supported by *in vitro* studies in which SV40-immortalized hepatocytes have undergone malignant transformation in response to overexpressed HBx. In one transgenic mouse line, HBx is thought to serve as a complete carcinogen, as these mice develop HCC without tumor promoters. However, this line is a singular exception, which suggests that other genetic factors may predispose that particular transgenic mouse line to hepatocarcinogenesis.

2. Biological Activities of X

The first biological activity associated with mammalian X proteins was that of a transacting factor. In this capacity, HBx can transactivate a wide variety of promoters upstream from many different genes in a wide variety of cell types. This initial activity led investigators to search for molecular mechanisms for the action of HBx and WHx and to characterize its cellular functions.

X gene functions have been and still are the subject of controversy, and extensive reviews have been presented on this topic. In recent years, convincing evidence has accumulated to suggest that the expression of X activates several cellular signal transduction pathways known to play a role in cell growth and transformation. Initially, HBx was shown to activate the Ras signal transduction pathway in a variety of hepatocellular and nonhepatocellular cell lines. Depending on the specific culture conditions, HBx may be pro- or antiapoptotic. An extensive series of reports in this area have focused on the Src signal transduction pathway, which can lead to the transactivation of important tumorigenesis genes, such as c-myc. The current challenge for researchers in the signal transduction area is to determine how these signaling pathways are altered in hepatocytes during persistent infections. Clearly, X expression alone is insufficient to fully transform hepatocytes. Thus, the mechanism of X action in the context of long-term persistent infection with its concomitant mutagenic effects is a critical importance.

The effect of HBx on tumor suppressor pathways has not escaped investigation. One of the most important tumor suppressors is p53, and a series of papers have provided a link between HBx and p53 action. Normally, p53 expression is upregulated in response to cell stress, and p53 sets in motion a set of gene activities that can lead to either apoptosis or cell cycle exit. Thus, knocking out p53 removes an important brake on the cell cycle and allows mutant cells to survive and progress to malignancy. Therefore, the finding that HBx binds to p53 and blocks some of its biological actions is significant. The initial reports have been confirmed in several cell culture systems; in one transgenic mouse line, however, interpretation of how these findings actually relate to hepatocarcinogenesis in carrier livers remains to be elucidated. One attractive hypothesis is that mutant or wild-type HBx proteins present in the cytoplasm bind to p53 and prevent it from translocating into the nucleus. This mechanism would require continuous expression of X proteins, which is not the case in many HCCs. However, a significant subset of HCCs that are nonpermissive for HBV replication continue to express HBx from integrated templates.

IV. SUMMARY

In light of the combination of procarcinogenic mechanisms briefly outlined earlier, it is understandable that in WHV carrier woodchucks there is virtually a 100% lifetime incidence of HCC and that in male HBV carriers there appears to be at least a 40% lifetime risk of HCC! The current therapies that limit HBV replication may also limit viral DNA integration and also reduce the rate of hepatocyte turnover in the liver. Thus, the triple threat may be significantly reduced. It is hoped that prospective studies of patients on long-term treatment protocols will reveal a reduced risk of HCC for these patients.

See Also the Following Articles

HEPATITIS C VIRUS • HEPATOCELLULAR CARCINOMA • LIVER CANCER: ETIOLOGY AND PREVENTION

Bibliography

Buendia, M. A. (1998) Hepatitis B viruses and cancerogenesis. *Biomed. Pharmacother.* **52,** 34–43.

Benn, J., and Schneider, R. J. (1994). Hepatitis B virus HBx protein activates Ras-GTP complex formation and establishes a Ras, Raf, MAP kinase signaling cascade. *Proc. Natl. Acad. Sci. USA.* **91,** 10350–10354.

Blumberg, B. S., Gerstley, B. J. S., Hungerford, D. A., London, W. T., and Sutnik, A. I. (1967). A serum antigen (Australai antigen) in Down's syndrome, leukemia and hepatitis. *Ann. Intern. Med.* **66,** 924–931.

Chisari, F. V. (1997) Cytotoxic T cells and viral hepatitis. *J. Clin. Invest.* **99,** 1472–1477.

Fourel, G., Trepo, C., Bougueleret, L., Henglein, B., Ponzetto, A., Tiollais, P., and Buendia, M. A. (1990). Frequent activation of N-myc genes by hepadnavirus insertion in woodchuck liver tumours. *Nature* **347**(6290), 294–298.

Fourel, G., Conturier, J., Wei, Y., Apiou, F., Tiollais, P., and Buendia, M. A. (1994). Evidence for long-range oncogene activation by hepadnavirus insertion. *EMBO J.* **13,** 2526–2534.

Guidotti, L. G., Rochford, R., Chung, J., Shapiro, M., Purcell, R., and Chisari, F. V. (1999). Viral clearance without destruction of infected cells during acute HBV infection *Science* **284**(5415), 825–829.

Ganem, D. and Schneider, R.J. (2000) The molecular biology of hepatitis B viruses. *In* "Fields Virology" (D. Knipe and P. Howley, eds.). Lippincott, New York.

Gong, S. S., Jensen, A. D., and Rogler, C. E. (1996). Loss and acquisition of duck hepatitis B virus integrations in lineages of LMH-D2 chicken hepatoma cells. *J. Virol.* **70,** 2000–2007.

Guo, J.-T., Zhou, H., Liu, C., Aldrich, C., Saputelli, J., Whitaker, T., Barrasa, M. I., Mason, W. S., and Seeger, C. (2000). Apoptosis and regeneration of hepatocytes during recovery from transient hepadnavirus infection. *J. Virol.* **74,** 1495–1505.

Hino, O., Shows, T. B., and Rogler, C. E. (1986). Hepatitis B virus integration site in hepatocellular carcinoma at chromosome 17:18 translocation. *Proc. Natl. Acad. Sci. USA* **83,** 8338–8342.

Kajino, K., Jilbert, A. R., Saputelli, J., Aldrich, C. E., Cullen, J., and Mason, W. S. (1994). Woodchuck hepatitis virus infections: Very rapid recovery after a prolonged viremia and infection of virtually every hepatocyte. *J. Virol.* **68**(9), 5792–5803.

Klein, N. P., Bouchard, M. J., Wang, L. H., Kobarg, C., and Schneider, R. J. (1999). Src kinases involved in hepatitis B virus replication. *EMBO J.* **18**(18), 5019–5027.

Nagaya, T., Nakamua, T., Tokina, T, Tsurimoto, T., Imai, M., Mayumi, T., Kamino, K., Yamamura, K., and Matsubara, K. (1987). The mode of hepatitis B virus DNA integration in chromosomes of human hepatocellular carcinoma. *Genes Dev.* **1,** 773–782.

Rogler, C. E. (1991). Cellular and molecular mechanisms of hepatocarcinogenesis associated with hepadnavirus infection. *Curr. Top. Microbiol. Immunol.* **168,** 103–141.

Rogler, C. E., Sherman, M., Su, C. Y., and Shafritz, D. A. (1985). Deletion in chromosome 11p associated with a hepatitis B integration site in hepatocellular carcinoma. *Science* **230,** 319–322.

Seeger, C., and Mason, W. S. (2000). Hepatitis B virus biology. *Microbiol Mol. Biol. Rev.* **64**(1), 51–68.

Sirma, H., Giannini, C., Poussin, K., Paterlini, P., Kremsdorf, D., and Brechot, C. (1999). Hepatitis B virus X mutants, present in hepatocellular carcinoma tissue abrogate both the antiproliferative and trasnsactivation effects of HBx. *Oncogene* **18,** 4848–4859.

Summers, J., and Mason, W. S. (1982). Replication of the genome of a hepatitis B-like virus by reverse transcription of an RNA intermediate. *Cell* **29,** 403–415.

Hepatitis C Virus (HCV)

Michael M. C. Lai

University of Southern California Keck School of Medicine

I. Hepatitis C Virus (HCV) Biology
II. Virus Structure
III. Virus Replication
IV. Epidemiological Evidence of Association between HCV and Hepatocellular Carcinoma (HCC)
V. Mechanism of HCV Oncogenesis
VI. Prevention of HCV-Associated HCC
VII. Perspectives

GLOSSARY

cryoglobulinemia A medical condition in which the presence of cold-precipitating immunoglobulins are present. These immunoglobulins are either monoclonal or polyclonal and have antibody activities against other immunoglobulins, thus forming immune complexes. This condition is found in lymphoproliferative, autoimmune, or infectious diseases.

interferon A natural antiviral glycoprotein produced by the cells in response to viral infections or other stimuli. Interferon binds to interferon receptors and triggers signal transduction and activates expression of many genes with antiviral activities.

internal ribosome entry site A special RNA structure at an untranslated region of a messenger RNA that allows the ribosome to bind directly to RNA without scanning through the 5' end of the RNA. Consequently, the protein is translated irrespective of the structure at the 5' end of the RNA. Several viral RNAs, such as poliovirus RNA, and some cellular RNAs have such a sequence.

liver cirrhosis Fibrosis and nodular degeneration and regeneration of the liver, usually as a result of chronic inflammation.

non-A, non-B hepatitis Hepatitis not caused by hepatitis A virus or hepatitis B virus. Conventionally, it refers to viral hepatitis caused by hepatitis C virus.

nonstructural proteins Proteins that are encoded by viral genomes but not found in the virus particles. These proteins typically perform functions in viral replication or modulate viral infection.

nuclear factor κB Originally discovered as a transcription factor binding to the enhancer region of the immunoglobulin κ light chain gene, but later found to regulate many other genes in response to inflammatory cytokines.

steatosis Fatty degeneration of the liver, characterized by the presence of lipid droplets in the liver cells.

H epatitis C virus (HCV), along with hepatitis B virus (HBV), is the major viral etiological agent of hepatocellular carcinoma (HCC) in many parts of the world. An estimated 100 million people in the world are infected with HCV, which has strong predilection for persistent infection, often leading to chronic hepatitis, liver cirrhosis, and HCC. HCV is an RNA virus, which encodes several proteins with potential oncogenic properties; however, the molecular mechanism of HCV oncogenesis is still poorly understood. The incidence of HCV-associated HCC has increased in recent years but may be reduced by interferon treatment of HCV infection.

I. HEPATITIS C VIRUS (HCV) BIOLOGY

HCV was discovered in 1989 by molecular cloning and subsequent immunoscreening of the nucleic acids from the serum of patients with transfusion-associated non-A, non-B hepatitis (NANBH). Prior to this discovery, HBV had been recognized as the major causative agent of HCC; however, NANBH was also known to be associated with a sizable number of HBV-free HCC cases. The discovery of HCV confirmed the strong association of this virus with HCC. HCV is an RNA virus belonging to the Flaviviridae family, which includes other well-studied human pathogens, such as yellow fever virus, Dengue virus, and Japanese encephalitis virus. These viruses have significant similarity in their genomic structure and replication strategy. HCV is transmitted by blood transfusion or other parenteral routes, such as intravenous drug use and contaminated needlesticks. Blood screening has minimized the risk of HCV infection through blood transfusion. HCV can infect chimpanzees, causing viremia and mild hepatitis, but no efficient cell culture system is yet available for growing this virus in culture. HCV can be divided into six major genotypes and multiple subtypes. Different genotypes may be associated with different biological properties of the virus and determines the efficacy of antiviral therapy. The viral RNA sequence is also characterized by the presence of multiple quasispecies, which represent slightly diverged sequences from a predominant RNA species. The nature of viral quasispecies often evolves during the course of viral infec-

tion and may allow the virus to escape the immune response of the host.

II. VIRUS STRUCTURE

HCV is an enveloped, spherical virus particle of 30–80 nm. It has a very low density because of its association with serum lipoproteins. The viral envelope contains two envelope proteins, E1 and E2, which form the spikes on the surface of the virus particles and are responsible for viral interaction with the receptors of the target cells. Inside the envelope is an icosahedral nucleocapsid, consisting of the core (C) protein and viral genome. The precise virion structure has not been elucidated.

The viral genome is a 9.5-kb, single-stranded RNA of positive polarity (Fig. 1). It contains a single open reading frame encoding a polyprotein of approximately 3010 amino acids. The polyprotein is processed into three to four viral structural proteins (C, E1, E2, and probably an additional protein p7 of undetermined nature) and six nonstructural proteins, ns2, ns3, ns4a, ns4b, ns5a, and ns5b, which are detected only in the infected cells, but not incorporated into the virus particles. At the 5' end of the RNA is a stretch (341 nucleotides) of untranslated region, which forms several stem–loop structures, collectively called an internal ribosome entry site (IRES). The IRES allows ribosomes to bypass the 5' end of RNA and initiate translation of the polyprotein. At the 3' end of the viral RNA is another stretch of untranslated region of approximately 200 nucleotides, which consists of (in the order from the 3' end) a 98 nucleotide highly conserved sequence (termed X region), a poly(U) and U/C-rich region of variable length, and another stretch of 30–40 nucleotides, which is variable between different genotypes but is conserved within the same genotype. The 5' and 3' end sequences likely interact with each other and are important for the regulation of translation and RNA replication. Both of them are the most conserved regions within the viral RNA.

The viral polyprotein is processed by both cellular and viral proteases into individual structural and nonstructural proteins. The C, E1, and E2 proteins are cleaved from each other by cellular signal peptidases

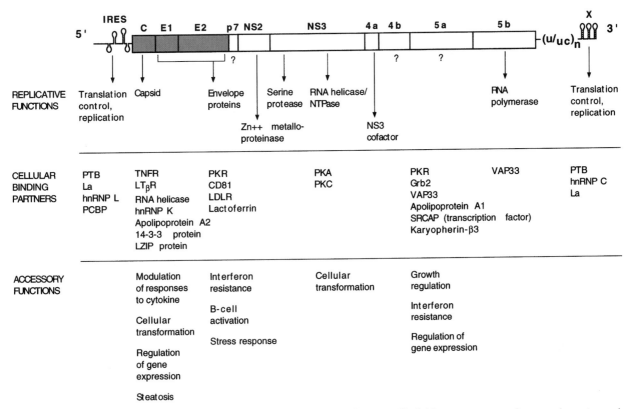

FIGURE 1 Schematic structure of HCV RNA, protein products, and their functions. Shaded boxes represent viral structural proteins, and open boxes represent nonstructural proteins. "Replicative functions" refer to the roles of RNA sequence or protein products in viral replication. Cellular binding partners are cellular proteins found to interact with viral RNA or proteins. Accessory functions are the effects of viral proteins on the functions of cells. PTB, polypyrimidine tract-binding protein; PCBP, poly(C)-binding protein; $LT_\beta R$, lymphotoxin-β receptor; TNFR, tumor necrosis factor receptor; PKR, double-stranded RNA-activated protein kinase; LDLR, low-density lipoprotein receptor; PKA and PKC, protein kinase A and C; Grb2, growth factor receptor-binding protein 2; VAP33, vesicle-associated membrane protein (VAMP)-associated protein of 33 kDa; hnRNP, heterogeneous nuclear ribonucleoprotein. The diagram is not drawn to scale.

during translation. The E2 protein displays the most heterogeneity, particularly in the two hypervariable regions (HVR1 and HVR2) at its very N terminus, among various HCV isolates. The ns2–ns5b are cleaved from each other by either ns2 protease (which cleaves the ns2–ns3 boundary) or ns3–ns4a protease (which cleaves all of the remaining protein boundaries, ns3/4a, ns4a/4b, ns4b/5a, and ns5a/5b). Ns2 is a metalloproteinase, requiring Zn^{2+} ions for its activity, but its protease activity is active only when it is linked to ns3. Ns3 is a serine protease, which also contains Zn^{2+} ions and requires ns4a as a cofactor. The ns3–4a protease can cleave protein substrates *in trans*. Ns3 also contains an RNA helicase/NTPase activity, which may participate in either translation or RNA replication. The functions of ns4b and ns5a are not yet

known. Ns5b is an RNA-dependent RNA polymerase, which is responsible for the replication of viral RNA.

III. VIRUS REPLICATION

HCV replicates primarily in hepatocytes in infected patients and chimpanzees. Increasing evidence, however, suggests that it may also infect cells of extrahepatic tissues, especially peripheral blood mononuclear cells. HCV can infect and replicate in various hepatocyte and T and B lymphoid cell lines in tissue culture. However, the viral RNA is present in these cell lines usually in very low titer and persists only for a very short time. The first step of viral infection is the binding of the virus particle to a receptor molecule on the surface of the target cells. Two normal cell surface molecules, CD81 (a tetraspanin molecule of unknown function) and low-density lipoprotein (LDL) receptor, have been implicated to be the receptor for HCV; however, whether they are the true and only receptors for HCV is not yet known. Both of these molecules are widely distributed, but not limited to the liver.

The binding of the virus to CD81 is mediated by the viral E2 protein; antibodies against E2 can block virus binding *in vitro*. The virus binding to the receptor triggers the internalization of the virus into cells, where the virus is uncoated to release the viral RNA. The RNA is first translated into a polyprotein, from which the viral RNA polymerase (ns5b) is released by proteolytic processing. The polymerase then initiates RNA synthesis to replicate the viral RNA into a negative-sense RNA, which, in turn, serves as the template for the synthesis of genomic RNA. No DNA intermediates are generated in the HCV replication process.

Additional viral polyproteins are translated from the newly synthesized genomic RNA and proteolytically processed. Some of the nonstructural proteins, in addition to the polymerase ns5b itself, may also be involved in viral RNA synthesis. The E1 and E2 proteins are anchored at the endoplasmic reticulum, where they interact with the viral nucleocapsid (C protein and viral genome) to assemble virus particles. Only positive strand, but not negative strand, RNA is incorporated into the virus particle. The completed virus particles are found in vesicles in the cytoplasm. Virions are probably secreted into extracellular space using cellular secretory pathways. The entire viral replication cycle occurs in the cytoplasm. It is not yet clear whether viral replication causes cytopathic changes. Viral RNA replication, but not virus production, can now be studied in cultured cells, using a subgenomic replicon system consisting of HCV nonstructural proteins and a selectable reporter gene.

IV. EPIDEMIOLOGICAL EVIDENCE OF ASSOCIATION BETWEEN HCV AND HEPATOCELLULAR CARCINOMA (HCC)

Although HBV remains the most important etiological agent of HCC in the high endemic areas for HBV,

such as southeast Asia and part of Africa, HCV has become the predominant cause of HCC in other geographical regions, including the United States, Japan, and European countries, where HBV is not endemic. The incidence of HCC in these regions has steadily increased in the last two decades. Epidemiological studies showed that 6–75% of HCC patients are infected with HCV (vs 1–2% for general populations), depending on the geographical regions. Case-control studies showed a relative risk of 15–50 for HCV carriers to develop HCC, which is even higher than that for HBV in non-HBV-endemic areas. Liver cirrhosis and alcohol consumption are significant risk factors contributing to the development of HCC among HCV carriers. There is a reported preferential association of certain HCV genotype (e.g., genotype 1b) with HCC, but this finding is controversial.

V. MECHANISM OF HCV ONCOGENESIS

The major characteristic of HCV infection is its strong tendency to establish persistent infection. Almost 85% of HCV infections result in persistent infections, and 70% of these infections will lead to chronic hepatitis; approximately 20% will develop liver cirrhosis and 1–5% overall may develop HCC. The chronic state of infection is likely one of the major contributing factors in the carcinogenesis of HCV. Chronic inflammation, with inflammatory cells and their associated cytokines, may cause chronic stimulation of hepatocytes, thereby altering the metabolic state of cells. Also, liver cirrhosis is typically accompanied by compensatory hepatocyte proliferation, which may increase the risk of abnormal cell growth. These nonspecific mechanisms caused by the cellular responses to chronic HCV infections may contribute to hepatocarcinogenesis.

HCV does not produce a DNA intermediate; thus, unlike HBV, it does not integrate into the chromosomes of infected cells. Therefore, HCV likely has innate and occasionally induced abilities to interfere with and evade the host immune response so that it can establish persistent infections. Studies have shown that several HCV proteins can interact with a variety of cellular proteins, resulting in the alteration of cellular gene expression, growth control, and responses to cytokines. Some of these interactions may contribute to the establishment of persistent viral infections and the development of HCC. In particular, three viral proteins have properties that suggest that they may directly or indirectly contribute to viral oncogenesis (Fig. 1).

A. Core Protein

The core protein forms the viral nucleocapsid, but also has other properties potentially capable of affecting viral pathogenesis. The core protein binds to the cytoplasmic domains of the tumor necrosis factor (TNF) receptor and lymphotoxin-β-receptor (LTβR). The binding sites correspond to those of the signal transduction molecules for these receptors. Therefore, the core protein likely affects the signal transduction of these receptors. The core protein also has been shown to enhance NF-κB activation either constitutively or in response to TNF. Cells expressing the core protein have been shown to have either enhanced or decreased sensitivity to TNF, Fas antigen, and lymphotoxins, probably depending on different cell conditions, as the core protein can also interact with several other cellular proteins, such as hnRNP K and RNA helicase, which may alter the expression of various cellular genes. It also has the ability to suppress the cytotoxic T-cell response. These combined effects likely contribute to the pathogenic potential of HCV. The core protein also binds apolipoprotein A$_2$, which may be linked to the occurrence of hepatic steatosis commonly observed in hepatitis C. The core protein has several other properties more directly related to the potential oncogenic potential. (1) The core protein can transform rat primary embryo fibroblasts, when cooperating with other oncogenes, such as *ras*, under some conditions. Furthermore, it can immortalize human primary hepatocytes. (2) Transgenic mice expressing the core protein may develop hepatocellular carcinoma. (3) It binds to a bZIP protein, which can activate CRE-dependent transcription and regulate cell proliferation. Binding of the core protein results in the loss of bZIP function, which correlates with the morphological transformation and anchorage-independent growth of cells expressing the core protein. (4) It binds to the 14-3-3 protein and activates Raf-1 kinase. This property may also enhance the trans-

forming ability of the core protein. The full-length core protein is located in the cytoplasm, whereas the C terminus-truncated core protein is located in the nucleus. The significance of the variable subcellular localization is not clear, but may allow the core protein to interact with various cellular proteins in both the cytoplasm and the nucleus.

B. Ns3 Protein

Ns3 contains serine protease and helicase/NTPase activity, both of which are required for viral replication. The N-terminal half of the molecule, which contains the protease domain, has been shown to have transforming activity for NIH3T3 cells *in vitro* and to cause tumors in nude mice. The precise mechanism of cellular transformation is not clear. Ns3 can bind to protein kinases A and C, affecting their nuclear translocation after stimulation with mitogens. This effect may alter cellular growth properties.

C. Ns5a

Ns5a protein does not appear to have functions that are required for viral replication; however, it binds to an interferon-inducible, double-stranded RNA-activated protein kinase (PKR). The binding sites are located within a region of ns5a termed the interferon sensitivity-determining region (ISDR), which has been demonstrated to correlate with the clinical sensitivity to interferon in some patients, particularly in Japanese patients. PKR activation can induce apoptosis and its inhibition may promote cell growth and facilitate the establishment of persistent viral infections. Correspondingly, the inhibition of PKR by ns5a has been shown to promote cellular proliferation; however, exactly the opposite result, namely the inhibition of cell growth, has also been reported. Ns5a also binds to a cellular growth regulatory protein Grb2 and either activates or inhibits the signal transduction cascades associated with growth factor stimulation. The truncated ns5a proteins lacking the N-terminal sequences have a *trans*-activating activity, capable of activating the transcription of some reporter genes in the cells. The variable and sometimes contradictory effects of ns5a may be linked to the different conditions of cells.

D. Other Genes

E2 protein is a viral envelope protein responsible for the initial contact between the virus and the target cells. In addition to its role in virus entry, E2 may exert other effects. First of all, E2 binds to CD81, a molecule on the surface of B cells, causing the aggregation of lymphoid cells and inhibition of B-cell proliferation under some conditions. Irrespective of the outcome of virus infection, this interaction triggers B-cell signaling. It is significant that HCV is strongly associated with type II mixed cryoglobulinemia (a B-cell proliferative disease) and with non-Hodgkin's B-cell lymphoma in some geographical regions. The E2–CD81 interaction may contribute to these disease manifestations. In addition, E2 shares some sequence similarity with protein kinase PKR, which is a mediator of the antiviral actions of interferon by inhibiting viral translation. As a result, PKR activity is inhibited by E2, and the antiviral effects of interferon are blocked. Furthermore, the inhibition of PKR may block apoptosis and facilitate the persistence of virus infection. E2 also activates stress response genes, such as glucose regulated protein grp78, probably because of the misfolding of the E2 protein in the endoplasmic reticulum.

Other viral proteins may also have effects in inhibiting interferon response. A cell line expressing the entire HCV proteins has been shown to interfere with the signal transduction (JAK-STAT pathway) of interferon receptors. However, the nature of the viral protein responsible for this effect has not been identified. Ns4b has also been reported to have oncogenic activities.

VI. PREVENTION OF HCV-ASSOCIATED HCC

Currently available therapy for HCV infection is interferon-α or interferon-α plus ribavirin as a combination therapy. The efficacy rate ranges from 20 to 60%, depending on the treatment regimen and, most importantly, the genotype of the virus. Genotype I HCV isolates are significantly more resistant than other genotypes to these therapies. The efficacy of the treatment is reflected in the lowering of virus RNA titer in the serum, normalization of liver functions (alanine aminotransferase values), and improvement of the histological index in liver biopsy. Significantly, interferon treatment has been shown to reduce the relative risk of HCC and delay its development among patients who responded to the treatment.

VII. PERSPECTIVES

Based on the epidemiological association, HCV has been shown to be an increasingly important cause of HCC in many parts of the world. Although several viral gene products have been shown to have oncogenic potential or have an ability to interfere with the antiviral responses of the host, the precise mechanism of HCV persistence and oncogenesis is still not clear. Anti-HCV therapy (interferon) has shown the promise of arresting or delaying the progression of liver cirrhosis and the development of HCC, but the overall efficacy of the treatment is still less than ideal. Understanding the mechanism of viral resistance to interferon and development of new anti-HCV therapy will be the urgent tasks in the near future.

See Also the Following Articles

HEPATITIS B VIRUSES • HEPATOCELLULAR CARCINOMA • LIVER CANCER: ETIOLOGY AND PREVENTION • TUMOR NECROSIS FACTORS

Bibliography

Agnello, V., Abel, G., Elfahal, M., Knight, G. B., and Zhang, Q. X. (1999). Hepatitis C virus and other flaviviridae viruses enter cells via low density lipoprotein receptor. *Proc. Natl. Acad. Sci. USA* **96,** 12766–12771.

Aoki, H., Hayashi, J., Moriyama, M., Arakawa, Y., and Hino, O. (2000). Hepatitis C virus core protein interacts with 14-3-3 protein and activates the kinase raf-1. *J. Virol.* **74,** 1736–1741.

Bronowicki, J. P., Loriot, M. A., Thiers, V., Grignon, Y., Zignego, A. L., and Brechot, C. (1998). Hepatitis C virus persistence in human hematopoietic cells injected in SCID mice. *Hepatology* **28,** 211–218.

Choo, Q. L., Kuo, G., Weiner, A. J., Overby, L. R., Bradley, D. W., and Houghton, M. (1989). Isolation of a cDNA clone derived from a blood-borne non-A, non-B viral hepatitis genome. *Science* **244,** 359–362.

Colombo, M. (1999). Hepatitis C virus and hepatocellular carcinoma. *Semin. Liver Dis.* **19,** 263–269.

Gale, M. J. J., Korth, M. J., Tang, N. M., Tan, S.-L., Hopkins, D. A., Dever, T. E., Polyak, S. J., Gretch, D. R., and Katze, M. G. (1997). Evidence that hepatitis C virus resistance to interferon is mediated through repression of the PKR protein kinase by the nonstructural 5A protein. *Virology* **230,** 217–227.

Heim, M. H., Moradpour, D., and Blum, H. E. (1999). Expression of hepatitis C virus proteins inhibits signal transduction through the Jak-STAT pathway. *J. Virol.* **73,** 8469–8475.

Jin, D. Y., Wang, H. L., Zhou, Y., Chun, A. C., Kibler, K. V., Hou, Y. D., Kung, H. F., and Jeang, K. T. (2000). Hepatitis C virus core protein-induced loss of LZIP function correlates with cellular transformation. *EMBO J.* **19,** 729–740.

Lai, M. M. C., and Ware, C. F. (1999). Hepatitis C virus core protein: Possible roles in viral pathogenesis. *Curr. Top. Microbiol. Immunol.* **242,** 117–134.

Laskus, T., Radkowski, M., Piasek, A., Nowicki, M., Horban, A., Cianciara, J., and Rakela, J. (2000). Hepatitis C virus in lymphoid cells of patients coinfected with human deficiency virus type 1: Evidence of active replication in monocytes/macrophages and lymphocytes. *J. Infect. Dis.* **181,** 442–448.

Lohmann, V., Körner, F., Koch, J.-O., Herian, U., Theilmann, L., and Bartenschlager, R. (1999). Replication of subgenomic hepatitis C virus RNAs in a hepatoma cell line. *Science.* **285,** 110–113.

Moriya, K., Fujie, H., Shintani, Y., Yotsuyanagi, H., Tsutsumi, T., Ishibashi, K., Matsuura, Y., Kimura, S., Miyamura, T., and Koike, K. (1998). The core protein of hepatitis C virus induces hepatocellular carcinoma in transgenic mice. *Nature Med.* **4,** 1065–1067.

Pileri, P., Uematsu, Y., Campagnoli, S., Galli, G., Falugi, F., Petracca, R., Weiner, A. J., Houghton, M., Rosa, D., Grandi, G., and Abrignani, S. (1998). Binding of hepatitis C virus to CD81. *Science* **282,** 938–941.

Ray, R. B., Lagging, L. M., Meyer, K., and Ray, R. (1996). Hepatitis C virus core protein cooperates with ras and transforms primary rat embryo fibroblasts to tumorigenic phenotype. *J. Virol.* **70,** 4438–4443.

Sakamuro, D., Furukawa, T., and Takegami, T. (1995). Hepatitis C virus nonstructural protein NS3 transforms NIH 3T3 cells. *J. Virol.* **69,** 3893–3896.

Taylor, D. R., Shi, S. T., Romano, P. R., Barber, G. N., and Lai, M. M. C. (1999). Inhibition of the interferon-inducible protein kinase PKR by HCV E2 protein. *Science* **285,** 107–110.

Yoshida, H., Shiratori, Y., Moriyama, M., Arakawa, Y., Ide, T., Sata, M., Inoue, O., Yano, M., Tanaka, M., Fujiyama, S., Nishiguchi, S., Kuroki, T., Imazeki, F., Yokosuka, O., Kinoyama, S., Yamada, G., and Omata, M. (1999). Interferon therapy reduces the risk for hepatocellular carcinoma: National surveillance program of cirrhotic and noncirrhotic patients with chronic hepatitis C in Japan. *Ann. Intern. Med.* **131,** 174–181.

Hepatocellular Carcinoma (HCC)

Paul F. Engstrom

Fox Chase Cancer Center, Philadelphia, Pennsylvania

I. Incidence and Mortality
II. Risk Factors
III. Pathogenesis
IV. Prevention
V. Diagnosis and Staging
VI. Management
VII. Summary

GLOSSARY

aflatoxin A toxic metabolite produced by aspergillus fungi and implicated as a contributing cause of hepatocellular carcinoma.

chemoembolization A technique that utilizes the placement of a catheter tubing in the hepatic artery to deliver chemotherapy agents plus clot inducers (thrombin) to selectively treat liver cancer to the exclusion of other organ systems.

chemoprevention Use of micronutrients or pharmaceutical drugs to neutralize a carcinogen or to interrupt progression of a precancer condition to an invasive cancer.

chemotherapy Utilization of orally or systemically administered pharmaceutical drugs (antimetabolites, alkylating agents, or biological agents) to treat cancer.

cholangiocarcinoma A malignant neoplasm of the liver arising from bile duct epithelium.

α-fetoprotein A circulating serum protein produced by fetal cells and specialized cancer cells normally pres-ent only at birth, but when elevated in an adult serves as a biomarker of liver cancer growth rate.

hemochromatosis An inherited iron metabolic condition resulting in iron deposits in the liver, which can cause cirrhosis and hepatocellular carcinoma.

hepatectomy A surgical resection of part (partial hepatectomy) or the whole liver (total hepatectomy) as treatment for liver tumor(s).

hepatitis An acute or chronic inflammation of the liver tissue usually due to viral infection but also associated with the ingestion of toxic chemicals, including alcohol.

hepatocellular carcinoma A malignant neoplasm arising from the liver cell (hepatocyte).

radiofrequency ablation Utilizing a percutaneous approach, a needle is placed into a liver tumor in order to kill cancer cells with a heat-generating current.

Hepatocellular carcinoma (HCC) rises in the hepatocyte of the liver and is one of the leading causes of death from cancer in Asia, Southeast Asia, and sub-Sahara Africa. HCC is associated with hepatitis B virus infection, hepatitis C virus infection, aflatoxin ingestion, and alcohol intake with cirrhosis. The most frequent form due to hepatitis B virus can be prevented with a safe, effective vaccine. Universal precautions against exposure to blood-borne infection agents are also protective. The disease is diagnosed in patients who develop liver enlargement, pain, and jaundice. The α-fetoprotein blood test, ultrasound of the liver, and imaging modalities including computed tomography and magnetic resonance imaging are useful in evaluating patients. Localized disease may be resected for cure. Some patients with locally advanced disease benefit from liver resection and orthotopic liver transplant.

I. INCIDENCE AND MORTALITY

Hepatocellular carcinoma (HCC) is a malignant condition of the liver hepatocyte. The American Cancer Society estimates that there were 13,600 deaths from liver and intrahepatic bile duct cancers in the United States in 1999, making it the 8th highest cancer mortality in men and 12th in women. The SEER registry shows that age-adjusted incidence and mortality rates for HCC in the United States are 2.4/100,000 in the period 1991–1995. This contrasts sharply with worldwide incidence and mortality rates; hepatocellular carcinoma is one of the leading causes of death from cancer in Asia, particularly in China, Japan, Taiwan, and southeast Asian countries as well as sub-Sahara Africa.

In all populations worldwide, there is a strong male predominance in HCC incidence. In the United States, the male to female ratio is 2.7 to 1. Worldwide, the risk for HCC is highest in areas endemic for hepatitis B virus (HBV), which are primarily in Asia and Africa. In the United States, Alaskan natives are a high-risk group because of high frequency of chronic HBV infection.

II. RISK FACTORS

A. Hepatitis B Virus Infection

In 1976, Baruch Blumberg was awarded the Nobel Prize in medicine for his discovery of HBV DNA virus particles in patients with chronic hepatitis and their subsequent relationship to HCC. In 1981, Beasley and co-workers established, in a prospective epidemiologic study in Taiwan, that male civil service workers who were HBV carriers had a 100-fold higher risk for HCC than noncarrier males in the same cohort. Although HBV DNA is present in the tumor tissues of the majority of HCC patients from endemic areas, there is no evidence of viral integration. Chronic infection with related viruses has been associated with liver cancer in the woodchuck and the ground squirrel. In the woodchuck model, the virus activates expression of the MYC oncogene by insertion into the host genome to cause hepatocellular carcinoma after 2–3 years of chronic infection in 90% of the animals. One major difference between human and animal forms of hepatitis B infection is that most human carriers cease active viral replication after several decades of infection. It is not known if patients who actively replicate virus for longer periods are at higher risk for HCC.

B. Hepatitis C Virus

The hepatitis C virus (HCV) was cloned in 1989; this was followed by reports of the association of chronic HCV infection with HCC. Although capable of causing chronic infection, HCV is a very different virus, i.e., a single-stranded RNA virus of approximately 9500 nucleotides, which does not integrate into the host genome. Although as few as 4–10% of infected persons develop symptoms of acute hepatitis, approximately 85% develop chronic infection. In studies of posttransfusion hepatitis, the mean interval between infection and chronic hepatitis is estimated to be 10–14 years, for cirrhosis 20 years, and for HCC 30 years. The proportion of HCC cases in a population associated with HCV infection is 70% in Japan, Italy, and Spain, whereas 30–50% of cases have this relationship in the United States.

C. Aflatoxin Ingestion

Aflatoxins are toxic metabolites produced by some species of aspergillus fungi, which can cause liver cancer in animals. A high consumption of aflatoxin contamination in moldy peanuts, corn, and soy products is associated with an increased risk of HCC in Asia and Africa. Studies in Shanghai, China, indicate that HBV carriers who have been exposed to aflatoxin have a 50-fold elevation in risk for HCC compared to the HBV carrier state alone. Data from case-control studies in China suggest that genetic polymorphisms in detoxification genes could contribute to this unusually high interaction.

D. Alcohol and Cirrhosis

In the United States, approximately 15% of HCC is associated alcoholic cirrhosis. In the absence of cirrhosis, however, alcohol has not been shown to be carcinogenic in animal models. Evidence suggests that alcohol exerts a promoting effect in the presence of HCV infection as a cause for chronic liver disease and hepatocellular carcinoma.

E. Hemachromatosis

Iron overload has been associated with a high risk of HCC and this risk can be lowered by iron depletion therapy if cirrhosis has not occurred. Hereditary hemachromatosis, which is the most prevalent autosomal recessive disorder in individuals of northern European descent, and African iron overload conditions are associated with increased HCC risk.

F. Other Factors

A relationship exists between oral contraceptive use and benign hepatic adenomas, but the relationship with hepatocellular carcinoma is tenuous at best. Numerous studies have shown that tobacco use, while high in HCC patients, probably has no direct carcinogenic effect on the liver.

III. PATHOGENESIS

If there is a common mechanism of pathogenesis in HCC, it is likely to be through chronic liver injury induced by viral and/or environmental factors. Although losses of chromosome regions 4q, 8p, 13q, and 16q are commonly reported in HCC tumor tissue, no clear pathogenic mechanism has been delineated to account for these changes. In geographic locations where there is high aflatoxin exposure, G-to-T trans-

versions of codon 249 of the p53 gene have been detected in human liver cancers. Therefore, the exact molecular pathogenic mechanism for human HCC awaits further research.

IV. PREVENTION

A. Primary Prevention

Based on the epidemiologic data discussed earlier, prevention of HBV and HCV infection and removing exposure to aflatoxin are the most effective ways of preventing HCC. A safe effective vaccine for HBV has been available since 1982. In Asia, the high prevalence of hepatitis among mothers requires that the vaccine be given as soon as possible after birth, preferably along with hepatitis B immune globulin to prevent perinatal transmission. In the United States, where 36% of chronic infections are acquired before adolescence, the CDC recommends universal infant HBV vaccination. In Taiwan, where universal vaccination of newborns has been practiced since 1984, HCC incidence rates have begun to decline in younger age groups. Prevention of HCV infection is more difficult because there is no vaccine or effective postexposure prophylaxis available. Therefore, universal precautions against exposure to blood-borne infection agents are the most effective strategy. Attempts to manage or suppress chronic HBV and HCV infection are underway. Interferon-α and, more recently, lamivudine have shown efficacy in reducing HBV viral replication. The most effective current therapy for chronic HCV infection appears to be the combination of interferon-α with ribavirin.

B. Secondary Prevention

Secondary prevention relies on early detection and resection of small tumors. α-Fetoprotein (AFP) is a fetal antigen produced by 40–75% of HCCs but not by normal adult liver. Patients with chronic viral hepatitis or cirrhosis of any etiology are candidates for screening with AFP. Subjects with AFP >20 ng/ml are studied with ultrasound or possibly computed tomography (CT) scan. Although such screening may pick up small neoplasms, there is no evidence that screening results in decreased HCC mortality.

C. Chemoprevention

Chemoprevention utilizes micronutrients or specific drugs to delay or prevent the onset of cancer. Polyprenoic acid, an acyclic retinoid, has been shown to inhibit chemically induced HCC in rats and suppress *in vitro* human hepatoma cell growth and AFP secretion. The exact mechanism of action of polyprenoic acid is unknown. Oltipraz, a synthetic dithiolthione, which induces glutathione S-transferase and DT-diaphorase expression, inhibits aflatoxin B_1-induced hepatic tumors in rats. Phase II clinical trials indicate that Oltipraz can reduce aflatoxin–DNA adduct formation in humans who consume aflatoxin-contaminated foods but had no impact on liver cancer incidence.

V. DIAGNOSIS AND STAGING

A. Clinical Presentation

Unfortunately, there are no early signs or symptoms for HCC. The most common complaints are right upper quadrant abdominal pain and distention of the abdomen plus anorexia with weight loss. Rarely, patients will present with jaundice, hematemesis, or evidence of metastatic disease. In a patient known to have cirrhosis, the development of unexplained upper abdominal pain, weight loss, fever, rapid enlargement of the liver, or ascites should alert the clinician to the possibility of HCC. The physical findings typically include hepatomegaly, ascites, jaundice, and possible splenomegaly secondary to portal hypertension. Other nonspecific findings include muscle wasting, fever, dilated abdominal veins, and other signs of cirrhosis. HCC may be associated with paraneoplastic manifestations, including hypoglycemia due to ectopic production of insulin growth factor, erythrocytosis due to ectopic erythropoietin, and hypercholesterolemia.

B. Pathologic Diagnosis

Grossly, HCC has four major growth patterns.

1. The expanding type, which compresses and distorts surrounding liver parenchyma.
2. The spreading type, which infiltrates surrounding

hepatic structures and forms a pseudonodular or invasive pattern.
3. The multifocal type with distribution of small tumors of similar size throughout both lobes of the liver.
4. An indeterminant pattern.

Histopathologically, HCC is graded from 1 to 4, depending on granularity and acidophilic quality of the cytoplasm, size and degree of hyperchromatism of the nuclei, and cohesive quality of the tumor cells. Classical or the usual form of HCC should be distinguished from the fibrolamellar form, which accounts for about 2–4% of cases but is often seen in young women who have an otherwise unaffected liver. These tumors are amenable to cure with surgical resection. Cholangiocellular carcinoma combines glandular elements of cholangiocarcinoma and hepatocellular elements in a noncirrhotic liver to produce a rapidly fatal course.

C. Staging and Prognosis

HCC is staged according to the TNM system (Table I) based on the size of the largest tumor nodule, the number of nodules, and vascular invasion. The prognosis is directly related to the stage or extent of involvement of the liver. Thus, patients with small tumor size, single vs multiple nodules, absence of cirrhosis, and location in the left lobe, where it may be totally resected, are likely to have longer survival.

D. Serologic Tests of HCC

AFP is normally produced by the fetal liver and the yolk sac; serum levels fall progressively after birth and in healthy adults are below 10 ng/ml. AFP is elevated in 50–90% of symptomatic HCC patients, and the positive predictive value of an elevated level in excess of 400 ng/ml exceeds 95%. However, transient and unsustained false-positive levels may occur in patients with cirrhosis, active hepatitis, or following partial hepatectomy.

E. Imaging Modalities

Hepatic ultrasound is the most useful and most cost-effective means of screening high-risk populations.

TABLE I
TNM Staging System in HCC[a]

Primary tumor (T)
  T_1 Solitary tumor 2 cm or less in greatest dimension without vascular invasion
  T_2 Solitary tumor 2 cm or less in greatest dimension with vascular invasion, multiple tumors limited to one lobe, none more than 2 cm in greatest dimension without vascular invasion, or a solitary tumor more than 2 cm in greatest dimension without vascular invasion
  T_3 Solitary tumor more than 2 cm in greatest dimension with vascular invasion, multiple tumors limited to one lobe, none more than 2 cm in greatest dimension, with vascular invasion, or multiple tumors limited to one lobe, any more than 2 cm in greatest dimension, with or without vascular invasion
  T_4 Multiple tumors in more than one lobe or tumor(s) involve(s) a major branch or portal or hepatic vein(s)

Regional lymph nodes (n)
  N_0 No regional lymph node metastasis
  N_1 Regional lymph node metastasis

Distant metastasis (M)
  M_0 No distant metastasis
  M_1 Distant metastasis

Stage grouping

I	T_1	N_0	M_0
II	T_2	N_0	M_0
IIIA	T_3	N_0	M_0
IIIB	T_1	N_1	M_0
	T_2	N_1	M_0
	T_3	N_1	M_0
IVA	T_4	Any N	M_0
IVB	Any T	Any N	M_1

[a]From American Joint Committee for Cancer Staging and End Results Reporting: Manual for Staging of Cancer, 3rd Ed.

Neoplasms in the liver may be more or less echogenic than surrounding normal hepatic parenchyma or may manifest a disorganized echoarchitecture. In patients with established cirrhosis, there is 78% sensitivity and 93% specificity for the detection of HCC. Color flow Doppler ultrasound can assist in preoperative assessment by identifying blood vessels, delineating their relationship to the tumor, and establishing the direction of blood flow within the portal vein.

Hepatic CT combines high sensitivity for focal lesions and high specificity regarding the nature of the lesions. Special arterial and venous phase CT scans can differentiate the predominant blood supply between normal liver parenchyma, which is from the portal vein, and the neoplastic lesion, which is nourished by the hepatic artery. CT portography enhances the diagnosis of portal vein obstruction and the localization of intrahepatic nodules.

Magnetic resonance imaging (MRI) is an important diagnostic tool in the detection of focal liver lesions. HCC is best detected with T2-weighted spin-echo sequences, which can distinguish fatty degeneration and vascular invasion of the tumor (Fig. 1). Reconstruc-

tion of vein and the biliary tree is possible with contrast techniques. Angiography is used to assess patients who are potential candidates for chemoembolization or candidates for partial hepatectomy.

VI. MANAGEMENT

A. Localized, Resectable Disease

Surgical excision is the treatment most likely to result in long-term survival. Eligibility for resection varies from 8 to 40% and depends on the size of the tumor, its location, and the degree of cirrhosis. Tumor resection with or without pre- or postoperative adjuvant therapy is the recommended management of patients with T1, T2N0 disease (Tables II and III). In a report detailing the results of 412 patients treated over a 6-year period at the Memorial Sloan-Kettering Cancer Center, patients with lesions <5 cm had a 57% five-year survival, whereas those with 10-cm or larger lesions had a 32% five-year survival. Factors associated with poor outcome included an AFP >2000 ng/ml, vascular

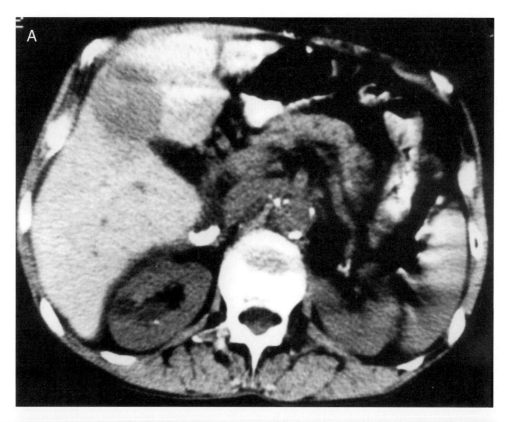

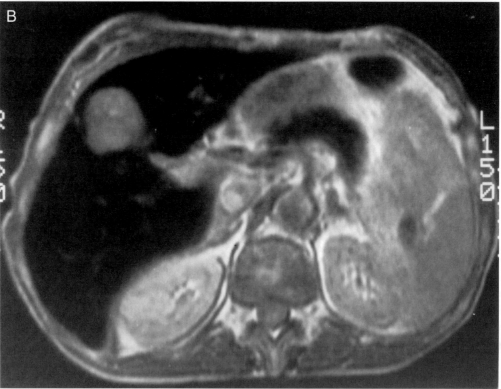

FIGURE 1 Hepatocellular liver cancer nodule: Gross pathology, CT scan, and MRI image. (A) CT scan showing lesion left lobe of liver. (B) MRI scan T2-weighted image of lesion, left lobe of liver. (C) Resected hepatocellular carcinoma from left lobe of liver; gross pathology.

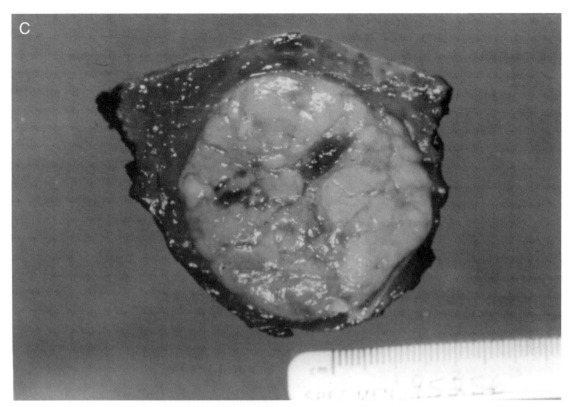

FIGURE 1 (*Continued*)

invasion, cirrhosis with low albumin levels, and poorly differentiated tumors with absence of capsule formation. Total hepatectomy and liver replacement or orthotopic liver transplant has been used to treat patients with small HCC and associated cirrhosis or hepatic failure. There are no phase III trials compar-

TABLE II
Treatment Outcomes for Hepatocellular Carcinoma

Surgical resection by tumor size	5-year survival
<2 cm	75%
2–5 cm	55–60%
>5 cm	30–40%

Intraarterial chemoembolization using doxorubicin + ethiodized oil gel pellets
Response rate: 30–50%
Median survival: 20–26 months

Systemic chemotherapy using fluorouracil and/or doxorubicin
Response rate: 10–15%
Median survival: 2–6 months

ing limited resection with total hepatectomy and liver transplantation. In an analysis of cases from Japan and the United States comparing hepatic resection to orthotopic liver transplant, the overall survival rate after transplant was significantly better than after hepatic resection when the tumor was <5 cm without microscopic vascular invasion. Patients with active HBV or HCV infection are not candidates for transplantation because of the high risk of recurrent infection and graft loss from hepatitis. The cost of the procedure and the scarcity of donated organs greatly affect the use of transplantation for this disease.

B. Localized Unresectable HCC

Ultrasound-directed percutaneous ethanol injection or percutaneous radiofrequency ablation may be used in patients with HCC tumors <5 cm in diameter. The 3-year survival was 63% in 162 cirrhotic patients with a single lesion and 31% in 45 patients with multiple but treatable lesions. Because HCC derives its

TABLE III
Guidelines for Liver Cancer Management

Clinical presentation	Liver mass ± cirrhosis Elevated AFP Normal CEA and CA 19-9	
Medical evaluation	History and physical examination Hepatitis antigen panel Liver function studies CT and/or MRI scans Liver biopsy	
Staged-based management	Localized resectable $(T_1T_2T_3N_0M_0) \Rightarrow$ No or minimal cirrhosis	Segmental resection or orthotopic liver transplant
	Localized inoperable $(T_2T_3T_4N_0M_0) \Rightarrow$	Percutaneous ethanol injection if <5 cm HAI Chemoembolization
	Metastatic (any $T, N_1 M_1) \Rightarrow$	Systemic chemotherapy; supportive care

blood supply primarily from the hepatic artery, whereas normal hepatocytes are sustained by portal vein, arterial infusion therapy has the theoretical advantage of increasing local drug delivery while lowering systemic and hepatic toxicity. Chemoembolization utilizing 50 mg of doxorubicin suspended in ethiodized oil followed by fibrin sponge microembolization of the tumor's blood supply has produced partial to complete tumor regressions in 30% of patients with a median survival of 13 months. This procedure is contraindicated in patients who have a thrombosed portal vein.

C. Metastatic Disease

Unfortunately, systemic chemotherapy has little effect on disseminated hepatocellular carcinoma. The refractoriness of HCC to chemotherapy is probably due to tumor heterogeneity and the inducible overexpression of multidrug resistance genes. The response rate to single agent doxorubicin is 16% with a median survival of only 3–4 months, and the response to combination cisplatin, mitoxantrone, and continuous infusion fluorouracil is 30% with a median survival of 6 months. Three-dimensional conformal radiation

treatment has been used to palliate patients with symptomatic masses in the liver.

VII. SUMMARY

Hepatocellular carcinoma is a possible model for understanding and approaching other adult cancers. The fact that hepatocellular carcinoma has several distinct environmentally associated causes (HBV, HCV, aflatoxin) in a background of genetic susceptibility makes it an ideal model for molecular epidemiology and chemoprevention studies. HCC is the first cancer to be successfully prevented through a vaccination program, which reduces the infectious agent associated with cancer. Lessons in hepatocellular cancer will undoubtedly be applied to the prevention of uterine cervix cancer (human papilloma virus infection) and possibly head and neck cancer (human simplex virus). Hepatocellular cancer is one of the few cancers with a reliable serum marker, which should help define better or improved systemic therapy. Finally, HCC patients benefit from a multidisciplinary evaluation by a team that includes a surgical oncologist, medical oncologist, interventional radiologist, pathologist, radiotherapist, and epidemiologist.

See Also the Following Articles

Bibliography

Beasley, R. P. (1981). Hepatocellular carcinoma and hepatitis B virus: A prospective study of 22 707 men in Taiwan. *Lancet* **2**, 1129–1133.

Bismuth, H. (1992). A primary treatment of hepatocellular carcinoma by arterial chemoembolization. *Am. J. Surg.* **163**, 387–394.

Centers for Disease Control (1991). Hepatitis B virus: A comprehensive strategy for eliminating transmission in the United States through universal childhood vaccination: Recommendations of the Immunization Practices Advisory Committee (ACIP). *Morbid. Mortal. Week. Rep.* **40**, 1–19.

Chang, M. H. (1997). Universal hepatitis B vaccination in Taiwan and the incidence of hepatocellular carcinoma in children: Taiwan Childhood Hepatoma Study Group. *N. Engl. J. Med.* **336**, 1855–1859.

Di Bisceglie, A. M. (1997). Hepatitis C and hepatocellular carcinoma. *Hepatology* **26**, 34S–38S.

El-Serag, H. B. (1999). Rising incidence of hepatocellular carcinoma in the United States. *N. Engl. J. Med.* **340**, 745–750.

Fong, Y. (1999). An analysis of 412 cases of hepatocellular carcinoma at a western center. *Ann. Surg.* **229**, 790–800.

Huang, C. (1992). Overexpression of the MDR-1 gene and P-glycoprotein in human hepatocellular carcinoma. *JNCI* **84**, 262–264.

Iwatsuki, S., and Starzl, T. E. (1993). Role of liver transplantation in the treatment of hepatocellular carcinoma. *Semin. Surg. Oncol.* **9**, 337–340.

Izumi, R. (1994). Prognostic factors of hepatocellular carcinoma in patients undergoing hepatic resection. *Gastroenterology* **106**, 720–727.

Kassianides, C. (1987). The clinical manifestations and natural history of hepatocellular carcinoma. *Gastroenterol Clin North Am* **16**, 553–562.

Kawai, S. (1997). Prospective and randomized trial of lipiodol-transcatheter arterial chemoembolization for treatment of hepatocellular carcinoma: A comparison of epirubicin and doxorubicin (Second Cooperative Study). *Semin. Oncol.* **24** (Suppl. 6), S6-38-S6-45.

Livraghi, T. (1992). Percutaneous ethanol injection in the treatment of hepatocellular carcinoma in cirrhosis. *Cancer* **69**, 925–929.

London, W., and Blumberg, B. (1982). A cellular model of the role of hepatitis B virus in the pathogenesis of primary hepatocellular carcinoma. *Hepatology* **2**, 10S–14S.

Mazzaferro, V. (1996). Liver transplantation for the treatment of small hepatocellular carcinomas in patients with cirrhosis. *N. Engl. J. Med.* **334**, 693–699.

McGlynn, K. A. (1995). Susceptibility to hepatocellular carcinoma is associated with genetic variation in the enzymatic detoxification of aflatoxin B1. *Proc. Natl. Acad Sci. USA* **92**, 2384–2387.

McHutchison, J. (1998). Interferon alfa-2b alone or in combination with ribavirin as initial treatment for chronic hepatitis C: Hepatitis Interventional Therapy Group. *N. Engl. J. Med.* **339**, 1485–1492.

Muto, Y. (1996). Prevention of second primary tumors by an acyclic retinoid, polyprenoic acid, in patients with hepatocellular carcinoma. *N. Engl. J. Med.* **334**, 1561–1567.

Nelson, R. C. (1989). Hepatic tumors: Comparison of CT during arterial portography, delayed CT, and MR imaging for pre-operative evaluation. *Radiology* **172**, 27–34.

Niederau, C. (1996). Long-term follow-up of HBeAg-positive patients treated with interferon alfa for chronic hepatitis B. *N. Engl. J. Med.* **334**, 1422–1427.

Nonami, T. (1996). Advances in hepatic resection and results for hepatocellular carcinoma. *Semin. Surg. Oncol.* **12**, 183–188.

Pateron, D. (1994). Prospective study of screening for hepatocellular carcinoma in Caucasian patients with cirrhosis. *J. Hepatol.* **20**, 65–71.

Resnick, R. H. (1993). Hepatitis C-related hepatocellular carcinoma: Prevalence and significance. *Arch. Intern. Med.* **153**, 1672–1677.

Sato, Y. (1993). Early recognition of hepatocellular carcinoma based on altered profiles of alpha-fetoprotein. *N. Engl. J. Med.* **328**, 1802–1806.

Sorensen, H. T. (1998). Risk of liver and other types of cancer in patients with cirrhosis: A nationwide cohort study in Denmark. *Hepatology* **28**, 921–925.

Wong, N. (1999). Assessment of genetic changes in hepatocellular carcinoma by comparative genomic hybridization analysis: Relationship to disease stage, tumor size, and cirrhosis. *Am. J. Pathol.* **154**, 37–43.

Hereditary Colon Cancer and DNA Mismatch Repair

Annegret Müller
Kang Sup Shim
Richard Fishel
Thomas Jefferson University

The DNA of all organisms is subject to continuous damage and repair. Because biology evolved coincident with most of the DNA-damaging processes, a multitude of repair mechanisms/pathways have emerged. This abundance of DNA repair process is responsible for maintaining the *stability* of genomes through succeeding generations. Gene alterations that escape DNA repair lead to new mutations, selection, adaptation, and the evolution of organisms.

Widespread genomic *instability* appears to be a common feature of human tumors. This observation is important because DNA damage repair and/or damage induced cell cycle arrest checkpoints are the ultimate culprits that lead to this genomic instability. A lack of appropriate repair processes has been proposed to result in an accumulation of numerous types of genetic alterations and is the foundation of the "mutator hypothesis." The mutator hypothesis posits that reduced DNA repair leads to increased mutation rates (mutator), the accumulation of multiple gene mutations, and ultimately the observation of genomic instability. One of the most commonly altered DNA repair pathways leading to genomic instability in human tumor cells is DNA mismatch repair (MMR). A mismatched nucleotide can arise in the DNA by at least three different processes: physical as well as chemical damage, genetic recombination between DNA parental strands, which lack perfect homology, and misincorporation errors during

Copyright 2002, Elsevier Science (USA).
All rights reserved.

DNA replication. Loss of MMR in prokaryotes and eukaryotes leads to an increase in mutation rates and has been the poster child of the mutator hypothesis.

Most hereditary nonpolyposis colorectal cancer (HNPCC) tumors display an easily identifiable form of genetic instability that results in length alterations of simple repeated (microsatellite) sequences. In addition to the approximately 5% of colorectal tumors that result from HNPCC, another 10–15% of sporadic tumors display microsatellite instability (MSI) (Fig. 1). In 1993, the MSI phenotype of human tumors was linked to defects in the human MMR system. Tumors characterized by MSI classically display an increase in the spontaneous mutation rate (mutator phenotype), which reflects the underlying MMR defect. Based on similar foundational observations in prokaryotes and lower eukaryotes, the hMSH2 gene (and later the hMLH1 gene) was identified and found to be causally associated with HNPCC. Although the exact molecular mechanism leading from the mutator phenotype to malignant transformation in HNPCC patients is not completely understood, it is generally assumed that tumors that arise from MMR defects are the result of the increased spontaneous mutation rate. However, studies have also demonstrated a direct link between the MMR system and damage-induced apoptosis. Such a link may explain the "selection" for MMR defects in sporadic tumors and the allelic distribution of the MMR genes in HNPCC, as well as the tolerance to DNA-damaging agents in some MMR-defective human cells.

I. DNA MISMATCH REPAIR IN BACTERIA

In *Escherichia coli* the DNA adenine methylation (Dam)-instructed MMR repair pathway is responsible for the repair of mismatched nucleotides arising from replication misincorporation errors. The Dam-instructed MMR repair pathway has been most widely studied *in vivo* and *in vitro*. The strand selection for Dam-instructed MMR is provided by a transient undermethylation of the GATC Dam sequence within the newly replicated DNA strand. Prior to replication, both strands are fully methylated. The repair

can include several thousand bases upstream or downstream of the mismatched nucleotides and is therefore designated a "long patch" repair pathway. In addition to the DNA adenine methylase, DAM-instructed MMR repair requires MutH, MutL, and MutS gene products, as well as the excision/resynthesis machinery, which includes mutU(uvrD), DNA polymerase III holoenzyme, DNA ligase, single-stranded DNA-binding protein, and at least one of the single-stranded DNA exonucleases, ExoI, Exo VII, ExoX, or RecJ. The DAM-instructed MMR repair pathway substantially increases the fidelity of replication, as mutations in *mutH*, *mutL*, and *mutS* genes cause an increase of spontaneous mutations of up to 1000-fold. Based on extensive biochemical studies, Modrich and colleagues have proposed a model for postreplication MMR that is based on ATP hydrolysis-dependent translocation from the mismatch site to a GATC site. MMR is initiated by the binding of MutS to mispaired nucleotides and is followed by interaction with the MutL protein. The MutS–MutL complex is then proposed to translocate to the hemimethylated GATC Dam site, which is bound by the MutH protein. The intrinsic endonuclease activity of MutH is then activated by the MutS–MutL complex, which results in a strand-specific incision of the newly synthesized DNA strand. The MutS–MutL–MutH complex provides the loading site for the UvrD helicase, which in concert with one of the four single-stranded exonucleases (RecJ, ExoI, Exo VII, Exo X) degrade the faulty DNA strand—unidirectionally back to the mismatch site. The resulting single strand gap is resynthesized by the Pol III holoenzyme complex and sealed with the DNA ligase. The largely unidirection excision/resynthesis is an important observation that must be accounted by a hypothetical mechanism and is one of the foundations of the hydrolysis-dependent translocation model. We have suggested an alternative mechanism in which MMR is controlled by a gradient of adenosine nucleotide molecular switches surrounding the mismatch site (see later; Fig. 1).

Homologues of the prokaryotic MutS and MutL proteins have been found in all organisms examined to date. In human cells, a set of five MutS homologues (hMSH2, hMSH3, hMSH4, hMSH5, and hMSH6) and four MutL homologues [hMLH1, hPMS1 (scMLH2), hMLH3, and hPMS2 (scPMS1)] have been

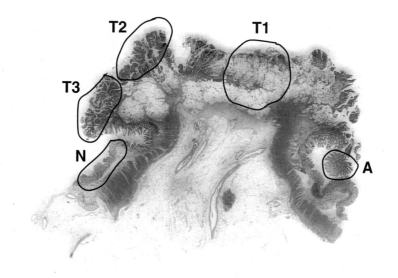

BAT 26

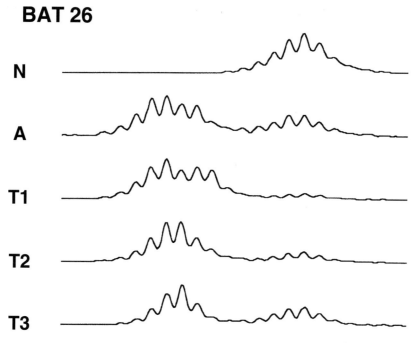

FIGURE 1 Microsatellite instability in a human tumor. MSI is determined by comparing the size of microsatellite sequences between normal and tumor tissue from the same patient. Microsatellite analysis was performed with DNA isolated from microdissected tissue of normal (N), adenomatous (A), and tumor (T) regions. While a panel of five microsatellites is normally used in the diagnosis of MSI, only the mononucleotid marker BAT26 is shown here. A normal distribution of peak sizes surrounding the actual size is expected because the polymerase chain reaction (a polymerase) will introduce MSI during the amplification process. Large additional size distributions and/or shifted size distributions that are different from the normal size distribution constitute MSI. In this example, MSI is present in the adenomatous and tumor DNA compared to normal tissue DNA. Moreover, continuous evolution of MSI appears to have occurred in the three pathologically different regions of the tumor (compare T1 with T3).

found that appear to function similarly to their original identified *Saccharomyces cerevisiae* (sc) counterparts.

While the bacterial MutS protein has been shown to recognize mismatched nucleotides as homodimers, eukaryotic MutS homologues (MSH) appear to function as heterodimers. For postreplication MMR, the relevant heterodimers are hMSH2 with hMSH3 or hMSH2 with hMSH6. The hMSH2–hMSH6 has been shown to primarily recognize single base pair and small insertion/deletion mismatched nucleotides, whereas the hMSH2-hMSH3 heterodimer has been shown to primarily recognize small and large insertion/deletion-mismatched nucleotides. The role and recognition substrates of the hMSH4–hMSH5 heterodimer remain enigmatic, but appear to be confined to meiosis.

Not all of the MMR genes are convertible to the human system. Of particular note is the fact that the mitochondrial-specific scMSH1 homologue has not been identified and there appears to be no MutH homologue outside of gram-negative bacteria, leaving the mechanism of the strand discrimination in eukaryotes (and gram-positive bacteria) as a major unknown.

II. RELATIONSHIP OF MISMATCH REPAIR TO HUMAN CANCER

Hereditary colorectal cancer falls into two subgroups: familial adenomatous polyposis (FAP) and hereditary nonpolyposis colorectal cancer. FAP patients have a large number of mostly benign intestinal polyps (adenomas), which by virtue of their numbers increase the probability of tumor development. HNPCC patients appear to develop intestinal polyps at the same frequency as the normal population, but display a dramatically increased adenoma-to-carcinoma transition. Approximately 90% of the tumors from HNPCC patients show MSI. MSI is determined by comparing the size of a panel of well-defined microsatellite sequences between normal and tumor tissue from the same patient (Fig. 1). These microsatellite sequences are generally distributed throughout the human genome and have been used for genetic linkage studies. The high frequency of MSI in HNPCC suggested

that there was likely to be a mutation in one of the human MMR genes previously described in bacteria and yeast. Defects in one of four human MMR genes (hMSH2, hMSH6, hMLH1, and hPMS2) have been found associated with HNPCC. Most of the germline mutations found in HNPCC are confined to hMSH2 and hMLH1. Mutations of hMSH6 and hPMS2 are rare and/or associated with atypical (late onset) families.

The HNPCC syndrome is the most common form of hereditary cancer and accounts for 2–7% of the total colorectal cancer burden. Because there are no single clinical features specific for HNPCC, diagnosis is based on family history (Amsterdam or Bethesda criteria) and is confirmed by the detection of a mutation in one of the MMR genes. For economic reasons, a diagnostic "stepladder" is recommended for HNPCC. The first step is evaluation of the family history related to clinical criteria (Amsterdam or Bethesda), followed by MSI analysis with an internationally recognized microsatellite markers. Tumors are then classified as MSI high (MSI-H) when they exhibit instability of at least two of five recommended microsatellite markers. In tumors with instability in only one marker, five additional microsatellite markers should be further tested in order to classify a MSH high (>40%) or MSI low (MSI-L) (<40%) status. Immunohistochemistry adds additional information, as a loss of expression of hMSH2 or hMLH1 correlates with MSI-H and can often specify the MMR gene, which is altered. In our ongoing experience, a clear germline alteration of hMSH2 or hMLH1 can be identified in ~60% of families diagnosed as a MSI-H tumor. In approximately 80% of the remaining families diagnosed as a MSI-H tumor, there was loss of expression of either hMSH2 or hMLH1, suggesting an uncharacterized germline genomic deletion or promoter mutation.

Two types of HNPCC families can be phenotypically distinguished. In type I patients, the tumors are exclusively located in the colon, whereas in type II patients they acquire extracolonic cancer in the endometrium, stomach, ovary, and/or urinary tract. The syndrome is clinically characterized by an autosomal-dominant mode of inheritance with an early age of onset (44 years). The location of the tumor is more often proximal to the splenic flexure and there are frequent metachronous and synchronous colon cancers. Histological examination has revealed a mucinous or solid cribriform and a solid medullary pattern, as well as an unusual lymphocytic infiltration called "Crohn's like lymphoid lesion." The prognosis and the outcome of HNPCC patients seem to be more favorable than in patients with sporadic colorectal cancers. Diploid DNA content in these tumors, as well as a nonmutated or overexpressed p53, may be one possible explanation for this clinical observation.

The risk of developing a cancer before the age of 70 for patients carrying a germline mutation is 91% for men and 69% for women. The colorectal cancer risk for male HNPCC patients is two times higher than for female HNPCC patients. However, the risk of developing an endometrial cancer in female HNPCC patients may be as high as 42%. There are general recommendations concerning lifetime cancer surveillance for HNPCC patients. A colonoscopy every other year should be started by the age of 20–25. The predominance of right-sided colon cancer in HNPCC patients requires examination of the entire colon. Colonoscopic examination should be repeated annually once the mutation carrier reaches an age of 40. For the endometrium, which is the most common extracolonic cancer in HNPCC patients, a gynecological examination, including a transvaginal sonography and a CA-125 measurement, is recommended every year starting by the age of 30–35. In case of stomach or urinary tract cancer patients with a family history, a gastroscopy/urine analysis is recommended every 2 years, starting by the age of 30–35. In the mutation carrier patient that developed tumors, a subtotal or total colectomy should be considered because there is a high risk developing synchronous and metachronous carcinomas.

Recommendations regarding colonic or gynecologic prophylactic surgery are still under debate. The major arguments for prophylactic surgery are the high risk of developing colorectal carcinoma during the lifetime and the more rapid progression of these tumors. An extenuated surgical treatment generally implies an extensive and individual decision as well as interdisciplinary discussion.

III. MECHANISM OF MISMATCH REPAIR IN HEREDITARY NONPOLYPOSIS COLORECTAL CANCER

There are two major questions regarding the mechanism of tumorigenesis by MMR gene defects in HNPCC patients. First, why are the vast majority of germline mutations found in hMSH2 and hMLH1 (allele distribution)? Second, what *selective advantage* do MMR defects present in the process of tumorigenesis? The most common explanation for allele distribution is the observation of overlapping and redundant MMR-binding activities, where hMSH2 and hMLH1 are thought to be the foundational players with transposable heterodimeric partners. The problem with this proposal is the increasing number of hMSH6 mutations and the observation that the hMSH2– hMSH3 heterodimer is capable of recognizing most of the same mismatched nucleotides as the hMSH2– hMSH6 heterodimer, yet there are no mutations in hMSH3 found in HNPCC (or even atypical families).

Both questions may be reconciled by the observation that MMR defects result in resistance to a wide variety of DNA-damaging agents. These results have been followed by the revelation that the MMR system efficiently recognizes a number of types of DNA damage. Moreover, the recognition of nucleotide methylation damage results in activation of the MMR system, which leads to apoptosis. Mutation of several MMR genes results in a lack of damage recognition, lack of damage-induced apoptosis, and a tolerance (resistance) to the DNA-damaging agent. With regard to methylation damage, only mutations in hMSH2, hMSH6, hMLH1, and hPMS2 lead to drug resistance and only the hMSH2–hMSH6 heterodimer is capable of recognizing methyl-damaged nucleotides within DNA. These seemingly disparate observations have led to a unique model for MMR and a novel role of MMR in HNPCC tumorigenesis.

IV. SIGNALING MISMATCH REPAIR

We have proposed a mechanism for MMR that is significantly different for the hydrolysis-dependent translocation model. The proposal is based on the observation that the function of the MutS homologues appears analogous to G protein molecular switches. Beginning in 1997, our laboratory demonstrated that mismatched nucleotides provoke ADP → ATP exchange by the human MSH proteins, which results in a large conformational transition and the formation of a hydrolysis-independent sliding clamp on the DNA adjacent to the mismatch (Fig. 2). It is the threshold number of sliding clamps associated with the DNA surrounding the mismatch that provokes MMR and provides enormous redundancy to this important repair system. The idea that human MSH proteins are "activated" by a mechanism that is similar to signaling G proteins, such as the Ras oncogene, has led to the concept of MMR signaling. Moreover, the MutL homologues (MLH and PMS) may also function as specialized "matchmaker molecular switches" that link the MSH sliding clamps to downstream effectors (e.g., the MMR excision-resynthesis machinery).

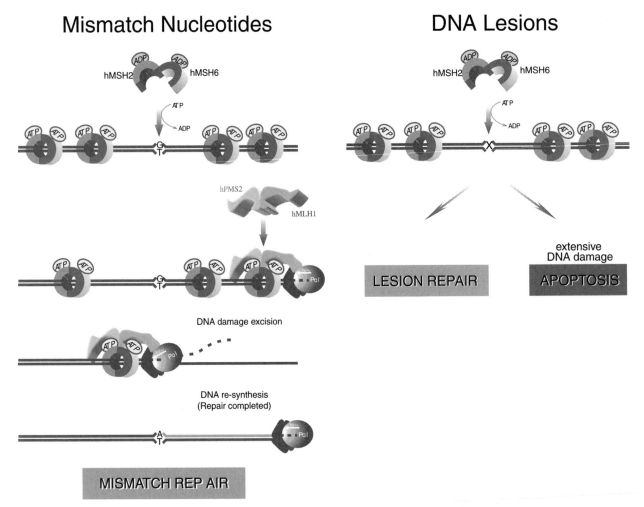

FIGURE 2 The sliding clamp signaling model for mismatch repair and apoptosis. (Left) DNA damage provokes ADP → ATP exchange by the hMSH2–hMSH6 heterodimer, resulting in conformational change and the formation of a hydrolysis-independent sliding clamp. Once the initial clamp leaves the mismatch, additional clamps may be loaded. Multiple clamps constitute a threshold signal for mismatch repair. The MutL homologues (hMLH1 and hPMS2), exonuclease, and DNA polymerase, as well as additional components, are likely to provide the function(s) that links the hMSH2–hMSH6 sliding clamps to downstream effectors in order to complete the repair of mismatched nucleotides. (Right) hMSH2–hMSH6 sliding clamps loaded onto the DNA surrounding a DNA damage lesion may provide a landing pad for other DNA metabolic machinery, which results in repair. Alternatively, in the absence of repair or when presented with an overwhelming amount of DNA damage, the hMSH2–hMSH6 sliding clamps signal to the apoptotic machinery.

V. ROLE OF APOPTOTIC MACHINERY IN DNA MISMATCH REPAIR

A signaling mechanism of the MMR system suggested that the damage-induced apoptotic response may be a specialized signaling pathway in the advent of overwhelming DNA damage (Fig. 2). This proposed is based on the idea that sliding clamps loaded around a mismatch or lesion would normally dissipate following repair. However, when the lesion numbers are too great for efficient repair, the sliding clamps would persist and result in a signal to apoptosis. This concept was solidified when it was shown that Msh2$^{-/-}$ and Msh6$^{-/-}$ mouse cells, but not Msh3$^{-/-}$ mouse cells, were resistant to alkylating agents, which correlated with the biochemical observation that only the hMSH2–hMSH6 heterodimer (not the hMSH2–hMSH3 heterodimer) recognized and was activated by alkylation DNA damage. Taken together, these studies linked the allelic distribution of HNPCC with DNA damage resistance and the lack of DNA damage-induced apoptosis. Based on these studies, we have suggested that the initial *selection* for MMR defects is likely to be the lack of damage-induced apoptosis and that the *bonus* of an MMR defect is an elevated mutation rate (mutator), which consequently accelerates the adenoma-to-carcinoma transition.

VI. SUMMARY

We have provided a new model of MMR in HNPCC in which the MSH proteins function as a signaling molecular switch. A direct link between this signaling molecular switch and damage-induced apoptosis appears to explain the allelic distribution in HNPCC as well as the resistance to some chemotherapeutic drugs.

Acknowledgments

The authors thank Dr. Tina Bocker for the photograph and MSI analysis shown in Fig. 1. This work was supported by NIH Grants CA56542, CA67007, and CA72027.

See Also the Following Articles

CELLULAR RESPONSES TO DNA DAMAGE • COLORECTAL CANCER: EPIDEMIOLOGY AND TREATMENT • HEREDITARY RISK OF BREAST CANCER AND OVARIAN CANCER • RESISTANCE TO DNA DAMAGING AGENTS

Bibliograph

Dietmaier, W., Wallinger, S., Bocker, T., et al. (1997). Diagnostic of microsatellite instability: Definition and correlation with mismatch repair protein expression. *Cancer Res.* **57**, 4749–4756.

Fishel, R. (1998). Mismatch repair, molecular switches, and signal transduction. *Genes Dev.* **12**, 2096–2101.

Fishel, R. (1999). Signaling mismatch repair in cancer. *Nature Med.* **5**, 1239–1241.

Jass, J. R., Stewart, S. M., Stewart, J., and Lane, M. R. (1994). Hereditary nonpolyposis colorectal cancer: Morphologies, genes, and mutations. *Mutat. Res.* **310**, 125–133.

Kolodner, R. (1996). Biochemistry and genetics of eukaryotic mismatch repair. *Genes Dev.* **10**, 1443–1442.

Loeb, L. A. (1991). Mutator phenotype may be required for multistage carcinogenesis. *Cancer Res.* **51**, 3075–3079.

Lynch, H. T., and Lynch, J. F. (1998). Genetics of colonic cancer. *Digestion* **59**, 481–492.

Lynch, H. T., Smyrk, T., and Lynch, J. F. (1998). Molecular genetics and clinical-pathology features of hereditary nonpolyposis colorectal carcinoma (Lynch syndrome): Historical journey from pedigree anecdote to molecular genetic confirmation. *Oncology* **55**, 103–108.

Modrich, P. (1987). DNA mismatch correction. *Annu. Rev. Biochem.* **56**, 435–466.

Peltomaki, P., and Vasen, H. F. (1997). Mutations predisposing to hereditary nonpolyposis colorectal cancer: database and results of a collaborative study: The International Collaborative Group on Hereditary Nonpolyposis Colorectal Cancer. *Gastroenterology* **113**, 1146–1158.

Rodriguez Bigas, M. A., Boland, C. R., Hamilton, S. R., Henson, D. E., Jass, J. R., Khan, P. M., Lynch, H., Perucho, M., Smyrk, T., Sobin, L., and Srivastava, S. (1997). A National Cancer Institute Workshop on Hereditary Nonpolyposis Colorectal Cancer Syndrome: Meeting highlights and Bethesda guidelines. *J. Natl. Cancer Inst.* **89**, 1758–1762.

Vasen, H. F., Mecklin, J. P., Khan, P. M., and Lynch, H. T. (1991). The International Collaborative Group on Hereditary Non-Polyposis Colorectal Cancer (ICG-HNPCC). *Dis. Colon Rectum* **34**, 424–425.

Vasen, H. F., Mecklin, J. P., Watson, P., Utsunomiya, J., Bertario, L., Lynch, P., Svendsen, L. B., Cristofaro, G., Muller, H., Khan, P. M., et al. (1993). Surveillance in hereditary nonpolyposis colorectal cancer: An international cooperative study of 165 families. The International Collaborative Group on HNPCC. *Dis. Colon Rectum* **36**, 1–4.

Hereditary Risk of Breast and Ovarian Cancer: BRCA1 and BRCA2

Thomas S. Frank

Myriad Genetic Laboratories, Salt Lake City, Utah

GLOSSARY

BRCA1 gene A breast cancer susceptibility gene located on chromosome 17q21, known to be mutated in families prone to a high incidence of early onset breast cancers and also ovarian cancers.

BRCA2 gene A gene mapped to chromosome 13q12-13; not yet fully characterized but believed to be involved in a significant number of familial breast cancers that are not associated with BRCA1.

The inheritance of a mutation in a tumor suppressor gene confers a greatly increased risk of cancer over the lifetime of an individual. Mutations in tumor suppressor genes that are inherited through the germline thus give rise to cancer susceptibility syndromes, in which a greatly increased risk of cancer is inherited in an autosomal-dominant fashion. Approximately 7% of breast cancer and 10% of ovarian cancer are attributable to such mutations, most of which occur in two specific genes: *BRCA1* and *BRCA2*. Although sometimes referred to as "breast cancer genes," *BRCA1* and *BRCA2* are also responsible for hereditary cancer of the ovary.

I. CHARACTERIZATION OF *BRCA1* AND *BRCA2*

Fifteen years of analysis of large multigenerational families with a strong history of breast cancer led in

1990 to the identification of a gene on chromosome 17q12-21 that conferred a greatly increased risk of breast cancer in an autosomal-dominant manner. The gene itself, BRCA1, was cloned in 1994 at Myriad Genetics. The discovery of the complete sequence of a second such gene, BRCA2 on 13q12-13, was reported in 1995, also by Myriad Genetics.

The protein-coding region of BRCA1 consists of 5592 bp in 22 exons that encode a protein of 1863 amino acids, and the protein-coding region of BRCA2 consists of 10,254 bp in 26 exons that encode a protein of 3418 amino acids. Studies of the interactions of these proteins led to the conclusion that they are involved in the regulation of genomic stability and DNA repair. The BRCA1 and BRCA2 proteins interact with each other, as well as with the Rad 51, RNA helicase A, and p53 proteins. Mice lacking Brca-1 and Brca-2 (the murine homologues of BRCA1 and BRCA2) undergo developmental arrest during embryogenesis. Furthermore, mice homozygous for a truncating mutation of Brca-2 that survive to adulthood have a wide range of defects, including improper tissue differentiation, absence of germ cells, and the development of lethal thymomas, and cultured embryonic fibroblasts from these mice were unable to repair radiation-induced DNA damage. Other studies have demonstrated that mouse embryonic stem cells deficient in Brca-1 are unable to carry out a transcription-coupled repair of oxidative DNA damage and are hypersensitive to ionizing radiation and hydrogen peroxide (but not ultraviolet light). Human BRCA2-defective cancer cells are also unable to repair double strand DNA breaks induced by ionizing radiation, although individuals with germline mutations in BRCA1 and BRCA2 do not appear to be hypersensitive to ionizing radiation.

II. CANCER RISK DUE TO MUTATIONS IN BRCA1 AND BRCA2

Mutations in BRCA1 and BRCA2 are responsible for increasing the risk of breast cancer by age 70 to between 56 and 87%. The lower estimate of risk was derived from an analysis of a general population with little or no family history of cancer, and the higher estimate was derived from families with multiple women affected by breast cancer. The increased risk of breast cancer is observed not only over a woman's lifetime, but particularly at a young age, to 33–50% before age 50 compared to the general population risk of 2%.

Mutations in BRCA1 also confer a greatly increased risk of ovarian cancer of up to 44%, by age 70, whereas mutations in BRCA2 increase this risk to approximately 27% compared to 1% for the general population of women. The age of onset of hereditary ovarian cancer is typically later than that of hereditary breast cancer, especially when associated with a BRCA2 mutation.

Women already diagnosed with breast cancer are at a greatly increased risk of a second cancer of breast and ovary if they carry a mutation in BRCA1 or BRCA2. Mutations in BRCA1 confer a 64% risk of contralateral breast cancer by age 70, or 20% within 5 years of the initial diagnosis, whereas mutations in BRCA2 increase these risks to about 50% by age 70, or 12% within 5 years of the first breast cancer. The risk of developing ovarian cancer after breast cancer is increased 10-fold to at least 16% compared to women with early onset breast cancer without such mutations.

Mutations in both BRCA1 and BRCA2 also confer increased (albeit low) risks of some cancers of men, particularly male breast cancer. Mutations in BRCA2 are responsible for an increased risk of prostate cancer (8% by age 70 and 20% by age 80), as well as an elevated but still low (2–3%) risk of pancreatic cancer. Early studies indicating that mutations in BRCA1 and BRCA2 might increase the risk of colorectal cancer have not been supported by subsequent studies.

III. ASSESSMENT OF HEREDITARY RISK OF BREAST AND OVARIAN CANCER

Genetic testing for mutations in BRCA1 and BRCA2 genes is no longer confined to research protocols, but is now clinically available to health care professionals. Sequence analysis is generally acknowledged as the most sensitive method of analyzing these genes because hundreds of mutations have been described throughout the lengths of each. While sequence analysis detects the majority of clinically significant abnormalities in BRCA1 and BRCA2, large duplications and deletions have also been reported for which clinical testing is largely unavailable.

Genetic testing for hereditary cancer risk is generally preceded by thorough assessment of an individual's family history in order to determine whether she (or he) is likely to carry a mutation responsible for hereditary cancer risk. The hallmarks of mutations in BRCA1 and BRCA2 include two or more family members with breast cancer at an early age of onset (usually before age 50) or ovarian cancer at any age. Breast and ovarian cancer in the same individual or male breast cancer at any age also indicates the possibility of hereditary breast and ovarian cancer. In evaluating a family history for the possibility of hereditary cancer risk, it is important to equally assess the father's side of the family as well as the mother's, as half of women with a hereditary risk of breast and ovarian cancer inherited it from their fathers.

Mutations in BRCA1 and BRCA2 have been described throughout the world but are more prevalent in some populations than others, such as individuals of Ashkenazi Jewish descent (i.e., central and eastern European origin). Evaluation of hereditary cancer risk may be warranted for any Ashkenazi Jewish woman with early onset breast cancer or ovarian cancer at any age regardless of family history.

Prior to genetic testing, a patient is generally provided pretest education and counseling regarding hereditary risk and genetic testing, including consideration of which relatives with whom the patient would share test results. Individuals who choose to be tested are at present asked to sign an "informed consent" form indicating that they understand the benefits and limitations of the test that they have chosen.

An identified mutation in either BRCA1 or BRCA2 can usually be assumed to have been inherited from one parent or the other, as spontaneous germline mutations in either gene are quite rare. An individual who does not have a germline mutation in BRCA1 or BRCA2 at the time of birth cannot acquire one later in life so tests for mutations in these genes are normally performed only once in a person's lifetime.

It is important to note that epidemiologic models (such as the "Gail model") that assess a woman's risk of sporadic breast cancer should not be used to assess the risk of cancer for women who may carry a muta-

tion in BRCA1 or BRCA2. Such mutations confer cancer risk in an autosomal-dominant fashion, and because epidemiologic models do not take into account whether the individual actually inherited the mutations, they greatly underestimate the cancer risk for mutation carriers and greatly overestimate the cancer risk for noncarriers within the kindred.

IV. HEREDITARY RISK OF BREAST AND OVARIAN CANCER: IMPLICATIONS FOR MEDICAL CARE

Evaluation for hereditary cancer risk should occur in the context of the medical interventions available to address that risk. Management options generally include increased surveillance, prophylactic surgery, and chemoprevention (medications that reduce the risk of cancer). The risks and benefits of these options should each be considered not only for women who do not themselves have cancer, but also women with breast cancer who are at risk of subsequent malignancy of the breast and ovary.

The "Cancer Genetics Studies Consortium" of the National Human Genome Research Institute has recommended that women with mutations in BRCA1 and BRCA2 undergo annual or semiannual clinician breast examinations, as well as annual mammography, to commence before age 35. Increased surveillance may be implemented in association with chemoprevention. Tamoxifen, a selective estrogen receptor modulator ("SERM"), reduces the risk of breast cancer in high-risk women and specifically reduces the risk of contralateral breast cancer by 50% in women with BRCA1 and BRCA2 mutations. It is thus likely, although not yet specifically demonstrated, that tamoxifen will reduce the occurrence of primary cancer in such women.

Prophylactic mastectomy has been shown to reduce the risk of breast cancer in "high-risk" women by at least 90% in women with mutations in BRCA1 or BRCA2. Because of the efficacy of surveillance in detecting most early stage breast cancer and the high cure rate of breast cancers detected at an early stage, prophylactic mastectomy is chosen by only a minority of women with mutations in BRCA1 and BRCA2. Prophylactic mastectomy may nonetheless be considered by women whose mammographic assessment is compromised by extensive fibrocystic change or by women whose perception of breast cancer has been affected by relatives or friends with the disease.

Oral contraceptives reduce the risk of ovarian carcinoma by 50% in the general population and have also been associated with a 60% reduction in the risk of ovarian cancer in women with mutations in *BRCA1* and *BRCA2*, although these findings were not confirmed in a subsequent study. Unfortunately, surveillance for ovarian cancer is often ineffective. Measurement of serum CA-125 is widely regarded as an unreliable screen for ovarian cancer and transvaginal ultrasound lacks specificity. Prophylactic oophorectomy should therefore be considered by women with mutations in *BRCA1* and *BRCA2* as recommended by a National Institute of Health consensus panel. Prophylactic oophorectomy is believed to reduce the risk of ovarian cancer in women with mutations in *BRCA1* and *BRCA2* by as much as 95% and also reduces their risk of breast cancer by nearly 50%.

A negative as well as a positive test result can have significant implications for patient care. If a mutation in *BRCA1* or *BRCA2* has previously been characterized in a relative, a negative result indicates that a woman is at the population risk of breast and ovarian cancer, despite having a strong family history of either or both diseases. It has also been shown that individuals who learn through genetic testing that they do not carry the mutation identified in their family have significant reductions in depressive symptoms compared to untested individuals.

V. SUMMARY

Inherited mutations in the genes *BRCA1* and *BRCA2* are associated with a significantly increased risk of breast cancer, particularly before age 50, as well as an increased risk of ovarian cancer. Laboratory analysis of these genes can determine whether a woman has inherited increased risks of breast and ovarian cancer. Identification of a hereditary risk of breast and ovarian cancer can facilitate the medical care of healthy mutation carriers, as well as those already diagnosed with cancer who are at risk of a second malignancy. Once a mutation has been characterized in a family,

a family member whose test indicates that he or she did not inherit the mutation has no elevated risk of cancer despite the strong family history, and can therefore avoid unnecessary interventions that might have previously been considered appropriate. Clinical laboratory analysis of *BRCA1* and *BRCA2* can be used to assist in the identification and management of individuals with a hereditary risk of breast and ovarian cancer.

See Also the Following Articles

Breast Cancer • Gastric Cancer: Inherited Predisposition • Genetic Alterations in Brain Tumors • Genetic Predisposition to Prostate Cancer • Hereditary Colon Cancer and DNA Mismatch Repair • Li-Fraumeni Syndrome • Ovarian Cancer: Molecular and Cellular Abnormalities

Bibliography

Armstrong, K., Eisen, A., and Weber, B. (2000). Assessing the risk of breast cancer. *N. Engl. J. Med.* **342,** 564–571.

Burke, W., Daly, M., Garber, J., Botkin, J., Kahn, M. J., Lynch, P., McTiernan, A., Perlman, J., Petersen, G., Thomson, E., and Varricchio, C. (1997). Recommendations for follow-up care of individuals with an inherited predisposition to cancer. II. BRCA1 and BRCA2: Cancer Genetics Studies Consortium. *JAMA* **277,** 997–1003.

Claus, E. B., Schildkraut, J. M., Thompson, W. D., and Risch, N. J. (1996). The genetic attributable risk of breast and ovarian cancer. *Cancer* **77,** 2318–2324.

Easton, D. F., Ford, D., Bishop, D. T., and Breast Cancer Linkage Consortium (1995). Breast and ovarian cancer incidence in BRCA1-mutation carriers. *Am. J. Hum. Genet.* **56,** 265–271.

Ford, D., Easton, D. F., Bishop, D. T., Narod, S. A., Goldgar, D. E., and Breast Cancer Linkage Consortium (1994). Risks of cancer in *BRCA1*-mutation carriers. *Lancet* **343,** 692–695.

Ford, D., Easton, D. F., Stratton, M., Narod, S., Goldgar, D., Devilee, P., Bishop, D. T., Weber, B., Lenoir, G., Chang-Claude, J., Sobol, H., Teare, M. D., Streuwing, J., Arason, A., Scherneck, S., Peto, J., Rebbeck, T. R., Tonin, P., Neuhausen, S., Barkardottir, R., Eyfjord, J., Lynch, H., Ponder, B. A. J., Gayther, S. A., Birch, J. M., Lindblom, A., Stoppa-Lyonnet, D., Bignon, Y., Borg, A., Hamann, U., Haites, N., Scott, R. J., Maugard, C. M., Vasen, H., Seitz, S., Cannon-Albright, L. A., Schofield, A., Zelada-Hedman, M., and Breast Cancer Linkage Consortium (1998). Genetic heterogeneity and penetrance analysis of the BRCA1 and BRCA2 genes in breast cancer families. *Am. J. Hum. Genet.* **62,** 676–689.

NIH Consensus Development Panel on Ovarian Cancer (1995). Ovarian cancer: Screening, treatment and follow-up. JAMA **273,** 491–497.

Ponder, B. (1997). Genetic testing for cancer risk. *Science* **278,** 1050–1058.

Struewing, J. P., Hartge, P., Wacholder, S., Baker, S. M., Berlin, M., McAdams, M., Brody, L. C., and Tucker, M. A. (1997). The risk of cancer associated with specific mutations of BRCA1 and BRCA2 among Ashkenazi Jews. *N. Engl. J. Med.* **336,** 1401–1408.

Welcsh, P. L., Owens, K. N., and King, M. C. (2000). Insights into the functions of Brca1 and Brca2. *Trends Genet.* **16,** 69–74.

Her2/neu

Patrick J. Brennan
Mark I. Greene
University of Pennsylvania School of Medicine

GLOSSARY

autophosphorylation or transphosphorylation Covalent modification, usually mediated by the activated intrinsic kinase or the associated receptor tyrosine kinse in order to serve as docking sites for downstream substrates.

disabled receptor Receptor whose normal signaling capacity has been abrogated through the action of another exogenous or endogenous peptide or pharmacologic agent. The disabled receptor can no longer respond to its normal ligand or stimuli.

growth factor Usually, a polypeptide molecule that binds specifically to its cognate receptor on the cell membrane. The intrinsic tyrosine kinase of the growth factor receptor is then activated to transduce the external signal to the cells, resulting in cellular proliferation and differentiation.

oncogenes Genes whose products mediate or increase transformation events, causing normal cells to become tumor cells. Certain oncogenes can be activated by the alteration of protooncogenes because of a critical point mutation, deletion, chromosomal translocation, or gene amplification and overexpression.

protooncogene A normal gene, or a cellular form of an oncogene, whose products are usually growth factor and their receptors, signal transduction molecules, or transcription factors.

receptor internalization or downregulation A process that takes place upon ligand binding in which the receptor that is diffusely distributed on the cell surface undergoes rapid lateral mobility, clusters in coated pits, and becomes internalized so that the expression of the receptor on the cell surface is reduced.

SH2 domain-containing proteins Proteins containing src homology domains, which are conserved, noncatalytic stretches of ~100 amino acids. These proteins can be either cellular substrates or serve as adapters for the assembly of additional proteins on the activated growth factor receptor complex.

The neu gene (also called Her2 or erbB-2) encodes a 185-kDa transmembrane glycoprotein with intrinsic protein tyrosine kinase activity. Her2/neu is homologous to, but distinct from, other members of the erbB family, which includes the products of the epidermal growth factor receptor (EGFR), erbB3, and erbB4. The binding of cognate growth factors to these structurally related proteins (termed class I receptors) regulates cellular growth, proliferation, and differentiation by activating receptor tyrosine kinases and triggering an incompletely defined signal transduction cascade. Consequently, a mitogenic or differentiation signal is delivered to the nucleus, completing the biological action of the growth factor. Overexpression of these receptors is often seen in various human tumor cells, and aberrant activation of their kinase activities is directly linked to tumorigenesis. The ability of one type of erbB family member to affect the activity of another via heterodimerization (such as EGFR and Her2/neu), a process described initially by Greene's laboratory, represents a general principle of receptor behavior and may result in cooperative biological effects leading to cellular transformation. Neoplasia can also result from genetic alterations (such as seen with rat p185^{neu}), causing constitutive activation of the protooncogene-encoded protein. Therefore, an understanding of the mechanisms by which Her2/neu and related growth factor receptors become activated may provide insight into how these receptor tyrosine kinases mediate oncogenic transformation.

I. DISCOVERY OF THE neu ONCOGENE

The neu oncogene was discovered in an interesting manner. Injection of pregnant rats with a chemical mutagen, ethyl nitrosourea (ENU) at day 15 of gestation, results in the appearance of neuroglioblastomas in the offspring. Cell lines established from these tumors were used by Shih and Weinberg to investigate whether the transformed phenotype of these tumors could be transferred to other cell lines. DNA was extracted from the tumor cell lines and transfected into NIH/3T3 cells (Fig.1).

Transfected cells formed malignant foci, indicating that the transfected DNA contained a gene(s) with oncogenic potential. Secondary NIH/3T3 transfectants were used to immunize mice; a crude antiserum was shown to precipitate a phosphoprotein of 185 kDa in the neuroglioblastoma cell lines, but not in control cells. This p185 phosphoglycoprotein was suspected to be the product of a rat oncogene and suggested that the malignant phenotype might be linked to a tumor cell surface antigen. Monoclonal antibodies (mAb) were then generated to the extracellular domain of p185 in order to characterize its biochemical and cellular behavior. The oncogenic product of p185^{neu} was shown to be associated with tyrosine kinase activity.

The neu gene was next shown to be transforming in a series of experiments by Schecter and colleagues. It was named "neu" for the neuroglioblastoma from which it was derived. Southern blot analysis of genomic DNA indicated a high degree of similarity with the v-erbB oncogene; using v-erbB-derived probes, the neu cDNA was cloned from a library constructed from the secondary NIH/3T3 transfectants described earlier. A comparison of cDNA clones isolated from both normal and transforming alleles showed that the rat c-neu protooncogene differs from its oncogene by a point mutation, an adenine to thymidine (A → T), that specifies a substitution of a negatively charged glutamic acid for a hydrophobic valine at position 664 in the transmembrane region of the protein. These studies showed that a carcinogen-induced point mutation was responsible for tumor induction in the rat.

Subsequently, the human homologue of c-neu, termed Her2 or c-erbB-2, was identified by several groups using molecular cloning techniques. Her2 was localized to the q12-q22 locus of chromosome 17. Sequence analysis of the neu cDNA revealed that the c-erbB-2 gene is highly homologous to, but distinct from, the c-erbB gene encoding the human EGFR, which was localized to chromosome 7. Thus, Her2/neu was believed to be a receptor for an unidentified ligand. These observations placed Her2/neu in a class

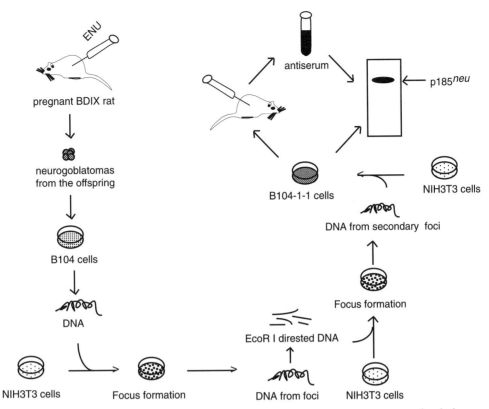

FIGURE 1 Discovery of neu oncogene and protein product. Pregnant BDIX rats were injected with the carcinogen ethyl nitrosourea (ENU) at day 15 of gestation. Neuroglioblastomas appeared in the offspring of BDIX rats, and tumor cell line B104 was established. Cells transformed by DNA from ENU-induced tumors developed malignant growth as recognized by focus formation EcoRI-digested DNA (but not other restriction enzyme-digested DNA) from the primary foci resulted in secondary foci when transfected into NIH/3T3 cells. At this point, secondary foci contain virtually no other foreign rat DNA besides the gene needed to transform the cells. Secondary transfectants (B104-1-1) were injected into mice, and crude antisera from tumor-bearing mice were shown to precipitate a phosphoprotein of 185 kDa, p185^{neu}.

of growth factor receptors involved in tyrosine kinase signaling and regulation of cellular growth.

II. PROTEIN STRUCTURE OF Her2/neu

The structure of all erbB family members is very similar. A comparison of the structures of EFGR and Her2/neu is presented in Fig. 2. The neu cDNA sequence predicts a 640 amino acid extracellular domain, containing a high proportion of cysteine residues clustered in two hydrophilic regions, facilitating the generation of specific conformation necessary for signal transduction through intra- or inter-disulfide bonds. The extracellular domains define

ligand specificity within the erbB family, and these poorly defined regions show limited homology between family members. For example, the EGFR binds, among other ligands, EGF, whereas the Her2/neu receptor, having only 43% homology to the EGFR in this domain, does not bind EGF as either a monomer or a homomer. A short extracellular juxtamembrane region is thought to be involved in ligand binding and dimerization in some ErbB family members. Saxon and Lee have demonstrated that mutation of this juxtamembrane region in the EGFR impairs ligand binding and receptor function. Gain-of-function mutations of this domain in the erbB-2 receptor, leading to constitutive signaling, have been observed in a mouse model of mammary tumorigenesis. The extracellular portion of the protein is anchored to the

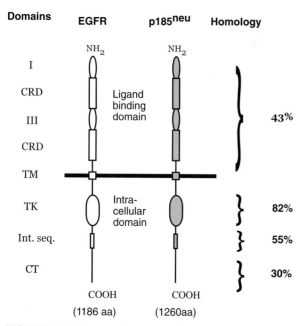

Domains   **EGFR**   **p185^neu**   **Homology**

FIGURE 2 Schematic illustration and comparison of amino acid (aa) sequence homology between p185/neu and human EGF receptor. Extracellular subdomains I and III, cysteine-rich domains (CRD), the transmembrane region (TM), the tyrosine kinase domain (TK), the putative internalization sequence (Int. seq), and the carboxyl terminus (CT) are indicated.

plasma membrane by a single transmembrane region consisting of 23 hydrophobic amino acid residues. This transmembrane region contains the site of the point mutation observed in rat neuroglioblastomas. This point mutation, discussed previously, endows the protein with the ability to cause cellular transformation. However, no similar mutation has been regularly observed in the transmembrane region of human erbB receptors. The transmembrane region is followed by a sequence of mostly basic residues, a feature common to many membrane proteins. The cytoplasmic domain harbors a 250 amino acid kinase domain that displays homology to the catalytic domain of the src family of protein tyrosine kinases. The neu kinase domain is 82% identical to that of the EGFR. A 60 amino acid region below the kinase domain shares 55% identity with the EGFR. This region has been shown to be important for protein trafficking. The extreme carboxyl terminus of Her2/neu, the carboxyl tail, contains 198 amino acids, including several tyrosine autophosphorylation sites, which serve as docking or attachment sites for cellular proteins. The re-

gion is the least conserved among erbB family members, and it is thought that the carboxyl termini of these proteins adopt a structure important for the specificity of signal transduction mediated by these kinases.

III. EXPRESSION OF Her2/neu IN NORMAL TISSUES

The early understanding of the biological functions of Her2/neu is derived from observations made in transformed cells. However, much less is known about its role in normal cell growth regulation and tissue development. Studies of human tissues have demonstrated the expression of p185 in secretory epithelia such as is found in the mammary gland, salivary gland, pancreas, intestine, gastrointestinal tract, ovary, thyroid, and skin. Expression patterns of Her2/neu in mammals suggest a biological role for the protein in tissue growth and mammalian development.

Several studies have been performed to determine the tissue-specific expression of p185 in normal mammalian fetal and adult tissues. These data are summarized in Table I. Some inconsistencies relate to differences in methods of analyses, tissue preparation, and

TABLE I
Comparison of Her2/neu in Fetal and Adult Tissues[a]

Tissues	Fetal	Adult
Central nervous system	+	−
Peripheral nervous system and vertebral column	+	N.D.
Cartilage and bone	+	N.D.
Muscle	+/−	−
Skin	+	+
Heart	+/−	−[b]
Lung	+	+
Gastrointestinal	+	+
Kidney	+	+
Liver	−	−
Pancreas	N.D.	+
Mammary gland	N.D.	+
Thyroid	N.D.	+

[a]N.D., not determined; +/−, variable results by different reports.
[b]Cardiac toxicity observed with Herceptin treatment may indicate an unappreciated low density of Her2/neu expression.

specificity of antibodies used. Analysis of 11 human fetuses, 6–12 weeks of age, by immunocytochemistry revealed expression of p185 in the peripheral and central nervous system. Staining was strongest within the neural processes and the ependymal and marginal layers of the developing brain. p185 expression has also been located in the epithelia of fetal human stomach and fetal rat and human intestines. It was noted that p185-specific staining was localized to epithelial cells at the villus tips and not in the crypts of the intestines. These data imply that p185 is relevant to the more differentiated cells. EGFR and Her2 show distinct, but possibly interrelated, expression patterns. Maguire and others have found a dramatic inverse distribution relationship of p185 and EGFR in normal secretory epithelial cells, such as renal, skin, and genital tract epithelia. These studies suggest that EGFR expression is limited to more immature cells, whereas p185 is observed in more mature cells. p185 also appears to be expressed in rat and human fetal lungs with persistence of expression at lower levels throughout adulthood. Human fetal epithelium of the female reproductive tract was positive for p185 expression, as was the adult vaginal epithelium. While follicular cells of the ovary were positive, there was no evidence of p185 in the oocytes. Quirke and colleagues found that the human placenta had significant levels of erbB receptor expression during all trimesters. Results of these studies imply that p185 has specialized functions in developmental and growth regulation of normal cells. The most consistent finding of these reports is that p185 is expressed in epithelial cells in the adult.

Additional evidence supporting a critical role for Her2/neu and other erbB family members has come from the generation of knockout mice. EGFR(-/-), ErbB2(-/-), ErbB3(-/-), and ErbB4(-/-) mice are not viable. The phenotypes of erbB knockout mice share many features, which is not surprising given their shared signaling roles, a consequence of heterodimerization between family members. EGFR-deficient mice display a variable phenotype depending on the genetic background of the mice in which these mutants are created; a common feature of these mice, however, is neurodegeneration.

Neural and cardiac defects are seen in ErbB-2-, -3-, and -4-deficient mice. ErbB2 mice die by day E11 (midgestation) from cardiac abnormalities. Birchmeier and others have demonstrated that even when this cardiac defect is rescued by cardiac-specific erbB2 expression, mice still die due to the failure of proper peripheral nervous system development, possibly related to the absence of Schwann cells.

IV. RECEPTOR DIMERIZATION LINKED TO CELLULAR TRANSFORMATION

Dimerization/oligomerization in response to ligands such as hormones, growth factors, and cytokines is a common receptor polypeptide signaling paradigm. While some ligands for protein tyrosine kinase receptors (e.g., PDGF and CSF-1) appear to be dimeric molecules containing two identical receptor-inducing epitopes, other ligands, such as EGF, appear to function as monomeric entities. Numerous observations support the idea that receptor dimerization/oligomerization is a central phenomenon in ligand-induced signaling.

A. Ligand-Dependent Dimerization

The EGFR was the first receptor tyrosine kinase proposed to dimerize upon ligand binding. Dimerization may permit the kinase domains to become positioned close to one another. These conformational changes might provide an allosteric signal that activates the receptor tyrosine kinase, resulting in receptor cross-phosphorylation, as well as substrate phosphorylation. Although it is now clear that dimerization is necessary for kinase signaling, Burke and colleagues have demonstrated that dimerization alone is not sufficient for productive kinase signaling. By mutating amino acid residues in the extracellular juxtamembrane domain, artificial dimers created through disulfide bonding were formed. While it might have been expected that the proximity effect created by the forced dimerization would have been sufficient to promote signaling, this was not the case; mutations were created that resulted in productive dimerization without tyrosine kinase activation. All mutations leading to the formation of an active dimer occurred with contacts on the same predicted face of the juxtamembrane α-helix, suggesting the importance of steric constraints to kinase activation. Therefore, kinase activation may require bringing the kinase domains into close proximity as well as positioning these domains in the correct relative orientation. Orientation may be influenced by the binding of ligand to the extracellular domains of erbB receptors.

The complexity of dimer formation between multiple erbB family members, in response to a growing list of ligands, constitutes a complex signaling network. The four members of the erbB family have been observed to form heterodimers in most combinations. Furthermore, with the exception of ErbB-2, which after exhaustive efforts to identify a ligand is now thought to be an orphan receptor, members of the erbB family bind multiple ligands with varying affinity, perhaps involving distinct binding surfaces. The EGFR is known to bind EGF, heparin-binding EGF-like growth factor, betacellulin, amphiregulin, and epiregulin. ErbB-3 and ErbB-4 bind to a family of ligands known as neuregulins. Although Her2/neu is thought to be an orphan receptor, it is the favored binding partner of all members of the erbB family; the basis for this preference is not well understood. Surprisingly, relatively little is known about the structural mechanism of ligand-induced dimerization, and what is known has been discovered recently. EGFR has been shown by multiple methods to bind EGF with a 2:2 stoichiometry. An attractive model of dimerization relies on the idea of ligand bivalence; in this model, the ligand has one high-affinity interaction with its receptor (i.e., EGF with EGFR) and a second, low-affinity interaction with a dimerization partner. Structural and biochemical studies seem to support this model, and it has been used as an explanation for the preference of Her2/neu as a binding partner; Tzahar and co-workers proposed that this second, low-affinity ligand–receptor-binding interaction site is found on the Her2/neu ectodomain.

B. Ligand-Independent Dimerization

Dimerization in the absence of ligand is seen with the Her2/neu receptor in two contexts: mutation leading to dimerization and spontaneous dimerization due to a mass action-like overexpression-dependent effect. The former has been observed in animal models,

whereas the latter is implicated in human carcinogenesis.

Central to the general principle linking kinase activation to cellular transformation was the discovery of ligand-independent dimerization of the oncogenic neu product p185. Weiner and colleagues used nonreducing electrophoresis to compare dimerization efficiency between normal and oncogenic p185 proteins; it was found that the majority (~70%) of oncogenic p185^{neu} appeared in a dimeric form, whereas the protooncogenic form p185^{c-neu} was predominantly in a monomeric state. Apparently, the single amino acid substitution (V644E) within the transmembrane region of p185^{neu} caused a shift in the molecular equilibrium from a monomeric to a dimeric form. In addition, oncogenic p185^{neu} in intact cells was shown to be more highly phosphorylated than the protooncogenic p185^{c-neu} on tyrosine residues and to be a more active kinase in immune complex kinase assays, resulting in increased phosphorylation of cellular substrates. To test the linkage between tyrosine kinase activity and cellular transformation, Weiner and co-workers mutated a part of the ATP-binding site within the kinase domain of oncogenic p185^{neu}, abolishing kinase activity. Cell lines transfected with this mutant protein were not transformed, demonstrating that a functional kinase is necessary for the transforming potency of p185^{neu}. These experiments demonstrated a connection between p185 dimerization and cellular transformation. It appears that the mutation in the transmembrane region of p185 results in dimerization, constitutive kinase activity, and transforming activity.

Several mutant proteins derived from p185^{neu} have been created with carboxy-terminal truncations, large cytoplasmic domain deletions, or ectodomain deletions to analyze the structural requirements for p185 dimerization; these mutant p185 proteins all underwent dimerization. Analysis of ectodomain-deleted neu products confirmed that the dimerization was ligand independent and was facilitated by the transmembrane mutation-containing region. Mutant neu proteins with carboxyl terminus or ectodomain deletions were still kinase competent, but the transforming efficiency was reduced when compared to full-length p185^{neu}. The phenotype of these mutant cells provided further evidence that the point mutation in the transmembrane region deregulated p185neu from ligand stimulation. Efficient dimerization of p185neu, in turn, constitutively activates the intrinsic tyrosine kinase, resulting in cellular transformation. Furthermore, the coexpression of two different types of mutant p185 proteins was studied in order to investigate whether functional complementation of p185 mutants occurs. Reduced transforming efficiency of kinase-active truncated neu was restored upon the coexpression of kinase-deficient full-length p185neu, a mutant incapable of ATP binding (see earlier discussion). The latter protein could be transphosphorylated by the associated active neu kinase that had either a C-terminal truncation or an ectodomain deletion. In addition, cellular signaling molecules known to interact with kinase-intact, activated p185neu were shown to associate with the kinase-deficient neu. This suggests that the kinase-deficient neu was transphosphorylated and activated by carboxy-terminal or ectodomain deletion mutants in a productive manner. In contrast, the constitutive activity of p185neu could be abrogated by codimerization with a cytoplasmic domain-deleted neu protein, decreasing the potency of cellular transformation and tumorigenicity (Fig. 3). We have argued that this is a consequence of the abrogation of the physical contact between intracellular domains required for kinase activation and transphosphorylation. These studies demonstrate the importance of dimerization of p185neu to the intermolecular mechanism of kinase activation and cross-phosphorylation.

A second form of ligand-independent dimerization seems to be dependent on the degree of expression of the Her2/neu protein. The oncogenic point mutation in the transmembrane region, which activates rat neu, has not been seen in the human neu homologue c-erbB-2. However, c-erbB-2 has been found to be amplified and/or overexpressed in a significant number of adenocarcinomas. The amplification was described in human gastric cancers by Akiyama and colleagues in 1986. As a follow-up, Slamon and colleagues examined the levels of Her2 RNA and DNA in breast and ovarian cancers and found that amplification of Her2/neu was apparent in 25–30% of primary cancer patients. A high copy number of c-erbB-2 correlated with shortened survival times for patients with these tumors. The issue of expression of p185 protein was

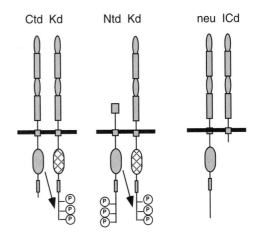

FIGURE 3 Interaction of mutant proteins derived from p185neu. All mutants contain a transmembrane point mutation and undergo dimerization. Coexpression of kinase-active deletion mutant p185neu (carboxyl terminus deletion, Ctd) with kinase-deficient p185neu (Kd, an ATP-binding mutant derived from p185neu) resulted in transphosphorylation and signal amplification. Deletion of the majority of the extracellular domain (amino-terminal deletion, Ntd) did not prevent kinase activation. However, dimerization of an intracellular domain-truncated p185neu (intracellular deletion, Icd) with full-length oncogenic p185neu resulted in kinase inhibition and reduced transforming potential.

argued by Maguire and Greene to be more relevant to human tumors than gene amplification. In further studies, Slamon indeed found increased protein levels to be a more reliable prognostic indicator than c-erbB-2 gene amplification. These results have been confirmed by other investigators. Overexpression of Her2 is associated with a number of other cancers, including some lung, colon, thyroid, and pancreatic adenocarcinomas.

Analysis of Her2/neu in NIH/3T3 cells has shown that transforming activity occurs once a critical expression level is reached. Studies to this end have utilized focus formation, anchorage-independent growth, and tumor formation in athymic mice as criteria for transformation. Expressing rat c-neu genomic DNA under the control of an SV40 promoter-driven expression vector led to a 10- to 20-fold higher expression of p185 compared to the normal rat fibroblast cell line Rat-1. This increased expression was not sufficient to cause cellular transformation. The transformed phenotype was achieved, however, independently of ligand stimulation, when either rat c-neu or human c-erbB-2 expression was driven by an LTR promoter-based expression system resulting in ~100-fold higher expression as compared to normal cellular levels. Moreover, the overexpression of rat c-neu under the control of the mouse mammary tumor virus (MMTV) LTR in a transgenic mouse model caused tumor growth in mammary tissue; as discussed earlier, mutations in c-neu cDNA leading to constitutive dimerization may be responsible for tumor formation in some cases.

The role of c-erbB2 amplification and overexpression of its protein product in human tumors can be explained by a shift in molecular equilibrium from predominantly monomeric to dimeric/oligomeric forms dependent on the level of Her2 protein. Dimer/oligomer formation results in increased tyrosine kinase activity and inappropriate cellular signaling leading to transformation. This hypothesis was supported by analyses of transfected cells expressing high levels of Her2/neu protein. Cell lines expressing Her2/neu under control of the LTR promoter displayed spontaneous dimerization and constitutive Her2 kinase activity. Furthermore, in a model of p185 oligomerization using purified proteins developed by our laboratory, a shift in equilibrium toward the aggregated state was demonstrated with increasing $p185^{c-neu}$ concentration. Moreover, analysis of enzyme kinetics indicated that the oligomerized protein forms had a significant increase in activity relative to the monomeric form. Taken together, these studies indicate that elevated expression levels of the protooncogenic Her2/neu can promote receptor dimerization, deregulating intrinsic kinase activity, mediating aberrant cellular signaling. Consequently, the role of Her2/neu overexpression links the *in vitro* transformation of mammalian cells to a phenomenon observed in human malignancy.

V. HETERODIMERIZATION OF EGFR AND Her2/neu

Although most, if not all, members of the ErbB family are capable of heterodimerization, and although multiple erbB/Her2 dimers may be important to human cancer, no receptor pairing has been studied as

thoroughly as the dimerization between EGFR and Her2/neu. EGF treatment increases the tyrosine phosphorylation of Her2/neu in an EGFR-dependent manner. Because EGF does not bind to Her2 neu monomeric or homomeric forms, these results suggest that EGF, acting through EGFR, can regulate the intrinsic kinase activity of Her2. The transregulation between EGFR and Her2/neu may have profound biological consequences.

Our laboratory found that to achieve a transformed phenotype and significant growth advantage *in vitro*, an increased level of expression (2- to 10-fold over normal) of either EGFR or $p185^{c-neu}$ was necessary. NIH/3T3 cells or NR6 (EGFR-deficient cells) expressing $p185^{c-neu}$ alone at a moderately high level (10^5 receptors/cell) were not transformed unless EGFR is expressed at an equivalent level. Downregulation of either EGFR or $p185^{c-neu}$ from the cell surface by antireceptor antibody treatment led to reversal of the transformed phenotype. These results suggested that two moderately overexpressed tyrosine kinases can synergistically interact, leading to cellular transformation. This hypothesis was verified by Wada and Greene, who provided direct evidence of heterodimer formation between EGFR and $p185^{neu}$ in transfected cells. Physical interaction of the two species was detected in the absence of chemical cross-linkers.

Noncovalent forces appear to predominate in heterodimerization. Multiple additional studies have confirmed that human EGFR and Her2 are associated in heterodimeric complexes in human breast cancer cell lines and transfected cells. Ligand binding to the EGFR promoted heterodimer formation over the basal level of heterodimer detected in unstimulated cells. Various deletion mutant p185 constructs were coexpressed with EGFR to examine the structural requirements for heterodimerization. Cytoplasmic domain mutants of either EGFR or p185 were still able to associate with full-length heterodimer partners. It is noteworthy that the association of EGFR with mutant p185 lacking the extracellular domain was undetectable. These data indicated that the extracellular domain was sufficient and necessary to stabilize heterodimerization. The predominance of heterodimer formation over either homomer revealed, unexpectedly, that heterodimerization is thermodynamically favored. Heterodimers, therefore, are more likely to represent physiologically important signaling assemblies than homomers.

The experimental model of p185 and EGFR interaction suggests that a causal relationship between heterodimeric kinase activities and malignant transformation may also have clinical implications. Several examples of human malignancies involve the aberrant expression of both EGFR and Her2, including the overexpression of EGFR and Her2 in a number of tumors of epithelial origin, e.g., thyroid tumors, pancreatic tumors, and endometrial carcinoma. There are numerous examples of tumors that overexpress Her2 on cell types that express EGFR, which, even if at normal levels, could contribute to transformation. All four members of the erbB family are expressed in some breast cancers (such as Sk-Br-3 cells), and overexpression of all four receptors may occur in some cases. These observations suggest that EGF and other ligands for erbB family proteins may contribute to the development and maintenance of the malignant phenotype of these tumors by mediating receptor interaction, recruitment, and subsequent activation of signaling cascades.

Consequences of heterodimeric association in living cells include tyrosine kinase activation, receptor autophosphorylation, and subsequent activation of downstream signaling molecules, resulting in the control of cellular behavior. As has been discussed previously, the functional activation of the receptor tyrosine kinase resulting from an intermolecular receptor–receptor mechanism is often followed by rapid cross-phosphorylation events involving the carboxyl termini of the receptors. This phenomenon seems to be a general mechanism, as it is observed in a number of other protein tyrosine kinase systems, such as pp60[c-src], the insulin receptor, and the PDGF receptor.

Transphosphorylation in the erbB family is observed not only among receptors of the same species, but between family members. This was demonstrated using a cell system coexpressing EGFR with a kinase-inactive p185[c-neu] deficient for ATP binding. The parallel experiment was performed using a kinase-inactive EGFR with a normal p185[c-neu]. In each case, the intact receptor was able to transphosphorylate the kinase-inactive binding partner.

An analysis of *in vivo* tyrosine phosphorylation and *in vitro* kinase activities measuring the incorporation of γ^{32}P-ATP into the receptor kinase and exogenous substrates indicated that the normal heterodimeric complex was a highly active kinase complex. Additionally, the intermolecular association and resultant tyrosine kinase activation involving the EGFR and p185[c-neu] demonstrated an upregulation of EGFR functions in transfected cells; these functions include an increased EGF-binding affinity and increased sensitivity to EGF stimulation.

Downregulation of p185 with a monoclonal antibody resulted in the loss of a very high EGF-binding subclass of receptors, supporting the notion that heterodimers were responsible for the previously observed increase in EGF affinity.

There are several possible explanations for the upregulated signaling functions and transforming ability observed with heterodimers. As described earlier, increased affinity for EGF may stabilize dimers and oligomers. Receptor trafficking may also provide an explanation; as will be discussed later, EGFR downregulation is inhibited by the presence of p185[c-neu]. Murali and co-workers provided a possible structural explanation through structural homology modeling; heterodimerization of kinase domains between EGFR and p185 was shown to be energetically favorable as compared to either homomeric pairing. Another possibility, which will be discussed in a subsequent section, is differential activation of signaling pathways. Understanding the basis for the increased transforming potential of heterodimers is crucial to the design of effective interventions.

VI. BIOSYNTHESIS AND DESTRUCTION OF Her2/neu

A. Different Forms of Her2/neu Proteins in Tumor Cells

The biosynthetic pattern of the p185 protein may affect the activation of the intrinsic tyrosine kinase and subsequent signaling. A number of investigators have characterized the presence of a soluble polypeptide fragment of p185 that is secreted into the cell culture medium. This phenomenon was initially observed in the sera of animals with p185-mediated progressively growing tumors by Kokai and Greene and then characterized in conditioned media from the breast cancer cell line SK-BR-3, which overexpresses Her2. A 130-kDa fragment was identified as an extracellular domain protein that was immunologically distinct from Her2/neu. In a number of experiments, the identity of the 130-kDa form fragment has been confirmed as a fragment of p185. Pupa and colleagues inhibited the release of soluble p185 from breast cancer cell lines by pretreatment with protease inhibitors, suggesting that the specific proteolysis results in the production of this fragment. In addition to cell lines, this proteolytic fragment has been detected in the sera of patients with Her2/neu-overexpessing tumors.

Truncated Her2 forms have also been observed. Scott and colleagues have demonstrated a truncated Her2 mRNA in various breast cancer cell lines. The truncated transcript apparently arises by alternative RNA processing and leads to the production of secreted and intracellular forms of a 100-kDa polypeptide. Doherty and co-workers described a second alternate transcript encoding a protein of 68 kDa that they have called herstatin. Expressed in normal human fetal liver and kidney, this protein consists of subdomains I and II of the extracellular portion of the Her2 receptor followed by an additional peptide sequence derived from an intron in the neu gene. The protein binds to Her2, inhibiting dimerization, disrupting existing dimers, and decreasing the phosphotyrosine content of full-length Her2 receptors. Studies of the differential processing of the p185 protein might have implications for the regulation of the activity of the receptor. A soluble form of the receptor may potentially compete with endogenous ligand, effectively lowering the physiologic response of those cells. Alternatively, a truncated intracellular form of p185 could have negative effects on the activity of full-length erbB complexes. The inhibitory nature of this alternate transcript raises the possibility of clinical utility.

B. Endocytosis and Turnover of Her2/neu

Endocytosis and protein turnover is a general mechanism that regulates signal strength and duration. The lack of a recombinant neu ligand has made internal-

ization studies of Her2/neu difficult. The best evidence of ligand-induced receptor endocytosis of erbB family members has come from the analysis of EGFR and dimers of EGFR and Her2/neu. Upon EGF binding, the EGFR that is diffusely distributed on the cell surface undergoes clustering in coated pits and becomes internalized. Subsequently, endocytic vesicles fuse with lysosomes to result in the degradation of both ligand and receptors. Thus, ligand-induced receptor internalization, then degradation, is a normal cellular routing of growth factors, resulting in signal attenuation, preventing long-term signaling. However, the erbB signaling network is more complicated than depicted earlier. EGFR homomers bound by TGF-α, another EGFR ligand, are internalized, but recycled to the cell surface. Failure to downregulate the receptor may explain an observed increased signal strength and duration.

While EGF-induced downregulation of heterodimers of EGFR and Her2/neu has been observed in some situations, the majority of studies have demonstrated an endocytosis defect for these heterodimers compared with EGFR homomers. Wang and colleagues demonstrated, in multiple cell lines, that overexpression of erbB-2 greatly inhibited EGFR endocytosis and completely abrogated erbB-2 endocytosis. Furthermore, when a chimeric protein consisting of the extracellular domain of erbB-2 and the intracellular domain of EGFR was overexpressed in cells, EGF-induced endocytosis was comparable to that seen with EGFR homomers. This suggests that protein trafficking is regulated by sequences in the intracellular domains of EGFR and erbB-2 proteins. Worthylake and co-workers suggest that it is not the rate of endocytosis of dimers of EGFR and erbB-2 that is affected, but rather the rate of lysosomal targeting. Surprisingly, heterodimers seem to be recycled, whereas homomers of EGFR are degraded, again implicating cellular trafficking in the control of downregulation.

We have previously suggested the importance of the intracellular domain through studies of antibody-induced p185 downregulation. Although EGF is not a potent inducer of p185 downregulation, certain antibodies are known to efficiently stimulate the endocytosis and degradation of this protein. To investigate the structural requirements for this antibody-mediated downregulation, two mutant p185 proteins were investigated; a truncation of the carboxyl terminus and an internal mutation of amino acid residues suspected to be involved in protein trafficking. The carboxy-terminal deletion did not affect downregulation, but the internal deletion showed greatly impaired downregulation. These experiments highlight the importance of ligand binding and protein internalization sequences to normal protein tyrosine kinase signaling. Inhibition of endocytosis and degradation caused by the overexpression of p185 may lead to increased surface protein levels, increased mitogenic signaling, and, hence, increased propensity toward transformation. Conversely then, downregulation of surface protein could serve to attenuate mitogenic signaling, an idea that has been investigated clinically through the use of immunotherapy.

In addition to intracellular sequences regulating membrane trafficking, numerous studies suggest the requirement of tyrosine kinase activity for a maximal rate of ligand-mediated receptor degradation as a general phenomenon for growth factor receptor endocytosis. Abolishing the intrinsic kinase activity of the EGFR by point mutation in the ATP-binding site renders it inactive in tyrosine kinase signaling. Unlike wild-type receptors, the mutant receptor undergoes diminished downregulation and degradation and appears to be recycled back to the cell surface. Similarly, studying antibody-mediated p185[neu] internalization, we have found that the endocytosis efficiency of a kinase-deficient mutant p185 was greatly reduced when compared to constitutively activated oncogenic p185[neu]. Therefore, these results suggest that tyrosine kinase activity influences receptor intracellular trafficking.

VII. RECEPTOR PHOSPHORYLATION AND CELLULAR SIGNALING

Receptor autophosphorylation/cross-phosphorylation of discrete tyrosine residues in the carboxyl termini is an initial consequence of receptor tyrosine kinase activation. The resultant phosphorylated tails of the receptor provide docking sites for cellular substrate binding and the subsequent transmission of signals to cause cell growth and differentiation.

A. Role of Tyrosine Phosphorylation in Substrate Binding and Receptor Specificity

Mutational analysis of tyrosine residues by site-directed mutagenesis has revealed a critical role of autophosphorylation in the cellular transforming activity of Her2/neu. Segatto and co-workers altered several tyrosine residues or made larger structural deletions in Her2 to examine the function of these residues. Individual amino acid substitutions at one of four individual positions failed to abrogate the transforming activity of overexpressed Her2 in NIH/3T3 cells. However, when multiple mutations were introduced, transforming activity was impaired as measured by a decrease in focal growth on monolayers. An overall decrease in Her2 phosphotyrosine content correlated with these observed effects.

Her2 phosphotyrosine-modified residues are required for mitogenic action because they serve as high-affinity binding sites for cellular proteins, such as those containing src homology 2 (SH2) domains or phosphotyrosine-binding (PTB) domains. The SH2 proteins can be either substrates themselves or serve as "adapters" for the assembly of additional proteins onto the activated growth factor receptor complex. Considerable specificity of SH2–growth factor receptor interaction is achieved by virtue of the sequence surrounding the phosphorylated tyrosine, suggesting a mechanism for signaling specificity. Direct analysis by tryptic peptide mapping of in vitro-labeled human Her2 protein led to the determination of several autophosphorylation sites. Specific sites of tyrosine autophosphorylation have been identified exclusively within the carboxy tail of the Her2/neu protein by multiple groups. Reasonable predictions of which SH2 domain-containing proteins are able to interact with an activated receptor on the basis of the amino acid sequences immediately following the phosphorylated tyrosine residues are now possible. This demonstrates that substrate binding requires more that just the phosphotyrosine moiety; considerable specificity of the interaction is achieved by virtue of the sequence motif surrounding the phosphorylated tyrosine as well. This suggests that the limited homology of the amino acid sequences of the carboxyl termini of EGFR and Her2/neu may define distinct signaling pathways. Although EGFR and p185 signaling does appear to converge at the nucleus, the observed patterns of tyrosine-phosphorylated proteins in NIH/3T3 cells transformed by these two tyrosine kinases are qualitatively and quantitatively different as demonstrated by DiFiore and colleagues.

Her2/neu has been shown to have a significantly higher transforming potency than EGFR in NIH/3T3 cells, whereas p185 had less transforming activity than EGFR in a hematopoietic cell line, suggesting that the two receptors are linked with different efficiencies to one or more signaling pathways. By creating chimeric molecules with different tyrosine kinase or carboxy-terminal domains, DiFiore and colleagues demonstrated that the tyrosine kinase domain of either receptor was responsible for the specificity of mitogenic signaling in 32D cells. A variety of studies indicated that p185 and EGFR have intrinsically different catalytic activities, as well as different substrate specificities, which lead to disparate mitogenic effects. These observations may help explain the tissue-specific alterations of different oncogenic growth factor receptors in different human tumors. Moreover, the aberrant coupling of two separate signaling pathways may also be involved in the synergistic transformation resulting from the simultaneous expression of both receptor tyrosine kinases as described elsewhere in this article.

In addition to specificity, which is engendered by an individual tyrosine kinase receptor, the ability of erbB family members to heterodimerize also appears to activate distinct signaling pathways. Although there is significant overlap in the signaling pathways activated by the erbB family of receptors, there are also signals specific to individual family members. c-Cbl is primarily triggered by activated EGFR. The p85 subunit of the phosphatidylinositol-3-kinase (PI-3-kinase) is activated very efficiently by erbB-3-containing complexes. A Csk homologous kinase binds mainly to Her2. Using tryptic phosphopeptide mapping, Olayioye and colleagues demonstrated that receptor tyrosine phosphorylation changes with distinct dimerization partners for EGFR and erbB-2. Furthermore, the downstream pathways activated depend on dimerization pairings. Muthuswamy and co-workers provided additional support for dimerization-dependent specificity through the use of chimeric erbB proteins for which dimerization could be regulated with a synthetic ligand. It was noted that while c-Cbl was associated with EGFR homomers, the protein was not associated with EGFR/Her2 heterodimers.

B. Pathways Activated by the Her2/neu Receptor

Receptor tyrosine kinase signaling is mediated by a number of SH2-containing substrates, including phospholipase C-γ (PLC-γ), PI-3-kinase, GTPase-activating protein (GAP), Shc, Grb2, src family kinases, and SH2 domain-containing phosphatases. Activation of kinase substrates by receptor tyrosine kinase leads to the release of second messengers, such as inositol phosphate and diacylglycerol intermediates. In addition, activation of the Ras pathway by receptor tyrosine kinases leads to the regulation of a serine/threonine protein cascade, including the Ras and the MAP kinase pathway. Eventually, signal transduction affects the nuclear transcription of genes or causes protein modifications, which regulate cell cycle progression and other cellular activities. A summary of several key signal transduction pathways involved in transformation driven by Her2/neu overexpression is presented in Fig. 4.

Tyrosine kinase signaling is known to activate multiple pathways controlling growth, proliferation, and survival. The relative contribution of each pathway is difficult to ascertain and may be cell type specific. Activation of the MAP kinase pathway, however, seems to be critical in many situations. We have shown in transfected cells of various types that transforming levels of erbB receptor complexes induce sustained, unattenuated activation of MAP kinase activities. Leder and colleagues have investigated the significance of different signal transduction pathways by examining the effect of pathway-specific pharmacologic inhibitors on tumor lines established from transgenic mouse models. Tumors lines derived from neu transgenic mice showed elevated activity in the MAP kinase pathway; furthermore, the growth of these tumor lines was inhibited by a pharmacologic inhibitor of the MAP kinase pathway, whereas mammary tumor lines of different origin were not affected by this agent. These data suggest that Ras activation of the MAP kinase pathway is a critical component of Her2/neu-induced growth.

We have demonstrated that the proteasome may

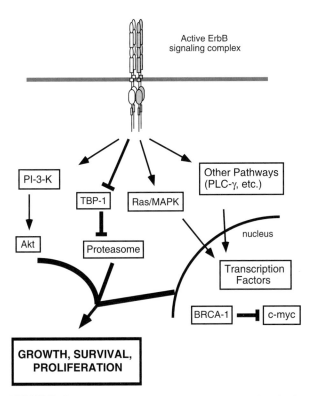

FIGURE 4 Signal transduction pathways, associated with the Her2/neu oncogene. Several signal transduction pathways, which are thought to contribute to the transforming potential of Her2/neu, are illustrated.

play a critical role in the regulation of cell growth and transformation in Her2/neu-expressing tumors. NIH/3T3 cells transformed by the overexpression of p185[neu] were treated with a monoclonal antibody known to lead to phenotypic reversion. These treated cells were compared to untreated cells using differential mRNA display, a screening technique that can identify mRNA species that differ in abundance between two samples. TBP1, originally cloned as a protein with high homology to the HIV Tat-binding protein-1, demonstrated elevated mRNA levels in antibody-treated cells. To test the significance of this result, TBP1 cDNA was used to transfect transformed cells. TBP1 expression led to reversion of the transformed phenotype as measured by diminished cell proliferation, reduced colony formation in soft agar, and greatly inhibited tumor formation in athymic mice. This identified a regulator of the proteasome as having a tumor suppressor-like activity. We expect that downregulation of proteasome functions will

limit the degradation of cell cycle inhibitors, thereby limiting cell growth.

Consistent with the idea that cell cycle regulation is critical to the transforming ability of Her2/neu, cyclin D1 has been recognized for its importance in neu transformation. Lee and colleagues noted that cyclin D1 protein levels were elevated in both neu transgenic mouse models and neu-transformed cell lines. Cyclin D1 induction could be abrogated by the mutation of critical residues within Her2/neu. Transformation was shown to be inhibited *in vivo* by cyclin D1 antisense, an experimental technique, which, theoretically, specifically prevents the synthesis of a target protein. Through the use of dominant-negative and pharmacologic inhibitors of cell cycle pathways, it was determined that the induction of cyclin D1 by p185[neu] was dependent on the Ras/MAP kinase pathway, but not on the PI-3-kinase pathway. These experiments reinforce the importance of the MAP kinase pathway and the critical regulation of cell cycle control by Her2/neu.

Although the MAP kinase pathway has been shown to be of great importance to erbB signaling, the significance of other major signaling pathways, such as the PI-3-kinase pathway, can by no means be discounted. A major downstream effector of the PI-3-kinase pathway, the importance of which has been revealed, is the Akt survival kinase pathway. As a downstream effector of many growth factor signals, this pathway provides an antiapoptotic signal. Mendelsohn and colleagues demonstrated a protective role for EGF from Fas-induced apoptosis in both a breast cancer cell line and normal immortalized human epithelial cells. The protection conferred by EGF stimulation was shown to rely on Akt signaling. Liu and colleagues demonstrated that Heregulin, an erbB family ligand, leads to the activation of Akt, and furthermore that Akt activation is blocked by an inhibitory antibody to Her2, revealing a role for Her2 in Akt activation. We have shown that the tumor suppressor BRCA1 is phosphorylated in response to erbB2 activation, and there is some evidence that this modification is also influenced by Akt signaling.

That erbB signaling leads to survival is not surprising given data concerning the effects of Her2/neu on chemosensitivty and radiosensitivity. It is now apparent that a major aspect of killing by both chemotherapeutic agents and radiation therapy is due to the induction of apoptosis. High-grade glial malignancies are particularly refractory to standard treatment strategies, and therefore, any method that might improve those treatment strategies would be of great clinical benefit. We have demonstrated that glial and other cells transformed by p185^{neu} overexpression can be phenotypically reverted by the introduction of a p185 mutant with an intracellular truncation just below the membrane, p185^{T691Stop}. In addition to causing phenotypic reversion, p185^{T691Stop}-mediated disabling of kinase signaling sensitized cells to apoptosis induced by γ-irradiation, a mediator of DNA damage. Furthermore, this apoptotic response was shown to be p53 independent, which is encouraging from a clinical standpoint, given the high proportion of human tumors for which survival is thought to be enhanced by loss of p53 function. Treatment with monoclonal antibodies to p185^{neu}, like expression of a truncated p185, can lead to phenotypic reversion and disabling of kinase receptors, and will be discussed later. Pietras and colleagues demonstrated that treatment with such an antibody leads to a decrease in DNA repair, possibly due to a failure in the induction of regulatory proteins such as p21^{cip}. While multiple groups have demonstrated that disabling of kinase receptors can enhance the effectiveness of antitumor agents, that Her2/neu overexpression provides an intrinsic chemoresistance remains controversial. Pegram and co-workers investigated this issue both in cell culture and in mouse models and found that Her2/neu overexpression alone was not sufficient to impart drug resistance and suggested that Her2/neu may appear to impart drug resistance due to more rapid regrowth of tumors. Collectively, however, studies of the role of Her2/neu and apoptosis suggest that survival pathways are a critical aspect of receptor tyrosine kinase signaling and that this component of receptor tyrosine kinase signaling is central to understanding the mechanisms of transformation and phenotypic reversion.

VIII. MONOCLONAL ANTIBODY-MEDIATED PHENOTYPIC REVERSION

The relationship of with either the oncogenic p185^{neu} or the overexpressed Her2 to cellular transformation

has been revealed using monoclonal antibodies (mAbs) directed against p185, intended to modulate the surface expression and activity of this protein. These data were consistent with a direct effect of antireceptor antibodies on p185^{neu} expression leading to a loss of surface p185 expression and targeted degradation of the oncogenic p185^{neu} protein. Taken collectively, these studies suggest that the continual expression of Her2/neu is necessary for the maintenance of the transformed phenotype of neu-transformed cells.

A. Monoclonal Antibodies against Her2/neu

Mouse monoclonal antibodies raised against B104-1-1 cells expressing p185^{neu} react with the extracellular domain of the p185 protein. These mAbs have also been used for cell surface staining and immunoprecipitation to analyze p185 proteins. Drebin and colleagues first described that the anti-neu mAb 7.16.4 caused a phenotypic reversion of transformed cells. Treatment of B104-1-1 cells with anti-p185 antibody 7.16.4 dramatically inhibited the anchorage-independent growth of these cells in soft agar, a characteristic of transformed cells. This effect was selective for p185^{neu}, as treatment with the same mAb did not affect the phenotype of Ras-transformed cells. Further experiments indicated that the reversion of transformation was correlated with the downregulation of p185^{neu} from the cell surface and the acceleration of its rate of degradation. Removal of the transforming receptor from the cell surface *in vitro* was associated with a reduction in the malignant phenotype and a conversion of the cellular phenotype into a more normal one. Downregulation of p185^{neu} and the transformed phenotype was dependent on the continual presence of the antibody and was reversible upon removal of the antibody. *In vivo* studies then demonstrated that treatment with anti-neu mAbs was able to significantly inhibit the tumorigenic growth of neu-transformed NIH/3T3 cells implanted into athymic mice. The use of two or more mAbs reactive with distinct epitopes of p185^{neu} resulted in an additive effect and complete tumor growth inhibition in 60% of the treatment animals. Our laboratory has also developed a transgenic model to study the preventative effects of antireceptor antibodies on incipient tumor development. In the transgenic model, animals that express the oncogenic neu, which develop tumors at about 30–35 weeks of age, were used. Studies indicated that the onset of tumor appearance can be delayed until 50 weeks by the administration of as little as 10 μg weekly of anti-p185 antibody. We have been able to entirely prevent tumor development in transgenic mice for over 100 weeks by doubling the amount of anti-p185 antibody administered. Therefore, incipient tumor development may be prevented by use of antibody cocktails early in disease treatment.

Although a wide array of potentially clinically useful biological effects have been observed with the use of monoclonal antibodies, the mechanisms of action are not well understood. To investigate this problem, Klapper and colleagues generated a large battery of mAbs directed against erbB-2. Most of the antibodies generated were able to stimulate tyrosine phosphorylation of erbB-2, a somewhat surprising result given the inhibitory nature of the antibodies. For most of the antibodies, the antitumor effect was correlated with enhanced receptor degradation, and hence decreased surface expression. Decreased surface expression of protein tyrosine kinase would lead, then, to decreased mitogenic signaling. Another class of antibodies appeared to exert antitumor effects through the inhibition of ligand binding and the inhibition of heterodimer formation.

B. Variations on a Theme: Humanized Antibodies, Antibody Fragments, Immunoliposomes, Bispecific Antibodies, and Small Peptide Mimics

Antibodies represent a potentially ideal method for imparting biologic specificity. Antibodies to Her2/neu have been observed in the sera of patients with tumors expressing Her2/neu, suggesting that an immune response may be a component of natural tumor resistance. A logical exploitation of this phenomenon, then, is to use immune-based therapies to target human tumors. Her2/neu, as a frequently overexpressed surface antigen, has the potential to be an ideal immunologic determinant.

A major limitation to the clinical use of rodent mAb is the development of an anti-idiotypic or antiglobulin response during therapy. To circumvent this potential problem, Carter and colleagues have developed a humanized antibody to Her2/neu, which has been named Herceptin. The development of Herceptin, based on earlier studies from our laboratory, represents the first oncoprotein-directed mAb therapy to be approved by the FDA. As will be discussed later, this antibody has been used clinically with a measure of success.

Another approach to immunotherapy involves the cloning and expression of recombinant antibodies as single chain Fv (scFv) fragments, which are monovalent and exclude the Fc regions of the antibody. Thus, these antibody-derived molecules cannot bind complement or interact with other effector cells. These molecules are slightly smaller in size, potentially leading to improved biodistribution, and may be less immunogenic. However, these molecules can be conjugated to immunoliposomes, providing a method of specific toxin or gene delivery. This approach has been employed by Park and co-workers using Her2/neu as a target. Immunoliposomes could be used to deliver high local concentrations of chemotherapeutic agents or to transfer specific antitumor genes. Taking advantage of molecular biology in order to express genes for two different Fv regions in one antibody-producing cell, it is possible to generate bispecific antibodies, where each arm of the antibody recognizes a different immunologic determinant. This approach has been used to create bispecific antibodies that recognize both Her2/neu and receptors present on cytotoxic immune cells, with the intention of inducing the specific lysis of Her2/neu-expressing cells. A second potential application for bispecific antibody technology is related to the increased transforming ability of EGFR/Her2 heterodimers. Extending the paradigm that two antibodies to these two erbB family members can inhibit transformation synergistically, it may be more efficient to target the two receptors with a single antibody species.

The use of large proteins, such as antibodies, as therapeutics, has some disadvantages. Large molecules have limited penetration into tissues and regulated body compartments, such as the brain and testis. In addition, large molecules such as antibodies are more likely to elicit an immune response, such as an anti-idiotypic response, that would limit the repeated use of a therapeutic agent. Another consideration is the cost of commercial preparation, which is extremely high for a molecule such as a monoclonal antibody. To address these potential problems, our laboratory has developed a method for the design of exocyclic peptide mimics based on the structure of antibody hypervariable loops. Evidence from biochemical and structural studies of antibody–antigen interactions suggests that an isolated CDR may be sufficient to bind an antigen and may retain bioactivity similar to its parental antibody. The mimic consists of a small peptide that is cyclized through a cysteine–cysteine disulfide bond. This type of compound is poorly immunogenic, resistant to peptidases, and nontoxic. Such a mimic, based on the structure of the Herceptin antibody, has been developed for Her2/neu. The anti-Her2 mimic shows potent activity in assays that measure the inhibition of tumorigenicity; we have observed decreased proliferation of cells *in vitro*, decreased formation of foci *in vitro*, the inhibition of tumor growth in athymic mice, and sensitization to ionizing radiation and chemotherapeutic agents. This anti-Her2 mimic, along with the general approach for the development of small peptide therapeutics, represents a promising potential clinical application.

IX. Her2/neu BIOLOGY AND BREAST CANCER TREATMENT

Her2/neu overexpression has been observed in a variety of human cancers and has come to the forefront of breast cancer treatment. This is not surprising, as Her2/neu amplification is observed in 25–30% of breast cancer. Studies into the basic mechanisms of transformation by this protein tyrosine kinase have already translated into useful clinical treatments for breast cancer, whereas additional and potentially superior therapeutics are under development.

A. Her2/neu as a Prognostic Indicator

Given the vast array of treatment options and the repercussions those options will have on the quality of patient life, it is critical to make informed decisions with regard to the choice of a treatment plan. Prog-

nostic indicators can be of great importance when making such a decision. Currently, lymph node status, which may indicate whether a neoplasm has undergone systemic invasion, is the standard prognostic indicator utilized for planning chemotherapeutic therapy. Node status, however, while of undeniable value, is by no means an error-free predictor. A large proportion of patients who have been judged to be node negative, and thus thought to harbor a cancer that has not progressed to systemic invasion, will go on to relapse. If these patients could be predicted, more aggressive, potentially life-saving therapy could be employed. For example, we have shown in a transgenic mouse model that anti-Her2 antibody administration can prevent tumor development; if patients who harbor Her2-driven disease and are at risk for relapse could be identified, such therapy could be of great benefit.

Numerous studies have looked at Her2/neu amplification and protein expression as a prognostic indicator in breast cancer. Results of these studies vary, which is not surprising given the different experimental methods employed; commonly utilized methods have included Southern blotting, polymerase chain reaction, *in situ* fluorescence hybridization, immunohistochemistry, Western blotting, and enzyme-linked immunosorbent assay. While there is a great deal of conflicting data, some clear trends have emerged. Her2/neu overexpression correlated with poor outcome and significantly worse overall survival in the vast majority of studies performed. Her2/neu seems to predict resistance to treatment with hormonal therapy, such as tamoxifen, as a single agent. Response to cytotoxic chemotherapy has not been convincingly correlated with Her2/neu amplification or overexpression. As previously mentioned, a proteolytically released soluble form of Her2 is observed in a subset of Her2-expressing tumors. The majority of studies measuring serum levels of this soluble Her2 fragment show a significant correlation with either disease recurrence or shortened survival. More studies are needed, however, to determine whether routine analysis of Her2 status in newly diagnosed breast cancer will be beneficial.

Knowledge of Her2 status is a necessary prerequisite, however, for Herceptin treatment, which is discussed next; if Herceptin becomes a standard treatment, so might routine screening for Her2 amplification or overexpression.

B. Clinical Experience with Herceptin

Herceptin (also known as Trastuzumab), an anti-Her2 mAb, is the first FDA-approved mAb therapy for the treatment of breast cancer. The basic science and rationale behind the use of this agent have been discussed in previous sections. More than 1000 women have been treated with Herceptin in clinical trials. Phase I, II, and III trials have been carried out to investigate the safety, efficacy, and the risks and benefits of this agent. Two clinical situations have been studied; Herceptin as a single agent for metastatic breast cancer refractory to cytotoxic chemotherapy and Herceptin in addition to standard chemotherapy as a first-line treatment. Herceptin is administered intravenously each week. The agent is generally well tolerated, as side effects in all studies were relatively minor as compared to standard chemotherapy. The development of anti-idiotypic antibodies, thought to be a potential problem with mAb therapy, has not been reported as a significant problem.

For the treatment of metastatic disease in which patients had relapsed following one or two regimens of cytotoxic chemotherapy, an overall response rate of 15–20% was observed. A complete response was seen in 4%, a partial response in 17%, a minor response in 7%, and stable disease in 30%. The median duration of response was 8.4 months. Studies involving Herceptin as a first-line treatment in combination with either anthracycline and cyclophosphamide (AC) or paclitaxel indicate an increase in both response rate and time to disease progression. The results of these studies are promising, suggesting that treatment directed at the abrogation of mitogenic Her2 signaling may become a standard consideration in the care of breast cancer patients.

The evolution of antibody therapy of either Her2- or EGFR/Her2-driven tumors is the use of cocktails of mAbs. Using an *in vivo* model, our laboratory has shown that the simultaneous administration of mAbs to two distinct domains of the extracellular portion of p185 is far more effective at downregulating p185 than use of a single mAb. Synergistic and curative effects are observed with the two mAb approach. Sim-

ilarly, antibodies to EGFR and Her2 are curative when transformation is driven by EGFR/Her2 heteromers.

C. Other Clinical Approaches

Our current understanding of the biology of the Her2/neu receptor has provided multiple clinical approaches, such as the Herceptin monoclonal antibody. Many other potential clinical approaches have been suggested, a few of which, such as small peptide mimics, intracellular-deleted neu forms, and soluble neu variants, have already been mentioned. Figure 5 summarizes current approaches to subversion of Her2/neu-mediated transformation.

Although clinical success has not yet been achieved, pharmacologic inhibitors of protein tyrosine kinases have been and continue to be developed, improving potency and specificity. The natural inhibitor herbimycin A irreversibly blocks the tyrosine kinases of Src, EGFR, and Her2. Some synthetic inhibitors, such as tyrophostin, also selectively inhibit tyrosine kinases. Tyrophostins also synergize with antityrosine receptor kinase antibodies in reversion of the transformed phenotype. The small molecular size of Laverdustin analogs such as AG957 allows them to permeate cells. AG1478 is highly selective for the inhibition of the EGFR kinase, whereas AG825 inhibits the Her2 kinase 60 times as efficiently as it inhibits EGFR *in vitro*. Irreversible tyrosine kinase inhibitors of EGFR and Her2, which work through the covalent modification of a cysteine amino acid residue in the ATP-binding pocket of the receptor kinase domain, have also been developed.

Receptor tyrosine kinase activities result in high levels of autophosphorylation and substrate phosphorylation. Tyrosine phosphorylation in the cell is a reversible, dynamic process. Protein tyrosine phosphatases (PTPs) are responsible for the removal of phosphate from tyrosine residues (dephosphorylation). An imbalance between these enzymes may impair normal cellular growth control, leading to cellular transformation. Several studies have reported the inhibitory effects of PTPs on cellular transformation in tissue culture systems. Expression of the human PTP1B gene has been shown to block Her2-mediated cellular transformation. The mechanism of suppression of transformation by PTP1B may be either

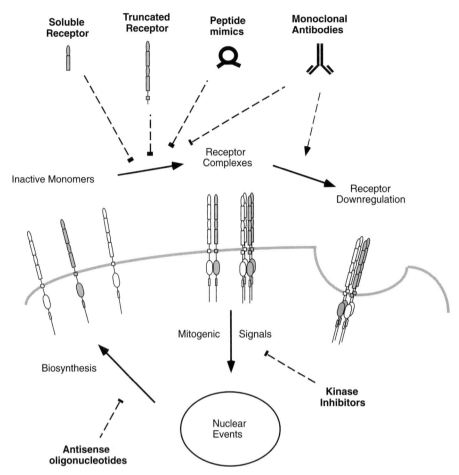

Soluble Receptor **Truncated Receptor** **Peptide mimics** **Monoclonal Antibodies**

Inactive Monomers

Receptor Complexes

Receptor Downregulation

Mitogenic   Signals

Biosynthesis

Kinase Inhibitors

Nuclear Events

Antisense oligonucleotides

FIGURE 5 Current approaches for the reversion of Her2/neu-driven neoplasia (see text for details).

through direct dephosphorylation of Her2/neu or through an effect on downstream substrates. More comprehensive studies are needed to define the substrates critical for the transformed phenotype and those that are regulated by protein tyrosine phosphatases.

Conceptually, the goal of Her2/neu-directed therapeutics is to block signaling from the receptor, either by directly blocking the enzymatic activity of the receptor tyrosine kinase or by downregulating the receptor from the cell surface altogether. One approach to downregulation, which is currently being investigated by Drebin and colleagues, involves the use of antisense oligodeoxynucleotides in an attempt to block expression of the Her2/neu protein at the RNA level. Antisense therapy was shown to be effective in the treatment of human tumor xenografts in athymic mice. Additionally, antisense oligodeoxynucleotides

in combination with chemotherapy led to a synergistic effect.

See Also the Following Articles

GASTRIC CANCER: INHERITED PREDISPOSITION • INSULIN-LIKE GROWTH FACTORS • MAP KINASE MODULES IN SIGNALING • PROTEIN KINASES AND THEIR INHIBITORS • PYRUVATE KINASES • SIGNAL TRANSDUCTION MECHANISMS INITIATED BY RECEPTOR TYROSINE KINASES • TGFβ RECEPTOR SIGNALING MECHANISMS

Bibliography

Dougall, W. C., Qian, X., Peterson, N. C., Miller, M. J., Samanta, A., and Greene, M. I. (1994). The *neu*-oncogene: Signal transduction pathways, transformation mechanisms and evolving therapies. *Oncogene* **9,** 2109–2123.
Di Marco, E., Pierce, J. H., Knicley, C. L., and Di Fiore, P. P.

(1990). Transformation of NIH 3T3 cells by overexpression of the normal coding sequence of the rat *neu* gene. *Mol. Cell. Biol.* **10**(6), 3247–3252.

Klapper, L. N., Kirschbaum, M. H., Sela, M., and Yarden, Y. (2000). Biochemical and clinical implications of the ErbB/HER signaling network of growth factor receptors. *Adv. Cancer Res.* **77,** 25–79.

O'Rourke, D. M., Qian, X., Zhang, H. T., Davis, J. G., Nute, E., Meinkoth, J., and Greene, M. I. (1997). Trans receptor inhibition of human glioblastoma cells by erbB family ectodomains. *Proc. Natl. Acad. Sci. USA* **94**(7), 3250–3255.

Park, B. W., O'Rourke, D. M., Wang, Q., Davis, J. G., Post, A., Qian, X., and Greene, M. I. (1999). Induction of the Tat-binding protein 1 gene accompanies the disabling of oncogenic erbB receptor tyrosine kinases. *Proc. Natl. Acad. Sci. USA* **96**(11), 6434–6438.

Park, B. W., Zhang, H. T., Wu, C., Berezov, A., Zhang, X., Dua, R., Wang, Q., Kao, G., O'Rourke, D. M., Greene, M. I., and Murali, R. (2000). Rationally designed anti-HER2/neu peptide mimetic disables P185HER2/neu tyro-sine kinases in vitro and in vivo. *Nature Biotechnol.* **18**(2), 194–198.

Press, M. F., Cordon-Cardo, C., and Slammon, D. (1990). Expression of the Her2/neu proto-oncogene in normal human adult and fetal tissues. *Oncogene* **5,** 953–962.

Qian, X., O'Rourke, D. M., Fei, Z., Zhang, H. T., Kao, C. C., and Greene, M. I. (1999). Domain-specific interactions between the p185(neu) and epidermal growth factor receptor kinases determine differential signaling outcomes. *J. Biol. Chem.* **274**(2), 574–583.

Ross, J. S., and Fletcher, J. A. (1999). HER-2/neu (c-erb-B2) gene and protein in breast cancer. *Am. J. Clin. Pathol.* **112**(Suppl. 1), S53–S67.

Wada, T., Qian, X., and Greene, M. (1990). Intermolecular association of the p185^{neu} protein and EGF receptor modulates EGF receptor function. *Cell* **61**(7), 1339–1347.

Weiner, D. B., Liu, J., Cohen, J. A., Williams, W. V., and Greene, M. I. (1989). A point mutation in the neu oncogene mimics ligand indution of receptor aggregation. *Nature* **339**(6221), 230–231.

HIV (Human Immunodeficiency Virus)

JoAnn C. Castelli
Jay A. Levy

University of California, San Francisco

GLOSSARY

acquired immunodeficiency syndrome A disease of the immune system caused by HIV infection and characterized by increased susceptibility to opportunistic infections, certain cancers, and neurological disorders.

CD4 A cellular surface protein found on T cells as well as other cells. It functions as a receptor for HIV binding and facilitates recognition of the T-cell receptor to antigens bound to MHC class II complexes.

chemokines A class of proinflammatory cytokines that have the ability to attract and activate leukocytes. They can be divided into at least three structural branches—C, CC, and CXC—according to variations in a shared cysteine motif.

cytokines Proteins secreted by leukocytes and some non-leukocytic cells that act as intercellular mediators. They are also produced by a number of tissue or cell types and generally act locally in a paracrine or autocrine manner.

dendritic cells Immune cells, derived from bone marrow, with long, tentacle-like branches called dendrites. Among dendritic cells are the Langerhans cells of the skin and follicular dendritic cells in the lymph nodes. Most dendritic cells function as antigen-presenting cells that digest extracellular pathogens and present segments of protein (antigen) on the cell surface to induce a primary immune response.

humoral immunity An antibody-mediated immunity involving secreted products of B cells that interact and neutralize extracellular pathogens.

lentivirus A genus of the family Retroviridae consisting of nononcogenic retroviruses that produce multiorgan diseases characterized by long incubation periods and persistent infection. Lentiviruses are unique in that they contain open reading frames between *pol* and *env* genes and in the 3' *env* region.

long terminal repeats (LTR) Identical DNA sequences, several hundred nucleotides long, found at either end of transposons and proviral DNA. LTRs are formed by reverse transcription of retroviral RNA. In proviruses, the upstream LTR acts as a promoter and enhancer, whereas the downstream LTR acts as a polyadenylation site.

macrophages Large white blood cells found mainly in connective tissue and in the bloodstream that ingest foreign particles and infectious microorganisms by phagocytosis.

retroviridae A family of viruses with a single-stranded RNA that, upon infection, generates a DNA copy via a viral reverse transcriptase; lentivirus is a subfamily.

simian immunodeficiency virus (SIV) Of the genus lentivirus that induces acquired immunodeficiency syndrome in monkeys and apes. SIV and HIV-2 exhibit close structural and immunologic properties and are 75% homologous.

T lymphocyte A subset of lymphocytes that develop in the thymus and circulate in the blood and lymphoid tissue. They orchestrate the response of the immune system to infected or malignant cells, either by lymphokine secretions or by direct contact. Helper T cells recognize foreign antigen on the surfaces of other cells, thus causing the stimulation of B cells to produce antibody and to cytotoxic T cells to destroy antigen-displaying cells.

T he human immunodeficiency virus (HIV), is a retrovirus that gradually destroys the immune system and has caused the worldwide epidemic of acquired immunodeficiency syndrome (AIDS). In 1983, HIV was first isolated from AIDS patients and was later identified as the infectious agent responsible for the disease. Other reports indicated the presence of this agent in many populations, including healthy individuals. Although HIV showed similarity to the human T cell leukemia virus (HTLV), HIV was cytotoxic to CD4$^+$ cells and did not transform them into malignant cells characteristic of HTLV infection. This infection of CD4$^+$ cells appeared to contribute to the dramatic decrease in CD4$^+$ cell numbers observed in AIDS patients. HIV can be transferred to individuals through sexual contact, blood products, or via mother-to-child transmission before or shortly after birth. Consistent with this observation, the levels of infectious HIV virions are significantly higher in the peripheral blood and genital fluids of individuals with the greatest chance of transmitting the virus.

I. STAGES OF HIV INFECTION

The typical course of HIV infection begins with an acute infection characterized by the presence of in-creasing levels of infectious viral RNA in plasma and a transient decrease in CD4$^+$ T lymphocytes. Within weeks to a few months, the amount of virus detected in the peripheral blood decreases as a result of immune responses, while the CD4$^+$ T lymphocyte count returns to a near-normal level. The initial infection is often associated with a flu-like syndrome that occurs within weeks and is followed by a quiescent period characterized by a healthy clinical state. The length of this asymptomatic latent period is influenced by environmental, genetic, and immunologic factors as well as by the predominant virus type. In the final stages of the infection, which takes place after an average of 10 years, the viral load increases in the peripheral blood and lymphoid tissues. This phenomenon is accompanied by a decrease in CD4$^+$ cell numbers and the occurrence of opportunistic infection or cancer leading to a fatal outcome.

II. GENETIC STRUCTURE AND PRODUCTS

HIV-1 and HIV-2 are grouped within the lentivirus genus as members of the Retroviridae family. The two types of AIDS viruses, HIV-1 and -2, share up to 50% overall nucleotide homology and are similar in structure and cellular tropism. The genomes of HIV-1 and HIV-2 consist of two identical single RNA strands enclosed within a cone-shaped core, surrounded by a glycosylated outer virion surface (Fig. 1). The 9.8-kb RNA genome contains a 5′ cap (Gppp), a 3′ poly(A) tail, and several open reading frames (ORFs). This genome codes for 15 major molecular products (Table I). The longest ORF encodes for viral structural proteins, whereas smaller ORFs encode regulators of viral binding, fusion, replication, and assembly.

A. Structural Proteins

1. Env

The Env structural polyprotein, gp160, is produced from a long ORF transcript. Gp160 is cleaved into gp120 and gp41 in the endoplasmic reticulum. These proteins are highly glycosylated and can be expressed on either the cell or the virion surface. Interaction of the viral gp120 with the cellular receptor CD4 causes

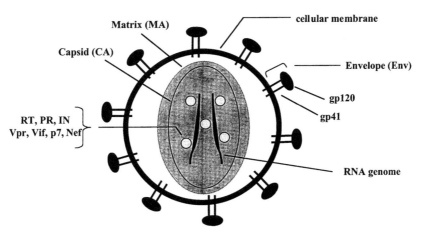

FIGURE 1 Structure of the HIV virion. The HIV RNA genome is encapsulated in a capsid (CA) composed of p24 and is stabilized by a matrix composed of MA. The cellular lipid bilayer containing envelope glycoproteins completes the outer structure. Several proteins located inside the capsid are required for maturation and infectivity of HIV.

a conformational change that facilitates virus binding and entry. The gp120 protein forms trimeric structures that are anchored to the membrane of the virion by the viral transmembrane protein gp41. The gp120 surface protein has several loops highly variable in amino acid sequence (V1–V5) among viral strains. These regions primarily regulate the efficiency of virus entry and cellular tropism. The envelope also con-

tains five constant regions (C1–C5) interspersed within its structure. Mutations in the V3 loop can decrease or alter infectivity and the fusion capabilities of HIV. One of the conserved regions of gp120, C4, has a complex folded structure that, if mutated, can affect conformational changes and thus the efficiency of binding to CD4. The C2 region of gp120 is important for interactions with CD4 and with gp41, to which

TABLE I
HIV Proteins and Their Functions[a]

Protein	Size (kDa)	Function
Gag	p24	Capsid (CA) structural protein
	p17	Matrix (MA) protein–myristoylated
	p6	Role in budding
	p7	Nucleocapsid (NC) protein; helps in reverse transcription
Polymerase (Pol)	p66, p51	Reverse transcriptase (RT); RNase H–inside core
Protease (PR)	p10	Posttranslational processing of viral proteins
Integrase (IN)	p32	Viral cDNA integration
Envelope	gp120	Envelope surface (SU) protein
	gp41	Envelope transmembrane (TM) protein
Tat	p14	Transactivation
Rev	p19	Regulation of viral mRNA expression
Nef	p27	Pleiotropic, can increase or decrease virus replication
Vif	p23	Increases virus infectivity and cell-to-cell transmission; helps in proviral DNA synthesis and/or in virion assembly
Vpr	p15	Helps in virus replication; transactivation
Vpu	p16	Helps in virus release; disrupts gp160–CD4 complexes
Vpx	p15	Helps in infectivity

[a]Adapted from Levy (1998).

gp120 binds by hydrophobic interaction. The gp41 protein mediates fusion and, along with gp120, cytotoxicity.

2. PR, RT, and IN

Another long viral ORF generates precursor Gag and Gag-Pol transcripts, which can be transported to the cytoplasm for translation by free ribosomes into polyproteins. A ribosomal frameshifting event produces the Gag-Pol polyprotein Pr160$^{\text{Gag-Pol}}$ that can be proteolytically processed by the viral protease, PR. The autocatalysis of PR, a product of Pol, is activated in the presence of high Pr160$^{\text{Gag-Pol}}$ protein concentrations. The PR-mediated cleavage of Pr55^{gag} and Pr160$^{\text{Gag-Pol}}$, during assembly of the virion, is necessary for the generation of infectious particles. In addition, PR processes the reverse transcriptase (RT) and integrase (IN) proteins from Pol and matrix (MA), p24, p9, and p6 proteins from Gag. Reverse transcriptase generates the complementary strand from the RNA genome producing the provirus cDNA form. Because RT is colocalized with the RNA genome in the capsid, some reverse transcription can occur in the viral particle before infection of the target cell. However, the completion of provirus production requires infection of the host cell and uncoating of the virion. Within the capsid, viral IN proteins are found along with MA and the accessory viral protein, Vpr. IN is required for integration of the provirus into the host genome.

3. MA, p24, p9, and p6

The Gag precursor protein Pr55^{gag} is responsible for generating structural proteins required for virus assembly. Due to myristoylation of Pr55^{gag}, the protein can be targeted to the plasma membrane for the regulation of viral assembly at the cell surface. Proteolytic processing of Pr55^{gag} by PR generates MA, p24, p9, and p6. MA is a myristoylated protein (p17) that forms a matrix assuring the structural integrity of the virion. The p24 protein is the major structural component of the cone-shaped core or capsid (CA) and can influence infectivity of the virion through interaction with cyclophilin A. The p9 protein is an RNA-binding protein in the core that protects viral RNA from nucleases and transports full-length viral RNA

to the assembly complex. The p6 protein can assist in budding of the virion and affect infectivity.

B. Regulatory Proteins

1. Tat and Rev

The smaller ORFs generate viral regulatory and accessory proteins. These viral gene products, Tat, Rev, Nef, Vpu, Vpr, and Vif, can be spliced in the nucleus by cellular splicesomes and transported to the cytoplasm for translation by membrane-bound ribosomes. Tat regulates viral transcription through interactions with specific cellular factors and TAR, the trans-activation response element in the 5′ stem–loop region of the HIV RNA genome. Tat can also enhance, but is not required for, virus replication. The Rev protein regulates nuclear export of transcripts by interacting with a Rev responsive element (RRE) located in the viral env-coding region. Rev controls the ratio of unspliced to spliced transcripts, which is important for initiating virus assembly.

C. Accessory Proteins

1. Vif, Vpu, Vpr, Nef

In addition to regulatory proteins, several accessory proteins have important functions in the HIV replicative cycle. Vif increases virus infectivity, and Vpu, found in HIV-1 only, mediates downregulation of the CD4 molecule and enhances infectious HIV virion release from the cell surface. Vpr, a nuclear protein found in most HIV subtypes, regulates transport of the preintegration complex. Both Vpr and Vpx, a cytoplasmic protein found only in HIV-2 and SIV, affect assembly and budding, as well as enhance viral replication. Nef is a pleiotropic protein that can positively regulate virus replication in quiescent cells and mediate pathogenicity. Nef appears to affect T-cell signaling activity, resulting in altered or lower levels of cytokines, particularly IL-2. The role for Nef in the regulation of viral infectivity and pathogenesis is supported by the recovery of Nef mutants of HIV-1 from infected individuals with no evidence of disease progression. However, the full mechanism of Nef activity remains unclear.

III. HIV REPLICATION CYCLE

The infection cycle of HIV can be divided into four major stages: binding and entry, reverse transcription and integration, transcription and translation, and assembly and budding (Fig. 2). (Step 1) In the binding and entry stage, the HIV envelope protein, gp120, has a high-affinity interaction with the cellular surface protein, CD4, and specific cellular coreceptors, which facilitate fusion with the cellular membrane. Once inside the cell, viral CA protein p24 and cyclophilins mediate the uncoating of the HIV core and release of the RNA genome. (Step 2) In association with several structural proteins, the RNA genome is primed by viral tRNA-lysine and is reverse transcribed into a double-stranded cDNA. The MA and Vpr viral proteins target the preintegration complex, com-

posed of viral cDNA and MA, Vpr, and IN, to the nucleus. Integration of the provirus occurs randomly in the cellular genome and is regulated by IN, which is capable of cleaving chromosomal DNA and mediating ligation of the provirus.

The HIV proviral cDNA is flanked by a 5' LTR and 3' LTR that regulate initiation of transcription and RNA termination, respectively, of regulatory enzymatic and structural genes. (Step 3) The 5' LTR is composed of several regulatory sites for the transcription of viral genes by RNA polymerase II. NF-κB, Sp1, and TATA binding protein (TBP) are among some of the cellular factors that bind upstream of the 5' LTR and assist in initiating viral transcription. The viral regulatory protein Tat is essential for increasing the rate of transcription. The regulation of splicing events, directed by the Rev protein, allows for the

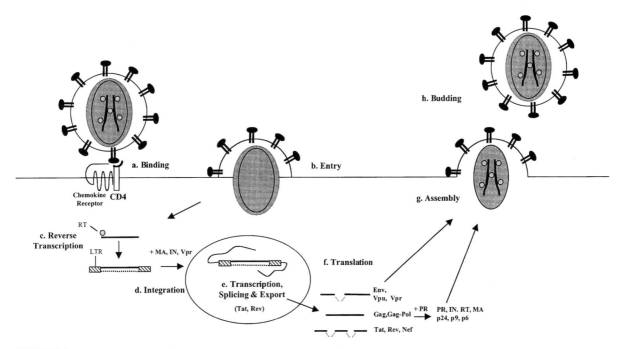

FIGURE 2 Steps in the HIV replication cycle. HIV infection proceeds through several stages involving binding, entry, reverse transcription, integration, transcription, translation, assembly, and budding. (a) The HIV gp120 envelope protein binds CD4 on the cellular surface and specific chemokine receptors facilitate fusion with the cellular membrane. (b) Entry involves uncoating of the virion, releasing the capsid containing the viral RNA genome and viral proteins into the cytoplasm. (c) Virally encoded reverse transcriptase generates the RNA genome into double-stranded cDNA. (d) MA, IN, and Vpr mediate nuclear transport of the cDNA preintegration complex, and IN completes integration of the HIV cDNA into random sites of the host genome. (e) Transcription of viral genes is initiated at the 5' LTR and requires Tat for optimal transcription. Splicing occurs in the nucleus, and the export of long viral transcripts is mediated by Rev. (f) Translation of viral transcripts in the cytoplasm produces viral products that assist in (g) assembly of the virion at the cell surface and the subsequent (h) budding from the cellular surface.

proper translation of many of the viral RNAs. Unspliced viral RNA can incorporate, at the cell membrane, into virus capsids that subsequently bud from the cell surface, incorporating the virus envelope expressed on the cell surface. (Step 4) During the budding process, proteolytic processing (mediated by the viral protease) brings about the maturation of the viral particle into an infectious virion.

IV. CELLULAR BINDING AND TROPISM

Cellular determinants of the host range include receptors for HIV binding and entry, such as the CD4 surface molecule, chemokine coreceptors, galactosyl ceramide, complement, and Fc receptors when virus is complexed with antibody. However, high levels of productive infection are predominantly observed in CD4$^+$ hematopoietic cells. The CD4 surface protein expressed by mononuclear phagocytes and helper T lymphocytes contains region D1 important for viral entry and cellular tropism. This CD4 molecule provides a docking site for, and induces a conformational change in, the envelope protein gp120, which exposes a site for virus binding to coreceptors on the cell.

A. Chemokine Receptors

Coreceptors are necessary for efficient HIV virion attachment that leads to viral fusion and entry. Two such receptors are the G protein-coupled seven transmembrane chemokine receptors CXCR-4 and CCR5. Chemokine receptors have important roles in the trafficking of T lymphocytes and macrophages. In HIV infection, chemokine receptors are essential for HIV entry after initial binding to the CD4 surface molecule and are determinants of cellular tropism.

A morphologic hallmark of productive HIV infection in cultured cells is the presence of syncytia, a fusion of infected cells resulting in multinucleated cellular complexes, and subsequent cell death. All HIV isolates can replicate in CD4$^+$ T lymphocytes and some are more cytopathic than others, as observed by the rapid formation of syncytia. Those HIV strains that replicate in established T-cell lines, as well as CD4$^+$ lymphocytes, are the syncytia-inducing (SI)

strains and utilize the CXCR-4 coreceptor, expressed on T lymphocytes. In contrast, nonsyncytia-inducing (NSI) strains that also infect CD4$^+$ lymphocytes grow well in macrophages using the CCR5 coreceptor. This receptor is expressed on monocytes, dendritic cells, T cells, and microglia. Additionally, some isolates are dual tropic and can infect both cell types. Therefore, the diversity of HIV isolates and coreceptor expression can affect cellular tropism.

Reports have shown that SDF-1, the natural ligand to CXCR-4, and the β-chemokines that bind to CCR-5 can suppress HIV replication in cell culture by blocking entry. These findings further support the importance of chemokine receptors in mediating HIV infection. Moreover, at the genetic level, homozygosity for a CCR5 allele with a 32-bp deletion, which prevents CCR5 surface expression, confers resistance in some HIV-infected individuals to the NSI virus strains.

HIV can infect CD4 negative cells, although with less replication capacity, through alternate receptors. In brain cells and bowel epithelium, gp120 interacts with surface galactosyl ceramide at a site distinct from its CD4 receptor-binding region. Another mode of entry may involve Fc and complement receptors. These receptors can interact with the Fc portion of nonneutralizing antibodies that attach to HIV and can transport the virus into the cell.

B. HIV Envelope

HIV envelope proteins act as viral determinants of cellular binding and host range. Both gp120 and gp41 appear important in regulating the rate and efficiency of virus entry through defined conformational changes or glycosylation patterns. Specific regions in the V3 loop also influence the pathogenicity or syncytia-inducing capability of the virion. The V3 loop is particularly important for determining the host range. Additionally, cleavage of gp120 by cellular proteases may be an essential step for viral entry and facilitate gp41 fusion with the cellular membrane.

V. VIRUS REPLICATION AND CYTOPATHOGENICITY

The difference in virus production and cytopathogenicity in T cells and macrophages may correlate with the state of activation. Quiescent T lymphocytes expressing CD4 on the surface are very susceptible to HIV infection. However, until activated, they cannot elicit a productive infection or permit integration of viral DNA. In nondividing $CD4^+$ macrophages, HIV infection can be productive with integration of viral DNA. Levels of virus replication are generally lower than in $CD4^+$ lymphocytes but some NSI strains can be produced to high levels in macrophages. In some CD4 negative cells, HIV can enter but generally replicates to low levels. Differences in the intracellular factors for early transcription and reverse transcription may account for the incapacity of some cell types to produce substantial amounts of virus. In addition, virus entry or envelope processing can vary among cell types and affect the extent of viral replication.

A. Cytopathic Effects

The loss of $CD4^+$ cells could be due to a variety of mechanisms, including antibody-dependent cellular cytoxicity, gp120-induced apoptosis, CTL lysis of infected cells or death of uninfected bystander cells by apoptosis, CTL activity, or necrosis. Syncytia formation is followed by membrane damage, leading to "balloon cell" degeneration, or necrosis. As noted earlier, SI viruses are generally more cytopathic than NSI viruses, and the appearance of SI isolates in infected individuals strongly correlates with progression to AIDS. Regions on CD4 and gp120 can regulate syncytia formation and, therefore, cytotoxicity of $CD4^+$ cells. Programmed cell death, or apoptosis, in response to virus infection appears to account in part for the decline in $CD4^+$ numbers in individuals progressing to disease. Direct infection of the cells is not needed to observe this effect. Many reports suggest that alterations in cytokine production can influence the rate of cell death by inhibiting survival cytokines (e.g., IL-2) or by directly inducing the death of uninfected bystander lymphocytes as well as infected cells. However, the pathway(s) leading to apoptosis *in vivo* is still unclear.

B. Cellular Latency

Cellular latency occurs following HIV provirus integration and is characterized by minimal transcrip-

tional or translational activity of viral genes. Virus activation from a latent state is often the result of stimulation by mitogens, cytokines, or DNA-damaging agents. The regulation of viral latency remains elusive. Some of the cellular factors recruited to the LTR for the active transcription of viral genes include NF-κB, Sp-1, and TBP. However, Rev, Tat, Vpu, and Nef have been implicated in mediating latency through their interactions with the LTR and replication cycle. Further understanding of the factors preventing induction of and reactivation from viral latency would be helpful for developing approaches to inhibit progression to disease.

VI. HOST IMMUNE RESPONSES TO HIV INFECTION

The effect of HIV on the immune system heavily influences the pathogenesis of the infection. A humoral response to the initial acute infection is reflected by the production of anti-HIV antibodies. As a host response to HIV infection, some of these antibodies are able to neutralize the virus, generally blocking the epitopes responsible for binding and/or fusion of gp120 or gp41 viral proteins to the target cell. Antibody-dependent cellular cytotoxicity (ADCC) is another host antiviral response that targets specific HIV epitopes for destruction by interactions of antibody-coated infected cells with effector cells such as natural killer (NK) cells or macrophages. In contrast, antibody-dependent enhancement (ADE) can potentiate HIV infection through complement or Fc receptors. A decreased concentration of inhibitors of complement in infected individuals suggests that the antibody-independent complement cascade pathway can be activated to lyse either the virus or the virus-infected cell. This and other innate immune responses may play a role in controlling HIV infection.

A. Natural Killer Cells

Another component of the innate immune system, natural killer cells, can directly eliminate virus-infected cells. The cytotoxic mechanism is not MHC-dependent and potentially involves ADCC. In individuals progressing to disease, a loss in NK cell number and function, partly reflecting direct infection of these cells by HIV, alters the production of proinflammatory cytokines such as interferon-γ. A decrease in interferon-γ production can also interfere with CD8$^+$ cell function.

B. CD4$^+$ Lymphocytes

The CD4$^+$cell number and proliferative responses are dramatically reduced during disease progression. Dysfunctional T helper cells and a loss of CD4$^+$ cells are characteristically observed during infection. Pronounced deficits in CD4$^+$ cell function are manifested by a decreased proliferative response first to recall antigens, then alloantigens, and, in later stages, mitogenic stimulation. Lower levels of IL-2 production in addition to decreased IL-2 receptor expression are observed with progression to disease. Generally, CD4$^+$ T helper cells produce higher levels of type 2 cytokines (IL-4, IL-5, IL-13) than type 1 cytokines (e.g., IL-2) during the course of symptomatic infection.

C. CD8$^+$ Lymphocytes

Unlike NK cells, CD8$^+$ cells with cytotoxic function require MHC restriction and are antigen-specific. These cytotoxic T lymphocytes (CTL) eliminate virus-infected cells through perforin or Fas/FasL-mediated pathways. CD8$^+$ T lymphocytes are critical for controlling the dissemination of HIV in stages early in infection and before the appearance of antibodies. Importantly, an increase of CD8$^+$ cells is observed during the asymptomatic stage of the infection, reflecting a response to infection as well as a compensatory reaction to the loss of CD4$^+$ T helper cells.

Both transient and long-lived CTL populations specific for viral proteins, Env, Nef, RT, and Gag gene products are found *in vivo*. However, during the progression to disease, a decrease in the frequency of HIV-specific CTLs has been observed along with a decline in cytotoxic responses. Proposed mechanisms for the loss of function include the generation of viral mutants that escape CTL recognition, downregulation of MHC I molecules (potentially through viral *tat* or *nef* gene products), and decreased T helper cell function.

CD8$^+$ cells can also exhibit noncytotoxic, non-MHC-dependent anti-HIV activity. This CD8$^+$ cell noncytotoxic antiviral response (CNAR), which acts on all strains of HIV-1 and HIV-2, is mediated at least in part by a factor secreted by CD8$^+$ cells. This CD8$^+$ cell antiviral factor (CAF) decreases HIV replication in CD4$^+$ cells and in macrophages by acting on the HIV LTR to block virus transcription. Lower levels of viral RNA and protein are observed in infected cells exposed to CAF. The activity of CAF is distinct from chemokines and other known cytokines; its identity remains unknown. CNAR activity correlates directly with a healthy clinical state; CD8$^+$ cells from asymptomatic individuals exhibit a greater capacity to suppress HIV replication than individuals progressing to disease. People infected for more than 10 years who are healthy and without therapy have a strong CNAR. Thus, this host immune response appears to be very important in controlling HIV infection.

D. Dendritic Cells

As dendritic cells and other antigen-presenting cells (APC) migrate in the peripheral blood and line mucosal surfaces, they are necessary, after interacting with infectious virus, for triggering subsets of effector cells. The replication of virus in these cell types is relatively low and stable and therefore they can remain for long periods of time as reservoirs releasing virus in the body. Because certain dendritic cells are believed to harbor virus, they can readily transfer HIV to T lymphocytes and contribute to the loss of CD4$^+$ cells. Many of the functions of APCs, including presentation capabilities and cytokine regulation for the differentiation, survival, and maintenance of memory and naive T cells, are compromised in HIV-infected individuals. Because dendritic cells are among the first cell subset to encounter infectious HIV and are capable of modulating a broad range of lymphocyte functions, a further understanding of their role in HIV pathogenesis is of particular importance.

VII. CONCLUSIONS

Current therapeutic approaches to block HIV replication involve targeting the viral enzymes reverse transcriptase and protease. These treatments have decreased plasma viral loads dramatically and increased the life expectancy for symptomatic individuals infected with HIV. Nevertheless, after about 4–5 years of treatment, many infected individuals develop resistance to the antiviral drugs, allowing the emergence of viruses that are difficult to control with current treatment. Also, because HIV infection often leads to the development of B-cell lymphomas and several central nervous system disorders, the extended life expectancies as a result of therapeutics could increase the prevalence of HIV-associated cancers and neuropathies.

Innovative approaches at enhancing antiviral immunologic responses can offer advantages to individuals infected with HIV, as the immune system can recognize a variety of viral subtypes and control infection in many different tissues of the body (e.g., bowel, brain). Further efforts to develop immune-modulating therapies that will enhance the cellular immune response of HIV (particularly CD8$^+$ cells) should provide promising approaches for long-term control of the infection.

The development of vaccines using antigenic components of HIV delivered through a variety of different modalities and with different adjuvants will be necessary for the prevention of infection. Because HIV can be transmitted by infected cells as well as by free virus, approaches for blocking an incoming infected cell raise a major challenge to the development of an effective vaccine. By studying the molecular, cellular, and biochemical pathways involved in HIV replication and the effective immune responses that can control the virus, particularly in long-term survivors, optimal therapies and strategies for the prevention of HIV and AIDS can be developed.

See Also the Following Articles

HUMAN T-CELL LEUKEMIA/LYMPHOTROPIC VIRUS • NEOPLASMS IN ACQUIRED IMMUNODEFICIENCY SYNDROME • RETROVIRUSES • T CELLS, FUNCTION OF

Bibliography

Banchereau, J., Briere, F., Caux, C., Davoust, J., Lebecque, S., Liu, Y.-J., Pulendran, B., and Palucka, K. (2000). Immunobiology of dendritic cells. *Annu. Rev. Immunol.* **18,** 767–811.

Barre-Sinoussi, F., Chermann, J.-C., Rey, F., Nugeyre, M. T., Chamaret, S., Gruest, J., Dauguet, C., Axler-Blin, C., Vezinet-Brun, F., Rouzioux, C., Rozenbaum, W., and Montagnier, L. (1983). Isolation of a T-lymphotropic retrovirus from a patient at risk for acquired immune deficiency syndrome (AIDS). *Science* **220,** 868–871.

Berger, E. A., Murphy, P. M., and Farber, J. M. (1999). Chemokine receptors as HIV-1 coreceptors: Roles in viral entry, tropism, and disease. *Ann. Rev. Immunol.* **17,** 657–700.

Cheng-Mayer, C., Seto, D., Tateno, M., and Levy, J. A, (1988). Biologic features of HIV that correlate with virulence in the host. *Science* **240,** 80–82.

Clerici, M., Stocks, N. I., Zajac, R. A. Boswell, R. N., Lucey, D. R., Via, C. S., and Shearer, G. M. (1989). Detection of three distinct patterns of T helper cell dysfunction in asymptomatic, human immunodeficiency virus-positive patients; Independence of CD4^1 cell numbers and clinical staging. *J. Clin. Invest.* **84,** 1892–1899.

Deacon, N. J., Tsykin, A., Solomon, A, Smith, K., Ludford-Menting, M., Hooker, D. J., McPhee, D. A., Greenway, A. L., Ellett, A., Chatfield, C., Lawson, V. A., Crowe, S., Merz, A., Sonza, S., Learmont, J., Sullivan, J. S., Cunningham, A., Dwyer, D., Dowton, and Mills, J. (1995). Genomic structure of an attenuated quasi species of HIV-1 from a blood tranfusion donor and recipients. *Science* **270,** 988–991.

Frankel, A. D., and Young, J. A. (1998). HIV-1: Fifteen proteins and an RNA. *Annu. Rev. Biochem.* **67,** 1–25.

Gupta, S. (1996). "Immunology of HIV Infection." Plenum Press, New York.

Harouse, J. M., Bhat, S., Spitalnik, S. L., Laughlin, M., Stefano, K., Silberber, D. H., and Gonzalez-Scarano, F. (1991). Inhibition of entry of HIV-1 in neural cell lines by antibodies against galactosyl ceramide. *Science* **253,** 320–323.

Homsy, J., Meyer, M., Tateno, M., Clarkson, S., and Levy J. A. (1989). The Fc and not the CD4 receptor mediates antibody enhancement of HIV infection in human cells. *Science* **244,** 1357–1360.

Jones, K. A., and Peterlin, B. M. (1994). Control of RNA initiation and elongation at the HIV-1 promoter. *Annu. Rev. Biochem.* **63,** 717–743.

Levy, J. A. (1998). "HIV and the Pathogenesis of AIDS," 2nd Ed. American Society of Microbiology, Washington, DC.

Levy, J. A., Hoffman, A. D., Kramer, S. M., Landis, J. A., Shimabukuro, J. M., and Oshiro, L. S. (1984). Isolation of lymphocytopathic retroviruses from San Francisco patients with AIDS. *Science* **225,** 840–842.

Levy, J. A., Mackewicz, C. E., and Barker, E. (1996). Controlling HIV pathogenesis: The role of noncytotoxic anti-HIV activity of CD8$^+$ cells. *Immunol. Today* **17,** 217–224.

Montagnier, L., Chermann, J., Barre-Sinoussi, F., Chamaret, S., Gruest, J., Nugeyre, M. T., Rey, F., Dauguet, C., Axler-Blin, C., Vezinet-Brun, F., Rouzioux, C., Saimot, A. G., Rozenbaum, W., Gluckman, J. C., Klatzmann, D., Vilmer, E., Griselli, C., Gazengel, C., and Brunet, J. B. (1984). A new human T-lymphotropic retrovirus: Characterization and possible role in lymphadenopathy and acquired immune deficiency syndromes. *In* "Human T-Cell Leukemia/Lymphoma Virus" (R. C. Gallo, M. E. Essex, and L. Gross, eds.), pp. 363–379. Cold Spring Harbor Laboratory, Cold Spring Harbor, NY.

Robinson, W. E., Jr., and Mitchell, W. M. (1990). Neutralization and enhancement of *in vitro* and *in vivo* HIV and simian immunodeficiency virus infections. *AIDS* **4,** S151–S162.

Starcich, B. R., Hahn, B. H., Shaw, G. M., McNeely, R. D., Morrow, S., Wolf, H., Parks, E. S., Parks, W. P., Josephs, S. F., and Gallo, R. C. (1986). Identification and characterization of conserved and variable regions in the envelope gene of *HTLV-III/LAV, the retrovirus of AIDS. Cell* **45,** 637–648.

Werner, A., and Levy, J. A. (1993). Human immunodeficiency virus type 1 envelope gp120 is cleaved after incubation with recombinant soluble CD4. *J. Virol.* **67,** 2566–2574.

Hormonal Carcinogenesis

James D. Shull
University of Nebraska Medical Center

GLOSSARY

allele One form of a gene for which different forms exist in a population.

allelic variant One of two or more forms of a specific gene existing within a population.

cytochrome P450 A large family of enzymes that catalyze oxidation/reduction reactions on a wide variety of endogenous and exogenous substrates.

genetic modifier A gene that through the actions of its protein product alters cancer risk in a quantifiable manner.

genotoxic DNA damage or mutagenesis.

inbred strain A mouse or rat strain in which genetic variation is eliminated through multiple generations of stringent inbreeding.

low penetrance A gene for which a specific allelic variant does not uniformly confer the specific phenotype.

polymorphism Genetic variability within a population.

xenoestrogens Exogenous chemicals that can bind to the estrogen receptor and mimic the actions of estrogens.

The endocrine system and its numerous hormones function to integrate genetically encoded developmental programs and environmental signals and regulate the myriad biochemical processes, such as cell proliferation, differentiation, and death, required to maintain homeostasis within boundaries compatible with life. It is becoming increasingly clear that aberrations in the control of these hormone-regulated processes contribute to the genesis of many forms of cancer. In specific instances, hormones also appear to act through nonreceptor-mediated mechanisms to contribute to carcinogenesis. Steroid hormones, in particular, are implicated in the etiology of cancers of the breast, female reproductive tract, and male reproductive tract, as well as benign tumors of the anterior pituitary gland. Both endogenous and exogenous steroid hormones appear to contribute to carcinogenesis. In addition, much effort is being focused on defining the potential of environmental chemicals, both naturally occurring and man made, to enhance or inhibit carcinogenesis via hormonal mimicry. This article summarizes our current knowledge of hormonal carcinogenesis, focusing on cancers of the breast and other tissues where hormones play primary, if not causative, roles in cancer etiology.

I. BREAST CANCER

A. Endogenous Estrogens, Progestins, and Breast Cancer Etiology

It is well documented that estrogens and progestins act through direct and indirect pathways to stimulate development of the breast at puberty and during pregnancy. In addition, the breast epithelium exhibits a cyclical pattern of cell proliferation and death throughout each menstrual cycle; cell proliferation is highest during the luteal phase of the menstrual cycle, when circulating estradiol is submaximally elevated and circulating progesterone is at its peak. Data from the study of mouse models in which the genes encoding either estrogen receptor (ER) α or progesterone receptor (PR) are disrupted through insertional mutagenesis indicate that ERα and PR are required for the growth-promoting actions of estrogens and progestins within the mammary epithelium.

The report of Cooper in 1836 that breast cancers regress in size at the beginning of each menstrual cycle and at menopause and the report of Beatson in 1896 that oophorectomy leads to regression of breast cancers are now recognized as providing the first demonstrated links between ovarian hormones and breast cancer. Subsequent epidemiologic and laboratory studies provide overwhelming evidence inextricably linking ovarian steroids to the genesis of breast cancer. Both early menarche and late onset of menopause are associated with an increased risk of breast cancer. Moreover, oophorectomy prior to menopause significantly reduces breast cancer risk, with the greatest reduction in risk being observed in women 35 years of age or younger. Several, but not all, studies have demonstrated a positive correlation between the level of circulating estrogens in postmenopausal women and breast cancer risk. Clinical trials have demonstrated that tamoxifen, a selective estrogen receptor modulator (SERM), reduces the risk of breast cancer in asymptomatic women at high risk of developing the disease. In addition, inhibitors of aromatase, the enzyme that catalyzes the production of estrogens from androgen precursors, are gaining use in the treatment of breast cancer and may provide additional effective agents for the prevention of these cancers. Together, these data indicate that lifetime exposure to endogenous ovarian hormones is directly correlated with breast cancer risk and demonstrate that these hormones, particularly the estrogens, play an important, if not causative, role in breast cancer development.

Several epidemiologic studies have attempted to identify associations between specific allelic variants of genes that encode enzymes involved in estrogen metabolism and breast cancer risk. The hypothesis being tested in these studies is that genes with variant alleles that impact expression and/or function of the encoded protein may be low penetrance, but high frequency, modifiers of breast cancer risk. Cytochrome P450c17 (CYP17) catalyzes two steps in the pathway leading to sex steroid biosynthesis. A variant allele encoding CYP17 has been identified that is associated with increased levels of circulating estradiol and progesterone. This variant *CYP17* allele has been associated with increased breast cancer risk in some, but not other, studies. Cytochrome P4501A1 (CYP1A1) catalyzes the hydroxylation of a variety of substrates, including polycyclic aromatic hydrocarbons and the estrogens, 17β-estradiol (E2) and estrone (E1). Variant alleles of *CYP1A1* have been identified that may differ in activity and/or inducibility. The m1 variant, which exhibits a single nucleotide polymorphism in the 3'-untranslated region, has been associated with an increased breast cancer risk in African-American and Chinese women. However, no risk modification was associated with the m1 allele in other studies. The m2 variant, a single nucleotide polymorphism that results in a single amino acid change, Ile462Val, in the heme-binding domain, did not significantly modify breast cancer risk in the general population, but was associated with an increased risk in specific subsets of smokers. Estrogens are also substrates for cytochrome P4501B1, which catalyzes the hydroxylation of E2 and E1 preferentially on C-4 of the aromatic A ring.

Two single nucleotide polymorphisms have been identified that impact amino acid sequence in the heme-binding domain of CYP1B1: m1, Val432Leu; and m2, Asn453Ser. Neither the m1 nor the m2 variant was observed to impact significantly breast cancer risk in Caucasian or African-American populations. However, homozygosity for the m1 allelic variant of *CYP1B1* was associated with an increased breast cancer risk in a Chinese population. Catechol-*O*-methyltransferase (COMT) catalyzes the methylation of various catechols, including the 2-hydroxylated and 4-hydroxylated metabolites of E2 and E1. A single nucleotide polymorphism in exon 4 of *COMT* results in an amino acid change, Val158Met, that reduces COMT activity. Two studies have associated homozygosity for the low-activity *COMT* allele with an increased breast cancer risk in postmenopausal, but not premenopausal, women; another study demonstrated an association between the low-activity *COMT* allele and increased breast cancer risk in premenopausal, but not postmenopausal, women; and yet another study did not associate the *COMT* genotype to breast cancer risk. The failure of these genetic epidemiology studies to produce consensus regarding the associations of variant alleles for genes encoding these different enzymes in the etiology of breast cancer most probably results from several factors, including (1) het-erogeneity within or between the populations studied; (2) gene–gene and gene–environment interactions that occlude modifier effects; and (3) modest population sizes in several of the studies. Additional studies will be required to establish firmly whether these genes act as low penetrance modifiers of breast cancer risk. In addition, it must ultimately be demonstrated that any associations between genotype at a particular genetic locus and cancer risk result from loss or gain of function of the gene residing at that locus or the protein encoded by that gene.

B. Exogenous Estrogens, Progestins, and Breast Cancer Etiology

Exogenous hormones also modify breast cancer risk. Several studies indicate that current or recent use of estrogen replacement therapies (estrogen alone) or hormone replacement therapies (estrogen and progestin) by menopausal women is associated with an increased breast cancer risk. The increase in breast cancer is greatest in women using regimens containing both estrogen and progestin. Breast cancer risk also appears to be slightly increased by the current use of oral contraceptives. Finally, use of the synthetic estrogen, diethylstilbestrol (DES), during pregnancy is associated with an increased breast cancer risk.

C. Estrogen Receptor and Breast Cancer Etiology

The ER, in particular ERα, is central to estrogen action in the breast. Much effort has been invested toward the identification of mutations and polymorphisms in the gene encoding ERα and attempts to correlate these genetic differences with breast cancer risk, pathology, ER status, or responsiveness to hormonal therapy. Although mutant forms of the ER have been identified that differ from the wild-type receptor in ligand-binding and/or transcriptional activation activity, little evidence exists to suggest that somatic mutations in the ER play a major role in breast cancer etiology. However, loss of ER expression does often occur during progression from a hormone-dependent to a hormone-independent stage. Specific ERα polymorphisms have been associated with an increased breast cancer risk in two of four published studies, suggesting that variant forms of ERα may act as low penetrance modifiers of breast cancer risk.

D. Potential Mechanisms of Hormonal Carcinogenesis in the Breast

It is well established that estrogens and progestins interact in the regulation of cell proliferation and cell survival in the breast. By stimulating cell proliferation and/or enhancing cell survival within the breast epithelium, ovarian steroids may increase the probability of somatic mutations, as well as enhance the growth and/or survival of transformed cells. These mutations could arise through the actions of environmental or endogenous mutagens, exposure to ionizing radiation, or replication errors during DNA synthesis. Mammographic density correlates with the proportion of the breast volume composed of the epithelial and stromal parenchyma as well as with breast cancer risk. Use of estrogens with progestins in menopausal hormone replacement regimens is associated with increased mammographic density, an increased rate of cell proliferation within the breast epithelium, and an increased risk of breast cancer. Moreover, the observation that the SERM tamoxifen significantly reduces breast cancer incidence in women at increased risk indicates that ER-mediated pathways play important roles in breast cancer etiology. Together, these studies strongly link the actions of ovarian steroids in the regulation of cell proliferation and/or survival in the breast epithelium to the genesis of breast cancer. At this time, the mechanisms through which ovarian hormones regulate proliferation and survival within the breast epithelium are not completely understood. Both estrogens and progestins induce expression of cyclin D1 in breast epithelial cells and may thereby directly stimulate progression of those cells through the G1 phase of the cell cycle. In addition, estrogens regulate the production of several growth factors, which in turn act through autocrine and/or paracrine mechanisms to stimulate cell cycle progression and/or enhance cell survival within the breast epithelium. It is becoming increasing clear that interactions between stromal and epithelial cells are required for normal development and function of the breast and that the estrogens and progestins act through the stroma to exert some of their stimulatory effects on the breast epithelium.

It is hypothesized that specific estrogen metabolites may be genotoxic carcinogens that contribute to the development of breast cancers and other cancers by inducing mutations in oncogenes and/or tumor suppressor genes. An often proposed mechanism of estrogen carcinogenesis is that E2 and/or E1 is hydroxylated at either the C-2 or the C-4 position to the corresponding catechol estrogen, which is subsequently oxidized through a semiquinone intermediate to the estrogen quinone, which could bind covalently to DNA. Alternatively, the catechol estrogen and/or estrogen semiquinone may undergo redox cycling and generate superoxide radicals, which could damage DNA. An enzyme(s) capable of generating the catechol estrogens 4-hydroxyestradiol and 4-hydroxyestrone is expressed in human breast cancers, and CYP1B1 has been identified as an estrogen-4-hydroxylase expressed in the MCF-7 breast cancer cell line. However, the carcinogenicity of catechol estrogens in the rodent mammary gland has yet to be established,

and estrone-3,4-quinone did not induce mammary cancers when injected directly into the mammary gland of female rats. In addition, several studies have demonstrated that estrogens and catechol estrogens lack mutagenic activity in standardized bacterial and mammalian cell assays. Therefore, the contribution of potentially genotoxic estrogen metabolites to the etiology of breast cancer remains to be defined.

Treatment of a mouse mammary epithelial cell line with 16α-hydroxyestrone induces anchorage-independent growth, suggesting that this estrogen metabolite has the potential to induce neoplastic transformation in this mammary cell model. The ability of estrogens and estrogen metabolites to induce neoplastic transformation in vitro has been extensively studied by T. Tsutsui and J.C. Barrett using Syrian hamster embryo cells. Transformation of Syrian hamster embryo cells is associated with the induction of aneuploidy, which may result from binding of estrogens or specific estrogen metabolites to β-tubulin and disruption of microtubule assembly during mitosis. More recently, the transforming potential of different metabolites of E2, including the 2-hydroxy and 4-hydroxy catechols of E2 and E1, as well as 16α-hydroxyestrone, in Syrian hamster embryo cells has been associated with the induction of mutations, chromosomal aberrations, and/or aneuploidy.

In summary, estrogens and progestins most probably act through multiple mechanisms to induce and/or promote the development of breast cancers (Fig. 1). Pathways dependent on the ER are clearly implicated by the ability of tamoxifen to reduce breast cancer incidence in women at increased risk. It is also clear that the actions of these hormones in regulating cell proliferation and survival within the breast epithelium contribute to the genesis of breast cancers. Data are emerging to suggest that genes encoding enzymes involved in steroid hormone metabolism may be low penetrance modifiers of breast cancer risk. In this regard, breast cancer risk could be impacted by genetic variation in (1) the amounts of active hormones produced; (2) the specific types of hormones or metabolites produced; (3) the timing of hormone production; and/or (4) the location of hormone production. Estrogens may be metabolized to genotoxic forms that can bind to DNA and induce mutations. Alternatively, estrogens may induce aneuploidy or other forms of genomic instability. Additional studies in validated

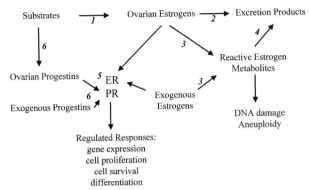

FIGURE 1 Possible pathways of hormonal carcinogenesis in the breast. Genetic variation in genes encoding enzymes involved in estrogen biosynthesis (1) or estrogen excretion (2) may impact the type or amount of steroidal estrogens acting on target cells. Endogenous and exogenous estrogens may be metabolized to reactive forms that can bind macromolecules, including DNA, and proteins such as tubulin (3). Genetic variation in genes encoding specific detoxifying enzymes may impact the clearance of potentially genotoxic estrogen metabolites (4). Genetic variation in the genes encoding ERα or ERβ may impact the binding of estrogens to its receptor, receptor levels, or receptor signaling. (5) Although not as intensely studied, genetic variability in progesterone metabolism or signaling may also contribute to breast cancer etiology.

animal models are required to define precisely the mechanisms through which hormones contribute to breast cancer etiology.

E. Animal Models of Estrogen-Induced Mammary Cancer

The first demonstration that estrogens induce mammary cancers in rodents was by Lacassagne in the 1930s. However, rodent models of estrogen-induced mammary carcinogenesis did not achieve the same degree of prominence in the research community as animal models in which mammary cancers are induced by carcinogens, such as dimethylbenz[a]anthracene (DMBA) or N-methyl-N-nitrosourea (MNU). Studies suggest that rat models of estrogen-induced mammary carcinogenesis can provide novel and physiologically relevant insights into the role of estrogens and other hormones in the etiology of breast cancer.

1. ACI Rat as a Model of Estrogen-Induced Mammary Cancer

The ACI rat was developed by Dunning and colleagues in 1926 from a cross between the August and the Copenhagen (COP) rat strains. Although these investigators first demonstrated the ability of DES to induce mammary cancers in the ACI rat in 1947, this model was used only sporadically over the next 50 years.

Data from our laboratory indicate that the female ACI rat exhibits a unique propensity to develop mammary cancers when treated continuously with physiologic levels of E2, released from subcutaneous Silastic tubing implants. Palpable mammary cancers begin to appear as early as 70 days following the initiation of E2 treatment, median latency is approximately 140 days, and virtually 100% of the treated animals exhibit palpable cancers within 210 days of treatment. Ovariectomy significantly inhibits the development of E2-induced mammary cancers, suggesting a requirement for another ovarian factor(s), possibly progesterone, in E2-induced mammary carcinogenesis. Focal regions of atypical epithelial hyperplasia are common in the mammary glands of E2-treated ACI rats, and these are probable precursors to carcinoma (Fig. 2). Relative to the surrounding mammary epithelium, cells within the focal regions of atypical hyperplasia and the mammary cancers exhibit an increased expression of progesterone receptor (PR). Carcinomas induced in ACI rats by E2 are estrogen dependent and commonly exhibit aneuploidy, two features that are common to breast cancers in humans.

Relative to the ACI rat strain, females of the COP strain, which is closely related genetically to ACI, and the Brown Norway (BN) strain, which is unrelated, are much less susceptible to E2-induced mammary cancers (Table I). These strain differences provide an avenue toward elucidation of the mechanisms through which estrogens induce mammary cancer development. For example, we have demonstrated that the proliferative response of the ACI mammary epithelium to E2 significantly exceeds that of the COP mammary epithelium, suggesting one possible mechanism for the differing susceptibilities of these rat strains to E2-induced mammary cancers. Genetic studies from our laboratory indicate that the highly susceptible ACI phenotype behaves as an incompletely dominant trait in crosses to either of the resistant COP or BN strains. Although most of the E2-treated ACI/COP F1 and ACI/BN F1 progeny develop mammary cancers when treated with E2, latency is significantly delayed relative to that observed in the parental ACI strain. We have mapped genetic

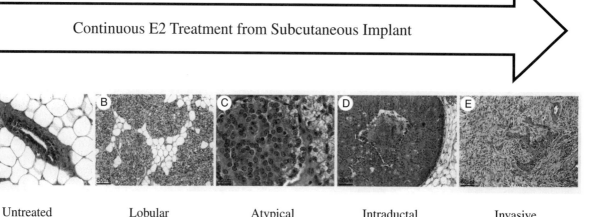

Continuous E2 Treatment from Subcutaneous Implant

| Untreated | Lobular | Atypical | Intraductal | Invasive |
| Ovary-Intact | Hyperplasia | Hyperplasia | Carcinoma | Carcinoma |

FIGURE 2 Histologic progression of estrogen-induced mammary carcinogenesis in the ACI rat. (A) The mammary gland of the ovary-intact, virgin female ACI rat is composed of ductal structures extending throughout the mammary fat pad. (B) Continuous treatment with E2 rapidly induces marked lobular development and hyperplasia. (C) Focal regions of atypical hyperplasia begin to appear within the hyperplastic epithelium following approximately 8 weeks of E2 treatment. (D) Palpable mammary carcinomas appear as early as 10 weeks following the initiation of E2 treatment, but the median latency to the appearance of the first palpable mammary carcinoma is 20 weeks. (E) Invasive features are observed in a fraction of the E2-induced mammary carcinomas.

modifiers of susceptibility to E2-induced mammary cancers to rat chromosome 5 in reciprocal crosses between ACI and COP rat strains and to chromosomes 5, 18, and 2 in a cross between ACI and BN strains. The gene encoding Cdkn2a is a candidate for the modifier residing on chromosome 5. Cdkn2a is an inhibitor of the cyclin D-dependent kinase Cdk4 and Cdk6 and would therefore be expected to inhibit the mitogenic actions of estrogens exerted through the cyclin D/Cdk/retinoblastoma pathway. We have demonstrated that the expression of Cdkn2a is markedly downregulated in both the focal regions of atypical hyperplasia and the mammary cancers in-

duced in ACI rats by E2, relative to the surrounding epithelium. We anticipate that the ultimate identification of the genetic modifiers of susceptibility to E2-induced mammary cancers in this rat model will reveal significant information regarding the mechanisms through which estrogens contribute to breast cancer in humans. These data strongly suggest that the ACI rat provides a unique and physiologically relevant animal model for investigating the mechanisms of estrogen-induced mammary carcinogenesis, as well as for studying interactions among hormonal, genetic, and environmental determinants of breast cancer susceptibility.

2. Noble Rat as Model of Estrogen/Androgen-Induced Mammary Cancer

The Noble (NBL) rat is another unique model for hormone-induced mammary carcinogenesis. Noble first demonstrated the ability of E1 to induce mammary cancers in males and females of this rat strain in 1940. In a subsequent study, Noble demonstrated that the susceptibility of the NBL rat to E1-induced mammary cancers declined markedly as a function of the age at which treatment was initiated. Whereas 100%

TABLE I

Unique Susceptibility of the Female ACI Rat to Estrogen-Induced Mammary Carcinogenesis[a]

Rat strain	Mean latency (days)	Incidence (%)	Palpable tumors/rat
ACI	141	100	3.9
COP	208	44	0.4
BN	369	20	0.2

[a]Silastic tubing implants containing 17β-estradiol were inserted subcutaneously when ovary intact rats of the indicated inbred rat strains were 9 weeks of age.

of the E1- treated NBL rats developed mammary carcinoma when treatment was initiated at 2 weeks of age, less than 10% of animals treated at 9 weeks of age were tumor positive following 13 months of E1 treatment. More recently, the combination of E2 and testosterone propionate has been demonstrated by S.A. Li and colleagues to induce a high incidence of mammary cancers in male NBL rats, whereas mammary cancers did not develop in the same time period in rats treated with E2 or testosterone propionate alone. Similarly, studies by Y. C. Wong and colleagues indicate that E2 benzoate plus testosterone propionate induces a high incidence of mammary cancers in female NBL rats. These studies, in conjunction with those on the ACI rat summarized earlier, suggest that the NBL is less sensitive to mammary cancer induction by E2 or E2 benzoate relative to ACI rats treated with E2. Moreover, the requisite for coadministration of androgen and estrogen for rapid development of mammary cancers in the NBL rat may illustrate a fundamental mechanistic difference between the NBL and ACI models of E2-induced mammary carcinogenesis. Therefore, each of these inbred rat strains may ultimately reveal different insights into the mechanisms of hormonal carcinogenesis in the mammary gland.

II. CANCERS OF THE FEMALE REPRODUCTIVE TRACT

A. Endometrial Cancer

Estrogens stimulate cell proliferation within the uterine endometrium, and most cell proliferation in this tissue occurs during the follicular phase of the menstrual cycle, when circulating estrogens are increasing. An increased risk of endometrial cancer is associated with late menopause and obesity, both of which are generally believed to result in prolonged exposure of the uterus to estrogens. Use of combination oral contraceptives decreases the risk of endometrial cancer, whereas use of sequential oral contraceptive formulations is associated with an increased risk. Estrogen replacement therapy to alleviate symptoms of menopause significantly increases risk. However, hormone replacement regimens containing both estrogens and a progestin do not increase the risk of endometrial cancer. Moreover, tamoxifen exhibits agonistic properties in the uterus, and use of tamoxifen has been strongly associated with an increased risk of endometrial cancers. A recent genetic epidemiology study provides suggestive evidence that allelic variants in the gene encoding ERα may modify the risk of endometrial cancer. Together, these data strongly implicate both endogenous and exogenous estrogenic hormones in the etiology of cancers of the uterine endometrium.

In the mouse, disruption of the gene encoding ERα, but not ERβ, drastically alters normal development of the uterus and eliminates responsiveness of the uterine tissues to estrogens. Treatment of newborn CD-1 mice with DES has been shown to induce a 90% incidence of uterine adenocarcinoma by 18 months of age. Development of uterine cancers in this model requires a functional ovary. More recently, the estrogens E2 and 17α-ethinylestradiol, as well as the catechol estrogens 2-hydroxyestradiol and 4-hydroxyestradiol, have been demonstrated to induce uterine adenocarcinoma in this CD-1 mouse model. Similarly, tamoxifen has been demonstrated to induce uterine adenocarcinoma when administered to neonatal Wistar rats. Data from these rodent models strongly suggest that estrogens play a direct role in inducing endometrial cancers and are consistent with the hypothesis that estrogens act through a genotoxic mechanism in the neonatal uterus to initiate carcinogenesis. Alternatively, the administered estrogens may act through an ER-mediated mechanism to trigger developmental changes in the neonatal uterine epithelium and/or stroma that predispose to adenocarcinoma in the adult animals.

B. Cervical and Vaginal Cancers

The synthetic estrogen DES has been inextricably linked to clear cell carcinoma of the cervix/vagina of young women who were exposed *in utero* when their mothers were treated with DES during the first trimester of pregnancy. This carcinogenic action appears to be quite specific because cancers at other sites are not significantly increased in women exposed to DES *in utero*. An association between exogenous estrogens and cervical cancers in mice has been demonstrated. For example, DES, administered prenatally or neonatally, induces vaginal adenocarcinoma in CD-1 mice. Endogenous ovarian steroid hormones, oral contraceptives, and hormone replacement regimens are not generally believed to be strong determinants of cervical cancer risk.

C. Myometrial Tumors and Cancers

Uterine leiomyoma is the most commonly observed uterine tumor in premenopausal women. Ovarian steroids have been linked to the genesis of these benign uterine tumors as well as to the development of malignant uterine leiomyosarcomas. Leiomyoma and, less frequently, leiomyosarcoma develop spontaneously in the Eker rat. Development of these tumors is markedly inhibited by ovariectomy or treatment with SERMs. Continuous treatment with E2 induces leiomyoma in guinea pigs. Ovariectomy increases the incidence of leiomyoma in this animal model and decreases the latency to tumor appearance. Tumor regression occurs in response to cessation of E2 treatment or treatment with the SERM raloxifene. Finally, treatment of Syrian hamsters with the combination of DES and testosterone propionate has been reported to induce uterine leiomyosarcoma. Together, these epidemiologic and laboratory studies indicate a role of estrogens in the development of tumors of the uterine myometrium.

III. PROSTATE CANCER

Abundant data link androgenic hormones to the etiology of prostate cancer. Orchiectomy leads to involution of the prostate and is recognized as an effective therapeutic regimen for the treatment of prostate cancers. Prospective studies have not demonstrated strong correlations between prostate cancer risk and circulating levels of testosterone, dihydrotestosterone, androstenedione, and several other androgenic hormones. However, several studies have demonstrated that variant alleles of the gene encoding the androgen receptor (AR) may modify prostate cancer risk. The *AR* gene contains within exon 1 a polymorphic CAG repeat that encodes a variable length glutamine tract that appears to impact the ability of the AR to activate gene transcription. Prostate cancer risk ap-

pears to be inversely correlated with the number of CAG repeats in the *AR*. A polymorphic GGC repeat in exon 1 of *AR*, encoding a variable length glycine tract, may also modify prostate cancer risk.

Evidence is emerging to suggest that genes encoding enzymes involved in androgen biosynthesis or catabolism may also modify prostate cancer risk. The enzyme 5α-reductase type 2 (SRD5A2) catalyzes the conversion of testosterone to the more active dihydrotestosterone, and the gene encoding this enzyme, *SRD5A2*, is expressed exclusively in the prostate. Finasteride, an inhibitor of SRD5A2, is currently being evaluated in a large cooperative trial for its ability to prevent prostate cancer. A variant *SRD5A2* allele, which encodes threonine in place of alanine at codon 49 (Ala49Thr), is associated with a significantly increased risk of prostate cancer in African-American and Hispanic men. In addition, the Ala49Thr variant is associated with a more aggressive disease phenotype and poorer prognosis relative to the wild-type allele. Interestingly, the Ala49Thr variant of *SRD5A2* encodes an enzyme with an increased capacity to produce dihydrotestosterone relative to the wild-type allele. Two other *SRD5A2* allelic variants, Val89Leu and a polymorphic dinucleotide repeat in the 3'-untranslated region, do not appear to significantly impact androgen metabolism or prostate cancer risk. As discussed in Section IA, CYP17 catalyzes two reactions in the biosynthetic pathway leading to androgens and estrogens. Data on *CYP17* as a modifier of prostate cancer risk are inconsistent, with two studies associating the A2 allelic variant of *CYP17* with an increased risk of prostate cancer and two studies associating the A1 allele with increased risk.

Epidemiologic studies associate vitamin D deficiency with prostate cancer, and numerous laboratory studies indicate a role of the hormonally active form of vitamin D, 1,25-dihydroxyvitamin D_3, in the regulation of proliferation and survival of prostate cancer cell lines. 1,25-Dihydroxyvitamin D_3 functions through a receptor that is a member of the nuclear receptor superfamily. Several allelic variants of the vitamin D receptor have been identified, and studies suggest that these variants may be associated with an altered prostate cancer risk. Although not all of these studies concur with regard to the associations between specific polymorphisms and risk, together they suggest that the gene encoding the vitamin D receptor may act as a low penetrance modifier of prostate cancer development.

Noble was the first to report that continuous treatment with either testosterone or testosterone in combination with estrogen induces the development of prostate cancers in the NBL rat. A series of studies by S.-M. Ho and colleagues indicates that treatment of intact NBL rats with testosterone and E2 for 16 weeks induces a high incidence of epithelial dysplasia in the dorsolateral lobe of the prostate. Relative to the surrounding epithelium, dysplastic lesions exhibit several changes in gene expression that may contribute to or result from their development, including increased expression of Ha-*ras* and progesterone receptor mRNAs. Induction of the dysplastic lesions is inhibited by treatment with bromocryptine, suggesting that prolactin contributes to their development. Interestingly, the location of the hormone-induced lesions within the prostate appears to be dependent on the amount and/or type of estrogen administered. For example, testosterone in combination with increased E2 induces atypical hyperplasia in the ventral lobe of the prostate. Similarly, treatment of NBL rats with testosterone plus DES induces dysplasia in the ventral prostate.

Studies by Bosland and colleagues indicate that long-term treatment of NBL rats with testosterone and E2 induces a 100% incidence of adenocarcinoma in the dorsolateral, but not ventral, prostate of the NBL rat. A DNA adduct of unknown structure was detected in the dorsolateral, but not ventral, prostate of NBL rats treated with testosterone and E2 for 16 weeks or longer. More recently, Y. C. Wong and colleagues have published a series of studies on the induction of carcinoma in the ventral prostate of the NBL rat by continuous treatment with testosterone and high-dose E2.

The mechanisms of prostate cancer induction by testosterone and estrogens are not currently known. It is clear that androgens play an important role in the regulation of cell proliferation and survival in the prostate gland of the human as well as rodent species, and it is probable that these actions contribute to the etiology of prostate cancers. For example, it is hypothesized that by stimulating proliferation within the prostate epithelium, androgens promote the development of cancers that are induced by endogenous or environmental carcinogens, possibly including genotoxic estrogen metabolites. The identification of specific mutations induced in the rat prostate as a consequence of combined testosterone and E2 treatment would provide strong support for this hypothesis. It is also hypothesized that the hormonal environment during embryonic development may contribute to the genesis of prostate cancers later in life. This hypothesis is based on data from numerous studies that indicate that prenatal exposure to naturally occurring estrogens, synthetic estrogens, or xenoestrogens impacts development of the male reproductive tract, including the prostate, in rats and mice. Each of these actions of androgenic and estrogenic hormones could contribute to prostate cancer development.

IV. PITUITARY TUMORS

Benign tumors of the anterior pituitary gland are common in humans, occurring in approximately 20–25% of individuals randomly evaluated at autopsy. Prolactin (PRL)-producing tumors, prolactinomas, represent the most common type of pituitary tumor. Estrogens have been implicated in the etiology of prolactinoma. The incidence of these tumors in females is approximately twice that of males, and several anecdotal observations link the development of prolactinoma to clinical or environmental exposures to estrogens. Supporting a role of estrogens in the etiology of prolactinoma are numerous reports that administered estrogens induce development of PRL-producing pituitary tumors in mice and rats. The literature on the role of estrogens in pituitary tumorigenesis in the human and rat has been reviewed by Spady and co-workers.

Different inbred rat strains exhibit marked differences in sensitivity to the pituitary tumor-inducing actions of estrogens. The Fischer 344 (F344) strain is the most sensitive of the inbred rat strains. Continuous treatment of male or female F344 rats with DES or E2 for 6 weeks or longer results in 10- to 20-fold increases in pituitary mass. This increase in pituitary mass results from increased proliferation and enhanced survival within the PRL-producing lactotroph population and correlates with both absolute lactotroph number and the level of PRL in the circulation. Estrogen-induced pituitary tumors are usually defined histologically as diffuse lactotroph hyperplasias, although adenomatous foci have been described in some studies. In our laboratory, we have only rarely observed a pituitary carcinoma in a rat treated continuously with estrogen for long periods of time. Although less sensitive than F344, the Wistar–Furth, ACI, NBL, and COP rat strains also develop PRL-producing pituitary tumors when treated with estrogens. In contrast, the BN rat strain is highly insensitive to the pituitary growth-promoting actions of estrogens.

The differing sensitivities of different inbred rat strains to the pituitary tumor-inducing actions of estrogens allow the underlying mechanisms to be studied using genetic techniques. The first studies of this type, by Wiklund and Gorski, indicated that the high sensitivity of the F344 strain to DES resulted from the actions of multiple, independently segregating genes. Wendell and Gorski have subsequently mapped within the rat genome the locations of several modifiers of DES-induced pituitary growth in F344 x BN intercrosses. Our laboratory has mapped additional modifiers of DES-induced pituitary growth in ACI x COP and ACI x BN intercrosses. Together, these genetic studies indicate that the actions of estrogens in the regulation of lactotroph proliferation and the survival and development of PRL-producing pituitary tumors are controlled by many genes. The ultimate goals of these genetic studies are to identify these genes and establish their functions. It is possible that at least some of these genes will impact carcinogenesis in other estrogen-responsive tissues.

V. OTHER HORMONE-INDUCED CANCERS

Numerous reports illustrate the ability of administered estrogens to induce cancers at a wide variety of tissue sites in rats, mice, hamsters, and other animal species. The incidence and type of cancers vary markedly as a function of species, genetic strain, type of estrogen used, route of estrogen administration, and timing of estrogen administration. For example, Noble described a wide variety of cancers or tumors

that develop in NBL rats in response to continuous treatment with E1. The affected tissues include the adrenal cortex, mammary gland, pituitary gland, ovary, uterus, cervix, vagina, testis, prostate, thymus, adipose, pancreas, and salivary gland, as well as lymphoid tissues. Noble recognized that dependence on estrogens for growth is a common feature of most estrogen-induced tumors.

Some studies suggest that exogenous estrogens may increase the risk of liver cancers in humans. Estrogens are potent tumor promoters in the rat liver, and the SERM tamoxifen acts as a complete carcinogen in the rat liver.

Several, but not all, estrogens induce renal cancers in orchiectomized Syrian hamsters. These cancers appear to be of epithelial origin, and their induction by estrogens is markedly suppressed by testosterone, progesterone, and SERMs. Continuous estrogen treatment is associated with histologically evident cytotoxicity and compensatory regeneration in the hamster kidney. It has been suggested that these actions contribute significantly to estrogen-induced renal carcinogenesis. A role of potentially genotoxic estrogen metabolites has also been suggested to initiate the development of kidney cancers in this animal model.

VI. CONCLUDING REMARKS

Based on a wealth of data from epidemiologic and laboratory studies, steroid hormones can be considered to be the cause of at least a subset of specific cancers in humans. The evidence that endogenous hormones cause cancer is most compelling for cancers of the breast and prostate. Consequently, strategies based on blocking the actions of estrogens and androgens are currently being used or are being evaluated for the prevention of cancers of the breast and prostate, respectively. Exogenous hormones contribute significantly to the etiology of cancers of the breast, uterine endometrium, and uterine cervix. Despite many years of intense study, the mechanisms through which these hormones exert their carcinogenic actions are not well defined. Possible contributory mechanisms include, but are not limited to the (1) stimulation of cell proliferation; (2) inhibition of apoptosis; (3) alteration of hormonally regulated developmental programs; (4) genotoxic actions of specific hormone metabolites; and (5) abrogation of genome stability. It is probable that multiple and/or different mechanisms contribute to the genesis of different cancer types and that genetic background impacts on these mechanisms.

Currently existing animal models of hormone-induced cancers should continue to serve as valuable tools for elucidating the mechanisms of hormonal carcinogenesis, and additional, physiologically relevant, animal models need to be developed. Genetics-based approaches can be utilized to compare different inbred strains of rats and mice that exhibit marked differences in susceptibility to specific hormone-induced cancers. Novel transgenic and knockout mouse models can be developed to evaluate the roles of specific genes as modifiers of susceptibility to hormone-induced cancers. It is critical to identify causative mutations for the different hormone-induced cancers to establish firmly whether hormones or their metabolites act through genotoxic mechanisms to initiate carcinogenesis. The ongoing human, mouse, and rat genome projects are providing vast information as well as new tools to support these efforts. It is hoped that significant improvements in the prevention and treatment of hormone-associated cancers are on the horizon.

See Also the Following Articles

Breast Cancer • Endocrine Tumors • Endometrial Cancer • Estrogens and Antiestrogens • Chemical Mutagenesis and Carcinogenesis • Hormone Resistance in Prostate Cancer • Prostate Cancer • Steroid Hormones and Hormone Receptors

Bibliography

Bosland, M. C., Ford, H., and Horton, L. (1995). Induction at high incidence of ductal prostate adenocarcinomas in NBL/Cr and Sprague-Dawley Hsd:SD rats treated with a combination of testosterone and estradiol-17β or diethylstilbestrol. *Carcinogenesis* **16,** 1311–1318.

Carthew, P., Edwards, R. E., Nolan, B. M., Martin, E. A., Heydon, R. T., White, I. N. H., and Tucker, M. J. (2000). Tamoxifen induces endometrial and vaginal cancer in rats treated in the absence of endometrial hyperplasia. *Carcinogenesis* **21,** 793–797.

El-Bayoumy, K., Ji, B.-Y., Upadhyaya, P., Chae, Y.-H., Kurtzke, C., Rivenson, A., Reddy, B. S., Amin, S., and Hecht, S. S. (1996). Lack of tumorigenicity of cholesterol epoxides and estrone-3,4-quinone in the rat mammary gland. *Cancer Res.* **56,** 1970–1973.

Harvell, D. M. E., Strecker, T. E., Tochacek, M., Xie, B., Pennington, K. L., McComb, R. D., Roy, S. K., and Shull, J. D. (2000). Rat strain specific actions of 17β-estradiol in the mammary gland: Correlation between estrogen-induced lobuloalveolar hyperplasia and susceptibility to estrogen-induced mammary cancers. *Proc. Natl. Acad. Sci. USA* **97,** 2779–2784.

Herbst, A. L. (1999). Diethylstilbestrol and adenocarcinoma of the vagina. *Am. J. Obstet. Gynecol.* **181,** 1576–1578.

Jaffe, J. M., Malkowicz, S. B., Walker, A. H., MacBride, S., Peschel, R., Tomaszewski, J., Van Arsdalen, K., Wein, A. J., and Rebbeck, T. R. (2000). Association of SRD5A2 genotype and pathological characteristics of prostate tumors. *Cancer Res.* **60,** 1626–1630.

Li, J., and Li, S. A. (1996). Estrogen carcinogenesis in the hamster kidney: A hormone-driven multistep process. *In* "Cellular and Molecular Mechanisms of Hormonal Carcinogenesis" (J. Huff, J. Boyd, and J. C. Barrett, eds.), pp. 255–267. Wiley-Liss, New York.

Liehr, J. G. (2000). Is estradiol a genotoxic mutagenic carcinogen? *Endocr. Rev.* **21,** 40–54.

Makridakis, N. M., Ross, R. K., Pike, M. C., Crocitto, L. E., Kolonel, L. N., Pearce, C. L., Henderson, B. E., and Reichardt, J. K. (1999). Association of missense substitution in SRD5A2 gene with prostate cancer in African-American and Hispanic men in Los Angeles, USA. *Lancet* **354,** 975–978.

Newbold, R. R., Bullock, B. C., and McLachlan, J. A. (1990). Uterine adenocarcinoma in mice following developmental treatment with estrogens: A model for hormonal carcinogenesis. *Cancer Res.* **50,** 7677–7681.

Newbold, R. R., and Liehr, J. G. (2000). Induction of uterine adenocarcinoma in CD-1 mice by catechol estrogens. *Cancer Res.* **60,** 235–237.

Noble, R. L. (1975). The development of prostatic adenocarcinoma in Nb rats following prolonged sex hormone administration. *Cancer Res.* **37,** 1929–1933.

Shull, J. D., Spady, T. J., Snyder, M. C., Johansson, S. L., and Pennington, K. L. (1997). Ovary intact, but not ovariectomized, female ACI rats treated with 17β-estradiol rapidly develop mammary carcinoma. *Carcinogenesis* **18,** 1595–1601.

Spady, T. J., McComb, R. D., and Shull, J. D. (1999). Estrogen action in the regulation of cell proliferation, cell survival, and tumorigenesis in the rat anterior pituitary gland. *Endocrine* **11,** 217–233.

Telang, N. T., Suto, A., Wong, G. Y., Osborne, M. P., and Bradlow, H. L. (1992). Induction by estrogen metabolite 16 alpha-hydroxyestrone of genotoxic damage and aberrant proliferation in mouse mammary epithelial cells. *J. Natl. Cancer Inst.* **84,** 634–638.

Tsutsui, T., Tamura, Y., Yagi, E., and Barrett, J C. (2000). Involvement of genotoxic effects in the initiation of estrogen-induced cellular transformation: Studies using Syrian hamster embryo cells treated with 17β-estradiol and eight of its metabolites. *Int. J. Cancer* **86,** 8–14.

Weiderpass, E., Persson, I., Melhus, H., Wedrén, S., Kindmark, A., and Baron, J. A. (2000). Estrogen receptor α gene polymorphism and endometrial cancer risk. *Carcinogenesis* **21,** 623–627.

Wong, Y. C., Wang, Y. Z., and Tam, N. N. (1998) The prostate gland and prostate carcinogenesis. *Ital. J. Anat. Embryol.* **103,** 237–252.

Hormone Resistance in Prostate Cancer

Samuel R. Denmeade
John T. Isaacs
Johns Hopkins University School of Medicine

GLOSSARY

androgen Male steroidal sex hormones, typically testosterone and dihydrotestosterone (DHT). Androgens are predominantly produced by the testes, but small amounts can also be produced by adrenal glands.

androgen dependent A prostate cancer cell type that requires androgen for growth and undergoes apoptosis in the absence of androgen.

androgen independent A prostate cancer cell type that neither requires androgen for growth nor undergoes apoptosis in the absence of androgen.

androgen receptor Nuclear receptor that preferentially binds DHT (conversion of testosterone by 5α-reductase produces this more active metabolite) as well as testosterone. Ligand binding results in conformational activation, allowing formation of a transcriptional complex that binds to androgen responsive elements in the promoter of androgen-regulated genes.

androgen sensitive A prostate cancer cell type that requires androgen for growth but does not undergo apoptosis in the absence of androgen.

hormone resistant Clinical status of a patient with progressive or worsening prostate cancer, even though the patient has castrate levels of serum testosterone (also termed hormone refractory).

luteinizing hormone-releasing hormone (LHRH) Released by the hypothalamus, stimulating the production of luteinizing hormone by the pituitary, which in turn stimulates the production of testosterone by testes. Synthetic analogs of LHRH are used to achieve medical castration in patients with metastatic prostate cancer.

Androgen ablation therapy has been an important modality for the treatment of disseminating prostatic cancer since the 1940s. Unfortunately, however, such therapy when given alone is rarely curative. The failure of this therapy to cure such tumors, even though it can induce an initially positive response, is not due to a change in the systemic effectiveness of such a treatment. Instead the development of resistance to such therapy is related to changes in the tumor itself. Experiments by a large number of investigators have identified several of the important tumor cell and host factors involved in these tumor changes. This article explores the problem of hormone resistance in the treatment of prostate cancer and new approaches for treatment.

I. THE PROBLEM OF HORMONE RESISTANCE IN THE TREATMENT OF PROSTATE CANCER

Prostate cancer cells, like normal prostate epithelial cells, depend on androgen for both growth and survival. It is on this basis that androgen ablation has been used as initial therapy for metastatic prostate cancer. Castration via surgical orchiectomy or through chronic treatment with luteinizing hormone-releasing hormone analogs has been the primary treatment modality used to lower serum androgen levels. More complete androgen blockade can be achieved with the addition of antiandrogens that inhibit binding of androgen to the androgen receptor or by inhibiting adrenal androgen synthesis. A total of 27 randomized studies have evaluated whether combined androgen ablation is superior to castration alone as treatment for metastatic prostate cancer. A meta-analysis conducted in 1995 by the Prostate Cancer Trialists' Collaborative Group included data from 22 of these randomized trials comparing monotherapy versus combination therapy and concluded there was no statistically significant difference between the two meth-

ods of treatment. Although androgen ablation therapy is very effective at palliating symptoms associated with metastatic prostate cancer, none of the patients with definitive metastatic disease are cured by such androgen ablation therapy regardless of how aggressively it was given. The therapy is palliative due to the presence of a subset of prostate cancer cells that depend on androgen for survival and which undergo apoptosis when androgen is removed (i.e., androgen dependent). In addition, androgen ablation can also slow the growth of a second subset of prostate cancer cells that grow faster in the presence of androgen but do not die when androgen is inhibited (i.e., androgen sensitive). Androgen ablation therapy is, for the most part, never curative due to the presence of a third subset of prostate cancer cells that are resistant to hormone therapy. These cells are termed androgen independent in that they do not rely on androgenic stimulation for growth, nor do they die in the absence of androgens. In 2001, approximately 31,000 American men will die from prostate cancer that is resistant to hormone therapy. In order to understand why prostate cancers develop "hormone resistance" and why androgen ablation is not curative, an understanding of the cellular basis for androgen responsiveness is necessary.

II. CELLULAR BASIS FOR ANDROGEN RESPONSIVENESS

Whether normal or malignant, the growth of any cell type is dependent on the relationship between its rate of cell proliferation and death. If these rates are equivalent, no net growth occurs, even though cellular turnover (i.e., steady-state replacement) occurs continuously. In contrast, if the rate of cell proliferation is greater than death, then continuous net growth occurs, and if the proliferation rate is lower than death, then cellular elimination occurs. Androgens are the major regulators of proliferation and death for the normal prostate. Androgens regulate the total prostate epithelial cell number by chronically stimulating the rate of cell proliferation (i.e., agonistic ability of androgen) while simultaneously inhibiting the rate of cell death (i.e., antagonistic ability of androgen) of specific subsets of androgen-sensitive and dependent epithelial cells and endothelial cells within the prostate. The normal prostate is heterogeneously composed of a limited number of androgen-independent stem cells (i.e., a subset of basal epithelial cells) that, in addition to maintaining their own limited numbers, give rise to a larger subset of progeny that differentiate into androgen-independent, but sensitive, amplifying cells (i.e., also located in the basal layer of prostate epithelial cells). When sufficient androgen is not present (i.e., following androgen ablation), the amplifying cells are maintained (i.e., rate of proliferation equals rate of cell death) but do not expand into transit (i.e., luminal epithelial) cells. In contrast, when physiologically normal levels of androgen are exogenously replaced in a previously castrated host, the majority of these basally located androgen-sensitive amplifying cells differentiate into luminally located androgen-dependent transit (i.e., glandular) epithelial cells. Once the normal number of these androgen-dependent transit (glandular) cells is reached, their rate of cell proliferation balances their rate of cell death such that neither prostatic regression nor continuous glandular overgrowth occurs. Thus, in the presence of physiological androgen, the normal prostate is in a steady-state, self-renewing, maintenance condition, heterogeneously composed of androgen-independent, sensitive, and dependent epithelial cells. Because of the clonally expansive nature of this hierarchical stem cell organization, the vast majority of the epithelial compartment is composed of androgen-dependent glandular cells, with lower numbers of androgen-sensitive basal cells and a limited number of androgen-independent basal stem cells.

III. ROLE OF ANDROGENS IN PROSTATE CANCER SURVIVAL VS APOPTOSIS

If a sufficient systemic androgen level is not chronically maintained (e.g., following androgen ablation), the entire subset of androgen-dependent prostatic glandular and epithelial subset of prostatic endothelial cells die rapidly via the activation of an energy-dependent cascade of biochemical and morphologic changes, collectively referred to as programmed cell death. Normally, this programmed death is actively

suppressed due to the androgen-dependent production of cell survival signals. These include the production of secreted peptide survival factors, such as insulin-like growth factors I and II (IGF-I and II), platelet-derived growth factor (PDGF), and vascular endothelial growth factor (VEGF). These survival factors initiate their effect by binding to their cell surface cognate receptor and inducing tyrosine transautophosphorylation, which functions to recruit intracellular signaling proteins to bind via their src homology (i.e., SH_2) domains to specific phosphorylated tyrosines in the ligand-occupied dimeric receptor complex. This autophosphorylation initiates three major kinase-dependent signaling cascades. These include (1) the ras/raf/Mek/srk cascade, (2) the phospholipase Cγ (PLCγ)/diacylgycerol (DAG)/inositol 3-phosphate (IP3)/protein kinase C cascade, and (3) the phosphoinosityl 3 kinase (PI3K)/protein kinase B kinase (PKBK)/protein kinase B (PKB also called Akt)/BAD/procaspase 9 cascade. Activation and/or inhibition of these pathways is a critically important determinant of cell survival, proliferation, or death. In the presence of androgen cells, survival/proliferation signals are produced, whereas following androgen ablation, levels of these factors decrease, leading to activation of apoptosis.

IV. RELATIONSHIP BETWEEN CELL OF ORIGIN FOR PROSTATE CANCER AND ANDROGEN RESPONSIVENESS

Based on the stem cell organization of the normal prostate epithelium, there are three distinct cells of origins possible for prostate cancer. The first alternative is that the prostate cancer is monoclonally derived from an androgen-independent stem cell. Even if the cell of origin is an androgen-independent stem cell, it is still possible for the resulting cancer to be responsive to androgen ablation. The malignant stem cell could retain the ability to progress down the hierarchical pathway described earlier, giving rise to larger subsets of androgen-sensitive amplifying and even larger numbers of androgen-dependent transit malignant cells. Such a heterogeneous cancer composed of these three cell types would respond to androgen ablation with the elimination of the largest subset of cancer cells (i.e., androgen-dependent malignant transit cells) and a reduction in the growth rate of the next largest subset of cancer cells (i.e., androgen-sensitive malignant amplifying cells). Such a response would not be curative because neither the malignant androgen-independent stem cell nor the androgen-sensitive malignant amplifying cell would be eliminated. A second alternative is that the original prostate cancer can be monoclonally derived from an androgen-sensitive amplifying basal cell. If this occurred, then the cancer would again be androgen responsive because it is composed of androgen-sensitive malignant amplifying cells that retain the ability of differentiating into androgen-dependent transit cell progeny. Again, due to clonal expansion, the major type of cancer cell present would be the androgen-dependent malignant transit cell. Such a heterogeneous cancer would be responsive to androgen ablation due to the elimination of the major subset of malignant transit cells; however, the cancer would not be cured by such therapy because the androgen-sensitive amplifying cells would not be eliminated.

A third alternative is that the original cancer is monoclonally derived from an androgen-dependent transit (glandular) cell. If this occurs, then the cancer would initially be highly androgen responsive to androgen ablation. If no further malignant progression occurred, the cancer theoretically could be cured by such therapy; however, as will be discussed, even if this third possibility occurs and the initial prostate cancer is homogeneously composed of androgen-dependent cancer cells, as these cells undergo sufficient cellular proliferation to produce clinically detectable prostate cancer (i.e., more than 30 population doublings), a series of mechanisms eventually lead to the heterogeneous development of malignant clones of androgen-sensitive or androgen-independent prostate cancer cells or both.

V. MECHANISM OF DEVELOPMENT OF ANDROGEN-INDEPENDENT PROSTATE CANCER CELLS

A. The Role of Genetic Instability

The exact mechanism responsible for the basic alteration of the cancer cell phenotype has not been completely resolved but involves changes in the structure, regulation, or both of the cancer cell genome. Regardless of the detailed mechanism, such a change in phenotype is inheritable. This requires that some type of basic genetic change occurs in these cells. Genetic change is defined here as a heritable alteration of phenotype, whether resulting from gene mutations, chromosomal alterations, or alterations in gene regulation. The ability of cancer cells to undergo such genetic changes demonstrates that these tumor cells are genetically unstable (i.e., genetically changeable). This genetic instability can lead to the addition of a series of genetically altered clones of cancer cells, each with a distinct phenotype. Only such newly developed clones in which the new phenotype allows these cells to proliferate without the requirement for androgenic stimulation (i.e., androgen-independent or sensitive cells) are important in the development of resistance to androgen ablation therapy. Once these androgen-independent or sensitive clones develop, they have a growth advantage following androgen ablation over all the other newly developed tumor clones that still retain androgen dependence, in addition to any original androgen-dependent cells still present in the tumor. Eventually, such a growth advantage leads via clonal selection to the development of resistance of androgen ablation therapy (i.e., hormonal refractory disease).

B. Causes of Genetic Instability

1. Microenvironmental Changes

The basic question becomes what causes the development of genetic instability of initially androgen-dependent prostate cancer cells? One possibility is that changes in the tumor microenvironment are critically involved in inducing the development of this genetic instability. Exactly how this could occur is not completely understood. The net result of this environmentally induced genetic instability is that genetically distinct androgen-independent or sensitive cells can be added to the tumor even before any androgen ablation therapy is given.

In addition to androgen ablation-independent changes in the tumor microenvironment, such change also can be directly induced by androgen ablation.

For example, the continuous growth and survival of any cancer critically require an adequate tumor blood supply. Because a critical tumor blood supply is continuously expanding (i.e., angiogenesis) with the net growth of the cancer, anything that inhibits tumor angiogenesis produces local (i.e., microenvironmental) hypoxia, acidosis, and toxic metabolic waste build-up. These microenvironmental changes could induce such instability of the cancer cells. Adequate tumor angiogenesis requires the continuous production of a series of angiogenesis factors, one of the most important of which is vascular endothelial growth factor. VEGF induces the migration, proliferation, and survival of endothelial cells and is also produced by prostate cancer cells themselves. Studies have demonstrated that VEGF secretion by androgen responsive and dependent prostate cancer cells is under androgen regulation. Thus, androgen ablation induces a significant decrease in VEGF levels within prostate cancers, which by inhibiting tumor angiogenesis could produce significant microenvironment stress on the prostate cancer cells, inducing their genetic instability.

2. Stochastic Increase or Decrease in Expression of Critical Genes

An alternative explanation is that changes in the host microenvironment, whether dependent or independent of androgen ablation, do not have a direct inductive role in the development of genetic instability of the initially androgen-dependent prostate cancer cells. Instead, it is possible that the development of genetic instability of the androgen-dependent prostate cancer cells occurs as a stochastic event related to the basic nature of the cancer cells. How such genetic instability could develop independent of microenvironmental factors is not entirely known. One possibility is that one of the earliest events in the malignant transformation of prostate epithelial cells could involve deactivation of a gene locus, which increases the likelihood of subsequent genetic errors. For example, in prostate cancer, the gene encoding for the phase II detoxification enzyme, the π isozyme of glutathione S-transferase, is extensively methylated in its promoter region in a completely cancer-specific fashion, with a concomitant absence of expression. Because this enzyme has a key

part in an important cellular pathway to prevent damage from a wide range of carcinogens, inactivation of its activity may result in increased susceptibility of prostate tissue to both tumor initiation and progression resulting from an increased rate of accumulated DNA damage (i.e., increasing its genetic instability).

Additional genetic changes may explain the progression to an androgen-independent phenotype. Bcl-2 is an oncogene located on chromosome 18q21 encoding a membrane-bound 26-kDa protein that prolongs cell survival by inhibiting apoptosis. Bcl-2 expression is localized to basal epithelial cells in the normal human prostate. Normal human prostatic secretory epithelial cells do not express the bcl-2 protein; however, a fraction of primary untreated prostate adenocarcinoma cells do express this apoptosis-suppressing oncoprotein at a significant level. With the use of immunohistochemical examination for bcl-2 expression in androgen-dependent and androgen-independent prostate carcinoma, bcl-2 is undetectable in approximately 60% of androgen-dependent cancers. In contrast, androgen-independent cancers displayed diffuse high levels of bcl-2 expression in 30–40% of cases. These findings suggest that enhanced bcl-2 expression is correlated with the progression of prostate cancer androgen dependence to androgen independence. The frequency of bcl-2 expression during the progression of human and rat prostate cancers from an androgen-sensitive non-metastatic phenotype to an androgen-independent metastatic phenotype is statistically significantly correlated. Such bcl-2 expression is not absolutely required for either androgen-independent or metastatic ability by human prostate cancer cells. Experimentally, overexpression of bcl-2 in human prostate cancer cells protects these cells from apoptotic stimuli *in vitro* and confers resistance to androgen depletion *in vivo*, and such protection correlates with the ability to form hormone-refractory prostate tumors *in vivo*.

C. Alterations in Androgen Receptor Expression or Function

The androgen receptor is a key mediator of androgen function within normal and malignant prostate cells. The androgen receptor is nearly universally expressed in primary and metastatic sites in untreated patients and in patients undergoing androgen ablation but with recurrent disease, suggesting that the androgen receptor is required for the progression of prostate cancer to the androgen-unresponsive metastatic stage. Molecular analysis has demonstrated that amplification of the Xq11-q13 region where the androgen receptor gene is located is common in prostate cancer recurring during androgen ablation therapy. Androgen receptor amplification has been detected in approximately 30% of recurrent prostate cancers but not in specimens taken from the same patients prior to therapy. Combining these results suggest that in approximately one-third of patients, failure of androgen ablation therapy may be caused by clonal outgrowth of prostate cancer cells with increased androgen receptor expression. In addition to amplification, mutations in the gene can cause androgen receptor dysfunction, including alterations of androgen receptor specificity, binding affinity, and expression. Androgen receptor mutations occur in low frequency in primary prostate cancer. In contrast, cells in distant metastases and recurrent prostate cancer after androgen ablation often contain androgen receptor mutations.

D. Alternative Signaling Pathways

A series of experimental studies have demonstrated that there is "cross talk" between the androgen receptor and the signaling pathway induced by peptide growth factors. These studies have demonstrated that when the androgen receptor is not expressed, certain peptide growth factors [e.g., nerve growth factor (NGF), keratinocyte growth factor, epidermal growth factor (EGF), and insulin-like growth factor-1 (IGF-1)] are unable to stimulate the transcription of androgen responsive genes by androgen-independent prostate cancer cells. In contrast, when the androgen receptor is expressed experimentally in these same androgen-independent cancer cells, these same peptide growth factors can now induce the expression of these androgen responsive genes in an androgen ligand-independent manner. Ligand-independent androgen receptor activation of transcription of specific genes can be induced by the costimulation of pathways involving protein kinase A or peptide growth factors.

VI. NEW APPROACHES FOR THE TREATMENT OF ANDROGEN-INDEPENDENT PROSTATE CANCER

The aforementioned results suggest that the androgen-regulated transcriptional pathways for growth and survival may be activated in an androgen ligand-independent manner by cross talk with the nuclear transcriptional machinery induced by peptide growth factors. This raises the interesting possibility that although certain prostate cancer cells can progress to become independent of androgen for growth and survival, these same cells may retain an androgen receptor dependence, independent of binding of the androgen ligand to this receptor. Thus, therapies targeted at decreasing androgen receptor expression within prostate cancer cells, independent of lower serum androgen levels, are a new approach. An additional new approach is to disrupt the ability of the androgen receptor to interact with a series of coactivator proteins (i.e., SRC-1) needed for the efficient transcription of androgen responsive genes.

In order for androgen-dependent prostate cancer cells to progress to a nonandrogen-dependent phenotype, these nonandrogen-dependent cancer cells must substitute alternative (i.e., nonandrogen dependent) mechanisms for activation of their survival pathways. There are a variety of growth factors and cytokines that could potentially provide activation of such survival pathways. Growth factors and cytokines vary in their ability to induce proliferation and survival (i.e., EGF and FGF are mitogenic factors, whereas insulin, IGF, PDGF, and NGF are survival factors), but they all function by binding to and thereby activating their cognate receptors, which in turn activates signal transduction pathways. Inhibition of these signal transduction pathways can activate apoptosis. Alternatively, inhibition of critical survival pathways may lower the "apoptotic threshold" and make treated cells more likely to undergo apoptosis following exposure to cytotoxic agents. In light of these findings, inhibitors of signal transduction pathways are under development. Currently, inhibitors of the PDGF and NGF signal transduction pathways are undergoing clinical testing as treatment for prostate cancer. The best use of these agents, however, may be in combination with androgen ablation or in combination with other cytotoxic agents.

VII. SUMMARY

Androgen ablation therapy has been an important modality for the treatment of disseminating prostatic cancer since the 1940s. Unfortunately, however, such therapy is rarely curative when given alone. The failure of this therapy to cure such tumors, even though it can induce an initially positive response, is not due to a change in the systemic effectiveness of such a treatment. Instead the development of resistance to such therapy is related to changes in the tumor itself. Experiments by a large number of investigators have identified several of the important tumor cell and host factors involved in these tumor changes. Through the identification of these factors, a concept has evolved that there may be multiple pathways for the development of resistance to hormonal therapy based on a stem cell model for the normal prostate. While such pathways can be described in phenomenological terms, the detailed molecular biology of such a process is still unknown. It is clear, however, that the essential feature of the development of androgen resistance is the emergence of androgen-independent and/or sensitive cancer cells. The critical question for future studies, therefore, is exactly how do androgen-independent cells develop? If this question can be answered, it might be possible to design therapies that prevent the development of these independent tumor cells.

Only under such conditions would androgen ablation therapy, used as a single modality, become potentially curative. However, even if therapeutic means can be developed to prevent the emergence of androgen-independent and/or sensitive tumor cells, this type of blocking therapy would have to be performed before such development had already occurred to be effective. Therefore, before such therapy was begun, some type of clinical test to determine that the tumor did not already have some androgen-independent and/or sensitive tumor cells present (i.e., the tumor was not already heterogencous androgen sensitive) would additionally be required. Because neither a method for determining the homogeneous vs hetero-

geneous nature of the androgen requirements of a particular tumor nor a method for prevention of the development of androgen-independent and/or sensitive tumor cells from dependent prostate cancer cells is available at present, these should be critical areas for extensive future study. Any advancement in either of these important areas would have profound consequences on the more effective issue of androgen ablation therapy.

See Also the Following Articles

Genetic Predisposition to Prostate Cancer • Hormonal Carcinogenesis • Insulin-like Growth Factors • Metabolic Diagnosis of Prostate Cancer by Magnetic Resonance Spectroscopy • Prostate Cancer

Bibliography

Culig, Z., Hobisch, A., Cronauer, M. V., Radmayr, C., Trapman, J., Hittmair, A., Bartsch, G., and Klocker, H. (1994). Androgen receptor activation in prostatic tumor cell lines by insulin-like growth factor-I, keratinocyte growth factor and epidermal growth factor. *Cancer Res.* **54,** 5474–5478.

Denmeade, S. R., Lin, X. S., and Isaacs, J. T. (1996). Role of programmed (apoptotic) cell death during the progression and therapy of prostate cancer. *Prostate* **28,** 251–265.

DeMarzo, A. M., Nelson, W. G., Meeker, A. K., and Coffey, D. S. (1998). Stem cell features of benign and malignant prostate epithelial cells. *J. Urol.* **160,** 2381–2392.

Hemmings, B. A. (1997). Akt signaling: Linking membrane events of life and eath decisions. *Science* **275,** 628–630.

Hobisch, A., Culig, Z., Radmayr, C., Bartsch, G., Klocker, H., and Hittmair, A. (1995). Distant metastases from prostate carcinoma express androgen receptor protein. *Cancer Res.* **55,** 3068–3072.

Isaacs, J. T. (1984). Antagonistic effect of androgen on prostatic cell death. *Prostate* **5,** 545–559.

Isaacs, J. T. (1999). The biology of hormone refractory prostate cancer. *Urol. Clin. North Am.* **26,** 263–273.

Isaacs, J. T., and Coffey, D. S. (1998). Etiology of BPH. *Prostate Suppl.* **2,** 33–50.

Isaacs, J. T., Wake, N., Coffey, D. S., and Sandberg, A. A. (1982). Genetic instability coupled to clonal selection as a mechanism for tumor progression in the Dunning R-3327 rat prostatic adenocarcinoma system. *Cancer Res.* **42,** 2353–2361.

Jain, R. K., Safabakhsh, N., Sckell, A., Chen, Y., Jiang, P., Benjamin, L., Yuan, F., and Keshet, E. (1998). Endothelial cell death, angiogenesis and microvascular function following castration in an androgen-dependent tumor: Role of VEGF. *Proc. Natl. Acad. Sci. USA* **95,** 10820–10825.

Lee, W. H., Morton, R. A., Epstein, J. I., Brooks, J. D., Campbell, P. A., Bova, G. S., Hsieh, W. S., Isaacs, W. B., and Nelson, W. G. (1994). Cytidine methylation of regulatory sequences near the p-class glutahione-S-transferase gene accompanies human prostate cancer carcinogenesis. *Proc. Natl. Acad. Sci. USA* **91,** 11733–11737.

McDonnell, T. J., Troncoso, P., Brisbay, S. M., Logothetis, C., Chung, L. W., Hsieh, J. T., Tu, S. M., and Campbell, M. L. (1992). Expression of the protooncogene bcl-2 in the prostate and its association with emergence of androgen-independent prostate cancer. *Cancer Res.* **52,** 6940–6944.

Prostate Cancer Trialists' Collaborative Group (1995). Maximum androgen blockade in advanced prostate cancer: An overview of 22 randomised trials with 3283 deaths in 5710 patients. *Lancet* **346,** 265.

Tilley, W. D., Buchanan, G., Hickey, T. T., and Bentel, J. M. (1996). Mutations in the androgen receptor gene are associated with progression of human prostate cancer to androgen independence. *Clin. Cancer Res.* **2,** 277–285.

Viskorpi, T., Hyytinen, E., Koivisto, P., Tanner, M., Keinanen, R., Palmberg, C., Palotie, A., Tammela, T., Isola, J., and Kallioniemi, O. P. (1995). *In vivo* amplification of the androgen receptor gene and progression of human prostate cancer. *Nature Genet.* **9,** 401–406.

Human T-Cell Leukemia/ Lymphotropic Virus

Gerold Feuer

SUNY Upstate Medical University, Syracuse, New York

Irvin S.Y. Chen

University of California, Los Angeles, School of Medicine

I. Clinical Syndromes
II. Genomic Organization and Virus Life Cycle
III. T-Cell Immortalization and Transformation by HTLV
IV. Oncogenesis

GLOSSARY

apoptosis Process by which cells are programmed to die.
clonal expansion Cells originating from a single infected precursor cell.
cytokines Proteins that stimulate and regulate the immune response.
etiology Causes or origins assigned to a disease.
human T-cell leukemia/lymphotropic virus-associated myelopathy/tropical spastic paraparesis Nonfatal neurological disorder characterized by progressive paralysis predominantly affecting the extremities.
oncogenes Genes capable of altering normal cell growth controlling processes resulting in the transformation of cells.
pathogenesis The origin and progression of disease.

retrovirus Positive-stranded RNA viruses, enveloped with unique morphology and means of replication.
transformation Process by which a normal cell becomes immortalized in culture, taking on characteristics of malignant cells.

Human T-cell leukemia/lymphotropic virus type-1 (HTLV-1) is the first human oncogenic retrovirus associated with malignancy and is recognized as an etiologic agent of diverse human diseases, most notably adult T-cell leukemia (ATL) and an immune-mediated neurological disorder termed HTLV-associated myelopathy/tropical spastic paraparesis (HAM/TSP). HTLV-1 infection affects several million individuals worldwide, and virus infection is endemic in southern Japan, regions of Central Africa, the Caribbean basin, and in South and Central America. Serological and epidemiological evidence initially revealed the association of HTLV-1 with the development of ATL, whereas subsequent investigations have linked HTLV infection with several inflammatory and immune-mediated conditions and disorders. Many aspects of HTLV-1 pathogenesis have remained obscure, predominantly due to the lack of viral molecular clones and the availability of suitable animal models. Because HTLV can transform and immortalize cells in culture, much emphasis has been focused on the characterization of viral genes involved in cellular transformation. In particular, the transcriptional activator gene (tax) has been implicated as a necessary component in cellular transformation, as well as in leukemogenesis induced by HTLV-1, and has been the target of much investigation. Although HTLV-1 infection is not considered to be a pressing health problem in the United States, understanding the pathogenic mechanisms of the virus provides a window for understanding the molecular events in the origin of cancers in humans.

I. CLINICAL SYNDROMES

A. ATL

ATL is a mature non-Hodgkin lymphoma characterized by leukemic cells of CD4$^+$/CD25$^+$ phenotype and was first described in 1977 in Japan. The etiological association between ATL in southwestern Japan and seropositivity for HTLV-1 was subsequently determined in the early 1980s. C-type retrovirus particles were first identified in a T lymphoblastoid cell line established from a patient with cutaneous T-cell lymphoma (CTLL). In 1981, an independently isolated cell line, MT-1, derived from a patient with ATL also harbored a retrovirus and produced antigens that reacted with sera from patients with ATL. Viruses produced from these distinct cell lines were subsequently named HTLV-1. Transmission of HTLV occurs primarily by three major routes: heterosexual and homosexual transmission, via contaminated blood products (i.e., transfusion or iv drug abuse), and vertical transmission from mother to child via breast milk. Although infection with cell-free HTLV-1 virions has been documented in vitro, efficient infection by HTLV-1 requires cell-to-cell contact between virally infected cells and recipient cells. Mother-to-child transmission was identified early in the investi-

gations of ATL, and transmission of the virus by infected lymphocytes in breast milk was ultimately identified as a leading cause of infection. Although the majority of HTLV-1-infected individuals are asymptomatic, an estimated 1 to 5% of individuals develop lymphoma over their life span. ATL generally occurs in early adulthood, 20 to 30 years following infection, suggesting that a long incubation period and additional mutational events are necessary for the manifestation of malignant transformation (Fig. 1). The HTLV-1 provirus is invariably integrated into the host genome of malignant cells, and many ATL patients display defective virus genomes. T lymphocytes isolated from the peripheral blood of HTLV-1-infected individuals show increased spontaneous proliferation when cultured in vitro. Over time, proliferation becomes independent of interleukin-2 (IL-2), and these cell cultures generally represent outgrowths of clones that do not predominate in the patient, but rather are selected for growth in culture.

The clinical course of ATL has been classified into four different subtypes: chronic, smoldering, acute, and lymphoma. Smoldering and chronic ATL are less aggressive than the acute and lymphoma forms of the disease. The smoldering subtype of ATL is often indolent and can last for years. Chronic and smoldering subtypes of ATL can progress to acute ATL at any time during the course of disease (an event termed "crisis"). This subtype is the most common form of the disease. ATL is a mature T-cell lymphoma, characterized by circulating, activated CD4$^+$/CD25$^+$ T cells and by prominent lymphadenopathy due to the expansion of HTLV-1-infected T lymphocytes in lymphatic tissues. Acute ATL is characterized by an expansion of a clonal population of HTLV-1-infected cells, as determined by a single TCR rearrangement. Diagnostic criteria for ATL include seropositivity for HTLV-1 proteins, the presence of morphologically unique T cells having a lobulated nucleus ("flower cells"), expression of the IL-2 receptor (CD25) on malignant cells, and the presence of all or part of the HTLV-1 genome integrated in neoplastic cells.

The histopathology of lymph nodes from ATL patients is identified most frequently as a large cell, immunoblastic classification. The most definitive evidence of ATL is the presence of monoclonal or oligoclonal T cells from the patient, with respect to

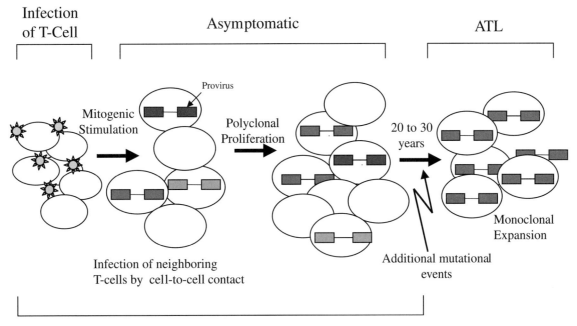

Modeled by *in vitro* infection and transformation

FIGURE 1   A model for HTLV-1-mediated tumorigenesis. Infection of T lymphocytes results in reverse transcription of virion RNA and formation of the provirus, which represents the viral genome integrated into chromosomal DNA. T cells are persistently infected for the life of the cell. Infected cells generate new virions, which infect neighboring cells by cell-to-cell contact. The production of virions has been shown to induce mitogenic effects, resulting in the further expansion of the pool of infected cells. Polyclonal proliferation of infected cells can be achieved by infection *in vitro* and is thought to simulate early infection processes *in vivo*. ATL occurs in a minority of HTLV-1-infected patients and only after decades following the initial infection event. ATL cells generally represent a clonal expansion of infected T cells, and additional mutational events are thought to be required for the manifestation of disease.

the integrated HTLV-1 provirus. Notably, although deletions of the HTLV-1 proviral genome are often detected in ATL cells, the *tax* gene is invariably maintained, implicating this viral gene product in leukemogenesis. Patients manifest unique characteristic symptoms, such as infiltration of leukemic cells into the liver, spleen, lung, and gastrointestinal track. Clinical features of the disease include hypercalcemia, skin lesions due to leukemic cell infiltration, lymphomatous meningitis, lytic bone lesions, and immunodeficiency.

Treatment

ATL is a highly malignant disease and is nearly 100% fatal, although rare cases of spontaneous remission have been reported. It should be noted, however, that only a small proportion of infected individuals progress from an asymptomatic to a disease state. Standard combination chemotherapy regimens have not proved effective for ATL. Recent regimens developed include using interferon-β and interferon-γ and administra-

tion of anti-Tac antibody, as ATL cells express high levels of CD25 (IL-2R). Combination therapy using zidovudine and interferon-α and the two in combination with etretinate have proven successful.

B. HAM/TSP

The involvement of HTLV-1 infection in progressive neurological disease was initially independently documented in the West Indies as well as in Japan in the mid-1980s. HAM/TSP has been described in all areas of the world known to be endemic for HTLV-1. HAM/TSP is a nonfatal, progressively disabling disorder whose symptoms include muscle weakness and spasticity of the extremities, hyperreflexia, and sensory disturbances. ATL and HAM/TSP development rarely coincide, suggesting genetic factors and/or the stage of development at the time of infection may be important in disease manifestation. The most prevalent initial symptoms of HAM/TSP are weakness and stiffness of the extremities, lumbar pain, hyperreflexia, clonus, Babinsky sign, and bladder disturbances, including urinary urgency and incontinence, and mild peripheral sensory loss is also present during the early onset of disease. The disease is reported to affect between 0.2 and 5% of infected individuals; however, in the case of infection via transfusion, development of HAM/TSP can occur within as little as 6 months. Patients with HAM/TSP generally display normal lymphocyte numbers, but morphologically atypical lymphocytes resembling ATL cells can be seen in peripheral blood or the cerebral spinal fluid. Although the pathogenesis of HAM/TSP is poorly understood, disease development can occur relatively rapidly following infection, in contrast to ATL, which develops decades after the initial infection event. In addition, HAM/TSP patients generally display significantly higher levels of proviral DNA in their peripheral blood lymphocytes (PBL) than asymptomatic HTLV-1 carriers. It is noteworthy that polyclonal integration of the virus is detected in patients with HAM/TSP, as opposed to the oligoclonal or monoclonal integration pattern seen in ATL.

The pathogenesis of HAM/TSP remains poorly understood. Central nervous system (CNS) damage may directly result from HTLV-1 infection of cells in the CNS or indirectly via cytokine-mediated mechanisms, resulting in neurotoxicity. In fact, the expression of cytokines including tumor necrosis factor-α (TNF-α), granulocyte–macrophage colony-stimulatory factor (GM-CSF), interferon γ (INF-γ) and IL-1α is higher in HAM/TSP patients than in asymptomatic carriers. Characterization of viral isolates from patients with HAM/TSP does not show any distinguishing features from HTLV-1 from those with ATL and provides no evidence that a variant virus is involved in disease. Although the exact mechanisms of HAM/TSP induction remains to be elucidated, it does appear that HTLV infection results in chronic activation and destruction of neuronal tissue by the cellular immune response. In that respect, it should be noted that high levels of cytotoxic T cells (CTLs) have been detected in HAM/TSP patients, which predominantly recognize HTLV-1-infected cells.

Treatment

Due to the inflammatory nature of HAM/TSP, systemic administration of oral corticosteroids has shown variable clinical efficacy. Danazol, an attenuated androgen with hormonal and immunomodulatory effects, has been proposed as an alternative to glucocorticoids. Significant progress in the treatment of HAM/TSP awaits a better understanding of the pathogenesis of this condition.

C. Other Diseases Associated with HTLV-1

Clinical reports have suggested a number of inflammatory conditions associated with the infection of HTLV-1. HTLV-1-associated uveitis and chronic inflammatory arthropathy have been linked in HTLV-infected individuals as a rare complication of infection. Animal models of HTLV-1 infection have reaffirmed the role of HTLV-1 in these diseases. Certain lines of transgenic mice for HTLV-1 have developed chronic arthritis resembling rheumatoid arthritis, suggesting an etiological link. Uveitis has also been observed in rabbits infected experimentally with HTLV-1.

Hematological malignancies other than ATL are associated with infection with HTLV-1. Sezary's syndrome and mycosis fungoides, another group of cutaneous T-cell lymphomas (CTCL), show clinical and histopathological features similar to ATL in that they are disorders of the CD4$^+$ T lymphocytes. These are generally of the small cell types and, in contrast to ATL, only infrequently express T-cell activation markers such as CD25. Sezary's syndrome is considered to be a leukemic variant of mycosis fungoides and is characterized by erythroleukemia, lymphadenopathy, and atypical lymphoctyes in peripheral blood. At present, the relationship of HTLV-1 infection and mycosis fungoides and Sezary syndrome development is unclear, as infection is only detected in a minority of cases.

D. HTLV-2

HTLV-2 was first identified from splenic tissue from a patient with hairy cell leukemia and is related to HTLV-1. Although a direct implication of the etiologic role of HTLV-2 in disease remains elusive, characteristics of HTLV-2 infection are similar in nature to those of HTLV-1. Like HTLV-1, HTLV-2 infects and transforms T lymphocytes in culture. Because

HTLV-1 and -2 have approximately 70% sequence homology, serological cross-reaction of HTLV-1 with HTLV-2 presents difficulties in identifying HTLV-2-infected individuals. HTLV-2 has been detected in a small number of patients with spastic myelopathy and variable degrees of ataxia. At least one patient has been identified with a chronic progressive neurological disease clinically indistinguishable from HAM/TSP, suggesting that HTLV-2 infection may be linked to the development of neurological disorders.

II. GENOMIC ORGANIZATION AND VIRUS LIFE CYCLE

HTLV is a member of Retroviridae, a family of RNA viruses having the unique ability to transcribe their RNA genome into double-stranded DNA (proviral DNA), which then becomes integrated into the host chromosomes. The genome of HTLV-1 shows features common to all retroviruses, including the 5' to 3' arrangement of the group-specific antigen (gag), reverse transcriptase (pol), and envelope (env) genes

(Fig. 2). In contrast to simple retroviruses, HTLV also encodes additional proteins termed Tax and Rex, which are involved in regulating gene expression. Tax, in particular, has the ability to modulate virus gene transcription and is involved in cellular transformation. After penetration of HTLV into the host cell, reverse transcriptase completes the synthesis of double-stranded DNA from the viral RNA. Double-stranded viral DNA is then integrated into the host genome, becoming the HTLV provirus. Cells carrying the provirus are persistently infected, and the infection is not cytolytic. Virion mRNAs are expressed from integrated proviral DNA.

A. Tax and Rex

The HTLV-1 genome contains a region located downstream of the env gene, termed the X region (pX). This region contains four different open reading frames (ORFs) numbered I to IV from 5' to 3' (Fig. 2). ORFs I and II encode proteins with unknown biological functions (p12^I, p13^{II}, and p30^{II}). These proteins are dispensable for the transformation of

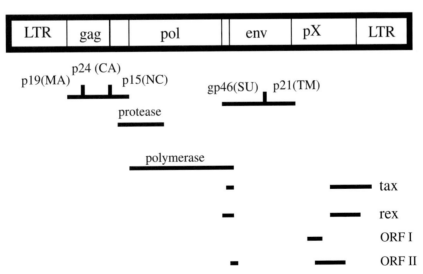

FIGURE 2 Structure and organization of the HTLV-1 genome. The HTLV provirus is illustrated schematically. Positions of the encoded viral proteins are shown below the provirus. The Gag protein is the precursor to the internal structural proteins, including matrix (MA), capsid (CA), and nucleocapsid (NC). Protease and polymerase (reverse transcriptase) are enzymes required for viral replication. Envelope (env) glycoproteins consist of a 46-kDa surface glycoprotein [gp46(SU)] and transmembrane protein [p21(TM)]. Tax and Rex are encoded at the 3' end of the provirus (pX). Proteins encoded within open reading frames (ORF) I and II have been identified only recently. Long terminal repeats (LTRs) flank either end of the provirus and contain sequences important for transcriptional initiation and termination.

lymphocytes *in vitro*. ORFs III and IV encode Rex and Tax, respectively, which regulate HTLV-1 replication and are expressed early following infection. The Rex protein controls HTLV-1 expression at the posttranscriptional level by directly binding to sequences present on unspliced and singly spliced viral mRNAs. The HTLV tax gene product is a nuclear protein translated from double-spliced viral mRNA that functionally transactivates expression from the HTLV LTR to increase viral RNA transcription. Tax is critical for HTLV-1 to establish productive infection and, furthermore, like many viral transcriptional regulatory proteins, has been linked to the perturbation of cell processes. The ability of Tax to promiscuously modulate cellular gene expression accounts for its role in transformation. Proteins with functions similar to Tax have been described in several DNA tumor viruses, such as papova viruses (SV40 large T antigen), herpesviruses (immediate early gene products), and adenoviruses (E1A). Tax plays a crucial role in cellular transformation and, importantly, is also capable of transactivating the expression of a multitude of cellular genes (Table I).

TABLE I
HTLV-1 Tax Effects on Cellular Genes

Genes induced by Tax	Genes repressed by Tax
Cytokines and cytokine receptors	Proapoptotic factors
IL-1	Bax
IL-2	p53
IL-2Rα	Caspase-8
IL-3	DNA repair enzyme
IL-4	β-polymerase
GM-CSF	Protein tyrosine kinase
G-CSF	lck
TGF-β	
TNF-α	
TNF-β	
Parathyroid hormone-related protein	
IFN-γ	
Lymphotoxin	
Antiapoptotic factors	
Bcl-X$_L$	
Protooncogenes	
c-fos	
c-myc	
c-rel	
c-sis	

III. T-CELL IMMORTALIZATION AND TRANSFORMATION BY HTLV

The growth potential of normal human peripheral blood T lymphocytes plated in culture is limited. T-cell transformation is defined as continuous cellular proliferation *in vitro* in the absence of IL-2. HTLV-1 transforms normal human T cells *in vitro*. HTLV-1 has a broad host range and can immortalize lymphocytes of other species in culture, including rabbits, cats, rats, and monkeys.

A. Immortalization of T Cells by HTLV-1

T-cell transformation in culture is initially characterized by a polyclonal expansion of infected T-cell subpopulations 4 to 8 weeks after infection by cocultivation with persistently infected, lethally irradiated HTLV-1-transformed cell lines. Cell-free HTLV-1 is generally noninfectious. Infected transformed T cells display an increased expression of IL-2 and IL-2Rα (CD25), suggesting that the initiation of an autocrine loop involving IL-2 activation of lymphocytes and stimulation of cellular proliferation via the IL-2 receptor may be relevant in the transformation process. Further passage of infected cell cultures results in the selective outgrowth of one or a few dominant clones. Transformed cells generally express the CD4 cell surface marker, although some cells may also express the CD8$^+$ marker. In ATL patients, tumor cells are almost invariably of CD4$^+$ types, although occasional CD8$^+$ tumors have been reported. HTLV-1-transformed cells typically display phenotypes and cell surface markers associated with activation, including the expression of IL-2R, transferrin receptor, and major histocompatibility complex class II molecules. Transformed cells also produce a wide spectrum of lymphokines, including IFN-γ and GM-CSF.

B. Transformation Associated with Tax

The HTLV-1 genome does not contain an oncogene derived from the cellular genome, the virus does therefore not belong to the acutely transforming retroviruses. No common proviral integration sites have been identified in ATL cells, suggesting that HTLV does not activate cellular oncogenes by insertional mutagenesis. Several lines of evidence implicate Tax as the oncogenic component of HTLV. These include (i) the induction of tumors in transgenic mouse models, (ii) immortalization of human T cells using *tax* transduction systems, and (iii) transformation of rodent cells using *in vitro* transformation assays. Data from infectious clones of HTLV-1 and HTLV-2 have shown that oncogenic cellular transformation requires expression of the Tax protein. The precise mechanism by which Tax initiates the malignant process is unclear, but likely involves several points of transcriptional and posttranscriptional dysregulation in the infected T cell (Table I). Although *in vitro* transformation by HTLV provides a model system for leukemogenesis in humans, there are limitations and differences inherent in the system. The process of *in vitro* transformation more likely reflects events ongoing early in the infection process, and cells transformed by HTLV in culture are distinct from cells of ATL patients (Table II).

The Tax protein acts indirectly by activation of transcription factors, including the cyclic AMP response element binding protein/activating transcription factor (CREB/ATF), NF-κB/Rel, serum response factor (SRF), NF-AT, and basic helix-loop-helix proteins. Activation of the NF-κB/Rel provides a critical proliferative signal early in the transformation process, whereas CREB/ATF activation promotes sustained cell growth and IL-2-independent cellular transformation. Expression of Tax is also associated with the accumulation of DNA damage. Tax medi-ates repression of cellular enzymes involved in DNA repair, including human β-polymerase and enzymes mediating nucleotide excision repair. Tax may facilitate transformation and leukemogenesis by decreasing the ability of cells to repair genetic damage. Leukemic cells of ATL patients often display chromosomal abnormalities, including deletions and translocations.

C. Perturbation of the Cell Cycle

Progression through the cell cycle is controlled through the modulation of key positive and negative regulators. Viral oncoproteins, including Tax, interfere with this regulation by increasing the expression of growth-promoting genes or by altering the function of cell cycle regulatory proteins. Tax can inhibit apoptosis by physically interacting with the p53 tumor suppressor protein (a cellular protein referred to as the "guardian of the genome"), effectively inactivating its transcriptional regulatory function. Tax also induces the expression of Bcl-X$_L$, a factor that inhibits apoptosis and represses the expression of Bax, a cellular gene involved in promoting apoptosis, thus effectively preventing cells from undergoing programmed cell death. Tax induces transition from the G_0/G_1 to S phase by altering activities of cyclin D, cyclin-dependent kinase (cdk) 4 and cdk 6, and the cdk inhibitor p21^{WAF} and p16^{INK4A}. Tax transcriptionally transactivates a subset of protooncogenes, which may also contribute to inappropriate progression through the cell cycle. Although the exact mechanisms of cell transformation by Tax have yet to be deciphered, dysregulation of cell cycle regulatory pathways is probably crucial in the transformation of T cells.

IV. ONCOGENESIS

Very little is known about the cellular progression events *in vivo* resulting in ATL. The molecular mechanisms by which HTLV transforms T lymphocytes *in vitro* may reflect the early polyclonal proliferation phase that occurs in humans. Subsequent selection processes result in the evolution of clones, which may ultimately develop into malignant cells (Fig. 1). Chromosomal abnormalities commonly exist in ATL cells, and the degree of cytogenetic aberration is often

TABLE II
Properties of ATL Cells and Cells Transformed
in Vitro by HTLV

ATL cells	*In vitro*-transformed T cells
CD4$^+$, CD25$^+$	CD4$^+$, CD25$^+$
No common viral integration site	No common viral integration site
Clonal	Oligoclonal
Little or no proviral gene expression	Proviral gene expression
20 to 30% display defective provirus	Provirus is replication competent
Difficult to propagate *in vitro*	Cultures in the absence of IL-2
Tumorigenic in SCID mice SCID	Decreased tumorigenicity in mice

related to the severity of the disease. HTLV transformation of T lymphocytes results in a pool of proliferating cells that are not oncogenic, but provide a population from which a malignant clone may subsequently arise. This extended process of selection may account for the long latent period between infection and manifestation of a tumor in HTLV disease. Tax may contribute to these later events as a result of its pleiotropic effects on proteins regulating mitosis, apoptosis, and DNA repair.

One of the distinguishing features of ATL cells is that although the viral genome is present as a provirus in all tumor cells, there is little or no viral gene expression in these cells. Paradoxically, if fresh ATL cells are placed into culture, viral gene expression can subsequently be detected, indicating that the block to expression is not a result of an intrinsic genetic defect in the virus genome. Lack of viral gene expression may relate to either a latent state of the virus or an immune selection against those cells that express recognizable viral antigens on their surface.

Pathogenesis and Animal Models

Development of animal models to study the initiation and progression of HTLV-1 infection and pathogenesis has aided in characterizing the virus and its ability to cause leukemia in humans. Transgenic mouse models containing either the HTLV-1 genome or the *tax* gene have been generated with limited success. Mice containing the *tax* gene expressed from the HTLV-1 LTR had a propensity for developing neurofibromatosis, a tumor of mesenchymal origin as well as an exocrinopathy resembling Sjogren's syndrome. More recently, the promotor targeting expression of *tax* to the mature T lymphocyte lineage using the human granzyme B promotor resulted in the development of large granular lymphocytic leukemia.

Severe combined immunodeficient (SCID) mice have been employed in the engraftment of ATL cells. Lymphoblastic lymphomas of human origin develop in SCID mice injected with PBL from ATL patients. The leukemic cells display the same genotype and phenotype as the original ATL clone from the patients, demonstrating expansion of the leukemic cells following injection into SCID mice. In contrast, cell lines transformed with HTLV in culture are less tumorigenic when inoculated into SCID mice, suggesting that inherent differences exist between ATL cells from patients and *in vitro* transformer cells.

Although HTLV-1 infection has been transmitted to rats and rabbits, no lymphoproliferative disorders occur in these systems. Infection in both of these animal models has been accomplished via inoculation of *in vitro*-infected T cells. Certain strains of rats infected with HTLV-1 have shown a propensity to develop a chronic progressive myeloneuropathy with paraparesis of the hind limbs, providing an *in vivo* model of HAM/TSP development. An elevated expression of cytokines was suggested to play a role in the neurotoxicity. Rabbits have been used to examine HTLV-1 and -2 viral replication and vaccine treatments. Most notably, rabbits infected with infectious molecular clones of HTLV-1 have been used to determine that HTLV-I ORFs I and II substantially contribute to viral infectivity and maintenance of viral load *in vivo*.

HTLV-1 was the first human retrovirus isolated and implicated as a likely causal agent for a form of human leukemia. Attempts to describe the pathogenic mechanism of HTLV in humans have been complicated by the extremely long latency between infection and development of disease. Further insights are needed to elucidate the pathogenic mechanisms of HTLV-1 and the selection events that occur *in vivo* after infection. Although initiation of the transformation process induced by HTLV can be mimicked *in vitro*, these events are probably more representative of early stages of infection in humans. The overall pathogenic mechanisms of HTLV and its role in human disease remain to be elucidated. The determinants of HTLV-1 that cause neurological disease rather than leukemia also remain to be defined. Genetic characteristics of individual hosts and the timing and route of infection may all prove to be important in the induction of HTLV disease.

See Also the Following Articles

ACUTE LYMPHOBLASTIC LEUKEMIA • CELL CYCLE CONTROL • CHRONIC LYMPHOCYTIC LEUKEMIA • HIV (HUMAN IMMUNODEFICIENCY VIRUS) • LYMPHOMA, NON-HODGKIN'S • RETROVIRUSES

Bibliography

Chen, I. S. Y., McLaughlin, J., Gasson, J. C., Clark, S. C., and Golde, D. W. (1983). Molecular characterization of genome of a novel human T-cell leukaemia virus. *Nature* **305,** 502–505.

Feuer, G., and Chen, I. S. Y. (1992). Mechanisms of human T-cell leukemia virus-induced leukemogenesis. *Biochim. Biophys. Acta* **1114,** 223–233.

Franchini, G. (1995). Molecular mechanisms of human T-cell leukemia/lymphotropic virus type-1 infection. *Blood* **86,** 3619–3639.

Gessain, A., Vernant, J. C., Maurs, L., Barin, F., Gout, O., Calender, A., and de The, G. (1985). Antibodies to human T-lymphotropic virus type-1 in patients with tropical spastic paraparesis. *Lancet* **ii,** 407–409.

Green, P. L., and Chen, I. S. Y. (1994). Molecular features of the human T-cell leukemia virus: Mechanisms of transformation and leukemogenicity. *In* "The Retroviridae" (J. A. Levy, eds.), Vol. 3, pp. 227–311. Plenum Press, New York.

Hinuma, Y., Nagata, K., Hanaoka, M., Nakai, M., Matsumoto, T., Kinoshita, K.-I., Shirakawa, S., and Miyoshi, I. (1981). Adult T-cell leukemia: Antigen in an ATL cell line and detection of antibodies to the antigen in human sera. *Proc. Natl. Acad. Sci. USA* **78,** 6476–6480.

Kalyanaraman, V. S., Sarngadharan, M. G., Robert-Guroff, M., Miyoshi, I., Blayney, D., Golde, D., and Gallo, R. C. (1982). A new subtype of human T-cell leukemia virus (HTLV-II) associated with a T-cell variant of hairy cell leukemia. *Science* **218,** 571–573.

Osame, M., Usuku, K., Izumo, S., Ijichi, N., Amitani, H., Igata, A., Matsumoto, M., and Tara, M. (1986). HTLV-I associated myelopathy, a new clinical entity. *Lancet* **i,** 1031–1032.

Poiesz, B. J., Ruscetti, F. W., Gazdar, A. F., Bunn, P. A., Minna, J. D., and Gallo, R. C. (1980). Detection and isolation of type C retrovirus particles from fresh and cultured lymphocytes of a patient with cutaneous T-cell lymphoma. *Proc. Natl. Acad. Sci. USA* **77,** 7415–7419.

Ratner, L. (1996). Animal models of HTLV-1 infection. *In* "Human T-Cell Lymphotropic Virus Type 1" (P. Holsberg, D. A. Hafler, eds.), p. 287. Wiley, Chichester.

Saxon, A., Stevens, R. H., and Golde, D. W. (1978). T-lymphocyte variant of hairy-cell leukemia. *Ann. Intern. Med.* **88,** 323–326.

Uchiyama, T., Yodoi, J., Sagawa, K., Takatsuki, K., and Uchino, H. (1977). Adult T-cell leukemia: Clinical and hematologic features of 16 cases. *Blood* **50,** 81–492.

Hyperthermia

Michael L. Freeman
Vanderbilt University School of Medicine

Kurt J. Henle
*University of Arkansas for Medical Sciences and
John L. McClellan Memorial Veterans Hospital*

Mark W. Dewhirst
Duke University Medical Center

GLOSSARY

differential scanning calorimetry A technique is used to detect thermotropic transitions.

heat shock proteins A group of highly conserved proteins that are transcriptionally induced by heat shock and other proteotoxic stresses. They play a role in protein folding, transport, assemby, and proteolysis.

protein denaturation A change in the spatial arrangement or configuration of a protein so that it approximates a disordered arrangement or random coil.

thermotolerance A transient increase in resistance to thermal damage.

This article discusses molecular mechanisms responsible for heat-induced cell death, hyperthermic radiosensitization, and thermochemotherapeutic drug sensitization. The proposed molecular mechanisms are related to tumor and tissue toxicity to provide an understanding for the rationale behind the use of hyperthermia as an adjuvant in cancer therapy.

I. TRANSITION TEMPERATURES FOR PROTEINS AND LIPIDS

Mammalian cells grow over narrow, species-specific temperature ranges. As temperatures exceed the maximum growth temperature, cell growth rapidly diminishes and cells die. The relationship between cell survival and temperature can be represented by dose–response curves; for convenience these are constructed by plotting the natural logarithm of surviving fraction versus time at the given temperature. Typically, survival curves for cell lines of human origin exhibit a "shoulder," followed by an exponential slope, a feature that may characterize cellular tolerance to reversible heat damage (Fig. 1). In contrast, survival curves characteristic of rodent cell lines are biphasic at temperatures below 42.5°C, suggesting that cells develop resistance in the course of mild hyperthermia. Above this temperature the survival curves also exhibit a shoulder and final exponential slope.

Reversible thermodynamic events are conveniently analyzed by Arrhenius plots and provide a measure of the activation energy required to accomplish an en-

ergy transition. Arrhenius analyses are also used for hyperthermic cell killing even though cell death is clearly not a reversible phenomenon. Over a limited temperature range of 43–57°C, the slope of the Arrhenius curve is linear, with a value of approximately 140 kcal/mol. This result has been interpreted to indicate that protein denaturation represents a "critical target" for cell killing. This hypothesis is supported by the knowledge that protein denaturation, proteolysis, and resynthesis are all temperature-dependent processes.

The concept of a "critical" temperature for cell killing implies that specific organelles or molecules can be identified that show critical temperature transitions, indicative of lethal events. A number of experimental techniques have been employed to identify such transitions, e.g., measurements of polarization anisotropy by spectrofluorometry, electron spin resonance studies of spin labels, and measurement of endothermic and exothermic transitions using differential scanning calorimetry (DSC). When applied to psychrotroph, mesophile, and thermophile bacteria, a good correlation was observed between the minimum growth temperature and the minimum temperature for detection of an irreversible transition for protein denaturation. In contrast, lipid phase transitions and DNA denaturation did not correlate with cell growth or cell survival.

Transition analysis applied to mammalian cells has focused on isolated mitochondria, microsomal membranes, nuclei, soluble cytosolic proteins, and plasma membranes, where irreversible transitions in protein structure occur near 40°C. The same threshold denaturation temperature was also obtained when whole cells were analyzed by DSC.

Membrane composition is also an important factor in protein stability. The fatty acid composition of cellular membranes can affect the temperature range over which organisms can grow and survive. Thermophilic bacteria grown over an increasingly higher temperature range modify their fatty acid membrane composition to increase the ratio of saturated to unsaturated fatty acids. Such changes affect lipid order and reduce viscosity. The transition from the gel state, dominant at low temperatures, into a liquid crystalline state at higher temperatures can be measured by both electron spin resonance and differential calorimetry

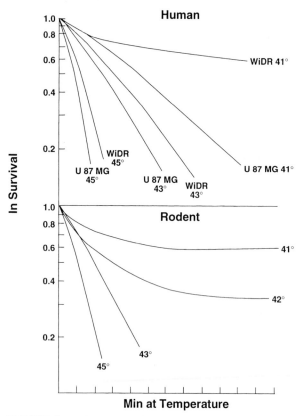

FIGURE 1   Cell survival curves for cell lines of human and rodent origin. Data illustrating the survival of human cell lines were adapted from E. P. Armour *et al.* (1993). Sensitivity of human cells to mild hyperthermia. *Cancer Res.* 53, 2740–2744.

as a reversible endothermic transition. This transition typically occurs at temperatures below the growth temperature and coincides with the minimum growth temperature, rather than the maximum one. Thus, the membrane can maintain a liquid crystalline phase over a wide range of temperatures. As the temperature is raised above the maximum growth temperature, a transition in viability occurs but without a corresponding transition in the parameters measuring lipid order or viscosity.

Both bacteria and mammalian cells can be grown in medium supplemented with either polyunsaturated or saturated fatty acids to modify their membrane lipid composition. Thermal sensitivity, inferred from cell survival curves, was found to increase with increasing membrane content of unsaturated fatty acids and increasing membrane fluidity. Conversely, increasing the saturated fatty acid content produced the opposite results. Although fluidity and membrane order changed as a function of temperature, no transition was observed in these parameters as the temperature was raised from a noncytotoxic to a cytotoxic one, as measured by fluorescence spectroscopy and electron spin resonance. These results have been interpreted to indicate that lipids, in and of themselves, are not a critical target. The effect of lipid composition on thermal sensitivity may reflect denaturation of membrane proteins whose stability is dependent on lipid composition, analogous to the influence that solvent composition has over water-soluble proteins.

II. IDENTIFICATION OF CRITICAL TARGETS IN MUTANT CELL LINES

Another approach to identifying the critical target(s) responsible for cellular lethality following heat shock is to compare heat-resistant and heat-sensitive cell lines. Human cell lines appear intrinsically more resistant to heat shock than cell lines of rodent origin. Examination of the thermal sensitivity of human (resistant)–hamster (sensitive) hybrid cells containing up to 20 human chromosomes indicates that heat resistance is a recessive trait. Heat-resistant variants, selected by repeated cycles of heat shock, have been produced in B16 melanoma, Chinese hamster, and RIF-I cells. Typically, resistant variants displayed nei-

ther ubiquitous changes in cholesterol nor phospholipid fatty acid content. In the RIF-1 system, an increase in the proportion of saturated fatty acids in the phospholipid fraction was found. Thus, changes in phosopholipid composition can occur, but this is not a universal phenotype in resistant cells.

The heat shock protein (Hsp; Section V) composition was also analyzed in variant cells. Hsp 70 was not increased in B16 variants; however, increased expression of Hsc 70 was found in Chinese hamster variants and a novel Hsp 70 was observed in the RIF-1 variant system. Because heat shock proteins act as molecular chaperones (Section V), their increased expression in heat-resistant variant cells is consistent with the critical target being protein denaturation.

III. THERMAL SENSITIZERS AND HEAT PROTECTORS

Numerous exogenous compounds have been evaluated as potential probes for identifying a critical target(s). Aliphatic alcohols and anesthetics such as procaine have long been recognized as thermal sensitizers and have been used at times to support the argument that lipids are a critical target. However, increased cellular heat sensitivity in the presence of alcohols can also support the concept of proteins as a primary target for heat damage because alcohols can alter protein stability, as measured by either solubility or DSC.

Other methods for modifying cellular sensitivity to temperatures below 43°C include intracellular acidification (sensitization), replacement of water with D_2O to decrease thermal sensitivity, and increased hydrostatic pressure. Inhibition of protein synthesis as a result of exposure to cycloheximide or puromycin also increases cellular heat resistance, but requires a cellular response that is not well understood. These observations can be interpreted in view of protein folding and unfolding data using DSC and high-resolution proton magnetic resonance spectroscopy that demonstrate protein denaturation to be critically affected by changes in pH, replacement of water with D_2O, and pressure. Furthermore, DSC of whole cells has directly demonstrated that inhibition of protein synthesis leads to increased thermal stability of cellular proteins.

An additional factor in the thermal stability of proteins is the osmolyte composition of cells. Osmolytes can be defined as low molecular weight molecules or solutes in a cell. Examples include amino acids, ions such as potassium and sodium, and polyhydric alcohols (polyols), such as glycerol. The composition and regulation of osmolytes during and following a hyperthermic exposure can affect the viability of a cell. Of special relevance is the intracellular ion concentration following heat shock. The consensus is that cells grown in suspension experience changes in potassium and sodium, but that cells grown in monolayer do not exhibit changes that correlate with loss of reproductive integrity. One rationale is that suspension cultures include both live and dead cells, whereas dead cells are often excluded from monolayer systems. However, heat shock does increase intracellular calcium ion concentrations possibly as a result of plasma membrane perturbations. These changes may be part of the signals involved in the induction of heat shock proteins and initiation of thermotolerance development. However, thermal sensitivity does not appear to be directly related to calcium homeostasis.

Many organisms that are subjected to wide temperature fluctuations use high concentrations of osmolytes to maintain protein stability. Glycine-based osmolytes are an example of molecules that may accumulate to high intracellular concentrations and increase the temperature at which proteins denature without affecting its function. Polyols, glycerol, glucose, and sucrose represent other examples. Exposure to exogenous polyols can result in sufficient intracellular accumulation to mediate decreased thermal sensitivity and increased thermal stability of cellular proteins. These studies support the concept that protein denaturation is a critical target for thermal cytotoxicity and form the mechanistic basis of thermotolerance in some yeast; however, mammalian cells appear to use other mechanisms for reducing intrinsic sensitivity in the thermotolerant state (see later). Finally, it may be wise to remember a quote by G.M. Hahn, "One always has to keep in the back of one's mind the possibility that many targets may be of approximately equal sensitivity, and that heat death is determined primarily by the environmental parameters of the particular experiment, (and) involves different organelles or macromolecules depending upon the particular cell line examined."

IV. THERMOTOLERANCE

One of the most intriguing aspects of a cell's response to heat shock is the development of thermotolerance (Fig. 2). In the broadest sense, thermotolerance is "any heat-induced increase in heat resistance, whether the shoulder or the terminal slope of the survival curve is affected." Thermotolerance is transient, i.e., most of the resistance decays in approximately 24 to 48 h and is distinct from intrinsic heat resistance. Tolerance is initiated by events that occur during the initial heat shock, or functionally equivalent stress such as ethanol, hypoxia/reoxygenation, glucose starvation, thiol oxidants (e.g., diamide), or heavy metals (e.g., arsenite). Development of thermotolerance requires an incubation at or near 37°C. Rodent cells can develop thermotolerance while incubated at temperatures as high as 42.9°C. This type of tolerance, which develops during continuous heating, is termed

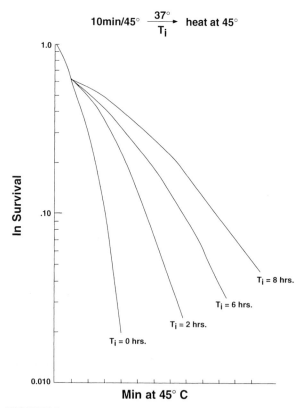

FIGURE 2 Development of thermotolerance. The figure illustrates the survival of cells exposed to a 10-min/45°C heat shock followed by incubation at 37°C for varying durations prior to being reheated at 45°C.

"chronic" thermotolerance and may be related to a heat-induced cell cycle delay in some cell lines. The expression of chronic tolerance may be the basis for the differential sensitivity observed between rodent and human cells at temperatures between 39 and 42°C.

The expression of thermotolerance appears to be ubiquitous and protects a diverse number of biochemical and cellular functions that are normally heat sensitive. Examples include Na^+,K^+-ATPase activity, cytoskeletal organization, RNA synthesis, RNA processing, protein synthesis, and cell growth. Tolerance-induced resistance is also observed at the level of protein denaturation, as demonstrated by DSC analysis; similarly, the expression of thermotolerance affects the accumulation and removal of proteins onto the nuclear matrix. In the latter case, heat-denatured proteins, which coisolate with the nuclear matrix, are removed at a faster rate in tolerant cells. The expression of thermotolerance also protects cells from protein denaturation produced by nonheat shock stresses, such as oxidation stress. Oxidation of protein thiols results in improper disulfide bond formation, protein denaturation, and aggregation. Thermotolerant cells exhibit less oxidation-induced protein denaturation.

Experimental evidence suggests that protein denaturation can initiate thermotolerance development. Improper formation of protein disulfides represents one specific example where incorrectly formed protein disulfides destabilize cellular proteins to thermal denaturation. Improper disulfides activate the heat shock transcription factor and induce heat shock transcription and Hsp synthesis with a concomitant development of thermotolerance. Finally, thermotolerance decreases the cytotoxicity produced by the oxidation of protein thiols.

The development of thermotolerance normally requires cellular protein synthesis. Mammalian cells can also express a protein synthesis-independent form of tolerance. However, the contribution of the synthesis-independent form of tolerance diminishes as the temperature is increased. These results are interpreted to indicate the induction of two separate thermotolerant states. The requirement for protein synthesis in the development of thermotolerance is emphasized in studies with cells defective in leucyl-tRNA synthetase activity. Synthetase activity is inhibited when temperatures exceed 39°C in these mutants and protein synthesis is arrested; thus, incubation at nonpermissive temperatures results in protein synthesis inhibition. If wild-type and mutant cells are exposed to an acute heat shock (e.g., 10 min at 45°C) and then incubated at a nonpermissive temperature (e.g., 40°C), wild-type cells will exhibit thermotolerance, but mutant cells will not. Mutant cells, however, develop thermotolerance when incubated at a permissive temperature of 34°C.

An interesting phenomenon, termed step-down heating, occurs in all types of cells when they are exposed to an acute heat shock (e.g., 45°C for 10 min) and then immediately incubated at a lower, but still hyperthermic temperature (e.g., 42°C). This treatment serves to reduce the development of thermotolerance while increasing the rate of cell killing produced by the second, lower temperature (in this case the 42°C heat shock). This phenomenon is not fully understood. At the subcellular level it is marked by selective inhibition of Hsp synthesis and profound inhibition of cellular protein glycosylation (see later).

The development of thermotolerance probably involves processes of ubiquitination. Ubiquitin has been shown to be a heat shock protein. Cells normally respond to the presence of denatured proteins by a covalent attachment of ubiquitin to N-terminal and lysine amino groups. This targets the protein for proteolysis. Cellular ubiquitin is maintained in pools of free and conjugated forms. The conjugated form may be important for chromatin organization and regulation. In yeast, thermal sensitivity is increased by deletion of a ubiquitin gene. During hyperthermic treatment, free ubiquitin levels fall in ubiquitin-deficient mutants, but not in wild-type cells. In mammalian cells, mildly lethal heating also results in decreased levels of free ubiquitin and its conversion into high molecular weight conjugates. These effects are reversible. However, they are irreversible following a lethal heat shock. The ts85 cell line is a temperature-sensitive mutant derived from FM3A mouse cells that is defective in ubiquitination of protein at temperatures above 39°C. This mutant cell line is also more heat-sensitive compared to wild-type cells. If mutant cells are exposed to an acute heat shock and then incubated at a nonpermissive temperature, such as 39°C, thermotolerance fails to develop, in contrast to wild-type cells. However, neither thermotolerance nor intrinsic heat sensitivity correlates with the rate, or the extent of protein degradation. Taken together, these results indicate that ubiquitin metabolism is an important factor in heat killing and in the development of thermotolerance, but its underlying mechanism is not well understood.

Trehalose (α-D-glucopyranosyl α-D-glucopyranoside) is a nonreducing disaccharide found in many organisms, including bacteria, fungi, nematodes, and plants. Trehalose is synthesized from UDP glucose and glucose-6-phosphate in a two-step reaction involving trehalose-6-phosphate synthase/phosphatase complex. Hydrolysis of trehalose occurs via enyzmes known as trehalases located in vacuoles and the cytosol. In the yeast *Saccharomyes cerevisiae*, the genes that code for the subunits that compose the trehalose-6-phosphate synthase/phosphatase complex have been cloned. These genes contain canonical heat shock elements and are induced by heat shock. Furthermore, heat shock increases the activity of the trehalose-6-phosphate synthase/phosphatase complex and decreases the activity of the cytosol trehalase. The end result is that heat shock results in a rapid increase in trehalose. The accumulation of trehalose produces significant thermal protection because it acts as an osmolyte. That is, high concentrations increase the thermal stability of proteins, as well as prevent heat-induced protein aggregation, thereby increasing cell survival.

Selectively enhanced protein glycosylation appears to be another feature associated with thermotolerance in possibly all mammalian cells. A major 50-kDa heat-induced glycoprotein, GP50, correlates with the expression of thermotolerance in many cell lines. GP50 has been shown to be identical to a retinoic acid-inducible gene product, J6, but its function is not known. In many cell lines, a 62-kDa glycoprotein has been shown to correlate with cellular heat resistance. Stress-inducible glycopeptides are not glycosylated forms of "classical" Hsps and appear in response to a variety of stress conditions. During the development of thermotolerance, the activity of specific glycosyltransferases is known to increase, e.g., *N*-acetylgalactosaminyltransferase. Chinese hamster variant cell lines, which are thermotolerant deficient,

exhibit a reduction in activation of glycosyltransferase activity and a reduction of labeling of the 50-kDa polypeptide. Furthermore, cellular protein glycosylation rates appear to correlate with basal heat resistance. These results suggest that protein glycosylation is probably an important determinant or predictor of cellular heat sensitivity. Functions of the stress-inducible glycopeptides may be related to the observation that glycosylation can enhance protein folding at hyperthermic temperatures because it prevents aggregation of denatured proteins and may regulate their interactions with Hsp chaperones.

V. HEAT SHOCK PROTEINS

Heat shock and many other stresses that cause protein denaturation can induce the synthesis of a set of proteins known as heat shock proteins. These proteins are highly conserved and rapidly induced. Examples of Hsp-inducing stress conditions include heat, amino acid analogs, transition heavy metals, oxidants, inflammation, and ischemia/reoxygenation. Together with glucose-regulated proteins, heat shock proteins comprise a family of stress proteins that function as chaperones. Chaperones "bind to and stabilize an otherwise unstable conformer of another protein and, by controlled binding and release of the substrate protein, facilitates its correct fate." The binding of denatured proteins to a chaperone is ATP independent, whereas release is ATP hydrolysis dependent. Binding and release of unfolded or denatured proteins to chaperones may occur multiple times before a stable conformation is established. This process is governed by several chaperones interacting with each other and by other cytosolic factors that regulate ATP binding and hydrolysis.

Denaturation of protein induces the synthesis of heat shock proteins. This has been directly demonstrated by microinjection of heat denaturation and chemically modified proteins. Induction is regulated by the binding of a protein known as heat shock transcription factor 1 (HSF1) to a DNA sequence, termed the heat shock element (HSE). The HSE is composed of adjoining 5-bp sequences, nGAAn. The number of these sequences is variable (there must be a minimum of two) and can appear in alternating orientations (head to head or tail to tail). Hsp 90, together with a multichaperone complex, binds monomers of Hsf1, keeping them in a non-DNA-binding form. Denatured proteins are thought to compete with Hsf1 for Hsp 90 binding. Because the affinity of Hsp 90 for denatured protein exceeds the affinity for Hsf1, Hsp 90 binds the destabilized protein and allows Hsf1 to undergo three-stranded α-helical coiled coil oligomerization resulting in DNA-binding activity. Phosphorylation and transcriptional activation follow. Hsf1 phosphorylation is complex. Phosphorylation of Ser 230 is required for stress-induced transcriptional activity. The molar ratio between positive-acting phosphorylation (Ser 230) events and phosphorylation events (Ser 303, 307, 363) that repress activity determines the magnitude of Hsf1 transcriptional activity.

Heat shock proteins are classified by subunit size determined by SDS–PAGE. Mammalian proteins include the Hsp 110, 90, the 70 family, Hsp60, 47, 40, 27, and ubiquitin. Hsp 110 exhibits significant chaperone activity and tumor vaccine potential. Yeast also contain a high molecular weight stress protein, Hsp 104. Hsp 104 exhibits ATPase activity and is homologous to ClpA/ClpB proteins, which display similar nucleotide-binding domains. In *Escherichia coli*, ClpA regulates ClpP protease activity. Expression of Hsp 104 is very important for the development of thermotolerance. Mutant yeast strains lacking Hsp 104 develop only a limited amount of tolerance. For example, wild type and mutant cells were shifted from 25 to 37°C for 30 min and then to 50°C, and the time required to reduce survival to 1% was determined. Thirty minutes at 50°C was required for wild-type cells, but only 10 min at 50°C was required for cells lacking Hsp 104. Survival was reduced to 1% in 2 min if either mutant or wild-type cells were shifted from 25°C directly to 50°C. A very important finding is that the Hsp 70 family (discussed later) cooperates with Hsp 104 in the development of tolerance. There are eight Hsp 70 associated genes in *Saccharomyces cerevisiae* divided into four groupings (SSA to SSD). The development of thermotolerance is unaffected in cells containing wild-type Hsp 104, but carry deletions in SSA1, SSA3, and SSA4. Site-directed mutagenesis of Hsp 104 in these cells decreases the development of thermotolerance to levels less than that displayed by cells containing wild-type SSA genes,

but a mutated Hsp 104. Further studies have shown that Hsp 104 is involved in the recovery of mRNA splicing following its disruption by heat shock.

Hsp 90 participates in the regulation of steroid receptor binding and also binds casein kinase II. Hsp90 exhibits ATPase activity, is found in the cytosol, and can be highly phosphorylated. The chaperone function of Hsp 90 is cooperative in nature and can be isolated from complexes with Hsp 70 and p59 (an immunophilin).

The Hsp 70 family consists of Hsp 70 (A), Hsp 70 (B), Hsc 70, the glucose-regulated protein, Grp 78, otherwise known as BIP, and Grp 75. In unstressed cells, Hsc 70 and Hsp 70 bind to newly synthesized proteins and assist in their folding. Hsp 70 can also participate in posttranslational membrane translocation. Hsp 70 proteins protect the mRNA splicing apparatus from heat shock disruption and keep proteins from heat-induced denaturation and/or aggregation. Enhanced synthesis of Hsp 70 is rapidly observed following heat shock. The majority of Hsp 70 is found in the nucleus, where it is associated with the nucleolus. Hsp/Hsc70 is thought to play an important role in protein synthesis-dependent thermotolerance. A strong correlation is found between synthesis and the nucleolus association of Hsp/Hsc 70 and the development or decay of thermotolerance. With few exceptions, nonheat stresses that initiate the development of thermotolerance also induce enhanced expression of Hsp/Hsc 70. Evidence that thermal sensitivity is dependent, at least in part, on the intracellular concentration of Hsp 70 was acquired by insertion of the heat shock element into a plasmid that was then transfected into Chinese hamster cells. The copy number was then elevated about 20,000-fold using methotrexate selection. The heat-induced expression of Hsp 70 was reduced 90% in cells containing elevated copy numbers of heat shock elements that competed for binding with HSF. As a result, cellular heat sensitivity was increased dramatically. Microinjection of affinity-purified monoclonal antibodies to Hsp 70 immediately prior to a heat shock inhibited the translocation of Hsp 70 into the nucleus and converted a nonlethal heat shock into a lethal one. Specific inhibition of Hsp 70 expression was accomplished by transforming cells with plasmids carrying an antisense Hsp 70 gene. In these cells, reduced Hsp 70 expression also increased cellular heat sensitivity, possibly through diminished development of thermotolerance. Conversely, the stable transfection and overexpression of Hsp 70 confer higher levels of heat resistance, although the overexpression of Hsp 70 caused a concomitant overexpression of GP62 (see earlier discussion) as well.

Hsp 60 proteins are termed chaperonins. As a functional unit, they form a 14 subunit double toroid. In mammalian cells, Hsp 60 is located in the mitochondria and functions in conjunction with Hsp 10, which forms a seven subunit ring. The ring attaches to the toroid to promote folding in an ATP-dependent fashion. Protein folding in the central toroid cavity may require several cycles after which the correctly folded protein and the recycling chaperonins separate.

Hsp 27 is related to the α-crystallin proteins and may also participate in the development of thermotolerance. Heat-resistant variants were isolated, characterized, and found to exhibit increased levels of Hsp 27 and altered phosphorylation profiles when compared to wild-type cells. Transfection and stable expression of Hsp 27 into rodent cells resulted in expression of a thermoresistant phenotype. However, concomitant cellular adjustment, such as the selectively increased protein glycosylation in HSP70-transfected cells (see earlier discussion), cannot be ruled out.

VI. MODES OF CELL DEATH AND CELL CYCLE EFFECTS

It is difficult to identify the cause of heat-mediated cytotoxicity, given the pleiotropic cellular effects produced by hyperthermia. The cell killing model of Roti Roti and Laszlo tries to incorporate many of these effects. The model is composed of five steps: (1) disruption of the plasma membrane and loss of cytoskeleton attachment points; (2) collapse of the cytoskeleton; (3) absorption of protein onto the nuclear matrix; (4) damage to critical nuclear structures, e.g., nucleolus; and (5) damage to chromatin. The rate-limiting step appears to be step 3, the absorption of protein onto the nucleus. Accumulation of protein occurs immediately after heating, and the amount of protein accumulated appears to be directly related to

thermal dose and correlates with the degree of cell killing. Protein accumulation is the result of a thermal alteration in nuclear protein solubility and leads to the migration of proteins into the nuclear matrix from the cytoplasm. Factors such as cell type, cell cycle position, and the signals produced from steps 4 and 5 apparently trigger the specific mode of cell death (i.e., intermitotic or apoptosis).

Cell survival is dependent both on the rate and on the amount of energy absorbed; decreasing the rate of heating generally promotes higher survival. This observation may be important for understanding heat-induced cell cycle effects. If Chinese hamster cells, synchronized in G_1, are exposed to a hyperthermic treatment, which kills a total of 50% of the cells, the majority of the cells that die will enter mitosis, divide, and then undergo multinucleation as a result of multipolar spindles caused by altered pericentriolar material. The remainder of the cells die a division-independent death in either G_1 or S phase. In contrast, the division-independent mode of cell death dominates if G_1 phase Chinese hamster cells are exposed to hyperthermic doses, which kill 90% or more of the cells. These results suggest that there are two modes of cell death and that their expression depends on the degree of cell killing caused by the administered thermal dose. Not all cell lines exhibit both modes of cell death. Mouse 10TI/2 cells only exhibit division-independent cell death. Further complicating the discussion of cell cycle effects is the fact that cells heated in S phase are highly sensitive and die by a distinct mechanism apparently related to the formation of chromosome aberrations. G_1 cells, in contrast, are the most heat-resistant cells in the cycle with an uncertain mode of cell death.

Analysis of other end points supports the argument that thermal dose and dose rate are important to the expression of heat damage. Lipid peroxidation is a consequence of oxidative damage to cellular membranes and has been observed in systems such as VX2 tumors grown in rabbits, C3H tumors grown in mice, perfused livers, and in the organs of rats or dogs exposed to hyperthermia. Peroxidation does not appear to occur until after a threshold dose is exceeded. The oxidative damage, which causes lipid breakdown, is at least partially the result of superoxide and hydrogen peroxide generation. These damaging species have been detected directly in such diverse systems as *Dictyostelium discoideum* and indirectly in rat lung tissue or by using GSSG formation as an index of oxidation damage in perfused rat liver. The reduced form of glutathione, GSH, is used as a cofactor to reduce and detoxify peroxides. Depletion of the mitochondrial GSH pool increases thermal sensitivity, but only if the hyperthermic temperature remains below 43°C. The interpretation of this observation is generally focused on oxidants generated in the mitochondria that are no longer detoxified. During hyperthermic treatment, protein denaturation is therefore increased as a result of oxidant attack. The most susceptible proteins at that time are newly synthesized proteins. Survival is independent of GSH concentration at higher temperatures where an acute heat shock inhibits protein synthesis and mitochrondrial function.

Conversely, acute high-temperature heating causes another phenomenon, "prompt" glycosylation that is not visible at lower temperatures. This effect leads to the selective glycosylation of a mature 67-kDa protein, recently identified as calreticulin. The functional significance of this effect is not yet known.

VII. EXPRESSION OF THERMAL DAMAGE IN NORMAL AND TUMOR TISSUE

Initial studies of the *in vivo* heat response of tumors indicated that transplantable rodent tumors were much more sensitive to hyperthermia than surrounding normal tissue. This difference in heat sensitivity is now believed to be largely the result of tumor physiology: e.g., differences in microvascular response, intratumor pH, and a deficient nutrient supply. Nutrient availability and pH may vary within the tumor volume as a result of improper vascularization, hypoxic foci, and increased glycolysis. Cells that are in an acidic environment (pH ≤ 7.0) or under nutrient-deprived conditions generally exhibit increased thermal sensitivity; oxygen per se may be one of the few exempt nutrients.

Microvasculature can affect heated tumor sensitivity in a number of ways. The perfusion rate and volume can affect the tissue temperature distribution: rapid blood flow can remove heat, whereas stasis cou-

pled with increasing energy input from microwave heating, for example, can lead to increasing temperatures. During the initial portion of a heat treatment, blood flow usually increases. This is observed in normal tissues, and often to a lesser extent in tumor tissues where the vasculature tends to be fully dilated. The increase in perfusion is both temperature and duration dependent. Once a critical thermal dose has been surpassed, blood flow deceases and can stop altogether with wide-spread thrombos formation and endothelial injury. The critical dose for statis is tissue specific and appears to be lower for tumor tissues compared to normal ones, reflecting a typically fragile tumor vasculature. The lower tumor blood flow may also be related to a high interstitial tumor tissue pressure. These observations may explain why large tumors generally exhibit increased thermal sensitivity when compared to smaller tumors of the same histology. As for cells in culture, the empirical relationship between temperature and heating time states that for every 1°C rise in temperature, a twofold reduction in heating time is required to produce the same degree of microvascular damage. This is true for both tumor and normal tissue, even though normal tissues typically exhibit a higher flow rate than tumors at a given temperature and therefore are more resistant to heating.

In normal rodent tissues (e.g., skin, cartilage, small intestine, kidney, and spinal cord), hyperthermia can cause a typical inflammatory response: rapid redness and swelling. The severity of erythema is dependent on thermal dose, where intense hyperthermia will obviously cause burns. Rapid expression of thermal damage in normal tissues may be the result of induction of apoptosis and is reduced by the development of thermotolerance; conversely, step-down heating increases the expression of damage. These findings highlight parallel features of thermal injury expression *in vivo* in normal tissues, in tumor tissues, and in culture experiments *in vitro* and provide a link with molecular interpretations of how hyperthermia produces cytotoxicity at the subcellular level.

One important reservation to consider is the potential difference in tumor physiology between rodent and human tumors, where the latter appear to be more heat resistant than the former. Data obtained from human tumors indicate that flow rates in these spontaneous, generally slow-growing tumors may be similar to that of normal liver, heart, or brain tissues. Further, there appears to be considerable heterogeneity within tumors. Thus, tumor size is not necessarily an indicator of the perfusion flow rate. Unlike rapidly growing transplantable rodent tumors, blood flow in human cancers does not necessarily decrease during clinical hyperthermia treatments.

VIII. THERMAL RADIOSENSITIZATION

The biological rationale for using hyperthermia as an adjuvant to radiation therapy relates to the fact that radioresistant cells are sensitive to hyperthermia and that heat shock has the characteristics of an excellent radiosensitizer. Sensitization is defined as an increase in the slope of the radiation dose–response curve. As discussed later, the increased slope of the radiation cell survival curve is the result of inhibition of DNA repair and not a consequence of increased formation of DNA damage. The most effective radiosensitization occurs when hyperthermia is administered simultaneously with X-irradiation. Separating the two modalities in time diminishes the degree of radiosensitization. The question of whether heat should precede or follow irradiation appears to depend on the cell and tissue type, as well as the specific temperature or thermal dose. This reflects the differences in molecular repair processes and their sensitivity to hyperthermia. It is commonly assumed that DNA double strand breaks represent potentially lethal lesions; if converted into chromosomal aberrations, these breaks become lethal lesions. Thus, formation of aberrations is the result of either unrepaired or misrepaired double strand breaks. Cytotoxic heat shock can result in unrepaired lesions, whereas exposure to hyperthermic temperatures, at or below 42°C following irradiation, can increase misrepair of DNA strand break rejoining, leading to an enhancement in the formation of chromosome aberrations.

Hyperthermia can inhibit the repair of sublethal and potentially lethal radiation damage, as measured by cell survival experiments. However, hyperthermia does not increase the radiation sensitivity of high LET particles, such as carbon or helium. This can be explained by the fact that high LET particles are so densely ionizing that damage produced is generally not repairable. These experiments are consistent with the concept that hyperthermia can inhibit DNA repair.

Hyperthermic temperatures below 45°C do not produce single or double strand DNA breaks, do not cause depurination, or do not affect nucleosome structure. At higher temperatures, a small degree of DNA damage can be observed. In S-phase cells, heat shock inhibits the initiation of replicons, reduces the rate of replication fork displacement, and increases the amount of single-stranded DNA in the replicating regions. Furthermore, hyperthermic treatment does not appear to increase radiation-induced thymine base damage or single or double strand DNA break formation. However, a major effect of hyperthermia is the inhibition of DNA repair. Heat shock can inhibit the rejoining of radiation-induced single and double strand breaks and inhibit excision of radiation-induced thymine base damage. The inhibition of DNA repair produced by heat shock appears to be the result of pleiotropic effects related to protein denaturation. Heat has also been shown to inhibit DNA polymerase activities, in particular, that of polymerase β. Heat further caused the accumulation of nonhistone proteins in nuclei and in the nuclear matrix, which appears to inhibit repair enzyme access to sites of DNA damage via decreased accessibility of enzyme to substrate. The end result of inhibition of repair of radiation-induced DNA damage is an increase in chromosomal aberrations. Whether cells are heated and irradiated in G_1, S phase, or in mitosis, a plot of the log survival versus aberration frequency always yields a straight line with the D_o value equal to about one aberration per cell, suggesting these events to be causally related to cell killing.

Work with a radiation-sensitive mutant cell line, xrs-5, which is deficient in rejoining radiation-induced DNA strand breaks, confirms the hypothesis that hyperthermia acts mainly by inhibiting repair. This cell line repairs radiation induced single strand breaks equally as well as the parental Chinese hamster ovary (CHO) line. However, xrs-5 cells are deficient in the repair of DNA double strand breaks and in the repair of chromosomal breaks. It should be pointed out, however, that there is not 100% inhibition; residual activity remains around 40%. A 45.5°C heat shock produced significant radiosensitization in CHO cells, but little or none in xrs-5 cells measured within the first decade of cell survival. The 45.5°C heat shock did not affect the number of radiation-induced single or double strand breaks that were formed per Gy per dalton in either cell line. Heat shock inhibited rejoining of DNA single strand breaks to a greater extent in xrs-5 compared to CHO cells. These observations indicate that repair of single strand DNA breaks does not significantly contribute to cell lethality. The important point is that the cell line deficient in double strand break rejoining did not exhibit hyperthermic radiosensitization, i.e., double strand break rejoining is a prerequisite for thermal radiosensitization.

The question concerning the effect of thermotolerance development on radiosensitization produced by a heat shock remains to be settled. At least 14 studies have been undertaken and no clear-cut answer has evolved. One possibility is that equitoxic heat doses yield equal degrees of radiosensitization; however, parameters, such as the radiation dose rate and the thermal dose rate, may well affect the biological outcome. For example, long duration mild hyperthermia (e.g., 41°C for up to 24 h) can induce thermotolerance, but the expression of tolerance does not diminish the degree of radiosensitization produced by the mild hyperthermic exposure (Table I).

TABLE I
Analysis of Radiation Therapy (RT)
versus RT plus Hyperthermia

End point	RT[a] (%)	RT + heat[b] (%)
Complete response	41	83
Partial response	41	6
Progressive disease	18	11
5-year actuarial probability of node control	24	69
5-year actuarial survival	0	53

[a]Radiation therapy alone, data taken from Valdagni and Amichetti (1994).

[b]Radiation therapy plus hyperthermia, data taken from Valdagni and Amichetti (1994).

IX. PHASE III CLINICAL TRIAL RESULTS

During the period from 1970 to 1984, the results of several phase I/II trials were published that indicated the potential for hyperthermia to increase the radiation response of superficially accessible tumors. Of particular interest was the series of studies that compared responses of matched lesions. Although there was some variation from one study to the next, the overall improvement in response averaged a factor of two over what was achieved with radiation alone. Largely based on these results, the Radiation Oncology Therapy Group initiated a phase III trial in 1981 (RTOG 81-04) that compared radiation alone to the combination of radiation therapy and hyperthermia. Unfortunately, the results of that trial were negative. A second phase III trial testing interstitial radiation therapy (brachytherapy) ± hyperthermia was also negative. Consequently, interest in the modality subsequently waned, particularly in the United States. Socioeconomic factors contributed to the loss of interest as well. Primarily this related to commercial marketing and use of hyperthermia devices that were not designed well enough to heat most tumors. The failure of RTOG 8104 to show a therapeutic advantage for hyperthermia may have been related to substantial problems with quality assurance. This issue was addressed in later publications by the RTOG. In 1984 the European Society of Hyperthermic Oncology (ESHO) recognized the limitations of the RTOG trial and adopted new quality assurance procedures that are quite similar to those now recommended by the RTOG. These quality assurance guidelines were used in the conduct of several subsequent phase III trials, all of which showed a therapeutic advantage for the use of hyperthermia in combination with radiation therapy, as compared with the use of radiation therapy alone. Positive trials have been reported for neck nodes from head and neck cancer and chest wall recurrences of breast cancer, melanoma, and esophagus. A North American phase III trial for previously untreated high-grade gliomas showed a survival advantage for adjuvant hyperthermia when combined with brachytherapy as compared with brachytherapy alone. The most recent study, from a cooperative group in Holland, demonstrated a survival benefit, as well as improved local control for carcinoma of the cervix treated with thermoradiotherapy compared with radiotherapy alone. Other pelvic disease sites treated in that trial were not shown to benefit from the combination treatment.

The outlook for application of hyperthermia for treatment of locally advanced diseases has never looked brighter. At this time, additional international phase III studies are underway, sponsored by the EORTC for soft tissue sarcomas and by ESHO for locally advanced colorectal cancer. In addition, a follow-up cervix trial is under development by a multinational consortium to compare chemothermoradiotherapy to chemoradiotherapy, as the combination of drugs and radiation is now considered standard therapy for carcinoma of the cervix.

The primary challenge facing the development of hyperthermia for more broad-based use in oncology is the difficulty of doing it. This is a multifactorial problem that starts with the lack of a noninvasive thermometry system. Systems are under development to use magnetic resonance imaging for noninvasive thermometry, and some studies have been done in humans to validate this method already. Once such systems are established, it will become much easier to use this technology and it will more likely be adopted by others.

X. THERMAL CHEMOSENSITIZATION

Thermochemotherapy represents an exciting research area. The cytotoxicity of several chemotherapeutic drugs has been shown to increase during hyperthermic treatment (e.g., nitrosoureas, melphalan, cisplatinum complexes, cyclophosphamide, bleomycin, and adriamycin). The molecular mechanisms responsible for increased cytotoxicity depend on the specific drug in question. However, some generalizations can be applied. Heat has been shown to increase DNA damage produced by specific chemotherapeutic drugs, inhibit the repair of DNA lesions, and inhibit drug efflux. It also has been shown to increase drug uptake and increase drug influx. In some cases, hyperthermia is effective for reversing multidrug resistance, which is a major treatment complication. Additional excit-

ing innovations have been developed in the past few years, including the purging of bone marrow for selective tumor cell killing, encapsulating anticancer drugs in temperature-sensitive liposomes, treating sarcomas and melanoma with hyperthermic isolated perfusion, combined with the infusion of tumor necrosis factor α, and treating benign prostate hypertrophy by transurethral thermotherapy. Biological mechanisms underlying some of these agents may be closely related to the cellular stress response, as evidenced by the observation that exposure to some drugs, e.g., adriamycin, can induce the development of thermotolerance. Conversely, the expression of thermotolerance can inhibit drug uptake.

In summary, hyperthermia represents an exciting potential for adjuvant treatment of cancer. Clinical hyperthermia can be used to help overcome radiation and drug resistance. The biology of hyperthermia has the potential for applications in all areas of medicine and biotechnology and favors continued research for improving its combination with conventional cancer treatment modalities.

See Also the Following Articles

CELL CYCLE CONTROL • HYPOXIA AND DRUG RESISTANCE • MOLECULAR ASPECTS OF RADIATION BIOLOGY

Bibliography

Hahn, G. M. (1982) "Hyperthermia and Cancer." Plenum Press, New York
Hendrick, J. P., and Ulrich, Hartl, F. (1993). Molecular chaperone functions of heat shock proteins. *Annu. Rev. Biochem.* **62,** 349.
Henle, K. J. (ed.) (1987). "Thermotolerance," Vols. I and II. CRC Press, Boca Raton, FL.
Holmberg, C. I., Hietakangas, V., Mikhailov, A., Rantanen, J. O., Kallio, M., Meinander, A., Hellman, J., Morrice, N., MacKintosh, C., Morimoto, R. I., Eriksson, J. E., and Sistonen, L. (2001). Phosphorylation of serine 230 promotes inducible transcriptional activity of heat shock factor 1. *EMBO J.* **20,** 3800.
Kampinga, H. H., and Dikomey, E. (2001). Hyperthermic radiosensitization: Mode of action and clinical relevance. *Inter. J. Radiat. Biol.* **77,** 399.
Morimoto, R. I., Tissieres, A., and Georgopoulos, C. (eds.) (1990). "Stress Proteins in Biology and Medicine," Cold Springs Harbor Laboratory Press, Cold Spring Harbor, NY.

Nielson, O. S., Horsman, M., and Overgaard, J. (2001). A future for hyperthermia in cancer treatment? *Eur. J. Cancer* **37,** 1587.

Peters, W. A., Liu, P. Y., Barrett, R. J., Stock, R. J., Monk, B. J., Berek, J. S., Souhami, L., Grigsby, P., Gordon, W., Jr., and Alberts, D. S. (2000). Concurrent chemotherapy and pelvic radiation therapy compared with pelvic radiation therapy alone as adjuvant therapy after radical surgery in high-risk early-stage cancer of the cervix. *J. Clin. Oncol.* **18,** 1606.

Pirkkala, L., Nykanen, P., and Sistonen, L. (2001). Roles of the heat shock transcription factors in regulation of the heat shock response and beyond. *FASEB J.* **15,** 1118.

Urano, M., and Douple, E. (eds.) (1988). "Hyperthermia and Oncology," Vols. 1 and 2. VSP BV, Utrecht, The Netherlands.

van der Zee, J., Gonzalez Gonzalez, D., van Rhoon, G. C., van Dijk, J. D., van Putten, W. L., and Hart, A. A. (2001). Comparison of radiotherapy alone with radiotherapy plus hyperthermia in locally advanced pelvic tumours: A prospective, randomised, multicentre trial. *Dutch Deep Hyperthermia Group* **355,** 1119.

Zou, J., Guo, Y., Guettouche, T., Smith, D. F., and Voellmy, R. E. (1998). Repression of heat shock transcription factor HSF1 activation by HSP90 (HSP90 complex) that forms a stress-sensitive complex with HSF1. *Cell* **94,** 471.

Hypoxia and Drug Resistance

Sara Rockwell
Yale University School of Medicine

<table>
<tr><td>

I. Microenvironmental Heterogeneity in Solid Tumors
II. Mechanisms of Hypoxia-Induced Drug Resistance
III. Oxygen as a Chemical Sensitizer
IV. Direct Effects of pH on Drug Resistance
V. Physiologic Effects of Adverse Environments
VI. Distribution of Drugs within Solid Tumors
VII. Genetic Changes Induced in Tumor Cells by Hypoxia
VIII. Implications of Microenvironmentally Induced Drug Resistance

</td></tr>
</table>

GLOSSARY

angiogenesis The formation of new blood vessels.

hypoxia A lack of adequate concentrations of oxygen. Oxygen tensions in healthy normal tissues are generally above 20 torr; hypoxic regions in solid tumors frequently have oxygen tensions as low as 1 torr, or may have no measurable oxygen.

hypoxic fraction The proportion of viable tumor cells that are hypoxic.

microenvironment The extracellular environment in a very small region of a solid tumor. Cells in different areas of solid tumors will have markedly different microenvironments.

pH Measurement of the hydrogen ion concentration. Healthy tissues generally have a pH of about 7.2–7.4; the pH in tumors tends to be lower (more acidic).

stress response A defined and consistent set of changes that occur in the physiology of cells exposed to potentially toxic environmental factors.

Solid tumors have abnormal, deficient vascular beds and lymphatics. As a result, blood flow within these malignancies is inadequate and chaotic, and the cancers contain regions that are chronically or transiently exposed to severe hypoxia, low pH, and nutrient deprivation. Cells in these unperfused, unphysiologic regions become resistant to drugs and other therapeutic modalities. This resistance reflects several different mechanisms and processes, some of which result in transient resistance that is lost when the region is reperfused and others of which reflect the induction of permanent genetic alterations that have led to the development of drug-resistant tumor cell populations. This article discusses the nature of the microenvironmental deficits in solid tumors, the mechanisms by which these deficits induce drug resistance, and the implications of environmentally induced drug resistance for cancer therapy.

I. MICROENVIRONMENTAL HETEROGENEITY IN SOLID TUMORS

A. Causes

The healthy normal tissues of the body are supported by a rich bed of blood vessels and lymphatics that bathe the cells continually, providing oxygen and nutrients and removing toxic metabolites. No cell in these tissues is more than a few cells away from a capillary. Precise homeostatic control mechanisms continually adjust the perfusion of each area of tissue to maintain the blood flow needed to provide appropriate oxygen tensions, physiologic pH, and adequate levels of glucose and other critical nutrients.

This balance is lost in solid tumors. The vascular and lymphatic beds within solid tumors are abnormal and deficient. Although the tumor cells are continually secreting angiogenic factors, which elicit the growth of new blood vessels, the resulting arterioles and venules are abnormal in structure and are unresponsive to the physiological signals that normally regulate the flow of blood through such vessels. Moreover, the patterned web of arterioles, capillaries, and venules that support healthy tissues is replaced by a chaotic network of randomly growing vessels. Shunts, loops, sinusoids, blind vessels, and open-ended vessels are common. Moreover, the blood vessels are often tortuous and are leaky. Lymphatics are similarly defective and may be absent. In addition, as the malignant cells within the tumor grow, they invade, compress, and obliterate blood vessels, further compromising the microcirculation. As a result, blood flow within solid tumors is chaotic, and these malignancies contain regions that are transiently or chronically exposed to conditions of severe hypoxia, unphysiologically low pH, and nutrient deprivation.

B. Hypoxia Is an Early Event in Tumor Development

These microenvironmental inadequacies are present from the earliest point in the development of solid tu-

mors. When an incipient tumor grows to a diameter of about 200 μm, it will outgrow the blood supply provided in the surrounding normal tissues. At this diameter, the consumption of oxygen by the cells near the periphery of the tumor will be sufficient to utilize all of the oxygen that diffuses in from the surrounding tissues, and the cells in the interior of the mass will become severely hypoxic. Two things must happen for this microscopic nodule to grow further: (1) the tumor cells must mutate to be able to survive in an unfavorable environment in which they would normally die and (2) the cells must induce the formation of new blood vessels that will support their further growth. Hypoxia is the primary trigger for angiogenesis; tumor cells become hypoxic before they begin to induce the formation of new blood vessels. Hypoxic cells are therefore present in primary neoplasms at the very earliest stages of their evolution to malignancy and in metastases at the earliest stages of their development.

C. Nature and Extent of Hypoxia in Solid Tumors

Macroscopic solid tumors contain large numbers of hypoxic cells. Some of these cells will be found in regions of the tumor where the blood vessels have been damaged or obliterated. These cells may remain in a state of chronic hypoxia until they die and are absorbed into the necrotic regions of the tumor. However, they may be rescued if the tumor is treated with subcurative treatments that lead to cell death, tumor shrinkage, or altered perfusion, which reoxygenates the areas in which they are located. Other tumor cells will be transiently hypoxic for seconds, minutes, or hours because of fluctuations in blood flow through individual tumor blood vessels. Because malignant cells are more resistant than normal cells to the cytotoxic effects of hypoxia, these cells will remain viable and will contribute to the subsequent growth and metastasis of the neoplasm. Tumor cells may experience extremely unphysiological conditions. While the oxygen tensions of normal venous blood are generally in the range of 20–40 torr and oxygen tensions of 5 torr are considered low in normal tissues, oxygen tensions of less than 1 torr are common within solid tumors. Similarly, measurements of extracellular pH within solid tumors show pH values as low as 5.8–6.0, and mean extracellular pH values well below the values of 7.2–7.4, which are considered normal. Because the diffusion distances of glucose and many other critical nutrients through metabolizing tissue are similar to that of oxygen, hypoxic cells also experience severe nutritional deficits.

Hypoxia is a common feature of solid tumors. Measurements of the "hypoxic fractions" have been made in dozens of experimental rodent tumor lines and human tumor cell lines xenografted into immune-deficient mice. In most of these experimental model systems, 10–20% of the viable, clonogenic tumor cells are severely hypoxic. In some systems, the proportions are much higher. Hypoxic regions have also been found in spontaneous rodent tumors and in solid malignancies in veterinary patients. Polarographic electrodes have been used to measure the spectrum of oxygen tensions within human tumors. Metabolic markers have also been used to identify areas of severe hypoxia in human malignancies. Although data on human tumors are still accumulating, it is now clear that many solid tumors in human patients, including carcinomas of the head and neck, primary brain tumors, carcinomas of the prostate, soft tissue sarcomas, breast cancers, and carcinomas of the cervix, contain regions of severe hypoxia. Within a tumor type, there is considerable patient-to-patient variability in the proportion of hypoxic cells and in the severity of the hypoxia. In some types of cancer, it appears that extensive, severe hypoxia is a prognostic factor, independent of stage and grade, that predicts for poor outcome after therapy.

II. MECHANISMS OF HYPOXIA-INDUCED DRUG RESISTANCE

There are several mechanisms by which hypoxia induces resistance to drugs and other therapeutic modalities. Some of these reflect direct effects of the hypoxia per se. Others reflect the indirect effects of hypoxia and the environmental perturbations that accompany hypoxia on the metabolism of the tumor cells. The resistance induced by these processes will be lost when the cells are returned to a normal envi-

ronment, or soon thereafter. In addition, hypoxia may produce and select for genetic changes in the tumor cells; these will produce permanent changes in the phenotypes of the cells and in the sensitivity of the cells to treatment.

III. OXYGEN AS A CHEMICAL SENSITIZER

The effect of oxygen levels on the response of malignant cells to therapy was first demonstrated for X rays. Oxygen is a radiosensitizer. The radiosensitizing effects of oxygen are independent of the role of oxygen in energy metabolism and instead reflect the fact that O_2 is an extremely reactive chemical. When O_2 is present during irradiation, this electron-affinic molecule participates in the chemical reactions that lead from the absorption of radiation energy to the production of DNA damage, increasing both the number and the severity of the lesions produced in DNA. Cells and tissues irradiated in the presence of oxygen are three times more sensitive to radiation than those irradiated under severe hypoxia. Very low levels of O_2 are needed: the sensitization reaches half of its maximal level at a concentration of about 3 torr and plateaus at its full effect at concentrations of less than 20 torr. Because most normal tissues in the body have oxygen tensions above this value, the radiation biology of normal tissues reflects the response of cells irradiated while fully radiosensitive. As described earlier, however, tumors have areas of severe hypoxia; cells in these areas are resistant to radiation. Survival curves measured for cell in solid tumors show the effect of the radioresistant hypoxic cells: at low doses of radiation, the radiosensitive aerobic cells are killed; as the dose increases, only the radioresistant hypoxic cells survive, and the survival curve for the tumor cells at high doses therefore resembles that seen for cells made hypoxic *in vitro*. Hypoxic cells dominate the response of solid tumors to the large single doses of radiation needed to cause complete regression and cure.

Oxygen can have similar effects for those drugs for which the mechanism of action involves the reactions of free radicals or other indirect chemical reactions to produce cytotoxic damage. Bleomycin, for example, induces redox cycling reactions, producing reactive free radicals, which in turn produce both single and double strand breaks in DNA. Oxygen appears to be involved in these reactions, altering the number and type of DNA fragmentation products from those found in hypoxia and increasing the cytotoxicity of the drug. Oxygen is also thought to be involved in the interactions between etoposide and topoisomerase II, which lead to the protein-associated DNA breaks that result in cytotoxicity from this drug. Oxygen may also be involved in the chemical reactions that lead to the cytotoxicity of adriamycin, armsacrine, mitoxantrone, and certain other anticancer drugs. Oxygen is also important to the chemical reactions occurring during photodynamic therapy and is therefore important to the therapeutic effects of this modality.

IV. DIRECT EFFECTS OF PH ON DRUG RESISTANCE

The activity of many anticancer drugs is pH dependent. Drugs that are unstable at low pH may not reach cells in poorly perfused, acidic regions of tumors in an active form. Moreover, passive diffusion of drugs into cells occurs more readily when the molecules are in the nonionized form; drugs that become ionized at low pH will therefore enter cells less readily, and be less toxic, at low pH. Extracellular pH therefore has direct effects on anticancer drugs, which can influence their effectiveness and can lead to drug resistance at low pH.

V. PHYSIOLOGIC EFFECTS OF ADVERSE ENVIRONMENTS

A. Proliferative Changes

Prolonged exposures to hypoxia, and to the low pH and poor nutritional status that accompany hypoxia in solid tumors, produce numerous changes in the metabolism and behavior of the tumor cells. Cells in these adverse environments cannot continue proliferating at their maximal rate. When subjected to moderate microenvironmental inadequacies, cells

may continue proliferating at a slower rate than normal or may continue through the cell cycle until the transition point in G_1, where they will arrest until the environment improves. Very severe environmental deficits will cause cells to arrest at whatever point of the cell cycle they are in when the deficit occurs; solid tumors therefore contain cells that have S or G_2 phase DNA contents, but which are not actively progressing through the cell cycle. These nonproliferating, or quiescent, cells can remain viable for long periods of time. If their microenvironment improves, they will resume proliferation and will then contribute to subsequent tumor growth and metastasis.

A great many of the drugs used in cancer therapy, including hydroxyurea, methotrexate, the purine analogs, and the pyrimidine analogs, interfere with critical steps in cell proliferation and are therefore selectively toxic to proliferating cells. Hypoxic cells in solid tumors will be extremely resistant to these drugs because they are quiescent. Many other drugs, including alkylating agents and microtubule-directed agents, as well as certain antimetabolites, are not uniquely effective against proliferating cells, but have greater effects on proliferating cells than on resting cells. Nonproliferating hypoxic cells in solid tumors will have an increased resistance to these drugs. The poor response of many solid malignancies, especially slowly growing malignancies, to anticancer drugs reflects the fact that only a very small fraction of the malignant cells in these tumors are actively proliferating. The vast majority of the cells are quiescent, either because they are held from proliferation by the remnants of the homeostatic control mechanisms that regulate proliferation in normal tissues or because they are inhibited from proliferating because of their inadequate environment.

B. Energy Metabolism

Severe hypoxia, low extracellular pH, and deficiencies in glucose and other critical nutrients all lead to the disruption of normal pathways of energy metabolism, and therefore to the inhibition of a wide range of energy-dependent biochemical pathways. These metabolic derangements can influence the activity of many anticancer drugs. The activity of drugs that require active transport into or within the tumor cells will be diminished if energy-dependent transport processes are inhibited. The toxicity of prodrugs that require activation by energy-dependent enzymatic pathways will also be decreased. Hypoxic cells will also be protected against the effects of those fraudulent nucleotides that must be phosphorylated or incorporated into DNA via energy-dependent pathways to produce cytotoxicity.

C. Induction of Stress Responses

Exposure of cells to hypoxia, energy deprivation, low pH, heat, or other environmental insults induces a generalized "stress response." The stress response coordinates cellular signaling pathways that induce resistance to and the repair of injuries produced by common environmental stresses. These physiologic changes can also induce resistance to anticancer drugs. If extensive injury has occurred in normal cells, the stress response pathways would lead to the initiation of programmed cell death; however, as described earlier, malignant cells have developed an enhanced ability to avoid the induction of apoptosis in adverse environments, and therefore may also undergo programmed cell death less readily after induction of the stress response by drugs. The cellular changes induced by the stress response may enable malignant cells in adverse environments to survive treatments with anticancer drugs, as well as environmental insults, leading to increased drug resistance.

D. Other Metabolic Perturbations

Severe microenvironmental insufficiencies, especially if prolonged, also have a plethora of secondary metabolic effects that influence the response of the cells to chemotherapy. Changes in the fluidity of the cell membranes in hypoxia and at low pH lead to changes in passive drug uptake and intracellular drug distribution. Changes in receptors and cell surface antigens lead to alterations in response to hormones, biological therapies, and immunologic therapies and to resistance to many of these agents. Changes in enzyme activities can alter the rates and pathways of drug activation. Changes in levels of glutathione and other nonprotein sulfhydryls alter chemical reactions and

therefore modulate the effects of many anticancer drugs. The implications of these pervasive perturbations in cell physiology for the activity of anticancer drugs remain to be fully explored.

VI. DISTRIBUTION OF DRUGS WITHIN SOLID TUMORS

Hypoxic cells will also be protected against anticancer drugs by the same perfusion deficits that rendered them hypoxic. Some drugs, such as adriamycin, penetrate only very poorly through avascular tissue; distribution of these drugs will be limited to areas within a few cell diameters of those blood vessels that are actively perfused at the moment of treatment. Many antibodies, gene therapy vectors, and other large biological molecules suffer from the same problem of distribution and can reach only the most well-perfused areas of solid tumors. The diffusion of drugs within tumors is further compromised by the deficiencies in the lymphatic drainage within neoplasms, which lead to unusually high interstitial pressures within tumor tissue and thereby inhibit the diffusion of molecules from the blood vessels into tissue. In addition, some drugs will be rapidly metabolized by tumor cells, further limiting their penetration through the tumor, whereas others will be unstable at acid pH and rapidly inactivated within the acidic regions of the tumor. Studies of the microscopic distribution of anticancer drugs within solid tumors show that many drugs are heterogeneously distributed within tumor tissue and that therapeutic drug concentrations are often attained only in the most well-perfused areas of the malignancies. Physical barriers to drug delivery within solid malignancies represent a major problem in the successful treatment of these cancers with drugs and biological macromolecules.

VII. GENETIC CHANGES INDUCED IN TUMOR CELLS BY HYPOXIA

The mechanisms of resistance described earlier are all relatively transient; the sensitivity of the cells will be restored when the circulation is restored to the region, or soon afterward as the physiology of the cells returns to normal. However, hypoxia may also have genetic effects, which produce permanent changes in the genomes of the tumor cells and may contribute to the development of genomic instability, genetic heterogeneity, and genetically based drug resistance in the malignant cell population.

Transient exposures to hypoxia have been shown to result in a wide range of stable genetic changes in cells in culture. Exposure to hypoxia can induce DNA over-replication and gene amplification. Amplification of the dihydrofolate reductase gene induced by hypoxia produces resistance to methotrexate. In addition, single and repeated exposures to hypoxia increase the mutation frequencies of cells *in vitro*. Hypoxia also induces chromosomal fragile sites, triggering genomic rearrangements. Decreased repair of DNA has been observed in cells under hypoxic and acidic conditions. Hypoxia and low pH also induce stable changes in gene expression, as well as transient changes in gene expression; these include changes in the expression of genes which offer growth or survival advantages when upregulated. Exposure to adverse microenvironments in tumors therefore produces a wide variety of genetic changes that can foster the development of genomic instability and cell populations having genetic changes that cause drug resistance.

In addition, hypoxia selects for the aggressive cell populations that have developed mutations in p53 or other genes that control cell proliferation. Many normal cells respond to prolonged exposure to severe hypoxia by activating apoptotic pathways that lead to programmed cell death. The repeated induction of hypoxic stress in mixed cell populations has been shown to select for those cells that have mutations that inactivate this apoptotic response. Exposure to hypoxia likewise selects for cells that express high levels of proteins or receptors that confer growth advantages under adverse conditions. As a result, cell populations subjected to repeated exposures to severe hypoxia become increasingly enriched in cells that are mutated in critical cell cycle regulatory proteins or that overexpress genes that increase their chance of survival or their rate of proliferation.

Hypoxia is an early event in the development of solid tumors, occurring before the microscopic pre-malignant population has begun to induce angiogenesis. The genetic changes and selection pressures induced by hypoxia may be critical in producing the development of the genomic instability and genetic heterogeneity characteristic of solid tumors and in causing the evolution of relatively benign cell populations to increasingly malignant, increasingly aggressive phenotypes. Evidence from studies in mice shows that tumor cells exposed to hypoxia have an enhanced potential for producing metastases. Ongoing studies at several institutions are measuring hypoxia in human tumors. Studies with carcinoma of the cervix and with soft tissue sarcomas both suggest that those patients whose tumors contain extensive, severe hypoxia are at greater risk of relapse after therapy. Evidence suggests that an increased resistance of the primary tumor to therapy with drugs and radiation is not the sole cause of this increased risk and that hypoxic tumors may be more aggressive and have greater potential for metastatic spread. The implications of hypoxia and its associated microenvironmental insults for the development of genetic heterogeneity, genomic instability, aggressive genotypes, and drug-resistant genotypes in solid tumors remain to be fully explored.

VIII. IMPLICATIONS OF MICROENVIRONMENTALLY INDUCED DRUG RESISTANCE

Hypoxia and its associated microenvironmental inadequacies develop in solid malignancies, both primary and metastatic, while these neoplasms are still microscopic. By the time solid tumors are detectable, regions of transient and chronic hypoxia are found throughout the tumor mass, not only in and near regions that are manifestly necrotic, but also in areas that have visible blood vessels and show no necrotic features. Cells in these areas are resistant to many chemotherapeutic drugs, to many biological therapies, and to radiation. A variety of mechanisms contribute to this resistance, including direct effects of anoxia, indirect effects of hypoxia on the proliferation, physiology, and metabolism of the cells; and problems of drug distribution. In addition, exposures to hypoxia can induce genetic changes in the tumor cells and will also select for cell populations with mutations in the genes that normally control proliferation. Hypoxia therefore contributes to the development of genomic instability and genetic heterogeneity in the tumor cell population and fosters the evolution of the tumor cell population to an increasingly aggressive, increasingly malignant phenotype. These processes result in the development of subpopulations of genetically altered tumor cells, which can have drug-resistant genotypes and therefore would be resistant to chemotherapy whether they are aerobic or hypoxic at the time of treatment. Microenvironmental heterogeneity in solid tumors therefore plays a major role in producing the physiologic and genetic drug resistance that is characteristic of solid malignancies.

See Also the Following Articles

ANGIOGENESIS AND NATURAL ANGIOSTATIC AGENTS • BLEOMYCIN • CARCINOGENESIS: ROLE OF ACTIVE OXYGEN SPECIES • FOLATE ANTAGONISTS • PURINE ANTIMETABOLITES • PYRIMIDINE ANTIMETABOLITES • TUMOR CELL MOTILITY AND INVASION

Bibliography

Durand, R. E. (1994). The influence of microenvironmental factors during cancer therapy. *In Vivo* **8,** 691–702, 1994.
Jain, R. K. (1994). Barriers to drug delivery in solid tumors. *Sci. Am.* **271,** 58-65.
Moulder, J. E., and Rockwell, S. (1987). Tumor hypoxia: Its impact on cancer therapy. *Cancer Metast. Rev.* **5,** 313–341.
Rockwell, S. (1997). Oxygen delivery: Implications for the biology and therapy of solid tumors. *Oncol. Res.* **9,** 383–390.
Teicher, B. A. (1994). Hypoxia and drug resistance. *Cancer Metast. Rev.* **13**(2), 139–168.
Wike-Hooley, J. L., Haveman, J., and Reinhold, H. S. (1984). The relevance of tumour pH to the treatment of malignant disease. *Radiother. Oncol.* **2,** 343–366.
Yuan, J., and Glazer, P. M. (1998). Mutagenesis induced by the tumor microenvironment. *Mutat. Res.* **400,** 439–446.

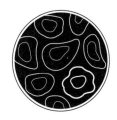

Immune Deficiency: Opportunistic Tumors

Harry L. Ioachim
Columbia University and New York University

I. Introduction
II. Neoplasms in Primary (Congenital) Immune Deficiencies
III. Neoplasms in Secondary (Acquired) Immune Deficiencies
IV. Neoplasms Most Commonly Associated with Immune Deficiencies

GLOSSARY

acquired immune deficiency syndrome A severe deregulation and ultimate failure of the immune system caused by the progressive destruction of cellular immunity in the course of infection with the human immunodeficiency virus.

autoimmune disease A deregulation of the immune system causing lymphoid cells and antibodies to attack and damage tissues and organs of their own organism.

dysplasia A precancerous stage of cells manifested by morphologic and biochemical abnormalities.

immune competent An organism with a normally functioning immune system that is capable of protecting it from pathogenic agents.

immune deficient An organism with a malfunctioning immune system that makes it vulnerable to pathogenic agents.

immunosuppressive therapy Ionizing radiations and cytotoxic drugs used to destroy neoplastic cells also affect components of the immune system, leading to its deregulation and deficiency.

non-Hodgkin's lymphoma A lymphoma that is unrelated to Hodgkin's disease.

opportunistic infectious agents Environmental pathogenic agents (viruses, bacteria) that may induce infections in immune-deficient but not in immune-competent organisms.

posttransplant lymphoproliferative disorders Lymphoid proliferations, both benign and malignant, occurring under the simultaneous immune stimulation caused by the transplant and the immune suppression caused by the chemotherapy.

primary immune deficiencies Immune deficiencies that are present at birth, either congenital or hereditary.

secondary immune deficiencies Immune deficiencies that are acquired later in life.

The immune system is a complex network of multiple specialized components able to potentiate, regulate, suppress, and compensate each other under various conditions. Different components may malfunction or fail entirely due to congenital defects or to acquired diseases. The result is an immune system that is functionally deficient. Due to the complexity of the system, immune deficiencies vary considerably according to the particular components involved.

Organisms affected by immune deficiency are vulnerable to environmental agents, particularly pathogenic microorganisms. Thus infections with a wide spectrum of viruses, bacteria, fungi, and protozoa, collectively referred to as opportunistic infections, may develop in immune-deficient persons. They range from occult asymptomatic lesions to severe, sometimes lethal infectious diseases. The immune deficiency that favored the infection also determines for it an unfavorable course with a resistance to treatment, tendency to dissemination, and fatal outcome.

I. INTRODUCTION

Immune-deficient organisms are susceptible not only to infections, but also to neoplasms. A relationship between immune deficiency and the occurrence of tumors has been suspected for a long time based on single case reports and experimental animal work. Solid documentation has been collected since the 1980s with the initiation of cancer registries for neoplasms occurring in persons with congenital immune deficiencies (Minneapolis, 1973) and for cancers occurring in relation to organ transplantation (Denver/Cincinnati, 1971). Tumors arising in individuals with immune deficiencies exhibit features similar to those characteristic of opportunistic infections. Like these, the tumors display increased aggressiveness and a tendency to early dissemination, resistance to treatment, frequent relapses, and short survivals. To emphasize the analogy of causes and manifestations, we refer to immune deficiency-associated neoplasms as opportunistic tumors. The opportunistic tumors, like the opportunistic infections developing as a result of immune deficiency, are not uniform because they reflect the deregulation or failure of various compartments of the immune system. Thus different infections are associated with the congenital deficiencies of the T- or B-cell systems, and viral or bacterial infections are predominant when, respectively, cellular

or humoral immunity is affected. In the case of opportunistic tumors, the relationships between different types of immunity and tumors are not as well defined. However, it is apparent that not all types of tumors occur with equal frequency in persons affected by immune deficiency. Some tumors occur early and others late in the course of immune deregulation depending on the severity of immune deficiency or perhaps on the variable intervals between oncogenesis and the clinical appearance of tumors. So far, several types of tumors, which will be further detailed, have shown a particular predilection for immune-deficient organisms. In persons with immune deficiencies, these tumors occur with unusually high frequency and severe manifestaions. Classification of an immune deficiency disorder presents multiple difficulties due to the great variability of immunologic findings in various cases. Two major categories—primary or congenital and secondary or acquired immune deficiencies—are recognized.

II. NEOPLASMS IN PRIMARY (CONGENITAL) IMMUNE DEFICIENCIES

The primary immune deficiencies represent developmental failures of the various components of the immune system. Most of the primary immune deficiencies are congenital and therefore the majority of patients are children. Primary immune deficiencies form a large group of syndromes of great diversity named and classified in 1971 by a special committee of the World Health Organization. According to the cell type predominantly affected, primary immune deficiencies were initially divided into cellular or T-cell and humoral or B-cell types. More recent classifications are more complex and comprise a greater number of specific subtypes. Immune deficiencies involving the B-cell system expressed as antibody immunodeficiencies are the most common, representing about 50% of all primary immune deficiencies. T-cell deficiencies comprise about 40% of the total; however three-fourths of these have associated B-cell deficiencies and are therefore far graver as, for example, severe combined immunodeficiency. Phagocytic immune deficiencies represent 6% and include impairments of polymorphonuclear leukocytes and monocyte macrophages. Disorders of the complement system make up the remaining 4% of the total. Severe combined immunodeficiency or Swiss-type agammaglobulinemia is the most severe form of congenital immunologic failure because it includes deficiencies of both the T- and the B-cell systems. The thymus is undeveloped and depleted of T lymphocytes, resulting in the lack of maturation of both T and B cells. The disease becomes apparent soon after birth and consists of recurrent septic episodes caused by a variety of agents to which no immune reaction is mounted. Children usually do not survive beyond 2 years of age. Notwithstanding the short life span, neoplasms may develop in these children. By 1987 there were 42 cases of neoplasms recorded in children with combined immune deficiency. Of these, 31 were non-Hodgkin's lymphomas (NHL), which is in sharp contrast with the virtual absence of lymphomas in immunocompetent children. In infantile X-linked agammaglobulinemia of Bruton's type, the defect involves B cells, which fail to differentiate, resulting in the absence of plasma cells. Malignancy, mostly leukemia and lymphoma, may develop in as many as 6% of boys with this sex-linked recessive abnormality. Dysgammaglobulinemia more common than agammaglobulinemia in which defects of the B-cell system are expressed by a decrease or total absence of one or two classes of immunoglobulins has also been associated with neoplasia. Thus, in IgA deficiency, adenocarcinomas of the stomach, lung, and colon, as well as leukemias and lymphomas, have been recorded. The Wiskott–Aldrich syndrome, which is genetically transmitted and X linked, is the result of mutations in the WASP gene. It consists of eczema, thrombocytopenia, and severe recurrent infections, which kill children in the first years of life. Females are carriers and appear healthy, whereas males have thymic hypoplasia and depleted T-cell zones in the lymph nodes. Before the introduction of antibiotics, the average survival was 8 months. As patients treated with antibiotics lived longer to a median survival of 10 years, neoplasms began to be reported. The Wiskott–Aldrich syndrome is presently associated with an estimated incidence of malignant tumors of more than 10%, the highest of all immune deficiencies. The majority of these tumors are lymphomas,

which like in acquired immune deficiencies are more often extranodal, predominantly gastrointestinal, and cerebral. The histologic types are of high grade malignancy and frequently, as in AIDS, are preceded by persistent, indolent lymphadenopathies.

Ataxia-telangiectasia is an autosomal recessive disorder with a mutant kinase gene. It comprises profound immunologic abnormalities, a predisposition for cancer, and other systemic manifestations, principally cerebellar degeneration. Clinically, ataxia-telangiectasia is characterized by the triad: cerebellar ataxia, mucocutaneous telangiectasia, and recurrent infections of sinuses and lungs (Fig. 1). The immunological deficiency involves both T and B-cell systems and is manifested by a lack of development of the thymus, depletion of T-cell areas, and Ig abnormalities. The registry in 1987 included 145 tumors associated with ataxia-telangiectasia, about half of which were lymphomas, the others, a variety of gliomas and carcinomas. The X-linked lymphoproliferative (XLP) syndrome transmitted by females and affecting males exclusively consists of a specific congenital T-cell defect, which causes an inability to control Epstein–Barr virus (EBV)-infected B cells. As a result, the patients

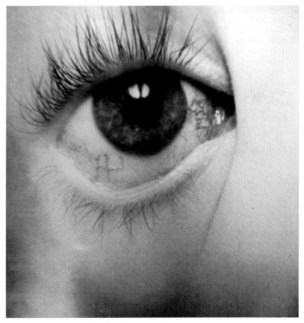

FIGURE 1 Marked vascular hyperplasia in the conjunctiva of a 9-year-old girl with ataxia-telangiectasia. Courtesy of Dr. Renate Dische.

are affected by malignant lymphoproliferative diseases, such as in the original observation of six boys in the Duncan family who all died within a 13-year period of severe forms of infectious mononucleosis and lymphomas (Fig. 2).

III. NEOPLASMS IN SECONDARY (ACQUIRED) IMMUNE DEFICIENCIES

A. Autoimmune Diseases

The medical literature contains many reports of neoplasms, particularly of the lymphoid system occurring in patients with a history of Sjögren disease, rheumatoid arthritis, scleroderma, dermatomyositis, systemic lupus erythematosus, and other autoimmune diseases. The increased risk of cancer may be related to the activation of lymphoid cells, an excessive production of antibodies, and deregulation of the immune system, all noted to occur in autoimmune diseases. However, large, controlled series of cases are difficult to assemble because of the low incidence and protracted course of most autoimmune diseases. Notwithstanding, a

number of more recent studies have confirmed earlier observations showing an elevated risk of lymphoma, leukemia, and myeloma in patients with rheumatologic and other autoimmune diseases. While these diseases are generally associated with immune deficiencies, their treatment with immunosuppressive agents makes it difficult to assess the respective contributions of these factores to the origin of the lymphoproliferative disorders. Whether the deregulated immune system of autoimmune diseases represents a predisposition to malignancy or simply renders organisms more susceptible to the oncogenic potential of therapeutic agents has not been determined.

Specific therapies for rheumatologic and related diseases include methotrexate, azathioprine, cyclosporine, prednisone, and combinations thereof. A similar association of lymphoproliferative disorders, benign and malignant, including Hodgkin's disease and non-Hodgkin's lymphomas, with Dilantin (Hydantoin) used in the long-term treatment of seizures, has been also identified. In all these cases of lymphoid neoplasms associated with immunomodulatory therapy for a variety of medical diseases, cases of spontaneous regression of tumors following the cessation of treatment were recorded. A majority of iatrogenic

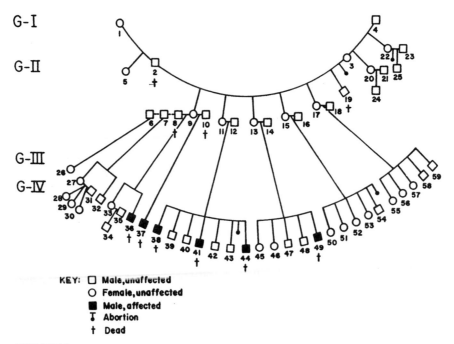

KEY: ☐ Male, unaffected
       ○ Female, unaffected
       ■ Male, affected
       Ŧ Abortion
       † Dead

FIGURE 2 Pedigree of Duncan kindred affected by the X-linked lymphoproliferative syndrome. From Purtilo *et al.* (1975) *Lancet* **1**, 935.

lymphoproliferative disorders contain occult EBV, which can be identified by immunohistochemistry for EBV-latent membrane protein (LMP) or by *in situ* hybridization for EBV-encoded RNA (EBER). Among the cases reported to have regressed on the discontinuation of methotraxate therapy were non-Hodgkin lymphomas with clonal immunoglobulin gene rearrangements as well as the clonal EBV genome.

B. Immunosuppressive Therapy

The treatment of various types of cancers by ionizing radiation and cytotoxic drugs has become increasingly complex and efficient. Long-term, disease-free survivals as well as complete cures, are currently achieved in neoplasms that are uniformly fatal in the absence of treatment. This remarkable success in the treatment of cancer, however, has been accompanied by an increasing occurrence of new tumors in the longer surviving patients. Because series of untreated patients to serve as controls are no longer available, it has been difficult to assess the intrinsic risk for second tumors of cancer patients. Equally difficult to separate in the origin of new tumors are the respective roles played by carcinogenicity and immune deficiency, which are both side effects of chemotherapy and radiation treatments. Regardless of the mechanisms involved, a high incidence of malignancy associated with immunosuppression is well documented. Thus the risk of developing acute myeloid leukemia was increased 78 times over that expected in a large series of patients with ovarian carcinoma and 100 times in patients with multiple myeloma after treatment with alkylating agents. An epidemiologic study of 1028 patients treated for Hodgkin's disease at Memorial Sloan–Kettering Cancer Center in the 1950s and 1960s revealed the occurrence of 44 other primary cancers of various types representing a frequency of 4%. The risk was greater for those treated in later years, which was apparently related to the introduction of combination as compared to single-drug chemotherapy. In a study at Stanford University, non-Hodgkin's lymphoma developed in 6 of 579 patients with Hodgkin's disease. The global actuarial risk of developing non-Hodgkin's lymphoma at 10 years was 4.4%, but in the group of patients receiving both radiation and chemotherapy, the risk increased to 15.2%.

The lymphomas were of high grade, large cell type, involving mainly the gastrointestinal tract and the brain. The features of high histologic grade and extranodal location are characteristic for the lymphomas arising on the background of immune deficiency. Cyclosporine, a cyclic polypeptide substance, is extensively used in organ transplantation as the most powerful immunosuppressant agent for the prevention of graft rejection. It acts at an early stage of T-cell differentiation and inhibits specifically T-helper cells. This activity, however, is inducive of severe viral and protozoal infections, as well as of lymphomas. Not infrequently, lymphomas develop after unusually short periods of time, 4 to 11 months in one series. In a survey of renal transplants, three lymphomas developed among 142 patients treated with cyclosporine, whereas none was observed among 149 patients treated with less powerful immunosuppressive drugs. Of special interest is the increase in antibodies to Epstein–Barr virus, particularly to the viral capsid antigen (VCA), which is not noted after conventional chemotherapy. It appears that cyclosporine depresses a specific population of T cells that is active against EBV-infected B cells, which may thus provide the source of EBV-associated B-cell non-Hodgkin's lymphomas.

A remarkable phenomenon observed in relation to the lymphomas induced by immunosuppression is their potential reversibility upon the cessation of treatment. Thus in various series of patients receiving transplants of kidney, liver, lung, or heart and severely immunosuppressed, particularly with cyclosporine and prednisone, NHL developed in 2 to 68 months after transplantation. The large majority of lymphomas were of B-cell type, and active infection with EBV was demonstrated by the presence of nuclear antigen (EBNA) or by DNA hybridization studies in 88% of cases. Although the lymphomas did not respond to conventional treatments with radiation or chemotherapy, they regressed spontaneously and, in most cases, disappeared when the immunosuppressive treatment was reduced or discontinued.

C. Organ Transplant Recipients

Malignant tumors occur three to four times more often in recipients of organ transplants than in the age-matched general population. The types of tumors, their incidence, and times of occurrence vary with the transplanted organs and the regimens of immunosuppression. Overall, neoplasms arise in 4 to 18%, an average of 6% of transplant recipients. As the survival of patients has increased due to improved treatments, the numbers and variety of malignant tumors have also augmented. By 1999, the Transplant Tumor Registry in Cincinnati, the largest worldwide database, had recorded about 12,000 posttransplant malignancies. The incidence of tumors increases with the length of time after transplantation. In one study of 124 cardiac transplant patients, the risk of developing cancer was 2.7 at 1 year and 25.6 at 5 years. The time intervals for the development of various tumors are different. Kaposi's sarcoma (KS) appears at an average of 21 months, lymphomas at 34 months, skin cancers at 75 months, and perineal tumors at 115 months average. The tumors affect relatively younger patients than in the general population, with an average age of 43 years at transplantation and 50 years at tumor presentation. The tumors most commonly observed were carcinomas of the skin and lip, showing a 4- to 29-fold increased incidence over the general population, Kaposi's sarcoma 400 to 500 times more common, non-Hodgkin's lymphoma 28 to 49 greater frequency, and carcinomas of vulva and perineum with a 100-fold increase. In contrast to the surprising high incidence of rare tumors, such as KS, the common cancers of the general population—lung, colon, breast, and prostate—are not more frequent in transplant recipients. The malignancies most frequently seen in these patients are cancers of the skin and lips. Skin cancers promoted by sunlight show a 4- to 7-fold increase in transplant patients over the general population, even in regions with limited sun exposure. The types of skin tumors in transplant recipients are different from those in normal individuals. While basal cell carcinoma, a tumor of low malignant potential, outnumbers the more invasive squamous cell carcinoma in the general population 5 to 1, this ratio is reversed in transplant recipients, with squamous cell carcinomas being twice as frequent as basal cell carcinomas. In immune-deficient hosts, squamous cell carcinomas of the skin, usually seen in 70- to 80-year old patients, appear in 40 to 50 year olds. They are multiple, more invasive, and more

likely to metastasize to the regional lymph nodes. Melanocytic tumors, benign and malignant, are also more frequent. Melanomas show an increase of up to 5-fold over the general population. Melanomas that develop after renal transplantation are different in that they occur more often on the unexposed skin of the back and tend to be more aggressive and deeply invasive. Merkel cell carcinoma, a rare but highly malignant cutaneous tumor, also occurs more often in transplanted patients. Tumors of smooth muscles have been also reported in association with immune suppression and transplantation. A rare but significant event is the appearance of leiomyosarcomas after heart and liver transplantation in adults and particularly in children. In three children who received liver transplants at 1 to 2 months of age, multiple malignant smooth muscle tumors developed 18 months to 5 years after treatment. In all cases, EBV antigens were identified in the tumors.

A spectrum of lymphoid neoplasms from benign to malignant tumors may develop in the recipients of transplanted organs. The incidence and type of tumors vary with the organ transplanted and the intensity or immunosuppression. Of all the tumors developing in recipients of renal transplants, lymphoid neoplasms compose a disproportionately large percentage, 26% as compared with 3% of all the tumors in the general population. As allotransplantation expanded to include other organs and the immunosuppressant regimens became more intensive, a considerable increase in the incidence of lymphoid neoplasms was recorded. Kidney recipients have the lowest (1%) and heart and lung recipients have the highest (9.4%) rate of lymphoproliferative disorders. These differences are most likely related to the introduction of more powerful immunosuppressant therapy, such as cyclosporin A and OKT3, an anti-T-cell antibody for the prevention of graft rejection. The latency period from the administration of treatment to the appearance of tumors is also related to the chemotherapy treatments used, showing a decrease from 4 to 5 years with azathioprine to only 5 to 7 months with cyclosporin A and OKT3. Lymphoid neoplasms encompass a variety of lesions from benign lymphoid hyperplasia at one end of the spectrum to high-grade malignant lymphoma at the other. Virtually all lesions are of the B-cell type and almost all are associated with a primary or reactivated EBV infection. The whole group is referred to as posttransplantation lymphoproliferative disorders (PTLD). The lymphoid lesions may present soon after transplantation in the form of an indolent lymphadenopathy or an infectious mononucleosis-like illness with mild or severe symptoms. Alternately, tumor masses, single or multiple involving lymph nodes or the gastrointestinal tract, may develop. Extranodal locations in up to 70% of cases and often the transplanted organs, liver or lung, may be the site of lymphomas. A unique feature of PTLD is that some may regress when the immunosuppressive treatment is reduced or discontinued. Others may progress rapidly despite intensive treatment. The clinical behavior does not always correlate with the histologic appearance or the clonality of the tumor. The histologic patterns range from mixed cell populations of lymphocytes, plasma cells, and immunoblasts that are polyclonal to the monomorphous monoclonal cellularity of lymphomas. Because of the rapid progression of lymphoid proliferation, frequently more than one pattern is found when multiple lesions are biopsied at the same time. Sometimes, nodules of apparent lymphoma cells can be seen in a lymph node that otherwise shows a pattern of reactive or atypical hyperplasia. This unusual appearance has been also noted in other lymphoproliferative lesions associated with immune deficiency. Genotypic studies have shown that multiple clones may arise concomitantly in one or different organs in the absence of regulatory T cells and under the stimulation of EBV, which is uniformly present in these cells. Presence of the EBV genome is demonstrated by immunohistochemical studies with antibodies to EBNA showing positive cells in 38 to 100% of cases or by *in situ* hybridization using a radiolabeled fragment of EBV-encoded DNA or EBER (Fig. 3), which identifies EBV in most of the lymphoid lesions. There are cases of PTLD in which the EBV genome cannot be identified. Such EBV-negative tumors tend to appear later and have a worse prognosis. The pathogenesis of PTLD seems to be an exaggerated proliferation of EBV-carrying B cells released from the control of the immunosuppressed T cells. B-cell proliferation progresses from polyclonal to monoclonal in a relatively short time, which ex-

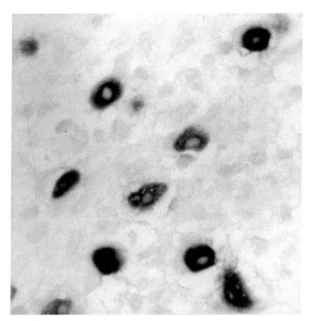

FIGURE 3 Large B-cell lymphoma in an immunosuppressed patient. *In situ* hybridization for EBV-encoded RNA shows nuclei of lymphoma cells positive for EBV genome.

plains the coexistence of hyperplastic and neoplastic histologic patterns and the difficulty of separating benign from malignant lesions.

D. Acquired Immune Deficiency Syndrome (AIDS)

The worldwide epidemic of HIV infection and the AIDS complex of diseases associated with it have brought to general attention the relationship between immune deficiency and opportunistic infections and tumors. The initial infection with HIV is followed by viremia and HIV dissemination throughout the lymphoid system. The HIV-specific immunity that takes place during this early phase is manifested by serum conversion and a marked decrease in circulating virus. However, the immunity is inadequate to completely eradicate the virus, which persists indefinitely in the lymphoid system. In most patients the acute phase of infection is followed by a long period of clinical latency that lasts for years (median 10 years). Although the patients may be symptomless during this time, HIV continues to proliferate and to cause the progressive depletion of CD4$^+$ T cells and the gradual deterioration of the immune system. As the decrease in CD4$^+$ T cells reaches critical values, the infectious diseases of AIDS begin to appear. In the classification system for HIV infection, an absolute value of less than 200 CD4$^+$ T lymphocytes per microliter or a CD4$^+$ T lymphocyte percentage of total lymphocytes of less than 14 in an HIV-positive patient is a defining criterion for AIDS.

Since the late 1990s, the disease patterns of AIDS have shown significant changes. The survival of AIDS patients has increased as a result of antiretroviral combination therapy and a better control of infections by specific treatments. However, a longer survival appears to be associated with an increased risk of malignancies. It is now estimated that more than 40% of all patients with AIDS will be diagnosed with malignant disease in the course of their HIV infection. Children infected by HIV may be also victims of cancers, showing a 100-fold higher incidence of tumors than their noninfected counterparts. Not all types of neoplasms, just as not all kinds of infectious diseases, have increased their occurrence in the population of long survivors. Numerous reports in the literature have described cases of malignant tumors in persons with HIV infection or AIDS. Some were tumors commonly occurring in the general population and therefore difficult to attribute to the status of AIDS, such as lung carcinomas, anal carcinomas, or basal cell carcinomas. Population-based studies have shown so far significant increases in incidence in only three types of neoplasms: Kaposi's sarcoma, non-Hodgkin's lymphoma, and squamous cell carcinoma of uterine cervix, which were included by the CDC in the list of AIDS-defining diseases. More recently, leiomyosarcomas, extremely rare tumors in children, have been frequently observed in HIV-infected children. The inclusion of new kinds of tumors as AIDS-defining conditions at different times during the epidemic reflects the relationship of various tumors with the lengths of survival and the continuous lowering of the total amounts of CD4$^+$ T lymphocytes. In the future, new treatments, lengthened survivals, and broader population surveys may reveal yet other neoplasms that are significantly associated with the HIV infection and the profound immune deficiency of AIDS.

IV. NEOPLASMS MOST COMMONLY ASSOCIATED WITH IMMUNE DEFICIENCIES

A. Kaposi's Sarcoma

In the 130 years since its original description, KS was considered a rare dermatologic condition that attracted only limited attention. In the United States and western Europe, KS occurs in a sporadic form with an incidence of only 0.02% of 10,000 tumors, although endemic areas are known to exist in sub-Saharan Africa, where KS accounts for 9% of all cancers. A relationship with immune deficiency was suggested by the occurrence of KS in about 0.6% of all patients undergoing renal transplantation, which is an incidence 150 to 200 times greater than would be expected in the general population. The high frequency of KS in patients with AIDS was noted from the very first reports of cases in 1981. In the following years the recorded incidence of KS in AIDS patients climbed as high as 40% and although it has since markedly decreased, it remains the most common AIDS-associated cancer in the United States. Even more unexpected are the great variations in the frequency of KS occurrence between the risk groups of AIDS. Thus KS may be as frequent as 36% among homosexual AIDS patients, whereas its occurrence is only 4.3% among intravenous drug addicts and 1% among hemophiliacs with AIDS. Similar differences between the incidence of KS in various AIDS risk groups are reflected in the epidemiologic data of various countries.

Depending on the characteristics of various populations, KS can present as one of four forms, each with different epidemiologic and clinical manifestations, although morphologically they are all identical. (1) Sporadic Kaposi's sarcoma affects elderly men of east European or Mediterranean origin. It appears as purple-blue plaques or nodules on hands and feet and progresses slowly over the years, eventually involving internal organs. (2) Endemic Kaposi's sarcoma is now the most frequently occurring tumor in central Africa, highly aggressive and responding poorly to treatment. Children are also affected, with KS representing up to 10% of all pediatric cancers in endemic areas. (3) KS associated with immunosuppression and transplantation may develop months after transplantation and behave aggressively, involving mucosae, lymph nodes, and viscera. Some ethnic groups are more susceptible. Thus in a group of transplant recipients in Toronto, KS developed in 12 persons, 9 of whom were of Italian origin. (4) Epidemic Kaposi's sarcoma, characteristically associated with the HIV infection, has an early tendency for dissemination and involvement, sometimes fatal, of internal organs. Characterized by its disproportionately high incidence in homosexual AIDS patients, it has decreased from its 40% peak in the early 1980s to less than 20% in the 1990s due to effective treatments and prevention. The peculiar epidemiology of KS has suggested an infectious cause and sexual transmission. The search for an etiologic agent produced a large number of studies, which, for a long time, ended inconclusively. In 1994, Chang and colleagues, using new techniques of genomic analysis, identified DNA sequences of a new herpes virus, named KS-associated herpes virus (KSHV) or human herpesvirus 8 (HHV8) in a skin lesion of an AIDS patient. With the use of standard polymerase chain reaction (PCR) or Southern blot hybridization assays, HHV8 viral DNA can be detected in virtually all KS lesions, regardless of their source or clinical type. In addition to KS, HHV8 was found to be associated with primary effusion lymphoma, a rare form of B-cell lymphomas arising in body cavities such as pleura and peritoneum and with some forms of multicentric Castleman disease. Specific HHV8 antibodies are detectable in up to 100% of patients with KS. Serologic studies of HHV8 among blood donors in various countries indicate that the spread of this virus is not ubiquitous. The infection rates are variable and parallel the incidence of KS. In Japan, where KS is very rare, only 0.2% of blood donors have antibodies to HHV8, in the United States, about 10%, in Central Africa, up to 50 percent have positive serology, and in Italy and other Mediterranean countries the values are intermediate. Close to 40% of homosexual men, regardless of HIV status, have circulating anti-HHV8 antibodies, even when asymptomatic.

Kaposi's sarcoma involves the skin, mucosal surfaces, lymph nodes, and internal organs. The skin lesions are more numerous and noticeable and are the most frequent presenting sign. The lesions range in size from 1–2 mm to 2–3 cm and in color from pink-red to purple-blue (Fig. 4). In form, they can be macules, papules, slightly elevated plaques, or prominent nodules. They can be single or numerous, and they can be widely spread over a single area or over the entire body. Patches are early lesions that are small, ovoid, pink-red, and flat. They may become elevated and indurated papules and eventually they may darken in color and increase in size to become prominent nodules. Occasionally, some lesions may flatten and regress spontaneously.

The location of KS lesions is more varied and widespread in AIDS patients than in patients with the classic form of disease in whom they tend to arise mainly on the legs and feet. On the face, favored sites are the tip of the nose, the medial third of the eyelids, the area behind the ears, and the earlobes. The trunk, the penis, and the dorsum of the feet are also common locations. In its new epidemic form, KS also involves mucosal surfaces, especially those of the gastrointestinal tract, lymph nodes, and viscera (Fig. 5). At autopsy, almost any internal organ may show Kaposi's sarcoma, with the exception of the brain, the involvement of which has not been documented. Early lesions in the mouth appear as macules or papules on the mucosa of the hard palate just above the level of the second molar. Similar red-purple

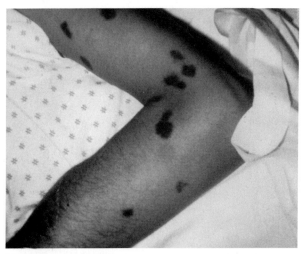

FIGURE 4 Kaposi's sarcoma purple macules and papules on the arm and forearm of an AIDS patient.

patches and plaques may develop on the tonsils, pharynx, esophagus, stomach, intestine, colon, rectum, and anus. Gastrointestinal involvement may cause bleeding and obstruction. The lungs may also be involved, in which case symptomatic pulmonary disease with dyspnea, hemoptysis, and pleural effusions may result. Advanced pulmonary involvement leads to short survival, usually less than 6 months. On histologic examination, all types of KS consist of exuberant proliferations of neoplastic spindle-shaped cells arranged in bundles or whorls, with capillary-like slits and clefts that contain a variable amount of red blood cells, a large part of which are extravasated (Fig. 5). The nuclei are large, but not markedly pleomorphic. Mitoses are usually present. The proliferation of neoplastic blood vessels is accompanied by infiltrates, sometimes abundant of plasma cells and lymphocytes. The neoplastic cells of KS originate in the endothelial cells of blood vessels, as indicated by their reactivity with monoclonal antibodies raised against the specific endothelial markers CD31 and CD34.

The classic lesions of KS in the sporadic form are treated with local radiation. For single lesions, even excisional surgery may be adequate. Extensive and recurrent KS can be treated with combinations of chemotherapy and radiotherapy. KS arising in immunosuppressed patients may regress simply by the discontinuation of therapy. In one study, KS regressed spontaneously in four of five renal transplant recipients after cessation of immunosuppressive treatment. Cutaneous KS in the setting of HIV infection is best treated with interferon-α, which results in remissions of lesions in 40 to 60% of patients. Response rates correlate with the levels of $CD4^+$ T cells and improve after vigorous antiretroviral therapy. Thus in the epidemic form, KS lesions are treated with interferon-α and/or appropriate chemotherapy, whereas background immune deficiency is amelio-

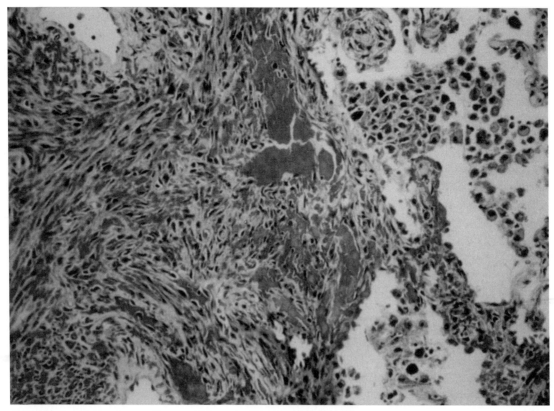

FIGURE 5   Kaposi's sarcoma of lung in AIDS. Pools of blood and fascicles of spindle-shaped sarcoma cells replace pulmonary alveolar spaces on the left side.

rated by the treatment of the HIV infection. Fortunately, KS has shown a steady decline to 10% in AIDS patients overall and 20% in homosexual AIDS, possibly as a result of preventive measures against sexually transmitted diseases.

B. Non-Hodgkin's Lymphoma

Lymphomas are the neoplasms most commonly associated with immune deficiencies of all types, congenital and acquired. In HIV-infected persons, non-Hodgkin's lymphomas are considered AIDS-defining illnesses. They occur in 3% of patients with AIDS, which are thus at a risk for NHL, 60 times greater than the general population. Studies show a continuing increase in the incidence of lymphomas among AIDS patients who now survive longer because of improved antiretroviral and antifungal therapies. In patients over 3 years on anti-HIV treatments the incidence of NHL may rise as high as 28%. In contrast to Kaposi's sarcoma, which is far more common among homosexual AIDS patients than other patients with AIDS, NHL affects equally all AIDS risk groups, including children. Hodgkin's lymphoma is also more frequent in AIDS patients, who carry a risk for this disease 10 times greater than non-AIDS patients (Fig. 6).

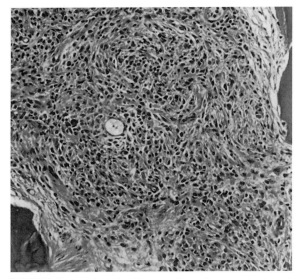

FIGURE 6 Hodgkin's lymphoma replacing hemopoetic tissues in the bone marrow of a HIV-positive patient.

AIDS-associated NHLs are a group of heterogeneous neoplasms that are virtually all of B-cell type, but differ in their histologic type, location, and pathogenesis. The HIV at the origin of AIDS is not involved in the malignant transformation of B cells, as no HIV sequences have been detected in the lymphoma cells. However, the HIV infection induces the production of a variety of cytokines and growth factors, which play an important role in the activation and differentiation of B cells. The intense follicular hyperplasia of HIV lymphadenitis shows the active proliferation of B cells, which provides opportunities for cellular instability and molecular alterations such as mutations, translocations, and deletions of tumor suppressor genes. Thus the excessive stimulation of B cells, the selection of B-cell clones carrying genetic alterations, and the cellular immune deficiency that inactivates the immune surveillance combine in the pathogenesis of AIDS-associated NHL. In the case of Burkitt's lymphoma, which accounts for 30% of AIDS-associated NHL, the molecular pathway involves infection with EBV, activation of the C-myc protooncogene, and inactivation of the p53 tumor suppressor gene.

In contrast to the lymphomas in the general population of young adults where Hodgkin's lymphomas are more common, among the lymphomas of AIDS, non-Hodgkin's lymphomas are by far more frequent. Also, contrary to the general population, lymphomas of AIDS more often originate in extranodal locations. In our study of 111 cases of AIDS-associated lymphomas, 11 were Hodgkin's lymphoma and 100 were non-Hodgkin's lymphoma. In the same study, of the 100 NHL, 61 originated in various internal organs, whereas only 49 were initially located in lymph nodes. Of these, the digestive tract, with 27 cases, and the central nervous system, with 15 cases, were the most common primary sites (Fig. 7). Unusual locations for primary NHL, such as the oral cavity, the anus, and the testis, are also involved (Fig. 8). Regardless of their location, AIDS-associated lymphomas, which are in almost all cases of high histologic grades, exhibit great clinical aggressiveness. Hodgkin's lymphomas in AIDS more often present in late stages III and IV, with the involvement of internal organs, including bone marrow dissemination (Fig. 6). Non-Hodgkin's lymphomas in AIDS are invariably of high

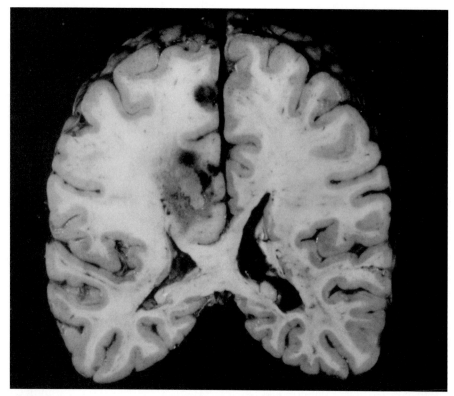

FIGURE 7 Non-Hodgkin's lymphoma of the brain in an AIDS patient. Large, partly hemorrhagic tumor nodules deep in the white matter of the left cerebral hemisphere compressing the corpus callosum.

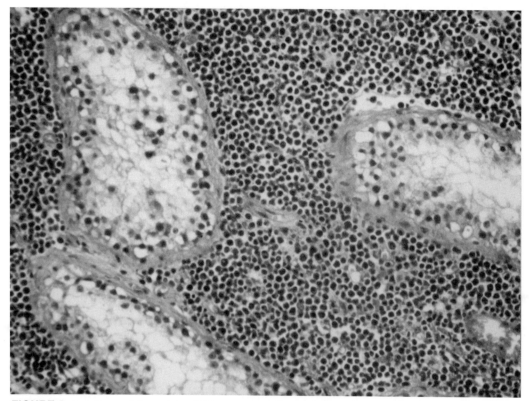

FIGURE 8 Lymphoma of the testis in a HIV-positive man. Few residual atrophic seminiferous tubules are seen within the sheets of lymphoma cells.

histologic grades, and high aggressiveness manifested by early dissemination, resistance to treatment, frequent relapses, and short survivals.

Lymphadenopathies, characteristic of the HIV infection, may precede lymphomas in AIDS patients. Sometimes, nodules of lymphoma cells can be seen in a lymph node that still shows a pattern of reactive hyperplasia. This observation is consistent with the reported finding of monoclonal rearranged bands in HIV lymphadenopathies possibly representing the emergence of lymphoma clones in lymph nodes that still have a benign histologic appearance.

Histologically, AIDS-associated NHL are a heterogeneous group composed of Burkitt's lymphomas in about 30% of cases and diffuse large cell lymphomas in the remaining 70% of cases divided almost equally between immunoblastic and pleomorphic variants (Figs. 9 and 10). Virtually all lymphomas associated with immune deficiencies, regardless of histologic type, are of the B-cell immunophenotype (Fig. 11). Rare cases of primary effusion lymphomas located in the pleura or peritoneum are related etiologically to

the newly discovered human herpesvirus 8, which is present in over 95% of Kaposi's sarcomas. Burkitt's lymphoma is 1000 times more common in HIV-infected people than in the population at large where its frequency is only 1% of all lymphomas. In AIDS patients, Burkitt's lymphomas are predominantly located in lymph nodes, whereas large cell lymphomas are found more often in extranodal locations, particularly the brain, where Burkitt's lymphoma is infrequent. AIDS patients with the Burkitt's type of NHL are usually younger, have higher levels of T CD4$^+$ cells, and may not have had prior manifestations of AIDS, whereas patients with large cell lymphomas present with advanced AIDS symptoms and T CD4$^+$ counts below 100.

The signs of EBV infection are found in about 30% of AIDS–Burkitt's lymphomas and in over 70% of AIDS–diffuse large cell lymphomas. In common with all other Burkitt's lymphomas, ones associated with AIDS also exhibit the 8:14 reciprocal translocation, which juxtaposes the protooncogene c-myc to the Ig locus, thus causing its transcriptional deregulation.

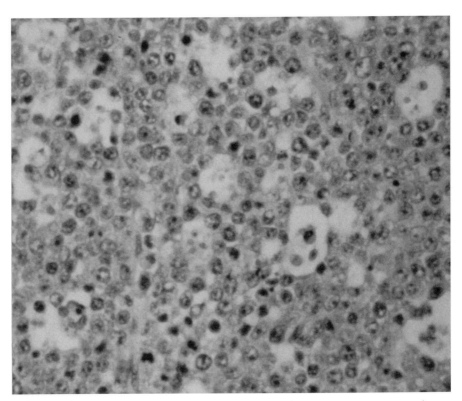

FIGURE 9 Burkitt's lymphoma with characteristic histologic pattern in an immunosuppressed organ transplant recipient.

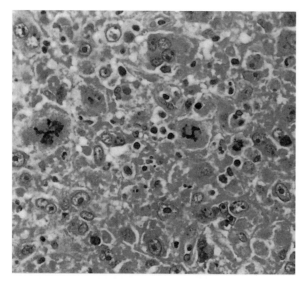

FIGURE 10 Non-Hodgkin's lymphoma, high grade, forming a peritoneal tumor mass in an AIDS patient. The cells are large with pleomorphic nuclei, prominent nucleoli, and multiple multipolar mitoses.

Mutations and deletions also result in the inactivation of the *p53* tumor suppressor gene in about one-third of cases. It may be postulated that a pool of previously EBV-infected B cells is activated in the course of the HIV infection and that multiple genetic lesions, including *c-myc* rearrangements and *p53* inactivation, are taking place. With the failing T-cell sys-

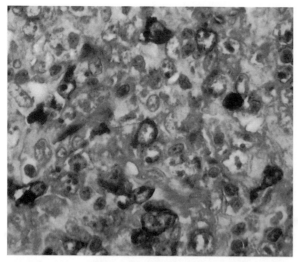

FIGURE 11 Non-Hodgkin's lymphoma large cell, immunoblastic type. A majority of cells show specific dark-brown staining of cell membranes with a monoclonal antibody directed against CD20, a B-cell marker.

tem unable to exercise normal surveillance, the transformed B cells may progress from polyclonal to oligoclonal and eventually to the monoclonal proliferations of the AIDS-associated B-cell NHL.

C. Anogenital Carcinoma

Individuals with immune deficiency are predisposed to infection with multiple serotypes of human papilloma virus (HPV). Some of these viruses are known to be associated with squamous cell carcinomas of the vulva and anus. Recipients of renal transplants have a 100-fold increase in the incidence of anogenital neoplasia over normal control subjects. More recently, it has become apparent that cervical squamous cell dysplasia, carcinoma *in situ*, and invasive carcinoma are more frequent in women with the HIV infection (Fig. 12). This observation led to the inclusion of cervical carcinoma as an AIDS-defining condition in the latest classification system for HIV infection by the Centers for Disease Control (1993). Infection with many types of HPV, particularly genotypes 16 and 18, has been implicated as a precursor to cervical neoplasia (Fig. 13). In one study, there was a 28% incidence of cervical intraepithelial neoplasia (CIN) grades 2 and 3 over the next 2 years after the first detection of HPV DNA in cervical tissues as compared to an incidence of 3% in patients negative for HPV. The risk for grade 3 CIN lesions was associated in 50% of patients with HPV types 16 and 18. The HIV infection increases considerably the risk of HPV infections and subsequently of cervical neoplasia. Thus HIV-infected women have a high prevalence of cervicovaginal cytologic abnormalities and genital HPV infections as compared to non-HIV-infected women. In one study, women matched for demographic and behavioral characteristics had detectable HPV genomic material in 49% of HIV-infected and in 25% of non-HIV-infected women. Women who had both HIV and HPV infections were 42 times more likely to have cytologic abnormalities on the Papanicolaou (Pap) smear than women who had neither virus infection. A study of prostitutes in Zaire in 1992 showed the presence of CIN lesions in 29% and of HPV DNA in 38% of 47 HIV-positive women as compared to 3% CIN lesions and 8% HPV DNA in 48 negative women. The degree of immunodeficiency is associ-

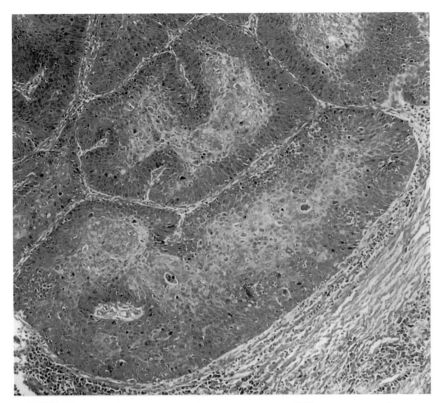

FIGURE 12 Condyloma acuminatum of uterine cervix in a HIV-positive patient. Large protruding masses of squamous cells with atypical nuclei, frequent mitoses, and koilocytotic dysplastic changes characteristic of HPV infection.

ated with cervical dysplasia and neoplasia. Thus women with CD4$^+$ T-cell counts of less than 400 have twice as frequent cervical cytologic abnormalities in their Pap smears. Not only is the risk of acquiring HPV-related malignancy higher in HIV-infected women, but the response to treatment and the prognosis are poorer. Patients with invasive cervical carcinoma have more advanced-stage disease, higher recurrence rates, and shorter survival when HIV infection is coexistent. In one comparative study, 49% of HIV-seronegative patients experienced relapse after treatment for invasive cervical carcinoma as compared to 100% of HIV-seropositive patients who had recurrent disease.

Anal dysplasia and carcinoma in homosexual men follow a similar course. Lower CD4$^+$ T cells in HIV-positive homosexual men are associated with more severe dysplasia and the presence of HPV DNA. Anal condylomata with the presence of HPV is more common in HIV-positive men. In addition to HPV-related lesions, herpes virus and CMV infections with

ulcers, Kaposi's sarcoma, and even primary NHL may involve the anorectal region. In general, in homosexual men with HIV infection, the extent of anorectal neoplasia correlates with the degree of immunodeficiency. In the early stages of HIV infection, when the levels of CD4$^+$ T cells are only moderately decreased, the HPV infection is only detectable by the polymerase chain reaction technique. As the CD4$^+$ T-cell counts decline, HPV DNA can be detected by hybridization techniques, and low-grade neoplasia, such as condylomata, becomes apparent. During the late stages of AIDS, when the very low CD4$^+$ T-cell levels are unable to provide immune surveillance, high-grade anal carcinomas *in situ*, such as Bowen disease and invasive squamous cell carcinomas, may develop.

D. Smooth-Muscle Tumors

Unexpected and unexplained is the increasing incidence of smooth muscle tumors in children with acquired immune deficiency (Fig. 14). In the

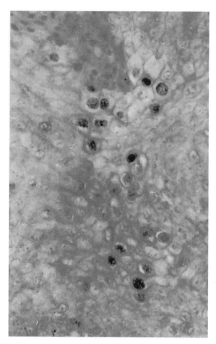

FIGURE 13 Condyloma acuminatum, anal lesion in a HIV-positive patient. Nuclei of cells infected with HPV are stained by anti-HPV antibodies.

HIV-infected pediatric population, often in very young children, multiple leiomyosarcomas arising in unusual locations—the liver, adrenal gland, lungs, and gastrointestinal tract—were reported. Similar tumors were seen in children and adults who were recipients of organ transplants and heavily immunosuppressed. In most cases the tumors were associated with the Epstein–Barr virus, as demonstrated by the detection of nuclear EBV sequences. Moreover, molecular genetic analysis showed the EBV genome to be clonal, thus suggesting an etiologic role for the virus in the oncogenic process. In contrast, EBV was not found in the smooth muscle tumors of non-HIV-infected and immunocompetent patients.

E. Other Tumors

In addition to the three malignant tumors—Kaposi's sarcoma, non-Hodgkin's lymphoma, and cervical carcinoma included by the Centers for Disease Control in the case definition of AIDS—a variety of other tumors have been reported to have occurred in HIV-infected individuals. They are generally referred to as non-AIDS-defining tumors. The more common of these, such as carcinomas of skin and lips, leiomyosarcomas of children, melanomas, and Hodgkin's disease, have been already discussed. Solid tumors that are the most common in the general population, such as carcinomas of the breast, prostate, and colon, do not appear to be more frequent in AIDS patients. There are numerous reports of lung cancers occurring in patients infected by HIV. These tumors tend to affect younger individuals, to exhibit high histologic grades of malignancy, and to display greater aggressiveness with earlier dissemination and shorter survival. However, a clear linkage between the two conditions is difficult to establish given that both are relatively frequent in the same male population. In a comparative study of nuclear changes in lung carcinomas of HIV-positive patients versus the general population, loss of heterozygosity (LOH) and microsatellite alteration (MA) were analyzed by polymerase chain reaction from extracted tumor DNA. It was found that LOH was similarly frequent in the two groups tested, whereas MA was six times more common in HIV-associated lung tumors. A search for viral sequences, HIV and HPV, in tumor tissues was negative. MA probably represents genomic instability

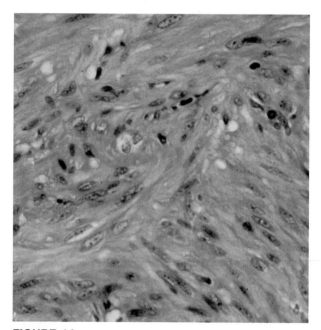

FIGURE 14 Large leiomyoma in the posterior mediastinum of a HIV-infected woman.

and has been also reported in other HIV-associated tumors; however, their pathogenesis and relationship with HIV infection remain unknown.

In conclusion, this article indicates that the various states of immune deficiencies with their impaired immune surveillance favor the occurrence of opportunistic infections.

See Also the Following Articles

ATAXIA TELANGIECTASIA SYNDROME • CELL-MEDIATED IMMUNITY TO CANCER • EPSTEIN–BARR VIRUS • HIV (HUMAN IMMUNODEFICIENCY VIRUS) • LYMPHOMA, HODGKIN'S DISEASE • LYMPHOMA, NON-HODGKIN'S • MOLECULAR BASIS OF TUMOR IMMUNITY • NEOPLASMS IN ACQUIRED IMMUNODEFICIENCY SYNDROME • T CELLS AGAINST TUMORS • T CELLS, FUNCTION OF

Bibliography

Abbondanzo, S. L., Irey, N. S., and Frizzera, G. (1995). Dilantin-associated lymphadenopathy-spectrum of histopathologic patterns. *Am. J. Surg. Pathol.* **19,** 675–686.

Antman, K., and Chang, Y. (2000). Kaposi's's Sarcoma. *N. Engl. J. Med.* **342,** 1027–1038.

Chadburn, A., Cesarman, E., and Knowles, D. M. (1997). Molecular pathology of posttransplantation lymphoproliferative disorders. *Semin. Diagn. Pathol.* **14,** 15–26.

Cleary, M. L., Warnke, R., and Sklar, J. (1988). Monoclonality of lymphoproliferative lesions in cardiac-transplant recipients: Clonal analysis based on immunoglobulin-gene rearrangements. *N. Engl. J. Med.* **310,** 477–482.

Filipovich, A. H., Heinitz, K. J., and Robison, L. L. *et al.* (1987). The immunodeficiency Cancer Registry: A research resource. *Am. J. Ped. Hematol./Oncol.* **9,** 183–184.

Georgescu, L., Quinn, G. C., and Schwartzman, S., *et al.* (1997). Lymphoma in patients with rheumatoid arthritis: Association with the disease state or methotrexate treatment. *Semin. Arthritis. Rheumat.* **26,** 794–804.

Ioachim, H. L. (1987). Neoplasms associated with immune deficiencies. *Pathol. Annu.* **22,** 177–223.

Ioachim, H. L. (1989). "Pathology of AIDS." Lippincott & Gower, New York.

Ioachim, H. L. (1990). The opportunistic tumors of immune deficiency. *Adv. Cancer Res.* **54,** 301–317.

Ioachim, H. L., Adsay, V., Giancotti, F., *et al.* (1995). Kaposi sarcoma of internal organs: A multiparameter study of 86 cases. *Cancer* **75,** 1376–1385.

Ioachim, H. L., Antonescu, C., Giancotti, F., *et al.* (1997). EBV-associated anorectal lymphomas in patients with acquired immune deficiency. *Am. J. Surg. Pathol.* **21,** 997–1006.

Ioachim, H. L., Antonescu, C., Giancotti, F., *et al.* (1998). EBV-associated primary lymphomas in salaivary glands of HIV-infected patients. *Pathol. Res. Pract.* **194,** 87–95.

Ioachim, H. L., Dorsett, B., Cronin, W., *et al.* (1991). Acquired immunodeficiency syndrome-associated lymphomas: Clinical, pathologic, immunologic, and viral characteristics of lll cases. *Hum. Pathol.* **22,** 659–673.

Irwin, D., and Kaplan, L. (1993). Clinical aspects of HIV-related lymphoma. *Curr. Opin. Oncol.* **5,** 852–860.

Knowles, D. M., Cesarman, E., Chadburn, A., et al. (1995). Correlative morphologic and molecular genetic analysis demonstrates three distinct categories of posttransplantation lymphoproliferative disorders. *Blood* **85,** 552–565.

Lipsey, L. R., and Northfelt, D. W. (1993). Anogenital neoplasia in patients with HIV infection. *Curr. Opin. Oncol.* **5,** 861–866.

Maiman, M., Fruchter, R. G., Guy, L., *et al.* (1993). Human immunodeficiency virus infection and invasive cervical carcinoma. *Cancer* **71,** 402–406.

McClain, K. L., Leach, C. T., Jenson, H. B., *et al.* (1995). Association of Epstein-Barr virus with leiomyosarcomas in young people with AIDS. *N. Engl. J. Med.* **332,** 112–118.

Monfardini, S., Vaccher, E., Pizzocaro, G., *et al.* (1989). Unusual malignant tumours in 49 patients with HIV infection. *AIDS* **3,** 449–452.

Pantaleo, G., Graziosi, C., and Fauci, A. S. (1993). The immunopathogenesis of human immunodeficiency virus infection. *N. Engl. J. Med.* **328,** 327–335.

Penn, I. (1983). Lymphomas complicating organ transplantation. *Transplant. Proc.* **15,** 2790–2797.

Penn, I. (1991). The changing pattern of posttransplant malignancies. *Transplant. Proc.* **23,** 1101–1103.

Pluda, J. M., Yarchoan, R., Jaffe, E. S., *et al.* (1990). Development of non-Hodgkin lymphoma in a cohort of patients with severe human immuno-deficiency virus infection on long-term antiretroviral therapy. *Ann. Int. Med.* **113,** 276–282.

Purtilo, D. T. (1976). Pathogenesis and phenotypes of an X-linked recessive lymphoproliferative syndrome. *Lancet.* **2,** 882–885.

Seiden, M. V., and Sklar, J. (1993). Molecular genetic analysis of posttransplant lymphoproliferative disorders. *Hematol/Oncol. Clin. North Am.* **7,** 447–464.

Starzl, T. E., Nalesnik, M. A., and Porter, K. A. (1984). Reversibility of lymphomas and lymphoproliferative lesions developing under cyclosporine-steroid therapy. *Lancet* **l,** 584–587.

Insulin-like Growth Factors

Derek Le Roith

National Institutes of Health, Bethesda, Maryland

Haim Werner

Sackler School of Medicine, Tel Aviv, Israel

GLOSSARY

apoptosis Programmed cell death.
insulin-like binding proteins Large molecular weight proteins found in the circulation and in the local tissue environment that bind IGFs and regulate their half-life and function.
insulin-like growth factors Polypeptides produced throughout the body; while their structures are similar to insulin, they act primarily as growth factors.
insulin-like growth factor-I receptor A large protein found on the surface of almost all cells that bind IGFs and are stimulated to affect cellular functions.
mitogenesis Proliferation of cells.
tumor suppressor gene Protein products of these genes normally affect the expression of other genes, thereby controlling the growth of cells and preventing unregulated or cancerous growth.

Insulin-like growth factors (IGFs) constitute a family of mitogenic ligands, receptors, and binding proteins that are intimately involved in the regulation of cell growth and transformation. IGFs, which were initially identified on the basis of their capacity to mediate the effects of growth hormone, are produced by many tissues and participate in a variety of physiological processes, including nervous system function, reproduction, and anabolic processes. Furthermore, members of the IGF family are key players in many transformation events and have therefore become a major focus of research in cancer. Activation of the IGF-I receptor by locally produced or circulating IGFs evokes potent mitogenic and antiapoptotic signals that are important steps in the progression of many tumors. As a corollary, targeting of the IGF axis constitutes a promising novel approach in cancer therapeutics.

I. INSULIN-LIKE GROWTH FACTOR (IGF) FAMILY OF LIGANDS, RECEPTORS, AND BINDING PROTEINS

The processes of growth, differentiation, and cellular death are tightly regulated by numerous cellular and secreted factors. These factors control the temporal and tissue-specific expression of a wide array of genes in a highly orchestrated fashion. Disruption of this finely tuned genetic program can result in a pathological phenotype, and possibly tumor formation. Insulin-like growth factors (IGF-I and IGF-II) are a family of mitogenic polypeptides that regulate diverse aspects of cellular function. The mature circulating IGF-I and IGF-II peptides contain, respectively, 70 and 67 amino acid residues and display a large similarity to proinsulin in that both peptides contain B and A domains that are analogous to the B and A chains of insulin. However, the B and A domains of IGFs are linked by a C domain that is slightly smaller than the C peptide of proinsulin, which, unlike that of proinsulin, is not removed during processing.

The mitogenic actions of IGFs are mediated largely through the IGF-I (or type 1 IGF) receptor (IGF-I-R), which, like the insulin receptor, is a heterotetrameric membrane-spanning glycoprotein. The receptor is composed of two α subunits, which are entirely extracellular and are mainly involved in ligand binding. The two transmembrane β subunits include a tyrosine kinase enzymatic domain in their cytoplasmic portion. The IGF-II receptor, which is identical to the cation-independent mannose-6-phosphate receptor, is mainly involved in enzyme recycling and its role, if any, in the transduction of IGF-mediated biological signals has not yet been elucidated.

The actions of IGFs are influenced by a family of IGF-binding proteins that are found in the circulation and in extracellular fluids; these proteins may have positive or negative effects on IGF action by controlling the availability of free IGFs. In addition, some IGFBPs exhibit biological effects that are independent of the IGFs and instead involve direct association between the IGFBP and specific cell surface-attached proteins or receptors. The IGFBP family includes six well-characterized members (IGFBP-1 to IGFBP-6). The actions of IGFBPs are modulated by IGFBP proteases that cleave the binding proteins into fragments with lower affinity for IGFs. Proteolytic cleavage of IGFBPs results in increased levels of free IGFs that can bind to and activate the IGF-I receptor.

II. PHYSIOLOGICAL ACTIONS OF IGFS: ENCOCRINE VS LOCAL EFFECTS

IGF-I was initially identified as a serum-borne peptide that is released mainly from the liver and that mediates the effects of growth hormone (somatotropin, GH) on longitudinal growth. It was therefore termed "somatomedin" and characterized on the basis of its ability to stimulate sulfate and thymidine incorporation into cartilage. Subsequent studies demonstrated that multiple extrahepatic tissues produce IGFs at both fetal and adult stages. This suggests that in addition to their endocrine role as mediators of growth hormone action, IGFs also have local activities (paracrine/autocrine effects). The important contribution of locally produced IGFs is illustrated by the fact that liver-specific disruption of the IGF-I gene in mice did not significantly affect growth, development, and sexual maturation, despite a marked reduction in circulating levels of IGF-I. Thus, autocrine/paracrine IGF circuits are sufficient for normal growth and development.

III. IGF ACTIONS AT THE CELLULAR LEVEL

At the cellular level, IGF-I functions as a progression factor during the cell cycle, being required for the cell to progress through G_1. Activation of the IGF-I receptor by IGF-I has been postulated to be sufficient for most cells to complete the cycle. According to this paradigm, the main role of competence factors (i.e., factors required by a quiescent cell to enter into G_1) is to induce enough IGF-I and IGF-I receptor to elicit the growth response. Support for this hypothesis comes from experimental evidence showing that classical competence factors such as platelet-derived growth factor and basic fibroblast growth factor increase the expression of IGF ligands and the IGF-I receptor.

In addition to their mitogenic action, IGFs exhibit a strong antiapoptotic activity that allows them to function as cell survival agents. The capacity of the IGF-I receptor to protect cells from apoptosis has been described in a variety of cells types, including hematopoietic cells, fibroblasts, and neurally derived cells. The implication of these findings is that activation of the IGF-I receptor can rescue apoptosis cells that, in the absence of IGFs, have been targeted for elimination.

The antiapoptotic activity of the IGF-I receptor is one of the key features of this receptor that confers it with potential transforming capability. Cells termed "R⁻ cells" (fibroblasts derived from IGF-I receptor "knockout" embryos) rapidly undergo apoptosis in a number of *in vitro* and *in vivo* models of programmed cell death. In contrast, fibroblasts overexpressing the receptor retain the capacity to multiply under the same experimental conditions. The primary factor controlling cell survival proved to be the concentration of IGF-I receptors on the cell surface. Furthermore, R⁻ cells could not be transformed by any of a number of oncogenes, including the SV40 large T antigen, bovine papillomavirus, and Ha-*ras*. If, however, R⁻ cells were stably transfected with a vector expressing the IGF-I receptor cDNA, cells became sensitive to the transforming abilities of these oncogenes and acquired a transformed phenotype. Thus, the presence of a functional IGF-I receptor is required for malignant transformation by most oncogenic agents.

IV. IGFS AND CANCER RISK: EPIDEMIOLOGICAL STUDIES

Epidemiological studies have linked elevated serum IGF-I levels to an increased risk of prostate, breast,

and colorectal cancer. In a nested case-control study within the Harvard's Physician's Health Study, levels of IGF-I and IGFBP-3 were determined in serum samples collected on average 7 years before 152 cases of prostate cancer were confirmed in a population of 15,000 men aged 40 to 82 years. The relative risk (RR) of prostate cancer in the upper quartile of IGF-I values was 2.4 compared with the lower quartile, and it increased to 4.3 when the concentrations of IGFBP-3 were included in the multivariate analysis. In men over 60 years the RR was 7.9. In a study including 121,700 women aged 30 to 55, 397 cases of breast cancer were confirmed on average 28 months after collection of serum samples. The RR of breast cancer in premenopausal women less than 50 years old was 4.6 in the upper tertile of IGF-I values compared to individuals in the lower tertile and increased to 7.3 when the concentrations of IGFBP-3 were incorporated into the analysis.

Unfortunately, the precise role of endocrine IGFs and IGFBPs in the etiology and/or progression of specific types of human cancer has not yet been clearly elucidated. Nevertheless, the idea that circulating IGF levels can serve as predictors of certain cancers has gained enormous support. Furthermore, the results of these epidemiological studies strengthen the rationale for clinical trials aimed at lowering IGF concentrations and/or at decreasing the sensitivity of the target organs to the mitogenic actions of IGFs.

V. EXPRESSION OF IGF AXIS COMPONENTS IN HUMAN CANCER

The abundant expression of IGF ligands, receptors, and IGFBPs by many cancers and transformed cell lines was recognized early on in the investigation in the IGF field. IGF-I is detectable in extracts of small cell lung cancer (SCLC) and non-SCLC cells and their conditioned medium (Table I). Ovarian carcinomas, central nervous system tumors, and thyroid cancers also express IGF-I. IGF-II is expressed by stromal tissues in breast cancer specimens, suggesting that IGF-II may act in a paracrine mode to stimulate cancer growth. Additional malignancies shown to express IGF-II include Wilms' tumor, rhabdomyosarcoma, and adrenal carcinoma. In general,

TABLE I

Expression of IGF-I and IGF-II in Some Common Neoplasms

IGF-I
  Central nervous system (CNS): glioblastomas, astrocytomas, meningiomas
  Gastrointestinal (GI) tract: Pancreatic, esophageal cancers
  Lung: Small cell lung cancer (SCLC) and non-SCLC
  Reproductive system: Ovarian, testicular cancers
  Thyroid
IGF-II
  CNS: Meningiomas
  GI tract: Colon, gastric cancers
  Reproductive system: Endometrial, cervical cancer
  Bone: Osteosarcomas

---

overexpression of IGFs in most tumors does not involve structural alterations, such as deletions or gene amplifications, but rather seems to result from a defective transcriptional control of the IGF genes.

The IGF-I receptor, which mediates the proliferative actions of IGF-I and IGF-II, is similarly expressed at very high levels by most tumors in comparison to normal adjacent tissue. The αIR-3 antibody, a monoclonal anti-human IGF-I receptor antibody, has been shown to inhibit the proliferation of numerous types of cancer cells, including breast, hematopoietic, colorectal, neuroblastoma, melanoma, osteosarcoma, and Wilms' tumor-derived cells. Comparable results were obtained in various cancer cell lines using antisense strategies against IGF-I receptor mRNA. A reduction in the number of cell surface receptors seems, therefore, to be a key step toward controlling IGF-mediated proliferation. Finally, alterations in the levels of the various IGFBPs have been shown to take place in many malignancies, with reports of both increases and decreases in the expression levels of specific BPs. Some IGFBPs are inhibitory, whereas others may be capable of enhancing IGF action. Thus, changes may occur in the level of free IGF, thereby enhancing tumor growth. Alternatively, some IGFBPs may actually directly enhance the growth of the cancer. However, an increased expression of certain IGFBPs may mediate the effects of inhibitors of cancer growth, such as retinoids, tumor necrosis factor, and certain interleukins.

VI. IGF-II: GENOMIC IMPRINTING, OVERGROWTH SYNDROMES AND CANCER

The IGF-II gene product, which is the most active IGF peptide during prenatal proliferative stages, is also an important autocrine/paracrine mitogenic factor for many tumors. IGF-II is expressed in most non-malignant tissues only from the paternal allele; the maternal allele is hypomethylated and thereby transcriptionally silent, presumably due to its easy access by transcriptional repressors. The process by which one allele is silenced is termed genomic imprinting. Genomic imprinting has been shown to be altered in certain tumors ("loss of imprinting," LOI); as a result, increased levels of IGF-II are present in the tumor microenvironment. Relaxation of imprinting has been reported, for example, in lung cancer, rhabdomyosarcoma, gliomas, cervical, and prostate cancer, as well as in Wilms' tumor. The molecular mechanism responsible for LOI involves the tumor suppressor gene H19, a gene that maps to the same chromosomal region as the IGF-II gene. H19 is also imprinted, being expressed from the maternal chromosome. LOI of IGF-II is linked to increased DNA methylation of the H19 promoter, suggesting that this abnormal methylation may result in IGF-II being turned on and H19 being turned off. The outcome of these opposite changes in gene expression is a net increase in cell growth. Other potential mechanisms that result in increased IGF-II activity include loss of heterozygosity with paternal duplication, excessive transcriptional activation and/or loss of transcriptional suppression, and deficiencies in modulation of IGFBPs. Interestingly, no significant correlation was observed between circulating IGF-II levels and increased RR of cancer, again suggesting a role as an autocrine/paracrine factor in tumor growth.

VII. IGF-II-SECRETING TUMORS AND HYPOGLYCEMIA

Nonislet cell tumors are intraabdominal or thoracic tumors of diverse etiologies that have been recognized for many years to be the cause of severe hypoglycemic conditions. The mechanism responsible for the reduction in blood glucose levels is the production of IGF-II by the tumors. Tumor IGF-II is mainly in its prohormone, high molecular mass (12–15 kDa), incompletely processed form, called "big" IGF-II. Normally, IGFs circulate in an inactive form, complexed to IGFBP-3 and an acid-labile subunit (ALS). However, "big IGF-II" cannot form this complex and is bound primarily to IGFBP-2, which is increased in these patients. Therefore, the IGF-II is more rapidly removed from the circulation and reaches the target organs. Interaction of IGF-II with insulin receptors and IGF-I receptors in muscle insulin and IGF-I receptors enhances peripheral glucose uptake, whereas its effect on hepatic insulin receptors results in inhibition of any potential compensatory liver glucose production. Following surgical removal of these tumors, big IGF-II disappears from the circulation, and only the normally processed liver-produced IGF-II is detected, usually in association with IGFBP3.

VIII. ONCOGENIC REGULATION OF COMPONENTS OF THE IGF AXIS

The expression of IGF ligands, receptors, and IGFBPs is controlled by a number of negative growth regulators (i.e., tumor suppressors), whose overall function is to inhibit proliferation and whose inactivation has been linked to the etiology of several tumors, and by cellular and viral oncogenes that positively stimulate cell transformation. For example, p53, the most frequently mutated tumor suppressor in human cancer, has been shown to inhibit transcription of IGF-II and IGF-I-receptor genes by suppressing activity of their respective promoters. However, wild-type p53 stimulated activity of the IGFBP3 gene that usually functions as an inhibitor of IGF action. Reduced expression of both ligand and receptor, and increased expression of IGFBP-3, may thereby mediate the effects of p53 on cell cycle arrest and apoptosis. In contrast, tumor-derived, mutant versions of p53 significantly stimulate activity of the IGF-II and IGF-I receptor promoters. This, in turn, leads to mitogenic activation of the overexpressed receptor by locally produced IGF-II.

Likewise, transcription of the IGF-II and IGF-I-R genes is negatively regulated by WT1, a zinc-finger transcription factor whose inactivation has been linked to the etiology of a subset of pediatric kidney cancers known as Wilms' tumor. The effects of WT1 on IGF-II and IGF-I receptor genes were associated with binding of WT1 and may result in transcriptional *de*repression of the IGF-II and IGF-I receptor genes. A particular case in which the WT1 gene is involved is desmoplastic small round cell tumor, an abdominal malignancy characterized by a recurrent chromosomal translocation, t(11;22)(p13;q12), that fuses the N-terminal domain of EWS (the Ewings' sarcoma gene product) to the C-terminal DNA-binding domain of WT1. The EWS–WT1 chimera is able to bind to WT1 consensus sites in the IGF-I receptor promoter and to activate transcription of this gene. Thus, translocation t(11;22)(p13;q12) converts WT1 from a tumor suppressor into a potential oncogene acting on the same target gene, the IGF-I receptor.

IX. TARGETING THE IGF AXIS AS A THERAPEUTIC STRATEGY

Because of the key role of the IGF axis in many neoplastic processes, it is a potentially important therapeutic target to suppress cellular proliferation. In general terms, potential therapies should be aimed at reducing the circulating levels of IGF-I (in view of the increased RR of certain cancers that was linked to high endocrine levels of IGF-I). Such therapies should also be aimed toward abolishing binding of IGF to its receptor, suppressing IGF-I receptor activity, and/or blocking IGF-mediated signal transduction pathways. Several approaches were employed for this purpose, including the use of ligand analogs, antireceptor antibodies, antisense strategies, and a number of chemical compounds.

Peptide analogs that compete with IGF-I binding to the IGF-I receptor, and therefore interfere with its activation, have been successfully employed in several cancer-derived cell lines, including a number of prostatic cell lines. Certain antineoplastic drugs have been shown to act, at least partially, by suppressing the IGF axis. For example, the antiestrogen tamoxifen exerts a potent cytostatic effect in breast cancer that is mediated, at least in part, by its inhibitory action of the IGF-I receptor. Similarly, the polysulfonated naphtylurea compound suramin has been shown to interfere with IGF-I binding to its receptor, a finding that may explain its antimitogenic activity in several cancers. Antisense stratagies have been employed to block IGF-stimulated proliferation using deoxynucleotides as well as stably transfected antisense IGF-I receptor mRNA. Very promising results have been obtained with this methodology both *in vitro* and *in vivo*.

In conclusion, there is an impressive volume of information of both a basic and clinical nature that is being generated in the IGF field. These and future studies will undoubtedly result in novel therapeutic approaches for those human malignancies in which the IGF axis is involved.

See Also the Following Articles

ANTIBODY-TOXIN AND GROWTH FACTOR-TOXIN FUSION PROTEINS • EWING'S SARCOMA (EWING'S FAMILY TUMORS) • HEMATOPOIETIC GROWTH FACTORS • STAT PROTEINS IN GROWTH CONTROL • WILMS TUMOR SUPPRESSOR WT1

Bibliography

Baserga, R., and Rubin, R. (1993). Cell cycle and growth control. *Crit. Rev. Eukary. Gene Express.* **3,** 47–61.

Chan, J. M., Stampfer, M. J., Giovannucci, E., Gann, P. H., Ma, J., Wilkinson, P., Hennekens, C. H., and Pollak, M. (1998). Plasma insulin-like growth factor-I and prostate cancer risk: A prospective study. *Science* **279,** 563–566.

Hankinson, S. E., Willett, W. C., Colditz, G. A., Hunter, D. J., Michaud, D. S., Deroo, B., Rosner, B., Speizer, F. E., and Pollak, M. (1998). Circulating concentrations of insulin-like growth factor-I and risk of breast cancer. *Lancet* **351,** 1393–1396.

Holly, J. M. P., Gunnell, D. J., and Davey Smith, G. (1999). Growth hormone, IGF-I and cancer: Less intervention to avoid cancer? More intervention to prevent cancer? *J. Endocrinol.* **162,** 321–330.

Karnieli, E., Werner, H., Rauscher, F. J., III, Benjamin, L. E., and LeRoith, D. (1996). The IGF-I receptor gene promoter is a molecular target for the Ewings Sarcoma–Wilm's tumor fusion protein. *J. Biol. Chem.* **271,** 19304–19309.

LeRoith, D., Werner, H., Beitner-Johnson, D., and Roberts, C. T., Jr. (1995). Molecular and cellular aspects of the insulin-like growth factor I receptor. *Endocr. Rev.* **16,** 143–163.

Lowe, W. L., Roberts, C. T., Jr., LeRoith, D., Rojeski, M. T., Merimee, T. J., Fui, S. T., Keen, H., Arnold, D., Mersey, J., Gluzman, S., Spratt, D., Eastman, R. C., and Roth, J. (1989). Insulin-like growth factor-II in nonislet cell tumors associated with hypoglycemia-increased levels of messenger ribonucleic acid. *J. Clin. Endocrinol. Metab.* **69,** 1153–1159.

Morison, I. M., and Reeve, A. E. (1998). Insulin-like growth factor 2 and overgrowth: Molecular biology and clinical implications. *Mol. Med. Today* **4,** 110–115.

Rechler, M. M. (1993). Insulin-like growth factor binding proteins. *Vitam. Horm.* **47,** 1–114.

Rininsland, F., Johnson, T. R., Chernicky, C. L., Schulze, E., Burfeind, P., Ilan, J., and Ilan J. (1997). Suppression of insulin-like growth factor type I receptor by a triple-helix strategy inhibits IGF-I transcription and tumorigenic potential of rat C6 glioblastoma cells. *Proc. Natl. Acad. Sci. USA* **94,** 5854–5859.

Rosenfeld, R. G., and Roberts, C. T., Jr. (1999). "The IGF System: Molecular Biology, Physiology, and Clinical Applications." Humana Press, Totowa, NJ.

Werner, H., Karnieli, E., Rauscher, F. J., III, and LeRoith, D. (1996). Wild type and mutant p53 differentially regulate transcription of the insulin-like growth factor I receptor gene. *Proc. Natl. Acad. Sci. USA* **93,** 8318–8323.

Werner, H., and LeRoith, D. (1996). The role of the insulin-like growth factor system in human cancer. *Adv. Cancer Res.* **68,** 183–223.

Werner, H., Re, G. G., Drummond, I. A., Sukhatme, V. P., Rauscher, F. J., III, Sens, D. A., Garvin, A. J., LeRoith, D., and Roberts, C. T., Jr. (1993). Increased expression of the insulin-like growth factor-I receptor gene, IGFIR, in Wilms' tumor is correlated with modulation of IGFIR promoter activity by the WTI Wilms' tumor gene product. *Proc. Natl. Acad. Sci. USA* **90,** 5828–5832.

Yakar, S., Liu, J.L., Stannard, B., Butler, A., Accili, D., Sauer, B., and LeRoith, D. (1999). Normal growth and development in the absence of hepatic insulin-like growth factor I. *Proc. Natl. Acad. Sci. USA* **96,** 7324–7329.

Integrin Receptor Signaling Pathways

Heinz R. Reiske
Jun-Lin Guan
Cornell University College of Veterinary Medicine

GLOSSARY

adapter proteins Adapter proteins form linkages between two other proteins, e.g., Grb2 binds to both FAK and SOS, effectively linking FAK with SOS.

extracellular matrix (ECM) The ECM is composed of proteins such as fibronectin and collagen. These proteins are secreted by cells, provide physical anchorage, and serve as a source of extracellular signals.

protein domains Protein domains usually refer to a module of a protein with a specific function. For instance, kinase domains catalyze the addition of a phosphate group to serine, threonine, and tyrosine residues. Src homology (SH) 2, SH3, and pleckstrin homology (PH) domains allow a given protein to physically associate with phosphotyrosines, proline-rich motifs, and phospholipds, respectively.

protein phosphorylation Addition of a phosphate group to the hydroxyl group of the amino acids tyrosine, serine, and threonine can modify enzymatic activity (stimulate or repress) of a given protein. Also, phosphorylation of tyrosine can create the binding site for proteins bearing SH2 domains. Often, a signaling cascade is propagated by the successive phosphorylation of a series of proteins.

recruitment and subcellular localization The proper functioning of signaling proteins depends in part on their subcellular localization. For example, PI3K is "active" when it is recruited to the membrane by binding by virtue of its SH2 and SH3 domains to proteins such as FAK.

During the past decade great strides have been made in accumulating knowledge pertaining to the signal transduction mediated by a class of cell adhesion molecules known as integrins. It has been appreciated that integrins regulate a number of cellular functions that play a role in pathological processes such as invasion and metastatis as well as physiological functions such as wound healing and tissue remodeling. The signal transduction pathways mediated by integrins have opened a view to these processes on the molecular level. Particularly important are the interactions between integrins and tyrosine kinases such as FAK as well as serine/threonine kinases such as ILK. Furthermore, the downstream effectors of integrins such as small G-proteins, MAPK family members, lipid kinases, and the products of oncogenes such as c-Abl and Akt are also of central importance in mediating cellular processes regulated by integrins.

I. INTRODUCTION

Integrins are a class of cell adhesion molecules that bind to components of the extracellular matrix (ECM). In addition to physically anchoring cells to the ECM, integrins transmit signals across the cytoplasmic membrane and initiate signaling cascades, which regulate a variety of cellular functions, including gene expression, cell proliferation, migration, and survival. These glycoproteins are heterodimers composed of an α and β subunit. Each subunit consists of three domains: An extracellular domain that binds to the ECM, a transmembrane region, and a cytoplasmic tail that associates with a litany of signaling molecules and mediates signal transduction pathways in response to cell adhesion. Currently, approximately 12 isoforms of each α and β subunit are known; these combine to form distinct receptors for specific ECM components. For example, $\alpha_5\beta_1$ associates with the ECM protein FN, whereas $\alpha_2\beta_1$ binds to collagen.

In vitro, integrins are localized to subcellular structures known as focal adhesions. Following adhesion, integrins activate tryosine kinases such as the focal adhesion kinase (FAK) and c-Src and serine/threonine kinases such as protein kinase C (PKC), as well as Rho family small G proteins. In addition, integrins recruit signaling molecules and structural proteins to focal adhesions to provide a scaffold for initiating signaling cascades and providing a physical link between the cytoskeleton and ECM, respectively. *In vivo*, integrins regulate many physiological processes, including embryogenesis, wound healing, and inflammation. These processes are regulated by the coordination of cell migration, proliferation, and survival, which are in turn mediated by signal transduction pathways emanating from integrins. Over the past decade, many of the signaling cascades responsible for the aforementioned processes have been well characterized. Integrins also play an important role in pathological processes such as accelerated cell growth, invasion, and metastasis and, like physiological processes, depend on the integration of migration, proliferation, and resistance to apoptosis. It is in this context that the signal transduction cascades mediated by integrins are discussed (Fig. 1).

II. SIGNALING PATHWAYS

A. FAK and Associated Proteins

1. FAK/PI3K Complex

FAK is a principle kinase in integrin signaling. FAK is activated (i.e., phosphorylated) following cell adhesion to several different integrins. The major phosphorylation event on FAK is the autocatalytic phosphorylation of tyrosine-397 (Tyr397). Tyr397 serves as the binding site for the Src homology 2 (SH2) domains of c-Src, phosphatidylinositol 3-kinase (PI3K), Grb7, and phospholipase C-γ1 (PLC-γ1). These molecules then phosphorylate their substrates localized to focal adhesions. Numerous lines of evidence show that FAK regulates cell migration. For instance, *in vitro*, FAK will promote the migration of fibroblast cell lines. *In vivo* FAK is overexpressed in highly invasive tumors. FAK also regulates cell proliferation and cell survival signals transmitted by integrins.

PI3K is a lipid kinase composed of an 85-kDa regulatory subunit (p85) containing two SH2 domains and one SH3 domain and a 110-kDa catalytic subunit (p110). p85 mediates the recruitment of PI3K to focal adhesions and growth factor receptors in the plasma membrane. PI3K phosphorylates the lipid phosphatidylinositol that serves as a second messenger to activate downstream targets of PI3K such as Akt.

PI3K associates with FAK, which is stimulated by adhesion and growth factor treatment. Formation of the FAK/PI3K complex is required for FAK-promoted cell migration. Disruption of this complex ablates the ability of FAK to stimulate cell migration *in vitro*. Treating cells with the PI3K inhibitors wortmannin and LY29004 also inhibits cell migration, demonstrating that the lipid kinase activity of PI3K is required in this process. Targeting p110 to the plasma

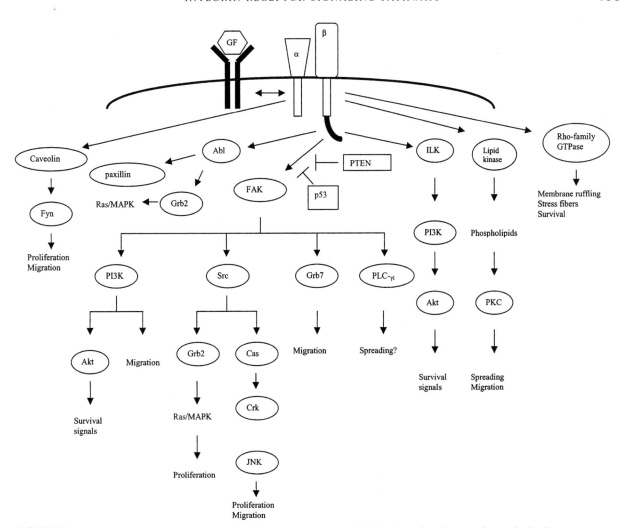

FIGURE 1   Diagram of signaling pathways emanating from integrins. Proteins highlighted in red are known to be involved in human cancers.

membrane artificially results in constitutive PI3K activity and cellular transformation. This result indicates that this pathway may hold relevance to invasion and anchorage-independent growth.

The serine/threonine kinase Akt (also known as protein kinase B) is activated by the phospholipid products of PI3K and is involved in propagating survival signals. Oncogenic forms of Akt result in cellular transformation *in vitro*. *In vivo*, v-Akt (product of the AKT8 retrovirus) is attributed to murine T-cell lymphoma. In some systems, FAK will stimulate Akt activity—activation that is dependent on the association of FAK with PI3K. Overexpression of FAK in Madin Darby canine kidney (MDCK) cells causes them to become resistant to anchorage-dependent

apoptosis or anoikis (i.e., cells held in suspension will undergo apoptosis). Disruption of the FAK/PI3K complex in this system abolishes FAK-promoted Akt activity as well as resistance to anoikis. This reinforces the notion that the FAK/PI3K complex plays a role in the ability of cancer cells to survive in the absence of adhesion to the ECM.

2. FAK/Src Complex

FAK also associates with the tyrosine kinase c-Src. c-Src, once bound to FAK, phosphorylates the adapter protein p130^{Cas} (Cas), which is also associated with FAK. Multiple phosphotyrosines on Cas now serve as binding sites for other proteins, principally Crk. Crk leads to the activation of the MAPK family member

JNK. JNK phosphorylates the transcription factor c-Jun, resulting in gene expression (Fig. 1). Studies have linked this signaling cascade to the regulation of cell migration and proliferation *in vitro*. The FAK/Src complex will also phosphorylate the cytoskeletal protein paxillin. Paxillin subsequently associates at these sites with Crk. This process has been implicated in regulating cell spreading on ECM proteins and may contribute to the control of migration and proliferation.

FAK-bound c-Src will phosphorylate FAK Tyr925. This phosphotyrosine serves as the binding site for the SH2 domain of Grb2. Grb2 in turn is complexed with an activator for Ras, SOS. The FAK/Grb2 complex is then capable of contributing toward activation of the Ras/MAPK cascade. This Src-dependent event is likely involved in the regulation of cell proliferation and possibly cell migration.

3. Additional FAK-Interacting Proteins

Tyr397 serves as the binding site for the adapter protein Grb7 and PLC-γ1. Evidence suggests a role for the FAK/Grb7 complex in cell migration. FAK association with PLC-γ_1 stimulates the enzymatic activity of PLC-γ_1, which results in the hydrolysis of phosphatidylinositol 4,5-bisphosphate to generate the second messengers diacylglycerol and inositol 3,4,5-trisphosphate, which activate PKC and mobilize intracellular Ca^{2+}, respectively.

FAK is rapidly dephosphorylated when cells in culture are held in suspension. FAK dephosphorylation would then block all integrin-initiated pathways mediated by FAK. This process, which often does not function properly in cancers, ensures *in vivo* that these cells cannot reattach aberrantly and proliferate on sites on different organs. Furthermore, focal adhesions are dynamic structures that must be created and disassembled during migration and cell division. It thus becomes necessary to activate and inhibit FAK-mediated pathways during these processes. FAK has intrinsic catalytic activity, which suggests that a phosphatase, activated by the disruption of integrin adhesion, may be responsible for this phenomenon. Thus far, studies have implicated two phosphatases in the negative regulation of FAK: Shp-2 will dephosphorylate Tyr397; this has been implicated in regulating focal adhesion turnover, and hence cell migration. The

tumor suppressor PTEN is mutated in glioblastoma, prostate, breast, and endometrial cancers. PTEN dephosphorylates FAK, inhibits cell migration and proliferation, and negatively regulates PI3K/Akt survival signals. Mutation of PTEN would allow growth, migratory, and survival-promoting pathways mediated by FAK to progress uncontrollably and contribute to invasion and metastasis.

4. Role of p53 in FAK Signaling

Mutations in the tumor suppressor gene p53 are common in many malignant cancers. Oftentimes, such cells have circumvented the requirement for cell adhesion to the extracellular matrix for survival. This anchorage-independent growth is a critical step in the progression of cancer to metastatic disease.

In a report by Ilic and co-workers, p53 was established as a mediator of apoptosis in response to a disruption in integrin signaling. FAK as a principal mediator of integrin signaling was implicated in a positive role for cell survival based on the observation that its inactivation resulted in apoptosis. Activated by cPLA$_2$ and PKCλ/ι, p53 promotes apoptosis in the absence of FAK function. Furthermore, inactivation of p53 suppresses the proapoptotic effect of inactivating FAK. Integrin signaling through FAK is therefore required for the propagation of cellular survival signals. An important part of the regulation of this process is the tumor suppressor p53, which is activated upon interference with integrin signaling. Stated differently, upon detachment from the ECM, FAK will become inactivated. Under these circumstances, p53 will ensure that aberrant cell growth does not take place by initiating apoptosis.

B. Protein Kinase C

PKC represents a family of serine/threonine kinases that consist of several isoforms. PKC isoforms have been implicated in regulating integrin affinity for ECM ligands. This "inside-out" signaling is not described in this article.

"Outside-in" signaling by integrins can activate PKC isoforms that results in the regulation of cell migration and spreading. For example, phospholipid products are potent activators of PKC isoforms. PI3K metabolites have been shown to activate PKC; this kinase then is capable of regulating cell migration through a pathway that may involve Rac. Given the ability of phospholipid metabolites to activate PKC isoforms, it remains likely that integrin-mediated pathways that involve PI3K may contain PKC as an intermediate.

C. Integrin-Linked Kinase

ILK is a serine/threonine kinase that binds directly to the β cytoplasmic domains of $\beta1$ and $\beta3$ integrins. Cell adhesion activates ILK in a PI3K-dependent manner, which then leads to Akt activation. Studies have implicated ILK in the promotion of tumorigenicity. Aberrant ILK activity can result in elevated Akt activity and thus resistance to apoptosis. In addition, studies show an increase in FN–matrix assembly, as well as a loss of E-cadherin expression, both of which can contribute to tumorigenicity.

D. Shc

Shc is an adapter protein that can associate with the Grb2/sos complex, which results in activation of the Ras/MAPK pathway. This adapter protein has been implicated in regulating both cellular proliferation and migration. Adhesion is capable of activating Shc, although the exact mechanism is currently unclear. One pathway involves the activation of caveolin, Src family member Fyn kinase, and subsequent activation of Shc. Another involves the activation of FAK and c-Src followed by Shc activation.

E. Rho Family Small G Proteins

Small G proteins are a family of low molecular weight GTP-hydrolyzing enzymes that cycle between a GTP-bound or active state and a GDP-bound or inactive state. Particularly relevant to integrin signaling is the Rho family of small G proteins: Rho, Rac, and Cdc42. All three enzymes have been implicated in regulating the dynamics of the cytoskeleton, including membrane ruffling, stress fiber formation, and focal adhesion assembly. These phenomena all play a role in cell spreading and migration, as well as cell growth. These G proteins also regulate integrin affinity and focal contact formation. This type of inside-out regulation is also beyond the scope of this article and will not be covered.

The formation of GTP-bound Rho, Rac, and Cdc42 can be stimulated by integrins. Active G proteins in turn activate downstream targets that include lipid, serine/threonine, and tyrosine kinases. Rho has been shown to interact with the lipid kinases PI3K and phosphatidylinositol 4-phosphate 5-kinase (PI4-5K), which cause the elevation of PI3-P and PI 4,5-P levels. These lipids then contribute to the polymerization of actin. PLC-$_{\gamma1}$ is also activated by Rho, resulting in the production of IP3 and DAG, which results in an increase in Ca^{2+} concentration and PKC activation, respectively, and hence changes in the cytoskeleton. Rho-kinase, a serine/threonine kinase, results in increased myosin light chain phosphorylation and thus cytoskeletal dynamics. The tyrosine kinase Akt, for instance, is activated by Cdc42, which renders the cell resistant to apoptosis.

F. BCR-ABL

c-Abl is a nonreceptor tyrosine kinase localized to both the cytosol and the nucleus. Nuclear c-Abl is rendered inactive in resting cells by the retinoblastoma protein. Cytoplasmic c-Abl is always active. Constitutively active variants of c-Abl, such as BCR-Abl and v-Abl, cause Abl to reside solely in the cytoplasm.

c-Abl is regulated by integrins. In suspended cells, c-Abl activity is reduced in both nuclear and cytoplasmic pools. Upon replated on FN, c-Abl is localized to focal contacts. This localization correlates with c-Abl export from the nucleus. Following adhesion, c-Abl translocates to the nucleus. Additional studies have shown that c-Abl will associate with the Ras/MAPK activator Grb2; kinase-dead c-Abl also blocks integrin-stimulated Erk2 activity, suggesting that integrins signal to MAPK through c-Abl. In addition, c-Abl has also been shown capable of phosphorylating and associating with the focal adhesion protein paxillin. These data further suggest that integrin intracellular signaling is mediated in part by c-Abl.

BCR-ABL is an oncogene formed by the Philadelphia chromosome translocation fusing the BCR and c-ABL genes to create a fusion protein known as p210BCR-ABL. Chronic myelogenous leukemia

(CML) is a myoproliferative disorder associated with BCR-ABL expression.

Integrin signaling is affected by BCR-ABL expression. One study has demonstrated that cell adhesion to the integrin substrate FN could be stimulated by BCR-ABL through a mechanism involving its tyrosine kinase activity. These data suggest that BCR-ABL is capable of positively modulating integrin function. Another study has also shown that BCR-ABL expression is capable of promoting cdk2 activity upon adhesion to FN, providing additional evidence that BCR-ABL modulates integrin function and has a positive effect on cell growth.

In hematopoetic cells, integrin-mediated cell adhesion has also been associated with cell cycle arrest. β1-integrins have been shown capable of upregulating p27Kip protein levels, which inhibits cdk2 activity and hence promotes cell cycle arrest. With the expression of BCR-ABL in CML CD34$^+$ cells, p27Kip protein levels are elevated, but cdk2 activity is not suppressed. This is due to BCR-ABL-induced mislocalization of p27Kip to the cytoplasm instead of the nucleus where it would have access to cdk2. With the sequestration of p27Kip to the cytoplasm, the inhibitory signal to cdk2 from integrins is blocked.

Inhibition of BCR-ABL expression using antisense oligonucleotides in CML hematopoietic progenitor cells results in the restoration of β1-integrin-induced cell cycle arrest. This study is another example of how BCR-ABL antagonizes the inhibition of cell proliferation mediated by integrins.

In the examples just given, BCR-ABL interferes with integrin function in a way that overcomes cell cycle arrest either by stimulating growth-promoting signals or by interrupting growth-inhibitory signals.

G. Cross-Talk with Growth Factor Receptors

Stimulation of integrins and growth factor receptors often synergize to produce various responses. Many parallels exist between growth factor and integrin-mediated pathways. For instance, PI3K phosphorylation and activity are induced by adhesion as well as treatment with growth factors. In addition, the tyrosine phosphorylation and tyrosine kinase activity of growth factor receptors serve to recruit adapter proteins such as c-Src and PI3K. Integrin activation by adhesion activates the tyrosine kinase FAK and results in the recruitment of both c-Src and PI3K to focal adhesions via the association with FAK.

In addition to parallels between growth factor and integrin signaling cascades, these also converge at points in their signaling pathways. For instance, MAPK activation, which is regulated by both adhesion and growth factor receptors, displays a different profile of activation in response to stimulation by adhesion alone or adhesion and growth factors. Integrin activation of MAPK alone results in rapid activation followed by a rapid return of activity to basal levels, whereas adhesion in the presence of growth factor results is sustained MAPK activity. This is one striking example of synergistic activation of signaling targets by adhesion and growth factors.

Clearly, the regulation of cellular processes is dependent on inputs from both stimuli. In the absence of adhesion, growth factor stimulation alone is not sufficient to promote growth or survival. One hallmark of cancer is the ability of cells to proliferate in the absence of adhesion; if the requirement for adhesion in integrin-mediated pathways is circumvented, then these cascades will constitutively promote cell growth in the presence of growth factors.

III. RELATIONSHIP OF BIOCHEMICAL PATHWAYS TO CANCER

Many of the biochemical pathways that emanate from integrins have been outlined. As shown in Fig. 1, the terminus of these pathways that begin with adhesion end with gene expression or the control of cellular processes such as migration, proliferation and survival—all of which play significant roles in the development of tumors and their invasion and metastasis to other tissues. These pathways, which regulate normal cellular and physiological functions, must be tightly regulated to properly coordinate the aforementioned phenomena. For example, FAK is overexpressed in cancer cells derived from highly invasive tumors. Not surprisingly, downstream targets of FAK (PI3K and Cas) are involved in regulating cell migration. Furthermore, the tumor suppressor PTEN, which negatively regulates FAK, is also mutated in highly invasive tumor lines. Here we can see how defects in gene expression (FAK overexpression) and mutation (loss of PTEN function) could play a role in the aberrant function of integrin-mediated signaling pathways and hence contribute to the development of cancer.

IV. FUTURE RESEARCH AND APPLICATIONS

Many of the intermediates in these signal transduction pathways remain to be discovered; indeed, additional pathways will likely be discovered in the near future. Having the molecular road maps of signal transduction pathways mediated by integrins will enable the design of better drugs and strategies to more efficiently treat different cancers. Knowing specifically what signaling cascades are behaving abnormally will also help in designing treatments for individual patients, as well as providing the framework for better cancer treatments in the future.

See Also the Following Articles

BCR-ABL • Extracellular Matrix and Matrix Receptors • Integrin-Targeted Angiostatics • MAP Kinase Modules in Signaling • Protein Kinases and Their Inhibitors • Signal Transduction Mechanisms Initiated by Receptor Tyrosine Kinases

Bibliography

Bhatia, R., and Verfaillie, C. (1998). *Blood* **91**, 3414–3422.

Bazzoni, G., Carlesso, N., Griffin, J. D., and Hemler, M. E. (1996). *J. Clin. Invest.* **98**, 521–528.

Clark, E. A., and Brugge, J. S. (1995). *Science* **268**, 233–239.

Datta, S. R., Dudek, H., Tao, X., Masters, S., Fu, H., Gotoh, Y., and Greenberg, M. E. (1997). *Cell* **91**, 231–241.

Chan, P.-C., Lai, J.-F., Cheng, C.-H., Tang, M.-J., Chiu, C.-C., and Chen, H.-C. (1999). *J. Biol. Chem.* **274**, 26901–26906.

de Klein, A., van Kessel, A. G., Grosveld, G., Bartram, C. R., Hagemeijer, A., Bootsma, D., Spurr, N. K., Heisterkamp, N., Groffen, J., and Stephenson, J. R. (1982). *Nature* **300**, 765–767.

Derman, M. P., Toker, A., Hartwig, J. H., Spokes, K., Falck, J. R., Chen, C-S., Cantley, L. C., and Cantley, L. G. (1997). *J. Biol. Chem.* **272**, 6465–6470.

Franke, T. F., Kaplan, D. R., and Cantley, L. (1997). *Cell* **91**, 435–437.

Guan, J.-L. (1997). *Int. J. Biochem. Cell Biol.* **29**, 1085–1096.

Han, D., and Guan, J.-G. (1999). *J. Biol. Chem.* **274**, 24425–24430.

Hurley, R. W., McCarthy, J. B., and Verfaillie, C. (1995). *J. Clin. Invest.* **96**, 511–512.

Hurley, R. W., McCarthy, J., and Verfaillie, C. (1997). *Exp. Hematol.* **25**, 321–328.

Ilic, D., Almeida, E. A. C., Schlaepfer, D. D., Dazin, P., and Aizawa, S. (1998). *J. Cell Biol.* **143**, 547–560.

Hynes, R. O. (1992). *Cell* **69**, 11–25.

Jiang, Y., Zhao, R. C. H., and Verfaillie, C. (2000). *Proc. Natl. Acad. Sci. USA* **97**, 10538–10543.

Juliano, R. L. and Haskill, S. (1993). *J. Cell Biol.* **120**, 577–585.

Lewis, J. M., Baskaran, R., Taagepera, S., Schwartz, M. A., and Wang, J. Y. J. (1996). *Proc. Natl. Acad. Sci. USA* **93**, 15174–15179.

Lewis, J. M., and Schwartz, M. A. (1998). *J. Biol. Chem.* **273**, 14225–14230.

Machesky, L. M., and Hall, A. (1996). *Trends Cell Bio.* **6**, 304–310.

Reiske, H. R., Kao, S.-C., Cary, L. A., Guan, J.-L., Lai, J.-F., and Chen, H.-C. (1999). *J. Biol Chem.* **274**, 12361–12366.

Renshaw, M. W., Lewis, J. M., and Schwartz, M. A. (2000). *Oncogene* **19**, 3216–3219.

Schlaepfer, D. D., Hauck, C. R., and Sieg, D. J. (1999). *Prog. Biophys. Mol. Biol.* **71**, 435–478.

Wang, J. Y. J. (1993). *Curr. Opin. Genet. Dev.* **3**, 35–43.

Welch, P. J., and Wang, J. Y. J. (1993). *Cell* **75**, 779–790.

Welch, P. J., and Wang, J. Y. J. (1995). *Mol. Cell Biol.* **15**, 5542–5551.

Wu, C., Keightley, S. Y., Leung-Hagesteijn, C., Radeva, G., Coppolino, M., Goicoechea, S., McDonald, J. A., and Dedhar, S. (1998). *J. Biol. Chem.* **273**, 528–536.

Zhang, X., Chattopadhyay, A., Ji, Q.-S., Owen, J. D., Ruest, P. J., Carpenter, G., and Hanks, S. K. (1999). *Proc. Natl. Acad. Sci. USA* **96**, 9021–9026.

Integrin-Targeted Angiostatics

Dwayne G. Stupack
David A. Cheresh
The Scripps Research Institute

I. Introduction
II. Angiogenesis Is an Invasive Process
III. A Physiological Context for
   Integrin-Targeted Activities
IV. Alternative Roles for Integrin Antagonism
   during Angiogenesis
V. Summary

GLOSSARY

angiogenesis The growth of new blood vessels from preexisting vasculature, usually in response to a local chemical cue.

apoptosis The activation of internal programs or proteolytic cascades within a cell that result in its death. Apoptosis occurs to eliminate unwanted, senescent, or inappropriately placed cells.

ECM The extracellular matrix of glycoproteins and proteoglycans that envelops cells and provides support and positional cues for cell and tissue growth, maintenance, and repair.

integrins Heterodimeric (α/β) transmembrane receptors that mediate cellular interactions with the surrounding ECM

components and transmit information into the cell regarding its physical environment.

ligation The binding of a ligand, or target molecule, to a receptor. However, in the case of integrins, productive ligation events generally occur only with immobilized ligands; soluble ligands typically act as antagonists.

MAP kinase A family of kinases that act as convergence points during cell signaling events, coordinating extracellular input with programmed cytosolic signaling and nuclear/transcriptional events.

Angiogenesis is the complex process by which new blood vessels grow. Like other tissues, the growth of tumors is dependent on the recruitment of a vascular bed, permitting the delivery of oxygen and nutrients while allowing the clearance of waste by-products. Endothelial cells in tumor-adjacent tissues are triggered by chemical signals from the tumor, causing them to become proliferative and eventually forming new sprouts into these areas. The growth of these vascular sprouts is a complex, invasive process, which involves local remodeling of the existing basement extracellular matrix (ECM) proteins and the deposition of new, provisional ECM components. Interactions with these ECM components are mediated largely by integrins, cell adhesion molecules that are mobilized or newly expressed on the surface of angiogenic endothelial cells. Integrins play a crucial role not only in facilitating the mechanical connection of endothelial cells to the ECM that is critical for cell migration into the vascular tissues, but also in potentiating the cellular response to growth factors and in the regulation of cell viability. Thus, the antagonism of specific integrin receptors during angiogenesis can lead to the blockade of cell migration, a reduced ability to respond to growth factors, and/or programmed cell death (apoptosis). Through these mechanisms, integrin-targeted drugs function as antiangiogenic agents. Importantly, these antagonists function against angiogenic endothelial cells, yet do not influence quiescent endothelium, thereby providing a means to target angiogenic tissues.

I. INTRODUCTION

A. Tissues Require a Blood Supply

Angiogenesis is the process by which new blood vessels sprout and grow into avascular tissue. While angiogenesis does not occur in normal adult tissues, it is induced during the process of tissue revascularization following wound healing and is integral to menstrual cycling and the formation of a placenta by a developing embryo. Not surprisingly, angiogenesis is also a central process during growth and development, allowing newly developed tissues to be served by the vascular system. In the embryo, this developmental angiogenesis follows vasculogenesis, which is the initial formation of a vascular bed from precursor angioblasts in the embryo.

Inappropriate or pathological forms of angiogenesis also exist in a variety of disease states, including retinopathies, arthritides, and during the growth of tumors. Although different neoplastic tissues may be vascularized to different degrees, it is generally acknowledged that the higher the degree of vascularization, the more aggressive the tumor. Thus, high levels of vascularization are associated with a poor prognosis.

An important concept, originally proposed by Dr. Judah Folkman, was that the inhibition of angiogenesis could block tumor growth indirectly, simply by blocking access of tumor cells to needed metabolites. This "siege" strategy would act to starve the tumor. In addition, it was noted that because the targets of this intervention are endothelial cells, this approach would also provide a means of bypassing the capacity to acquire drug resistance associated with transformed tumor cells.

B. Angiogenesis Is Initiated by Cytokines

In order to trigger an angiogenic response from quiescent endothelial cells, the cells must become activated by local cues. This generally occurs when stromal or neoplastic cells in the surrounding tissues respond to hypoxia, or other environmental cues, through the secretion of soluble proangiogenic factors. Upon reaching the local vasculature, these factors stimulate the local endothelium and foster new blood vessel growth. The ingrowth of this vasculature is ultimately important to the growth of the tumor. In elegant initial studies, Folkman demonstrated that thymic tumors could not progress beyond a millimeter or two in diameter without acquiring a blood supply. It was not initially clear what factors governed the *de novo* growth of blood vessels, although it was anticipated that if these factors and their receptors were identified, then antagonists might be designed that could interfere with angiogenesis.

The advent of molecular biology provided a means to isolate cDNAs encoding proteins that impacted angiogenesis. Surprisingly, the last two decades of the millennium revealed the existence of more than a dozen factors that promote angiogenesis. Most of the characterized proangiogenic factors are secreted proteins (growth factors) that bind to glycoprotein receptors on the endothelial cell surface, and thus activate these cells. While some of these factors, such as vascular endothelial growth factor (VEGF, also called vascular permeability factor) and angiopoietin-1, are relatively selective for effect on endothelial cells, many other angiogenic factors, such as basic fibroblast growth factor (bFGF) and transforming growth factor α, have receptors on a wide range of cell types.

As part of a normal cellular program, or as a result

of their transformed status, tumor cells develop the capacity to secrete one or more of these growth factors. It is important to note that, within a given tumor, different regions can exhibit different patterns of angiogenic factor production. Thus, even the analysis of a tumor biopsy may not provide an indication of the angiogenic potential of the tumor as a whole. This observation, combined with the ever-increasing list of angiogenic factors and the apparent redundancy of function of these factors, provided indications that the targeted antagonism of a single growth factor receptor might be insufficient to implement as a general antiangiogenic strategy. However, growth factor signaling is nevertheless crucial to the acquisition of an angiogenic phenotype by endothelial cells.

C. Signaling Events Occur Downstream of Angiogenic Growth Factor Receptors

An increased understanding of the cytoplasmic signaling events that occur in response to angiogenic growth factor binding has resulted from focused studies on the events following growth factor receptor ligation from a variety of cell types. The binding of growth factors commonly leads to dimerization of the growth factor receptors, bringing the individual receptors into close contact and forming a signal-producing complex. Subsequently, growth factor receptors that possess tyrosine kinase activity may phosphorylate each other as well as individual target proteins, or combinations of proteins. Receptors that lack kinase activity typically activate signaling pathways through the recruitment of cytosolic "adaptor" proteins (proteins with several protein interaction domains that direct the association of other proteins) and cytosolic kinases. Nevertheless, these initially different intracellular signaling pathways often converge on common intermediates at downstream stages of the signaling cascade. For example, activation of the mitogen-activated protein (MAP) kinases ERK1 (extracellular signal-regulated kinase) and ERK2 appears to be a required end event if angiogenesis is to occur, regardless of the initiating stimulus. ERKs are pleiotropic regulators of cell biology that influence gene transcription, initiate proliferation, and activate cell migration. In essence, the activation of ERKs serves to coordinate the induction of an invasive pro-

gram in endothelial cells. This downstream action of angiogenic growth factors on endothelial cells transforms them from quiescent, nonproliferative cells to highly proliferative and invasive. Whereas much less than 1% of quiescent endothelial cells are observed to be undergoing cell division at any given time, the majority of cells in an angiogenic vessel can exhibit mitotic markers.

Endothelial stimulation by angiogenic growth factors thus results in dramatic changes in the biology of these cells. This, in turn, renders the endothelium susceptible to many drugs that target proliferative cells. Initial antiangiogenic approaches exploited the observation that although angiogenic endothelial cells are highly proliferative, they are nonetheless untransformed and maintain a low mutation rate. Thus, these cells are much less likely than tumors to acquire drug resistance. Drugs such as tamoxifen, TNP-470 and Combrestatin A, which disrupt microtubule function, have increased activity against actively proliferating endothelial cells, as mitosis requires the action of microtubules and microtubule motors. These agents work selectively on the endothelial cells, yet are not endothelial cell specific and may impact other proliferative cells in the body.

However, a second profound effect of MAP kinase activation by angiogenic growth factors is to (1) induce the production of ECM proteins, (2) induce the production of ECM-degrading enzymes, such as metalloproteases, and (3) to alter the quantity and quality of ECM adhesion receptors expressed on the endothelial cell surface. These are crucial modifications that allow endothelial cell interaction with the altered ECM and facilitate the invasion of nearby tissues. Such invasive events are very rare in adults, and provide a second attractive opportunity for interventions that target angiogenesis.

II. ANGIOGENESIS IS AN INVASIVE PROCESS

Typically, quiescent endothelial cells interact tightly with each other through the action of cadherins and immunoglobulin superfamily members and are anchored to the underlying basement matrix components via the interactions of integrin receptors (Fig. 1).

Quiescent endothelium

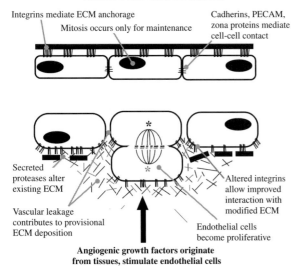

FIGURE 1 The activation of endothelial cells by angiogenic factors leads to proliferation and reorganization of endothelial cell adhesion molecules, as well as remodeling of the local ECM.

Cadherins are calcium-dependent receptors that mediate homophilic cell–cell contact. Endothelial cells may express at least three cadherins [vascular endothelial (VE) cadherin, neural (N) cadherin and truncated (T) cadherin], whereas immunoglobulin receptors, such as CD31 (platelet-endothelial cell adhesion molecule), engage in both homophilic interaction and heterophilic binding to other receptors, including integrins.

Integrins are a family of heterodimeric (α/β) adhesion receptors that mediate attachment to cell surface or ECM ligands in a divalent cation-dependent manner. In mammals, there are at least 18 different integrin α chains and about half as many β chains. Integrins pair in a limited number of α/β subunit combinations (about two dozen), and endothelial cells only express a fraction of these (Table I). Each of the integrin α/β subunit combinations demonstrates distinct characteristics with respect to ligand specificity, affinity and regulation of ligand binding, cytoplasmic signaling events elicited by ligation, and/or the capacity to facilitate cell migration or matrix contractile events. Thus, although different integrins may interact with the same ECM component, these interactions are not purely redundant.

For example, integrin $\alpha 5 \beta 1$ is principally a receptor for the ECM component fibronectin, which is

TABLE I
Relative Expression of Endothelial Integrins

Integrin	Ligands	Expression during angiogenesis
$\alpha 1 \beta 1$	Collagen	Increase
$\alpha 2 \beta 1$	Collagen, laminin	Increase
$\alpha 3 \beta 1$	Collagen, laminin, fibronectin, thrombospondin	Increase
$\alpha 5 \beta 1$	Fibronectin, fibrin	Increase
$\alpha 6 \beta 1$	Laminin	Maintain
$\alpha 6 \beta 4$	Laminin	Maintain
$\alpha v \beta 3$	Collagen type IV, XVII (NC domains), Del-1, denatured collagen, fibrin(ogen), fibronectin, laminin, MMP2-PEX PECAM, tenascin, thrombospondin, vitronectin, von Willebrand's factor	de novo
$\alpha v \beta 5$	Del1, fibronectin, vitronectin	Maintain

bound through an arginine-glycine-aspartate (RGD) sequence in the "cell-binding domain." Although integrin $\alpha v \beta 3$ similarly recognizes this region, it also binds at least 10 other ECM protein ligands, many of which are bound in an RGD-independent manner. Changes in integrin expression and activity play a central role in mediating the invasive behavior of cells. The formation of new integrin contacts, the release of neighboring cells (via relaxation of cadherin and similar links), and alterations to the local ECM are coordinated events that allow endothelial cells to invade nearby tissues.

A. Changes to the ECM during Angiogenesis

The vascular endothelium is supported by a basement matrix composed principally of laminin and type IV collagen. Quiescent endothelial cells interact with this ECM principally through clusters of integrins located in discrete adhesive patches or in stable cellular organelles termed hemidesmosomes (particularly $\alpha 6 \beta 4$) found on the abluminal face of the cells. This basolateral location reflects the role that integrins normally play in providing stable ECM anchorage. As mentioned, endothelial cells also interact laterally with each other, largely through interactions between clustered cadherin–cadherins and immunoglobulin superfamily members. Together, these elements present a stable, cohesive barrier that allows the diffusion of nutrients, oxygen, and small proteins into the underlying tissues but prevents the access of cells and larger plasma proteins.

Stimulation of endothelial cells with an angiogenic factor, such as VEGF, results in a dramatic remodeling of this vascular architecture. VEGF binding to its receptors (flk, flt-1, flt-4) leads to early signaling events within the cell that trigger the breakdown of cell–cell adhesion. This allows "leakage" of blood plasma proteins from the circulation directly into the underlying ECM. Many of these proteins are provisional ECM components, such as fibrinogen, fibronectin, and vitronectin, which are present in the plasma at very high concentrations (~300–400 μg/ml) as inert precursor forms. While some provisional ECM forms require proteolytic cleavage for activation, others may simply alter conformation upon contact with the underlying ECM. These provisional ECM proteins are modular in nature and interact with a variety of other proteins. For example, fibronectin is a dimer composed of two similar associated proteins, each of which may contain a total of 30–32 protein domains (the exact total varies with alternative splicing) of three distinct types. Collectively, these domains mediate interactions with heparin or other proteoglycans, fibrin, collagen, other molecules of fibronectin, and several different integrins. Thus, the ECM underlying the endothelial cells can change rapidly after the addition of VEGF through the deposition of new ECM proteins. A variety of other angiogenic factors (such as bFGF) do not induce this permeability immediately, yet accomplish similar events by inducing the synthesis of these provisional ECM components by the endothelial cells themselves, by inducing the expression of VEGF, or through gross leakage events (some of which are hemorrhagic) that can be associated with later stages of angiogenesis.

The original basement ECM of type IV collagen and laminin is not maintained intact through this process. Endothelial cell stimulation by angiogenic factors leads to the secretion or activation of several classes of proteases that act upon the perivascular ECM. Some proteases will cleave and activate the adhesive function of ECM proteins. Collagen contains cryptic sites that support cell binding after it becomes denatured or proteolyzed. The protease thrombin cleaves fibrinogen, allowing it to polymerize into insoluble fibrils, resulting in its deposition within the ECM. Other proteases, including urokinase plasminogen activator, plasmin, stromelysins, and other matrix metalloproteinases, also cleave existing ECM proteins and act to modify or eliminate components of the local ECM. However, ECM degradation is regulated by the presence of endogenous protease inhibitors such as the tissue inhibitors of metalloproteinases and plasminogen activation inhibitors (PAIs) and is directed by selective localization to invasive regions of the cell surface. Thus, local proteolysis of ECM during angiogenesis is a controlled process modulated by the presence of proteases and their associated inhibitors.

B. Changes in Adhesion Receptor Expression on Angiogenic Endothelial Cells

Coordinated with the changes occurring in the local ECM, growth factor-stimulated endothelial cells modify their adhesion receptor repertoire. During this process, cadherins may be downregulated or "shed" by the action of proteases. In contrast, many integrins, including $\alpha2\beta1, \alpha3\beta1, \alpha5\beta1,$ and $\alpha v\beta3$, are upregulated on the surface of angiogenic endothelial cells (Table I). These alterations in adhesion receptors reflect the onset of a program allowing decreased cell–cell contact and increased ability to interact with the underlying ECM, promoting cell invasion. Variation in the specific integrin heterodimers expressed probably reflects changes in the underlying ECM. However, it is clear that all integrins are not equal in their ability to support migratory or invasive processes and so these alterations in expression reflect a balance between integrins that provide anchorage and integrins that can best facilitate cell invasion of the tissue.

Among these alterations in integrin expression, the dramatic upregulation of integrin $\alpha v\beta3$ is particularly dramatic. Unlike the other integrins listed, $\alpha v\beta3$ is not expressed on quiescent endothelium, yet is highly expressed on angiogenic endothelial cells. In nonendothelial cells, integrin $\alpha v\beta3$ is associated with an invasive phenotype. For example, the exogenous expression of integrin $\alpha v\beta3$ is sufficient to induce tumor cell migration without a requirement for growth factor stimulation. Notably, integrin αvβ3 is absent from most adult tissues, but is present on invasive tumors, including melanoma and glioma, as well as on trophoblasts and placental tissue. The limited distribution of this integrin *in vivo*, and its specific upregulation on the surface of growth factor-stimulated endothelial cells, suggests that αvβ3 plays an important role in angiogenesis.

C. Antagonism of Selected Integrins Inhibits Angiogenesis

Because αvβ3 is selectively expressed on angiogenic endothelial cells, investigations have been conducted to determine the role for this integrin in angiogenesis. The disruption of integrin αvβ3 binding to ECM ligands by treatment with peptide antagonists, organic compounds, or monoclonal antibodies leads to the inhibition of angiogenesis *in vivo* in response to basic fibroblast growth factor in a variety of avian and mammalian models. Targeting αvβ3 also blocks angiogenesis in response to tumors, resulting in tumoristasis and, in many cases, leading to the regression of tumor. An important extension of these studies was the observation that antagonism of αvβ3 was, similarly, able to block tumor growth in human skin xenografted onto nude mice. Histologically, tumor regression was associated with cellular necrosis within the tumors and a dramatic reduction in the presence of vascular endothelial cells within the tumor tissue. The limited distribution and capacity to inhibit angiogenesis in animal models of disease led to the introduction of αvβ3-targeted therapies in human clinical trials.

The inhibition of other integrins can also influence angiogenesis. In the case of VEGF-induced angiogenesis, antagonists that targeted integrin αvβ3 were found to be relatively weak inhibitors. In contrast, antagonism of the related integrin, αvβ5, was found to potently block VEGF-induced angiogenesis. Interestingly, the expression of αvβ5 on endothelial cells does not change during angiogenesis. However, cellular stimulation by growth factors causes integrin αvβ5 to become "functionally activated" (it binds and releases ligand at an increased rate), leading to increased cell migration *in vitro*. This may be due to downstream effects of VEGF signaling, including functional

association of αvβ5 with other cell surface receptors, such as the urokinase plasminogen activator receptor. Alternatively, VEGF stimulation may result in increased interactions with a repertoire of cytosolic signaling proteins that are known to cluster with integrin cytoplasmic domains, including α-actinin, tensin, vinculin, p130cas, phosphorylated focal adhesion kinase, and actin. It is not entirely clear why a specific effect against angiogenic endothelial cells is observed after treatment with antagonists of integrin αvβ5, as αvβ5 is present on all endothelial cells. However, it is likely related to ongoing requirements for integrin-mediated signaling in cells that have activated an angiogenic program. Further, the dynamic nature of the αvβ5 on these cells provides increased opportunities for antagonists to bind, and therefore have effect, relative to quiescent cells. In quiescent cells, integrins are engaged in clustered multivalent ECM contacts that are relatively static and quite stable. These types of contacts are more difficult to antagonize and thus less likely to be influenced by the anti-integrin regimens used to block angiogenesis.

Additionally, it has become clear that the antagonism of other endothelial integrins, including α1β1, α2β1, and α5β1, may also interfere with neovascularization induced by certain angiogenic factors. These integrins are similar to integrin αvβ5 in the respect that they are present upon quiescent endothelial cells and appear to be activated functionally to some degree during angiogenesis. However, like integrin αvβ3, the expression of these integrins is also upregulated on angiogenic endothelial cells, although to a lesser degree. While the blockade of these integrins on vascular endothelial cells has not yet been demonstrated to inhibit tumor growth, results obtained from studies with antagonists of αvβ3 and αvβ5 suggest that this may be possible. Collectively, these observations underscore the importance of integrins in angiogenesis and also provide an impetus to determine why integrins should play such a major role in regulating angiogenesis.

III. A PHYSIOLOGICAL CONTEXT FOR INTEGRIN-TARGETED ACTIVITIES

Integrins play a central role in most aspects of endothelial cell biology, maintaining anchorage of quiescent cells while facilitating endothelial sprouting and tissue invasion during angiogenesis. Therefore, the antagonism of integrins, as discussed, could function through a variety of possible means.

A. Mode of Action

On the one hand, the antagonism of integrins could block activation of the angiogenic program in endothelial cells. Antagonism of integrin $\alpha v\beta 3$ results in the disruption of sustained signaling by angiogenic growth factors, such as bFGF, to the ERKs. Signaling mediated by growth factor receptors has been determined to be dependent on integrin-mediated contact with the ECM. Many growth factor receptors complex with, or near, integrin complexes during the initiation of signaling. The blockade of integrin ligation can disrupt these signals, essentially suppressing the invasive and proliferative program normally triggered by these growth factors. This might be expected to have a "calming" effect on the endothelial cells, suppressing the proliferative response, decreasing the expression of new ECM components and proteases, and disabling selected cytoplasmic elements of the migration machinery. Extracellularly, a more obvious function of integrin antagonism would be to disrupt the ability of integrin $\alpha v\beta 3$ to bind ECM ligands, preventing the physical link between the cytoskeleton and the ECM, thus blocking migration. Together, these effects would have a profound influence on the capacity of the endothelial cells to contribute to an ongoing angiogenic response.

On the other hand, the antagonism of integrins on angiogenic endothelial cells is also known to eventually result in the induction of programmed cell death, or apoptosis. This leads to the physical elimination of angiogenic endothelial cells. Invasive endothelial cells are crucially dependent on maintaining integrin-mediated interactions with the underlying ECM in order to maintain their viability. It is possible that this is a regulatory mechanism to prevent aberrant invasive events or uncontrolled endothelial proliferation. However, it is noteworthy that many integrins, which have increased expression on endothelial cells *in vivo*, especially $\alpha v\beta 3$ and $\alpha 5\beta 1$, have been demonstrated to have a crucial impact on cell viability in studies performed *in vitro*. In the case of integrin $\alpha v\beta 3$, antagonism has been shown to result in the apoptosis of angiogenic endothelial cells *in vivo* in a variety of models of angiogenesis. As might be expected, this has a significant effect not only on newly forming sprouts, but also on recently formed microvessels, as the elimination of even a portion of endothelial cells along a capillary can have significant disruptive effects on vascular integrity. Thus, at least in the case of integrin $\alpha v\beta 3$, antagonism leads to the induction of apoptosis.

These observations might be interpreted to suggest an obligate role for integrin $\alpha v\beta 3$ in mediating angiogenic events. However, this is not the case. Lack of $\alpha v\beta 3$ expression in humans is responsible for one form of Glanzmann's thrombasthenia, yet these patients develop an apparently normal vasculature. Similarly, the generation of $\alpha v\beta 3$-deficient mice supported the notion that $\alpha v\beta 3$ was not absolutely required for angiogenesis, as these mice have apparently normal vasculature. Despite this "lack of requirement" for $\alpha v\beta 3$, the *de novo* expression of integrin $\alpha v\beta 3$ occurs during angiogenesis on the endothelium of all mammalian and avian species that have been examined. Thus, although it is not absolutely necessary for angiogenesis, the induction of integrin $\alpha v\beta 3$ expression during angiogenesis has been evolutionarily conserved. However, the observations are not paradoxical, as it is clear that although integrin $\alpha v\beta 3$ is not required to promote angiogenesis, it nevertheless plays a crucial role in the regulation of this process.

B. Integrin Antagonists Are Produced during Angiogenesis

Largely due to studies focused on components of the ECM, it has become apparent that angiogenesis is a balance of local positive and negative regulatory cues and that both sets of cues are required for productive neovascularization. In some cases, the presence of a factor required for angiogenesis (e.g., PAI-1) may also inhibit angiogenesis at higher concentrations. With respect to this, established tumors have long been known to secrete or shed unidentified factors that suppress the growth of distant metastasis, and it has now become clear that a major means of accomplishing this is by preventing angiogenesis in these distant sites. Surprisingly, tumors shed a variety of angiogenesis

TABLE II
Endogenous Integrin Antagonists

Type	Examples	Integrins bound
Collagen NC domains	Collagen IV α1, α2, α3, α6 Endostatin (collagen XVIII α1) Collagen VII	α1β1, α2β1, α5β1, αvβ3
Protease domains	PEX, angiostatin	αvβ3
Altered ECM	Thrombospondin, Del1	αvβ3, α3β1
Proteolytic ECM fragments	RGD-containing peptides (e.g., laminin P1, thrombin 3 kDa, fibrin I9-D, fibronectin-CBD, L1-CAM)	αvβ3, α5β1, αvβ5
	Non-RGD peptides (e.g., laminin GD-6, Col DGEA)	αvβ3, α3β1

inhibitors. Many of the molecules that negatively influence angiogenesis are ECM proteins, ECM fragments, fragments of adhesion molecules, or fragments of proteolytic enzymes that bind to and antagonize integrins (Table II).

These antiangiogenic proteins may be produced as proteolytic by-products during angiogenesis. For example, the basement ECM that underlies quiescent blood vessels is principally composed of type IV collagen and laminin. Both of these proteins are subject to proteolysis during angiogenesis. Six different α chain genes (α1–α6) can be present in type IV collagen. Each chain is composed of a classic collagenous domain and a noncollagenous (NC) domain. NC domains from four of the six α chains (α1, α2, α3, α6) have been reported to bind to integrins. Although only one binds in an RGD-dependent manner, all four function as "natural" integrin antagonists and all are antiangiogenic. This may not be an uncommon property of collagen NC domains, as it is also present in endostatin, the NC domain of collagen type XVIII α1. Similarly, isolated laminin peptides have been described to possess antiangiogenic and/or integrin-binding activities, which may be RGD dependent or independent.

Interestingly, the nonproteolytic domains of several proteases also possess integrin-binding, antiangiogenic properties. Proteases are often secreted in an inactive, or zymogen, form, which is activated by autocleavage or the action of other proteases. The antiangiogenic drug angiostatin is composed of kringle domains 1–4 of plasminogen and is bound by integrin αvβ3 in an RGD-independent manner. Similarly, the hemopexin domain (PEX) of matrix metalloprotease 2 (MMP-2), a protease that cleaves both type IV collagen and laminin, also interacts with integrin and blocks angiogenesis. The hemopexin domains from other MMPs may possess similar activity. Importantly, all of the antiangiogenic products described, MMP-2 PEX, collagen IV NC1 domains, and laminin fragments, are produced perivascularly from physiologically localized, interacting proteins.

Adding to this complexity, local production of the new ECM components may also serve to regulate angiogenesis. Both thrombospondin (Tsp) and the product of the developmentally regulated endothelial locus-1, Del-1, can regulate angiogenesis. Like most of the provisional ECM components, these proteins bind to several cellular receptors, including integrins αvβ3 (Del1 and Tsp) and α3β1 (Tsp). A wide variety of proteins, which are locally produced during angiogenesis, can therefore act to antagonize endothelial integrins and can thus act to regulate angiogenesis as a process. Despite this apparent complexity, these observations nevertheless explain why integrin antagonists inhibit angiogenesis; they mimic a naturally occurring process.

IV. ALTERNATIVE ROLES FOR INTEGRIN ANTAGONISM DURING ANGIOGENESIS

In addition to supporting increased tumor growth through the delivery of required metabolites and the elimination of toxic catabolic products, the increasing vascular bed in the tumor also serves as an exit conduit for tumor cells. The vasculature in tumors is mosaic and includes endothelial cells as well as tumor cells in direct contact with the vascular flow. This direct access allows dissemination of the tumor through the simple shedding of tumor cells into the vasculature. This shedding can be substantial, resulting in millions of tumor cells being released on a daily basis from larger tumors.

Some of these cells metastasize to distant capillary beds via the circulatory system. There, they may lodge and/or subsequently extravasate. However, most of the distant metastases that survive will not immediately grow into viable tumors, in part due to the systemic presence of antiangiogenic factors, as discussed earlier. Therapies that target integrins, in addition to blocking angiogenesis, may also have anti-invasive effects on these tumor cells.

Antagonism of integrins may alternatively prevent cell recruitment into tumors. During angiogenesis, endothelial precursor cells may be recruited from the circulation. These cells become incorporated into developing vessels and can later be detected as part of the contiguous endothelial lining. The recruitment of these cells to angiogenic regions, and their ability to invade nearby tissues, certainly requires integrin-mediated events. Integrins are required for the recruitment of other circulating cell populations (leukocytes). By comparison, it is reasonable to assume that the antagonism of selected integrins will interfere with the ability of these endothelial precursors to be recruited to angiogenic sites, just as integrin-directed treatments have been shown to block leukocyte recruitment to inflammatory sites.

V. SUMMARY

A variety of strategies are currently being developed that target angiogenic endothelial cells. The central role of integrins in the complex process of angiogenesis makes them an attractive target for intervention (Fig. 2). Although investigations are revealing that different integrins may play slightly different roles in angiogenesis, it is clear that at any given time the ability to maintain viability and to sustain angiogenesis is dependent on integrin-mediated contacts with the ECM. In this respect, integrins such as $\alpha v \beta 3$ play several roles, modulating the activity of growth factors, providing an increased ability to interact with the newly remodeled ECM, and acting as an ECM biosensor that can govern cell viability in response to naturally occurring integrin antagonists.

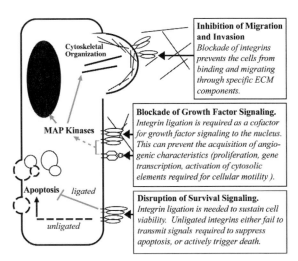

FIGURE 2 Integrin antagonists have pluripotent effects on activated endothelial cells, blocking adhesion, migration, cytosolic signaling events, and cell survival.

See Also the Following Articles

ANGIOGENESIS AND NATURAL ANGIOSTATIC AGENTS • ANTI-VASCULAR ENDOTHELIAL GROWTH FACTOR-BASED ANGIOSTATICS • EXTRACELLULAR MATRIX AND MATRIX RECEPTORS • INTEGRIN RECEPTOR SIGNALING PATHWAYS • MAP KINASE MODULES IN SIGNALING

Bibliography

Aplin, A. E., Howe, A., Alahari, S. K., and Juliano, R. L. (1998). Signal transduction and signal modulation by cell adhesion receptors: The role of integrins, cadherins, immunoglobulin-cell adhesion molecules, and selectins. *Pharmacol. Rev.* **50,** 197.

Boehm-Viswanathan, T. (2000). Is angiogenesis inhibition the Holy Grail of cancer therapy? *Curr. Opin. Oncol.* **12,** 89.

Cheresh, D. A., and Mecham, R. P. (eds.) (1994). "Integrins : Molecular and Biological Responses to the Extracellular Matrix (Biology of Extracellular Matrix)." Academic Press, San Diego.

Eliceiri, B. P., and Cheresh, D. A. (1999). The role of alphav integrins during angiogenesis: Insights into potential mechanisms of action and clinical development. *J. Clin. Invest.* **103,** 1227.

Folkman, J. (1995). Angiogenesis in cancer, vascular, rheumatoid and other disease. *Nature Med.* **1,** 27.

Mousa, S. A. "Angiogenesis Inhibitors and Stimulators: Potential Therapeutic Implications." Landes Bioscience, Georgetown.

Rubanyi, G. M. (ed.) "Angiogenesis in Health and Disease: Basic Mechanisms and Clinical Applications." Dekker, New York.

Interferons: Cellular and Molecular Biology of Their Actions

Dhananjaya V. Kalvakolanu
Greenebaum Cancer Center, Baltimore, Maryland

Ernest C. Borden
Taussig Cancer Center, Cleveland, Ohio

GLOSSARY

GAS IFN-γ activated site.
ICSBP IFN consensus sequence binding protein.
IFN Interferon.

ISG IFN-stimulated gene.
ISRE IFN-stimulated response element.
IRF IFN–gene regulatory factor.
ISGF IFN-stimulated gene factor.
JAK Janus kinase (just another kinase).
JH JAK homology domain.
SH *src* homology.
STAT signal transducing activator of transcription.
tyk2 tyrosine kinase 2.
PKR Protein kinase R.

Interferons (IFNs) are secretory proteins produced by virus-infected cells. The name interferon refers to their ability to interfere with viral replication. However, IFNs induce several pleiotropic responses, including antiviral, antitumor, immunomodulatory, antiparasitic, and antiproliferative activities. In addition to viral infection, double-stranded RNA (dsRNA), fungal cell wall products, and other cytokines also induce the production of IFNs. dsRNA may be a physiologically relevant regulator of IFN synthesis because it is thought to be an intermediate product of viral infection. It not only induces the expression of IFN and IFN-inducible genes but also serves as a cofactor for some IFN-induced enzymes.

I. INTERFERON GENES

Distinct cellular genes encode for various IFNs. The current IFN nomenclature is based on gene sequences. The major types IFN-α and -ω, IFN as IFN-β, and IFN-γ are produced by leukocytes, fibroblasts, and lymphocytes, respectively. There are 18 IFN-α nonallelic genes in humans among which four are pseudogenes. IFN-ω is represented as six nonallelic genes of which five are pseudogenes. Single genes encode for IFN-β and -γ. IFN-α, -ω, and -β genes are clustered on the short arm of human chromosome 9. An IFN-γ gene with three introns is located on human chromosome 12. All these genes are thought to have arisen from a single ancestral gene. A secretory signal sequence is present in all IFNs, which is cleaved off prior to their secretion. The mature forms of IFNs contain 165–172 amino acids.

Expression of IFNs is primarily regulated at the transcriptional level, although the rate of mRNA decay may also contribute. Among IFNs, regulation of the IFN-β gene is relatively well understood. Virus or dsRNA activated transcription factors, IFN-gene regulatory factor-1 (IRF-1) and NF-κB (nuclear factor-κB), bind to specific elements in the IFN-β gene promoter and stimulate transcription. A negative factor IRF-2, related to but distinct from IRF-1, inhibits gene expression. IFN-α genes are regulated by distinct promoter elements and the corresponding cognate factors. Although viruses induce both IFN-α and IFN-β, there are distinguishable differences between the patterns of induction of these genes. The virus-regulated element (VRE) of IFN-α contains IRF-binding elements but not NF-κB-binding sites. The exact sequence of IRF-1-like elements present in the IFN-α gene determines its inducibility by various agents such as virus infection or IRF-1. IRF3 and IRF-7, the recently discovered members of the IRF-family, also induce IFN-α gene expression.

The expression of IFN-γ gene is induced in T cells activated by antigens, mitogen anti-CD3, anti-CD28 antibodies, IL-2, IL-12, or IL-18. Unlike IFN-α/β, expression of the IFN-γ gene is regulated by elements both upstream of the transcription start site and those within the introns. Pregnant domestic ruminants express a novel type of IFN-ω called IFN-τ. These proteins are produced in the absence of any stimuli by the trophoectoderm of the concepti and appear to signal via specific receptors in the endometrium to maintain an appropriate milieu for the embryo.

II. INTERFERON RECEPTORS

IFN-α and IFN-β bind to a similar receptor(s), whereas IFN-γ binds to a different one. IFN-α and IFN-β receptors have high affinity for their ligand (10^{-10}M) with an abundance of $0.5–5 \times 10^3$/cell. After generating the necessary response, the ligand–receptor complexes are internalized and degraded. The exact composition of the IFN-α/β receptor is still controversial. The minimal receptor consists of two polypeptides, IFNAR1 and IFNAR2. Human IFN-α/β receptor genes are located on chromosome 21. Mice lacking IFNAR1 gene are highly susceptible to infectious agents.

The IFN-γ receptor is composed of two distinct polypeptides: the ligand-binding α chain and the signal transducing β chain. α chain genes are present on chromosomes 6 and 10 of human and murine species. Genes for the β chain have been localized on chromosomes 21 and 16 in humans and mice, respectively. Functional IFN-γ is a dimer. Therefore, two α and two β chains form the active receptor in a ligand-dependent manner. Mice lacking the IFN-γ receptor or patients with a mutant receptor are highly susceptible to mycobacterial infections.

III. INTERFERON-REGULATED PROMOTER ELEMENTS

IFN actions are mediated by IFN-stimulated genes (ISG). Some ISGs are exclusively induced by

IFN-α/β or IFN-γ. Other ISGs are induced by both IFNs. Specific response elements present in the promoters of the IFN-stimulated genes (ISGs) sense IFN-stimulated signals. Induction of ISGs by IFN-α/β is a rapid but transient process, which often lasts 3–4 h. The temporal control of IFN-γ-stimulated genes is variable. After the initial induction, ISG transcription declines and returns to basal level.

A conserved 15-bp element, the IFN-stimulated response element (ISRE), is essential for inducing ISGs by IFN-α/β. The consensus sequence for ISRE is AGGTTTCNNTTTCCT. In contrast, a variety of elements respond to IFN-γ. These include ISRE, the X and Y box elements of HLA class II genes, and the IFN-γ activation sequence (GAS). GAS-like sequences are present in the promoters of several cytokine or growth factor-inducible genes. The consensus sequence for GAS is TTNNNNNAA.

IV. INTERFERON-STIMULATED TRANSCRIPTION FACTORS

IFN-stimulated gene factors (ISGFs) bind to ISRE and regulate gene expression. Two such factors, ISGF1 and ISGF2, are constitutive, although ISGF2 is further induced by IFN treatment. ISGF1 and ISGF2 are not the primary regulators of several ISGs. ISGF2 is identical to IRF-1. ISGF3 is rapidly activated in the cytoplasm by IFN-α/β, which then translocates to the nucleus and stimulates ISG transcription. ISGF3 is composed of four proteins: p48 (ISGF3γ or IRF9), STAT1α (p91), STAT1β (p84), and STAT2 (p113). The acronym STAT (signal transducing activator of transcription) defines the bifunctional nature of these proteins. IFNs activate the STAT proteins using Janus tyrosine kinases (JAK). STAT1α and STAT1β are generated from the same gene. STAT1α and STAT1β are identical except that the former has an additional 38 amino acid long sequence at the C terminus. STAT1α alone can fully restore IFN responses in STAT1$^{-/-}$ cells. STAT2 is encoded by a distinct gene. p48 (IRF-9 or ISGF3γ) is a member of the IRF-*myb* family of DNA-binding proteins (see later).

V. STAT PROTEINS

These proteins not only transduce the signals but also act as transcription factors. The first two members of the STAT family, STAT1 and STAT2, specifically participate in the IFN-initiated JAK-STAT pathway. Five other STATs, discovered later, have been shown to participate in various cytokine-induced signaling pathways. Most STATs have the following characteristics: (1) interact with cytoplasmic tails of cytokine or growth factor receptors, (2) are tyrosine phosphorylated by JAKs, (3) contain SH2 and SH3 (SH = src homology) domains, (4) homo- or heterodimerize with other members of their family, (5) translocate to the nucleus after activation and dimerization, (6) bind to DNA in a sequence-specific and activation-dependent manner, and (7) induce gene transcription. SH2 domains are critical for homo- or heterodimerization in response to ligand-induced tyrosine phosphorylation and maintenance of the signal specificity. A conserved tyrosine residue at six to eight amino acids downstream of the SH2 domain is crucial for STAT dimerization. A transactivation domain (TAD) is present at the C terminus. Phosphorylation of a specific serine residue in the TAD is also crucial for deriving optimal transcription.

VI. JANUS TYROSINE KINASES

These enzymes are essential for cytokine signaling. Most JAKs have been isolated by polymerase chain reaction based on conserved oligonucleotides of protein tyrosine kinase domains. Because their physiologic functions were uncertain at the time of discovery, they were designated as just another kinases (JAK). JAKs are 120–130 kDa in size and contain seven conserved JAK homology (JH) domains. The functional tyrosine kinase activity is located in the JH1 domain. The JH2 domain, also known as the pseudokinase domain, is highly homologous to JH1 but does not have kinase activity (Fig. 1B). Therefore, the acronym JAK also refers to their structural analogy to Janus, the Roman god of gateways who possessed two heads. JAKs do not have SH2 or SH3 domains. JAKs do not have substrate specificity toward STATs. Most JAKs require another JAK to be

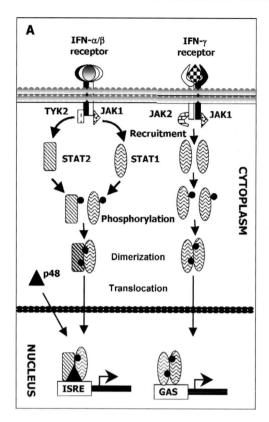

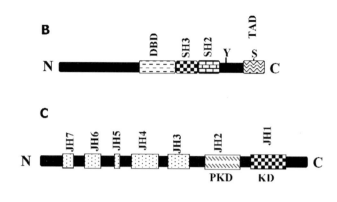

FIGURE 1 Signal transduction by interferons. (A) IFNs-α/β, employing *tyk-2* and *JAK1*, induce the tyrosine phosphorylation of STAT1 and STAT2 on binding to their receptor. STATs are ligand bond receptors recruited to the receptor, phosphorylated. Following this, a STAT1:STAT2 dimer is formed, which migrates to the nucleus, associates with the p48 subunit, and stimulates ISRE-dependent gene expression. Similarly, FN-γ induces the tyrosine phosphorylation of STAT1 using *JAK1* and *JAK2*, which binds to GAS and activates gene expression. (B) Structure of a typical STAT molecule. DBD, DNA-binding domain; SH, Src homology domain; Y, critical tyrosine; S, serine; TAD, transcription activating domain; N, amino terminus; C, carboxyl terminus. (C) Structure of a typical JAK. JH, JAK homology domain; PKD, pseudokinase domain; KD, kinase domain.

functional because the intermolecular tyrosine phosphorylation of the JH1 domain stimulates their action. To date, four JAKs—JAK1, JAK2, JAK3, and Tyk2—have been identified.

VII. SIGNAL TRANSDUCTION BY INTERFERONS

A. IFN-α/β Signaling

The IFN-α/β receptor is composed of two subunits, IFNAR1 and IFNAR2. The cytoplasmic tail of IFNAR1 is preassociated with Tyk2. JAK1 is associated to the intracellular domain of IFNAR2. Binding of IFN-α/β to the receptor causes mutual tyrosine phosphorylation of JAK1 and Tyk2. Activated Tyk2

then phosphorylates the tyrosine (at 466) of IFNAR1. This phosphotyrosine serves as a docking site for STAT2. Tyrosyl phosphorylation of STAT2 at position 690 creates a binding site for STAT1. STAT1 is then phosphorylated by JAK1 at tyrosine 701. The STAT2–STAT1 dimer dissociates from its receptor, migrates to the nucleus, and associates with p48 (ISGF3γ) to form ISGF3. STAT2, unlike STAT1, is not phosphorylated at serine. STAT2 contains a critical transcription-activating domain at the C terminus.

B. IFN-γ Signaling

The dimeric IFN-γ first interacts with two molecules of the ligand-binding IFNGR-α chain, associated with JAK1. Subsequently, two molecules of the signal-transducing IFNGR-β chain, preassociated with JAK2, are recruited into the complex. Neither JAK1 nor JAK2 is phosphorylated in the absence of the other. Thus, the JAK–STAT pathway does not involve classical kinase cascades as in the case of Ras–Raf–Map kinase pathways. Aggregation of receptor polypeptides brings the JAKs closer, leading to mutual phosphorylation and the phosphorylation of IFNGR-α at tyrosine 440 by JAK1. Tyrosine-phosphorylated IFNGR-α serves as a docking site for the SH2 domain of unphosphorylated STAT1α. JAK2 then phosphorylates STAT1α at tyrosine 701. Phosphorylated STAT1α serves as an anchor for the second STAT1α molecule, leading to its tyrosine phosphorylation. The STAT1 dimer then migrates to the nucleus, binds to GAS, and induces transcription. Mutant STAT1α (lacking tyrosine 701) is not phosphorylated and therefore cannot translocate to the nucleus. As mentioned earlier, serine phosphorylation at 727 is essential for strong transcriptional stimulation by STAT1α. The kinase responsible for this activity is unknown. A nuclear GTP-binding protein, Ran, facilitates the nuclear import of STAT1. Finally, the transcriptional activity of STAT1 is terminated by unknown tyrosine phosphatases. Thus, JAK1 and STAT1 are shared components of IFN-α/β and IFN-γ signaling pathways.

Discovery of the IFN-stimulated JAK–STAT pathway served a paradigm for most cytokine signal transduction pathways. Following this, five other STATs and four JAKs that govern the cellular responses of various cytokines and other growth factors were discovered.

VIII. INHIBITORS OF JAK–STAT SIGNALING

Studies have identified several cellular inhibitors of the JAK–STAT pathway. A family of proteins, SOCS (suppressor of cytokine signaling) or SSI (STAT-induced STAT inhibitor), inhibit the activation of STATs. These proteins contain a SH2 domain, bind to JAKs, and suppress their tyrosine kinase activity. They are induced by the same ligands that activate STATs. For example, SOCS-1 is inducible by GM-CSF, IL-3, IL-13, and IFN-γ. Overexpression of

SOCS-1 blocks the antiproliferative and antiviral actions of IFN-α. Certain ubiquitously expressed protein inhibitors of activated STATs (PIAS) also suppress STAT functions. PIAS1 inhibits STAT1. It appears that physical levels of PIAS and STAT molecules determine the outcome of cellular response to a given cytokine.

IX. BIOLOGICAL EFFECTS OF JAK–STAT GENE DISRUPTION

Targeted disruption of STATs and JAK genes in mice has been reported (Table I). STAT1$^{-/-}$ mice are normal, except for a loss of innate immunity against viral infections and high susceptibility to cancers. Disruption of STAT2 causes embryonic lethality, indicating its crucial role in the development. Disruption of the JAK1 gene causes postnatal lethality. JAK1$^{-/-}$ pups fail to nurse and die. Neurons from these mice undergo rapid apoptosis compared to those from wild-type mice. Thus, neuronal development seems to be incomplete in these mice. Disruption of JAK2 causes embryonic lethality due to defective embryonic hematopoiesis. Tyk2$^{-/-}$ mice are normal in their appearance but their physiological defects are unclear at this stage.

X. INTERFERON-STIMULATED GENES

A number of ISGs induced by IFNs-α/β and IFN-γ regulate the cellular responses (Table II). Nearly 250 genes are induced and 10 others are repressed by IFNs. This section discusses a few of the well-studied gene products that have influences on viral replication and neoplastic cell proliferation. For example, protein kinase R (PKR), a dsRNA-activated enzyme, phosphorylates several cellular proteins, including the eukaryotic protein synthesis initiation factor-2α (eIF-2α). Phosphorylation of eIF-2α results in the cessation of polypeptide chain initiation, thus leading to cellular and viral growth inhibition. PKR also activates transcription factor NF-κB by phosphorylating its inhibitor IκB. PKR is essential for certain cellular stress responses.

TABLE I
Defective IFN System and Pathogenesis

Gene product	Defects detected in knockout/human patients
IFN-γ receptor	Susceptibility to bacterial infections in mice and humans and carcinogens in mice
STAT1	Loss of innate immunity and susceptibility to carcinogens in mice
STAT2	Embryonic lethality in mice
JAK1	Postnatal lethality, neuronal development defects in mice
JAK2	Lack of hematopoiesis, leukemia in humans
IFNAR1	Loss of antiviral responses in mice
IRF1	Immunodeficiency, loss of tumor suppressor functions in mice and humans
IRF2	Loss of antiviral effects and B-cell proliferation
ICSBP	Immunodeficiency and chronic myelogenous leukemia in mice
p48	Loss of antiviral responses and immune system defects in mice
PKR	Loss of stress responses, antiviral functions, and signaling defects in mice
RNAseL	Loss of antiviral responses, defective thymic apoptosis in mice
CIITA	Loss of antigen presentation, bare lymphocyte syndrome
DAPK	Loss of antimetastatic function, loss of expression in human lymphomas

2′,5′-Oligoadenylate synthetases (2′5′ AS) are a family of unique enzymes induced by IFNs. Isoforms of 2′5′ AS, whose molecular masses range from 20 to 100 kDa, are either derived from a single gene due to alternate splicing or from different genes. Their subcellular location is also different. Using dsRNA as a cofactor, they polymerize ATP into 2′-5′-linked oligoadenylates [2′-5′ (A)$_n$]. These products activate an endoribonuclease, RNase L, which cleaves cellular or viral RNAs.

IFN-α and IFN-β also induce a number of GTP-binding proteins, including the Mx family, which inhibits the replication of several viruses. The IGTP protein is critical for antitaxoplasma responses *in vivo*. Inducible nitric oxide synthase is critical for macrophage-dependent antimicrobial and antitumor responses. MHC class I and II antigens and proteasome components are critical for antigen presentation and development of immune responses.

Cell Growth Regulators

In addition to regulating IFN and ISGs, IRF (IFN gene regulatory factor) proteins control cell growth and immune responses. IRFs are a family of proteins that include IRF1, p48 (ISGF3γ), IRF2, IRF3, IRF4 (Pip), IRF7, ICSBP, and v-IRF of Kaposi's sarcoma-associated herpes virus. All these proteins have a structurally similar DNA-binding domain at their N termini and nonconserved C termini. However, except for this similarity, these proteins are quite diverse in their functions. Both IFN-dependent and IFN-independent actions of IRFs are known.

IRF1$^{-/-}$ cells fail to undergo apoptosis and are transformed readily by activated oncogenes, indicating a tumor suppressor role for this protein. The IRF1 gene is deleted in myelodysplasia and myelocytic leukemia. IRF1$^{-/-}$ mice are immunodeficient due to defects in T cell, NK cell maturation. Mice lacking IRF1 are also defective in antigen presentation. p48 is critical for antiviral responses and antigen presentation. Cells lacking the p48 gene die rapidly upon exposure to cytotoxic drugs compared to wild-type cells. These results suggest that p48 plays other roles in cell growth control in an IFN-independent manner. In contrast, IRF2 induces cell proliferation and acts as an oncogene. ICSBP, lymphoid transcription factor, is also a tumor suppressor. ICSBP$^{-/-}$ mice develop a chronic myelogenous leukemia (CML)-like disease and immunodeficiency. ICSBP gene expression is suppressed in cells derived from patients with myeloid leukemia. ICSBP suppresses the expression of the BCR–ABL oncogene. IRF3 and IRF7 appear to be essential for IFN gene expression.

TABLE II
Mammalian Interferon-Regulated Genes

Gene	Function	Inducer
β2-Microglobulin	MHC class I light chain	α,β,γ
CIITA	Transcription factor	γ
C56,561,PIF-2	Unknown	α,β>γ,dsRNA
CRG-2	Monokine	α,β,γ
C/EBP-E	Transcription factor	γ>α,β
Cytochrome b	Mitochondrial gene product	α inhibits
Cytochrome c oxidase, subunit I	Mitochondrial gene product	α inhibits
2-5 (A)synthetase	Antiviral enzyme	α,β>γ,dsRNA
Inducible nitric oxide synthase	Macrophage effector	LPS, >γ ISG
54,PIF-2	Unknown	α,β>γ,dsRNA
FcγRI	Binds IgG-Fc	γ
GBP,γ67	GTP binding	γ>α,β
IGTP	Antitaxoplasma activity	γ
Indoleamine-2,3-dioxygenase	Protozoan inhibition	γ>α,β
ISG-15	Ubiquitin like	α,β>γ,dsRNA
ISG-20	PML nuclear body	α,β
ISG-43	Deubiquitinating enzyme	β α,>γ,dsRNA
IFP-35	Leucine zipper protein	α,β,γ
Invariant chain	MHC class II assembly	γ
IP-10	Platelet factor 4 related	γ>α,β
IP-30	Unknown	γ>α,β
IRF-1	Transcription factor, tumor suppressor	α, β, γ,dsRNA
IRF-2	Transcription factor, growth promoter	α, β,dsRNA
ICSBP	Transcription factor, tumor suppressor	γ; α/β inhibits
Leucine amino peptidase	Exopeptidase	γ
Mn-leucine amino peptidase	Mitochondrial superoxide scavenger	γ
Lysyl oxidase	Anti-ras activity	α,β
Tryptophanyl-tRNA synthetase, γ56	Trp-tRNA synthetase	γ>α,β
MxA	Antiinfluenza virus and VSV	α,β>γ,dsRNA
MxB	Unknown	α,β>γ,dsRNA
MHC class I	Antigen presentation	α,β,γ
MHC class II	Antigen presentation	γ
Phagocyte gp91-phox	NADPH oxidase cytochrome b subunit	γ, α inhibits
PKR	Inhibits protein synthesis, signaling	α,β>γ
RING 12	Proteasome complex	γ
RING 4	Putative peptide transporter	γ
γ.1	Unknown	γ>>α,β
202	Cell cycle regulator	α,β
204	Growth regulator	α,β
1-8/9-27	Unknown	α,β,γ
6-16	Unknown	α,β>γ,dsRNA
RNase L	Viral RNA degradation	α,β

A novel class of IFN-induced growth regulatory proteins is encoded by the gene 200 cluster of mouse chromosome 1. Murine p202, p203, p204, D3, and human MNDA and IFI16 genes belong to this family. These proteins share a characteristic 200 residue segment at their C termini. p202, a well-characterized member of this family, is a nuclear protein that inhibits cell proliferation. By binding to the pRb–E2F complex, p202 inhibits the action of transcription factor E2F, which regulates the expression of a number of genes involved in DNA synthesis and cell division. p202 also inhibits the action of a number of growth-promoting transcription factors, such as NF-κ B and AP1. A role for the 200 family of genes in growth control is suggested by the translocation of the MNDA gene in human myeloid leukemias. The role of other members of this family in cell growth control needs to be defined.

IFN-γ activates the expression of p21/WAF/Cip-1, a cyclin-dependent kinase inhibitor, to inhibit cell growth. IFN-β induces lysyl oxidase, a specific regressor of Ha-ras-induced transformation. IFN-α down-regulates c-myc gene expression and increases the levels or dephosphorylation of pRb to cause growth arrest.

A number of novel apoptosis-regulating genes are controlled by IFN-γ. These include thioredoxin, death associated protein-1(DAP-1), death associate protein kinase (DAPK), cathepsin D, and DAP-5, a homologue of eukaryotic translation initiation factor 4G. Among these DAPK is a potent tumor suppressor. DAPK, a calmodulin-dependent serine-threonine protein kinase, disrupts cytoskeleton during cell death. The DAPK gene is deleted in several carcinomas and lymphomas. It suppresses tumor metastasis. A number of DAPK-related genes have been identified. These enzymes also induce apoptosis.

XI. DYSFUNCTION OF INTERFERONS AND PATHOGENESIS

A number of studies have identified various aspects of IFN resistance and their roles in pathogenesis (see Table III). The following section discusses a few of these observations.

TABLE III
Viral Resistance to IFNs

Virus	Component	Target	Mechanism
Adeno	E1A	ISG induction	Blocks signaling
	VAI RNA	PKR	Blocks activation
Hepatitis B	TP	ISG induction	Blocks signaling
	ORF-C	IFN-β gene	Inhibits gene expression
Epstein–Barr	EBNA-2	ISG induction	Inhibits anticellular action
	EBER	PKR	Blocks activation
	BCRF-1	IFN-γ gene	Inhibits IFN-γ synthesis
Herpes simplex	2-5A analog	RNase L	Blocks activation
HIV-1	Tar RNA	PKR	Blocks activation
	Tat protein	PKR	Inhibits PKR
Influenza	Cellular p58	PKR	Inhibits PKR
Polio	Unknown	PKR	Degrades PKR
Reo	σ3	PKR	Sequesters dsRNA
Vaccinia	SKI	PKR	Sequesters dsRNA
	K3L	PKR	Analog of eIF-2α
	E3L	PKR	Inhibits PKR
Myxoma	MT2	IFN-γ receptor analog	Neutralizes IFN-γ
Polyoma virus	T antigen	ISG induction	Blocks JAK1
Papilloma virus	E6	IFN-D-induced genes	BLocks Tyk2

A. Inactivation of ISG Products

PKR regulates cellular or viral growth by inhibiting protein synthesis. A number of viral gene products inhibit PKR. These include the virus-associated I (VAI) RNA product of adenoviruses, Epstein–Barr virus (EBV)-encoded small molecular weight RNAs (EBERs), and HIV-TAR RNA, HIV-tat protein, reovirus σ3 protein. The influenza virus inhibits PKR using a cellular protein, p58. The vaccinia virus encodes several inhibitors, which either serve as pseudosubstrates or sequester dsRNA to prevent PKR activation. The polio virus targets PKR for degradation.

B. Disruption of JAK-STAT Pathway

Certain viruses inhibit ISG transcription by preventing ISGF3 formation. Adenoviral E1A and hepatitis B virus terminal protein (TP) mediate such effects. Consistent with this, biopsy samples from patients with HBV infection show a dramatic reduction in HLA class I expression. These data, in part, may explain the IFN-α resistance of a substantial subgroup of chronic HBV-infected patients. EBV nuclear antigen-2, an oncogene that immortalizes B cells, also inhibits the antiproliferative action of IFNs by repressing ISGs. Mouse polyoma viral T antigen, human papilloma viral E6 oncogene inhibit JAK1- and Tyk2-induced gene expression, respectively.

Similarly, deletion of JAKs and STATs leads to deregulation of cell growth. For example, tumor cells expressing a dominant-negative mutant of the IFN-γ receptor are not rejected upon transplantation. The chemical carcinogen 3-methylcolanthrene induces tumors at higher frequency in mice lacking STAT1 or IFN-γ receptor compared to normal ones. A constitutive activation of STAT1 by mutant fibroblast growth factor receptor-3 results in abnormal induction of WAF/Cip-1, an inhibitor of cell cycle, and growth stunting. This appears to be a mechanism in type II thanatophoric chondroplasia, a form of human dwarfism.

Hyperactivated JAK2 appears to play a role in acute lymphoblastic leukemia (ALL). Chromosomal translocation t(9;12)(p24;p13) in childhood ALL causes production of a chimeric protein consisting of TEL (a member of ETS family of transcription factors) and JAK2 genes. The resultant chimeric protein, TEL-JAK2, is a constitutively active oncogene.

C. Virokines and Viroceptors

Pox viruses evade the immune system by producing a number of secreted virulence-associated factors. These factors include homologues of cytokines or their receptors. These so called "virokines" include EGF-like growth factors, complement-binding protein, and serine protease inhibitors. Among the viroceptors, the homologues of cytokine receptors are secreted IFN receptors. These proteins bind to IFNs and inhibit their biological actions.

XII. THERAPEUTIC ACTIVITY IN HUMANS

Several clinical studies indicated the potential use of IFNs in therapy of human diseases. Leukocyte IFNs derived from blood donor units were introduced into clinical trials in the mid-1970s. Subsequently, recombinant IFNs have entered clinical trials. These studies have led to licensure in more than 50 countries for the treatment of neoplastic disease, viral diseases, multiple sclerosis, and certain microbial infections. IFN-α controls the disease in ~40% of patients chronically infected with hepatitis B and C viruses. Approximately half of these patients will remain virus free.

In more than a dozen malignancies, IFNs cause regression or control disease progression. In chronic myelogenous leukemia, more than 75% of patients experience complete regression of the disease with approximately one-third of these experiencing complete cytogenetic remission. IFNs, in combination with other systemic treatments, have been used successfully in hairy cell leukemia, B- and T-cell lymphomas, CML, and multiple myeloma. For some solid tumors, IFN treatment resulted in palliation equal to the best chemotherapeutic regimens. Metastatic melanoma and renal cell carcinoma are two refractory malignancies in which IFN-α is more effective than any available chemotherapeutic agent. IFN-α can also induce regressions in Kaposi's sarcoma, endocrine-pancreatic tumors, and metastatic colorectal, ovarian, and bladder carcinomas. In malignant melanoma, IFN-α delays recurrence following resection of primary disease. In relapsing multiple sclerosis, IFN-β reduces the frequency of relapse and inhibits demyelination of the central nervous system. IFN-γ is effective in chronic granulomatous disease and has been used in combination with chemotherapy for leprosy. IFN-γ may also be useful against chronic pulmonary fibrosis and antibiotic-resistant mycobacterial infections.

Preclinical and clinical findings form the basis for new therapeutic directions in chronic myelogenous leukemia, lymphomas, myelomas, melanoma, urologic malignancies, primary brain tumors, ovarian carcinoma, multiple sclerosis, chronic viral hepatitis, and papillomatous diseases. Major research challenges for full understanding and clinical application of the IFN system are (i) the diversity of the IFN family, (ii) the role of induction, (iii) molecular mechanism of action, (iv) cellular modulatory effects, (v) advantages of combinations, and (vi) identification of new therapeutic indications.

Clinical Effectiveness of Second-Generation IFNs

Quantitative differences exist between various IFNs in terms of their *in vitro* and *in vivo* effects. Pegylated IFN-α has a covalently linked polyethylene glycol (PEG) moiety. PEG reduces immunogenicity, sensitivity to proteolysis, and extends the serum half-life. It has been utilized advantageously for therapeutic proteins such as erythropoietin, thrombopoietin, and adenosine deaminase. Pharmacokinetic studies have demonstrated a dose-related increase in serum concentrations and delayed clearance of PEG–IFN-α2 compared to IFN-β. IFN-β has also been modified with various molecules, including PEG and the soluble portion of its receptor to enhance its stability *in vivo*. Although IFN-α binds to the same receptor on the cell surface as IFN-β, IFN-β does so with higher affinity. IFN-β has distinct effects on cell differentiation and proliferation in contrast to those of IFN-α2. IFN-β is a more potent of growth inhibition and apoptosis than IFN-α2. These advances suggest that the empirical combination of various IFNs with

other modalities will have an increasingly broad impact on clinical therapy.

XIII. CONCLUSIONS

IFNs have come a long way since their discovery. The IFN-stimulated JAK–STAT signal transduction pathway serves as a paradigm for most cytokines. These signal-transducing molecules have central roles in cell growth, differentiation, and tumorigenesis. Over the past decade, IFNs have been established as effective therapeutic molecules for malignant and viral diseases. Gene knockout studies in mice have established new animal models for studying pathogenic mechanisms. It is likely that the therapeutic spectrum of IFNs has just begun to be exploited. Knowledge of signal transduction mechanisms and the ISG actions may help in the development of novel combination therapeutic strategies in the near future.

Acknowledgments

The authors thank Daniel Lindner and Robert Freund for a critical reading of the manuscript. DVK is supported by research grants from the National Cancer Institute.

See Also the Following Articles

Acute Lymphoblastic Leukemia • Chronic Myelogenous Leukemia • Cytokine Gene Therapy • Epstein–Barr Virus • JAK/STAT Pathway

Bibliography

Boehm, U., Klamp, T., Groot, M., and Howard, J. C. (1997). Cellular responses to Interferon-γ. *Annu. Rev. Immunol.* **15**, 749–795.

Borden, E. C. (1997). Interferons. *In* "Cancer Medicine" (J. F. Holland, E. F. Frei, R. C. Bast, D. W. Kufe, D. L. Morton, R. R. Weischelbaum, eds.), pp. 1199–1212. Williams & Wilkins, Baltimore.

Borden, E. C., Lindner, D. J., Dreicer, R., Hussein, M., and Peereboom, D. (2000). Second generation of interferons for cancer: Clinical targets. *Sem. Cancer Biol.* **10**, 125–144.

Darnell, J. E., Jr. (1997). STATs and gene regulation. *Science* **277**, 1630–1635.

Gutterman, J. U. (1994). Cytokine therapeutics: Lessons from Interferon α. *Proc. Natl. Acad. Sci. USA* **91,** 1198–1205.

Kalvakolanu, D. V. (1999). Virus interception of cytokine regulated pathways. *Trends Microbiol.* **7,** 166–171.

Nguyen, H., Hiscott, J., and Pitha, P. M. (1997). The growing family of interferon regulatory factors. *Cytokine Growth Factor Rev.* **8,** 293–312.

Pfeffer, L. M., Dinarello, C. A., Herberman, R. B., Williams, B. R. G., and Borden, E. C. (1998). Biological properties of recombinant alfa interferons: On the 40th anniversary of the discovery of Interferons. *Cancer Res.* **58,** 2489–2499.

Sen, G. C., and Ransohoff, R. M. (1997). "Transcriptional Regulation in the Interferon System." Chapman & Hall and Landes Bioscience, Austin, TX.

Stark, G. R., Kerr, I. M., Williams, B. R. G., Silverman, R. H., and Schreiber, R. D. (1998). How cells respond to interferons. *Annu. Rev. Biochem.* **67,** 227–264.

Interleukins

F. Stephen Hodi
Robert J. Soiffer

Dana-Farber Cancer Institute, Boston, Massachusetts

GLOSSARY

interleukin A cytokine that influences the functional activity of immune effector cells.

Interleukins (IL) are a specialized group of cytokines identified by their ability to influence the function of lymphocytes (Table I). These proteins act as the primary means of signaling between cells of the immune system. They are produced by a variety of cells, including lymphocytes, phagocytes, and endothelial cells. There are currently 18 defined interleukins, and several substances undergoing physiologic identification will likely be added to this list.

I. INTRODUCTION

Interleukins are members of the broader group of cytokines that alter the behavior of cells. Cytokines may be grouped into hematopoietins, which include interleukins and colony growth factors, interferons (INF), and the tumor necrosis factor (TNF) family of molecules. Interferons are a class of molecules first found to interfere with viral replication in previously uninfected cells. There are three classes of interferons (α, β, and γ) produced by activated natural killer (NK) cells and effector T cells. The interferons influence expression of MHC class I molecules, as well as transporter and proteosome proteins involved with antigen presentation. All of the interferons have been developed for clinical use. Interferon-α is currently approved for the treatment of melanoma and CML; INF-α is also used for the treatment of hepatitis; INF-β is being used in the treatment of multiple sclerosis; and INF-γ has been found to be effective

TABLE I
Interleukins

Interleukin	Source	Targets
Il-1	Macrophages/epithelial cells	T-cell/macrophage activation
IL-2	T_H1/CTL	T-cell/NK cell proliferation/activation
IL-3	T-cells/thymic epithelia	Early hematopoiesis
IL-4	T_H2/mast cells	B-cell activation/IgE switch/suppress T_H1
IL-5	T_H2/mast cells	Eosinophil growth/IgA differentiation
IL-6	T cells; macrophages; endothelial cells	T-/B-cell growth/differentiation
IL-7	Non T cells	Growth of pre-B and pre-T cells
IL-8	Monocytes	Attracts neutrophils, basophils, and T cells
IL-9	T cells	Activates mast cells
IL-10	T_H2/macrophages	Inhibits T_H1/cytokine release; increases MHC class II; mast cell growth
IL-11	Stromal fibroblasts	Hematopoiesis; synergistic with IL-3/IL-4
IL-12	B cells/macrophages	NK-cell activation; T_H1 differentiation
IL-13	T cells	B-cell growth/differentiation; inhibits macrophage cytokine production; inhibits T_H1 cells
IL-15	T cells	Similar to IL-2; stimulates T/NK cells
IL-16	T cells/mast cells/eosinophils	Attracts CD4 T cells/monocytes/eosinophils; antiapoptotic for T-cells IL-2 stimulated
IL-17	CD4 memory cells	Cytokine production in epithelia/fibroblasts
IL-18	Activated macrophages/Kupffer cells	IFN-γ by T/NK cells; T_H1

Adapted from Jameway *et al.* (1999).

for scleroderma. The TNF family includes TNF-α and -β, as well as Fas ligand and CD40 ligand. Their effects include activation of macrophages, plasma cell isotype switching, T-cell, and NK-cell stimulation. Each class of cytokines has distinct as well as complementary effects. This article focuses on interleukins and their use in the clinical treatment of human malignancy.

II. INTERLEUKINS AND IMMUNE EFFECTOR CELLS

Interleukins exert powerful effects on T lymphocytes. T cells possess distinct effector functions that can be defined by the sets of cytokines they manufacture. Cytotoxic T lymphocytes (CTL) are CD8$^+$ cells that recognize antigenic peptides bound to MHC class I molecules. CTL release granzymes and perforin, which lyse target cells. In addition, their activation causes the release of interferon-γ, TNF-α, and TNF-β. T cells that express CD4 react with antigenic peptides bound to MHC class II and can be classified into two types: T_H1

and T_H2. T_H1 cells are characterized by their secretion of INF-γ, but also produce granulocyte-macrophage colony stimulating factor (GM-CSF), TNF-α, TNF-β, IL-2, IL-3, CD40 ligand, and Fas ligand. The expression of these molecules on T_H1 cells determines function. T_H2 cells manufacture IL-4, IL-5, and CD40 ligand principally, but also IL-3, IL-10, GM-CSF, TGF-β, and eotaxin. T_H1 and T_H2 cells exhibit complementary immunostimulatory activity.

The production of various interleukins influences multiple effector cells, resulting in a concerted response to targeted antigens. B cells, for example, are stimulated to proliferate in the presence of CD40 ligand and IL-4. The secretion of IL-4 occurs at the site of contact of the T_H2 cell with B cell, enhancing the clonal expansion of the antigen-specific target B cell. Following the clonal expansion of B cells, some will differentiate into antibody-producing plasma cells with the assistance of T_H2 secreted IL-5 and IL-6. Natural killer cells are effector cells that can kill certain target cells in an antibody-dependent manner without the need for prior activation. NK cell activity is increased severalfold by the presence of INF-α

and -β, as well as IL-2, IL-12, IL-8, and IL-15. IL-12 plus TNF-α elicits the production of significant amounts of interferon-γ by NK cells.

A. Interleukin-2

Interleukin-2 is the most studied of this group of molecules for the treatment of cancer. IL-2 was identified and cloned in the early 1980s as a T-cell growth factor. IL-2 is produced by activated T cells and promotes further growth and differentiation of activated T cells. Its effects include the proliferation of CTL, T-helper cells, and NK cells, while enhancing the secretion of IFN-γ and TNF-α. The IL-2 receptor has three chains: α, β, and γ. On resting T cells, the β and γ chains are expressed and bind to IL-2 with moderate affinity. Upon activation of T cells, the α chain is expressed, which forms a high-affinity receptor along with the β and γ chains. In genetic knockout studies of IL-2 in mice, animals developed decreased T-cell responsiveness to numerous antigenic stimuli and some subsequently developed a syndrome akin to inflammatory bowel disease.

Systemic administration of IL-2 in murine animal models has resulted in the regression of established pulmonary and subcutaneous metastases in a dose-dependent manner. Intraperitoneal administration of IL-2 every 8 h mediated the regression of established pulmonary metastases in MCA-105 and MCA-106 syngeneic sarcomas, as well as syngeneic B16 melanoma. Lymphocytes were visualized at sites of regressing tumors. Experience in the animal models ultimately led to the development of high-dose IL-2 regimens for clinical investigation.

Numerous clinical trials in humans with cancer have been performed with IL-2. IL-2 has been administered to patients via a variety of routes: intravenously, subcutaneously, intraperitoneally, and intrathecally. IL-2 has been given as a single agent or in combination with other cytokines such as interferon. It has been used with both autologous and allogeneic lymphocytes in adoptive transfer therapies and as an adjuvant to numerous vaccination strategies. While studied in a variety of tumor types, IL-2 has been most widely adapted in the treatment of renal cell carcinoma and metastatic melanoma.

High-dose bolus IL-2 treatments (600,000–720,000 IU/kg IV every 8 h at days 1–5 and 15–19; maximum 28 doses per course) as a single agent or in combination with lymphokine-activated killer (LAK) cells results in overall responses of 15–20% with complete responses in 4–6% of patients with renal cell carcinoma and melanoma. Durable responses observed in renal cell carcinoma led to FDA approval of bolus high-dose IL-2 in 1992. In a study reviewing the treatment of 270 patients in eight protocols with high-dose IL-2 for metastatic melanoma, the median duration of complete responses (CRs) was greater than 40 months and the median progression-free survival time for responding patients was more than a year. No relapses occurred in responding patients after 30 months. High-dose IL-2 regimens produce a significant clinical benefit for a minority of patients. However, given that a small subset of patients had a durable complete response, high-dose IL-2 was FDA approved for patients also with metastatic melanoma. The severe toxicities resulting from high-dose IL-2 administration have limited its use to patients with excellent performance status and intact end organ function.

In animal studies, LAK cells harvested from peripheral blood and subsequently activated *in vitro*, combined with IL-2, were found to be effective in shrinking tumors. Initial studies conducted with LAK cells in humans demonstrated up to a 35% response rate for renal cell carcinoma and a 21% response rate for melanoma with a duration of responses ranging from 1 to 5 years. Histologic examination of cutaneous metastases in responding melanoma patients demonstrated infiltrating lymphocytes. NK cells exposed to high doses of IL-2 become the predominant component of the adoptive LAK cells. The mechanism for the observed antitumor activity is still relatively poorly understood. Both T cells and NK cells may play a role. It is unclear whether there is any truly demonstrable benefit to the combination of LAK cells with high-dose IL-2 compared to high-dose IL-2.

Another program of adoptive immunotherapy involves tumor-infiltrating lymphocytes (TILs). TILs are cells found coursing throughout tumors. TILs that potentially offer antitumor antigen specificity can be expanded easily *in vitro* by the addition of IL-2. TILs expanded in the presence of autologous tumor and IL-2 demonstrate cytolytic activity against autologous and HLA-matched tumors. The most comprehensive clinical study by Rosenberg and co-workers treated 86 patients with metastatic melanoma with autologous TILs and high-dose bolus IL-2. Response rates were reported to be 34%, not significantly different from those observed with systemic IL-2 administration alone in both renal cell carcinoma and melanoma, with approximately 6% complete responses. The durability of these responses was approximately 6 months. Improved responses were seen when TILs had shorter doubling times, derived from subcutaneous tissues as opposed to lymph nodes, and were cultured for shorter periods of time. A randomized phase III trial in patients with metastatic renal cell carcinoma demonstrated a lack of efficacy for the addition of TILs to low-dose IL-2 following nephrectomy.

The toxicity from high-dose IL-2 regimens can be particularly severe and may include capillary leak syndrome, cardiac arrhythmias, pulmonary edema, catheter-related sepsis, and hypotension requiring pressor support, all which can lead to death. The induction of nitric oxide plays a principal role in IL-2 toxicity. In addition, secondary cytokines appear to contribute to the development of toxic manifestations of IL-2. IL-2 is a strong inducer of inflammatory cytokines, including IL-1, TNF-α, and IFN-γ. In animal models, there have been beneficial effects of adding soluble TNF or IL-1 inhibitors to diminish toxicites. Such agents were investigated in patients receiving high-dose IL-2. However, these agents did not permit higher doses of IL-2 to be administered or produce less toxicity at a given dose of IL-2. The use of dexamethasone with high-dose IL-2 administration has resulted in a marked decrease in TNF levels, as well as significant improvement of toxicity from fever and hypotension, permitting nearly a threefold increase in the maximum tolerated dose. Dexamethosone administration, however, may limit IL-2 antitumor efficacy by preventing the production of secondary cytokines. Identification of the neutrophil chemotactic defect with IL-2 administration has underscored the need for administration of prophylactic antibiotics. Such prophylaxis has made a positive impact on the risk of mortality with IL-2 administration due to bacterial sepsis.

Attempts to decrease IL-2 toxicity by administration via continuous infusion rather than bolus form have resulted in decreased side effects. However, this means of administration also led to response rates that were lower and of shorter duration than those noted with high-dose bolus therapy. Substitution of low-dose IL-2 for a high-dose bolus-containing regimen for the treatment of solid tumors has generally sacrificed responsiveness for decreases in toxicity. Lower dose and less toxic IL-2 regimens may have activity against renal cell carcinoma, but similar efficacy for melanoma has not been observed. The use of low-dose IL-2, however, does have a biologic effect in the ability to increase NK cell number.

IL-2 has been used in conjunction with both combination chemotherapy and with other cytokines. Most commonly, IL-2 has been combined with interferons. However, there is no convincing evidence that there are synergistic or even additive therapeutic effects. Attempts to add other agents to cytokine combinations of IL-2/interferon-α treatments for renal cell carcinoma such as 5-fluorouracil have not been demonstrated to improve efficacy. Results are a little more encouraging for studies that combine cisplatin chemotherapy regimens with IL-2. Additional chemotherapies combined with IL-2 are under investigation, including agents that range from fotemustine to arginine butyrate.

Biochemotherapy combinations in melanoma, typically a dacarbazine-based chemotherapy regimen with IL-2 and INF-α, have yielded the highest responses, up to 50–60%, albeit with significant side effects. Studies to decrease the toxicity of biochemotherapy through modified administration in a decrescendo dosing pattern or lower dose outpatient regimens have been somewhat successful in diminishing side effects. It is hoped that ongoing phase III clinical trials will determine whether significant differences in response rates and overall survival exist between biochemotherapy and chemotherapy alone.

IL-2 has also been used as an adjuvant in a number of vaccination strategies against cancer. With the premise of assisting in the activation and expansion of T cells, IL-2 has been used in conjunction with vaccination with dendritic cells, as well with synthetic peptides representing known MHC-binding motifs. Vaccination with an immunodominant gp100 nonapeptide manufactured to increase binding to HLA-A2 revealed successful immunization in 91% of melanoma patients. Objective responses were seen in 13 of 31 patients receiving peptide plus IL-2 with four other patients reporting mixed responses. Clinical results were superior to that of vaccination alone. Based on these preliminary results, prospective trials are being performed to delineate the efficacy of the peptide plus IL-2 treatment compared to IL-2 alone.

IL-2 has also been used as an immunomodulatory agent after stem cell transplantation. For patients undergoing bone marrow transplantation for hematologic malignancies, key determinants of outcome include reconstitution of immune competence against infectious agents and immune activity against tumor targets. Prolonged infusions of low-dose IL-2 in patients receiving both autologous and allogeneic bone marrow transplants have demonstrated that it is safe. In this setting, IL-2 can increase NK cell number and activity. Low-dose IL-2 does not appear to accelerate graft-versus-host disease (GVHD). There is some evidence that such therapy may improve disease-free survival, but this has not yet been confirmed in a randomized trial.

B. Interleukin-12

IL-12 was identified as a heterodimeric protein produced in significant quantities by professional antigen-presenting cells (APC) as a response to infection by bacteria, intracellular parasites, fungi, and viruses. It can be produced in a T-cell-independent manner as part of an early inflammatory response or in a T-cell-dependent manner via binding of CD40 ligand on activated T cells with the CD40 receptor on APC. Production of IL-12 is enhanced by IFN-γ and inhibited by IL-10. TGF-β and IL-4 inhibit T-cell and NK-cell responses to IL-12. The principal role of IL-12 is the activation of T cells and NK cells, leading to an increased production of INF-γ, proliferation, and cytotoxic potential. IL-12 also induces the production of TNF-α, IL-2, IL-3, IL-8, and IL-10, while stimulating the proliferation of hematopoietic precursors and B cells. It is a primary inducer of T_H1 type responses. IL-12 plays significant roles in combatting infections, induction of septic shock, tissue damage during inflammation, and autoimmunity, as well as antitumor immunity. IL-12 is important for

the effector phase of the immune response, particularly in augmenting CTL activity. It has also been identified to possess antiangiogenic activity.

In a number of animal models, IL-12 has demonstrated antitumor efficacy in reducing the size and number of metastatic lesions. In the nonimmunogenic B16 murine melanoma model, IL-12 has demonstrated significant preventative activity against spontaneous tumors resulting from protooncogene transfer and tumors resulting from methylchloranthine treatment. Transfection of IL-12 into dendritic cells or tumor cells has also been used in several vaccination strategies. Such studies have resulted in the prolonged survival of vaccinated animals or, in some cases, complete tumor regression. IL-12 has also been used in combination with other cytokines and costimulatory molecules, demonstrating a synergistic effect. Systemic delivery of IL-2 and local administration of IL-12 prevented tumor occurrences in a MCA-105 murine sarcoma model. This revealed improved effectiveness compared to a reduction in tumor sizes with IL-12 and partial protection (3/6 mice) with IL-2 alone. Tumor cells that are transfected to express the costimulatory molecule B7-1 are rejected with greater efficacy with the addition of systemic IL-12.

While the first clinical trial of IL-12 in cancer patients using a dose up to 500 ng/kg had acceptable levels of toxicity, a subsequent phase II trial produced some significant liver toxicities with several fatalities. IL-12 was noted to have a long half-life and perhaps a unique schedule dependency in its administration. This prompted the study of different schedules of IL-12 administration. A single dose given 2 weeks prior to consecutive doses significantly decreases the toxicity. The mechanism by which this occurs is poorly understood at the present time, but it is believed to be tolerizing to the subsequent production of cytokines. Whether this initial dose interferes with the efficacy of the drug has yet to be determined, but decreases of INF-γ have been noted with this schedule. Several studies with subcutaneous IL-12 administration revealed upregulation of the IL-12 receptor and expansion of a subset of CD8$^+$ T cells. Responses to IL-12 have been seen in cutaneous T-cell lymphoma, as well as in subsets of renal cell carcinoma and melanoma patients. Evidence for efficacy has also been demonstrated in Kaposi's sarcoma. While the toxicity observed with the systemic administration of IL-12 has dampened efforts for further clinical testing, efforts continue principally with its use in gene transfer studies. Studies have been undertaken utilizing intratumoral injections with fibroblasts secreting IL-12, as well as with vaccination with autologous tumor cells expressing IL-12.

C. Interleukin-4

IL-4 is a cytokine with pleiotropic functions. IL-4 plays a key role in the development of T_H2 responses. In mice that lack IL-4, there is significant abrogation of T_H2 cellular activity. IL-4 promotes the growth and activation of B lymphocytes that produce IgG1 and IgE classes of antibodies and increases MHC class II induction. Preclinical animal models have demonstrated modest antitumor efficacy for IL-4. In the nonimmunogenic B16 murine melanoma model, irradiated B16 cells engineered to express IL-4 induced antitumor protection against a wild-type B16 challenge.

Clinically, most groups have focused on the ability of IL-4 to propagate dendritic cells (DCs) *in vitro* for *in vivo* use. When combined with GM-CSF, IL-4 will increase the antigen-presenting capacity of DCs. Dendritic cells are the most potent professional APC. The use of autologous dendritic cells to target specific immune responses against cancer has gained widespread use in numerous clinical trials. Studies are underway in which dendritic cells are pulsed with known HLA-binding peptides of the antigenic target or are transfected with the full-length gene product. Such programs have been successful in inducing targeted immune responses; however, the clinical significance of such immunostimulatory activity in patients with cancer is not known.

D. Interleukin-6

IL-6 was originally identified as a substance that induced the production of acute-phase reactants in the liver along with IL-1 and TNF-α. IL-6 is involved in the polarization of T cells toward the T_H2 type. IL-6 has been identified as an essential factor for the growth of multiple myeloma cells. It has been shown to inhibit the apoptosis of myeloma cells and alter adhe-

sion molecules, tumor suppressor genes, and oncogenes. The Kaposi's sarcoma-associated herpesvirus encodes the viral homologue of IL-6. This in turn can promote hematopoiesis and angiogenic factors, such as vascular endothelial growth factor (VEGF), which contributes to the survival and growth of Kaposi's sarcoma cells. Considering the biologic effects of IL-6, efforts are currently underway to target IL-6 in therapeutic trials. Murine anti-IL-6 monoclonal antibodies have been combined with dexamethasone and high-dose melphalan in patients with multiple myeloma. This has led to inhibition of IL-6 activity and induced a relatively high complete remission rate. The use of a monoclonal antibody that neutralizes IL-6 was investigated in 10 patients with posttransplant EBV-related lymphoproliferative disease. Following a 15-day treatment regimen, 5 of the remaining patients had a complete remission and 3 had partial remissions. There is now some interest in studying anti-human IL-6 receptor antibodies, IL-6 antagonist proteins, and IL-6 antisense oligonucleotides in clinical studies.

E. Interleukin-1

IL-1 is a multifunctional cytokine in that it affects numerous other effector cells of the immune system. Biologic effects of IL-1 include increased synthesis of IL-2, IL-3, IL-4, IL-5, IL-6, IL-7, IL-10, and IL-12, increased IL-2 receptor synthesis, propagation of T_H2 responses, and increased antibody production. Many of the biologic effects of IL-1 are related to its induction of inducible nitric oxide synthase (iNOS). Synergistic actions have been seen with bradykinin, as well as with several cytokines and growth factors. There is synergism between IL-1 and TNF that leads to hemodynamic shock.

In models of inflammation and/or infection, IL-1 has been demonstrated to increase the production of G-CSF, GM-CSF, IL-3, and stem cell factor (SCF) by increasing their levels of transcription. IL-1 can protect approximately 90% of mice from a lethal dose of radiation through the propagation of both pluripotent stem cells and mature populations.

IL-1 is produced by a variety of leukemias. *In vitro* studies suggest that approximately 70% of acute myelogenous leukemia (AML) blasts exhibit autonomous growth, which is dependent on IL-1β expression. IL-1 production has also been associated with CML, acute lymphoblastic leukemia, Hodgkin's disease, and multiple myeloma. In these diseases, it stimulates IL-6 production, which is thought to be an important mediator of its proliferative effect. In solid tumors, IL-1 production has been reported in melanomas, hepatoblastomas, sarcomas, squamous cell carcinomas, transitional cell carcinomas, and ovarian carcinomas. In animal models, IL-1 production correlates with the ability of melanoma to metastasize to the liver. This is felt to be at least partially the result of IL-1's induction of adhesion molecules such as ICAM-1. *In vitro* addition of IL-1 to cultured melanoma and ovarian carcinoma cells increases their proliferative rate. Also supporting a role for IL-1 in propagating metastases are experiments in which mice with subcutaneous melanoma were given low doses of systemic IL-1. This led to an increase in the size of their tumors with greater vascularity and local invasion.

IL-1 has also been reported to actually inhibit tumor cell proliferation for some tumor types, including melanomas, gliomas, meningiomas, breast carcinomas, cervical, thyroid, and ovarian carcinomas. This effect may be due in part to the induction of other cytokines such as TNF-α, as well as an increased production of oxygen radicals. In a number of tumor models, IL-1 administered in relatively higher doses reduced tumor sizes in animals receiving both systemic and intratumoral injections, protecting some animals against tumor challenge for as long as 180 days. This protection was felt to be due to improved CTL responses, as IL-1 has been shown to increase the production of LAK cells in adoptive transfermodels.

IL-1α and IL-1β have been used in phase I/II immunotherapy trials to treat patients with cancer, including melanoma, breast, colon, renal cell, glioma, and cutaneous T-cell lymphoma. Side effects were greater when the drug was administered intravenously than subcutaneously and included fever, chills, generalized fatigue, headache, nausea, vomiting, myalgias, arthralgias, and hypotension. Infusions of IL-1 increased cortisol levels soon after administration, significant increases in IL-6 production, and increases in both white blood cell counts and platelet counts. A few responses have been reported, but, in general, results have been disappointing. Combinations of IL-1 and chemotherapy agents such as doxorubicin and cisplatin have been shown to be synergistic *in vitro*, but are yet to be tested definitively in clinical trials. IL-1 administered during autologous bone marrow transplantation has resulted in earlier hematopoietic recovery.

Efforts are also underway to utilize agents aimed at blocking IL-1 and/or its receptor as a treatment of cancer. Neutralizing antibodies to IL-1 or IL-1 receptor have been demonstrated to reduce the number and size of tumors in the B16 melanoma model. Due to their endogenous production of IL-1, which assists in propagation of the disease, IL-1 receptor blockade is currently being tried in patients with AML and CML.

F. Interleukin-3

IL-3 (also known as multispecific hemopoietin) is naturally produced by both T_H1 and T_H2 lymphocytes, mast cells, and eosinophils. IL-3 stimulates the production of macrophages, granulocytes, and dendritic cells from bone marrow precursors. The high-affinity IL-3 receptor shares a common β-subunit with GM-CSF and IL-5. In murine models, injection of tumors engineered to secrete IL-3 lead to the infiltration of inflammatory cells, which includes a striking percentage of macrophages. In clinical studies, IL-3 has been studied in the treatment of myelosuppression in patients receiving chemotherapy with minimal benefit. However, the use of IL-3 in patients with myelodysplastic syndrome and aplastic anemia has been more encouraging. For patients with aplastic anemia, 250–500 $\mu g/m^2$ of IL-3 increased platelet counts and reticulocyte counts in several patients. The combination of IL-3 and GM-CSF has demonstrated greater efficacy in reversing chemotherapy-induced myelosuppression than either alone. IL-3R agonists are being tested in the *ex vivo* expansion of stem cells and dendritic cell development. The IL-3 receptor has also been contemplated as a target for immunotherapy. The IL-3 receptor α chain is highly expressed in AML stem cells. Currently, *in vitro* studies utilizing diphtheria fusion proteins targeted against the IL-3 receptor have demonstrated selective cytotoxicity to myeloid leukemia cells. Clinical trials with such agents are being developed for the near future.

G. Interleukin-11

While initially characterized as a cytokine with thrombopoietic activity, IL-11 was later shown to offer a wider array of effects. It is expressed in numerous tissues, including spleen, thymus, connective tissues, heart, brain, spinal cord, lung, uterus, and bone. The production of IL-11 is upregulated by IL-1α and TGF-β. Both IL-11 and IL-6 use the gp130 common subunit. In a murine transgenic model, its overexpression leads to decreased eosinophilia, a diminished T_H2 response, and decreased production of IL-4, IL-5, and IL-13.

IL-11 is currently being marketed as a hemopoietic growth factor for chemotherapy-induced thrombocytopenia. IL-11 functions synergistically with IL-3, thrombopoietin, and stem cell factor to stimulate megakaryopoiesis and thrombopoiesis. It works synergistically with IL-4, IL-7, IL-12, and IL-13 while also improving thrombopoiesis indirectly by increasing the production of IL-6 and GM-CSF. In addition to its profound effects on thrombopoiesis, IL-11 also stimulates pluripotent stem cells from bone marrow and cord blood, as well as peripheral blood. In a number of animal models, IL-11 administration reduces mortality from infection with *Pseudomonas aeruginosa* as well as improves the recovery of platelets and neutrophils following bone marrow transplantation. IL-11 has been approved for treating patients at risk for developing treatment-related thrombocytopenia. At doses ranging from 25 to 100 μg/kg/day, IL-11 appears to limit the incidence of severe thrombocytopenia and decreases the need for platelet transfusions. Toxicities, however, have included a 20% increase in plasma volume from renal sodium reabsorption with fluid retention resulting in peripheral edema, dyspnea, and tachycardia. Given the side effect profile and limited clinical efficacy, the true clinical utility of IL-11 remains unknown.

H. Interleukin-18

IL-18 is one of the newest cytokines, which was first identified by its ability to induce IFN-γ. It was for-

merly called IFN-γ-inducing factor. IL-18 plays a principal role in T_H1 responses through IFN-γ production in T cells and NK cells. It is similar to IL-1 in both amino acid sequence and activity in terms of signal transduction and proinflammatory properties. IL-18 is also similar to IL-12 in its effector function. The role of IL-18 in antitumor immune responses has been investigated in murine models alone and along with IL-12. IL-18 treatment posttumor challenge prevented tumor growth in approximately 50% of mice. IL-18 increased tumor immunogenicity, enhanced NK cell activation and production of IL-2, and decreased levels of IL-10. In a murine mammary tumorigenicity model, carcinoma cells expressing IL-18 were less tumorigenic, forming tumors more slowly than wild-type cells. The injection of IL-18-producing cells and a nontransfected tumor revealed approximately a 70% reduction in tumor growth, with evidence that this was the result of IFN-γ production. IL-18-expressing tumor cells also demonstrated systemic inhibition of angiogenesis, similar to the function of IL-12. IL-18 activity, however, is still present in IFN-γ receptor-deficient mice, as opposed to IL-12, which is dependent on IFN-γ. As a result, IL-18 most likely possesses effector influences that are independent of IFN-γ. Measurement of IL-18 serum levels in patients with various forms of leukemia revealed higher levels in leukemia patients as compared to a group of apparently healthy individuals. Patients with acute lymphoblastic leukemia and chronic myelogenous leukemias possessed the highest levels. Studies to test the efficacy and tolerability of these cytokines are needed before implementing into human clinical trials.

I. Interleukin-10

While much of the discussion surrounding cytokines involves the activation of effector mechanisms, IL-10 (also known as cytokine synthesis inhibitory factor) is primarily involved in inhibiting macrophage activation by limiting the production of IL-1, IL-6, and TNF-α. IL-10 indirectly prevents antigen-specific T-cell activation, associated with the downregulation of antigen presentation and accessory cell functions of monocytes, macrophages, Langerhans cells, and dendritic cells. IL-10 directly inhibits T-cell expansion by inhibiting IL-2 production. Its source is the T_H2 cell. Its production increases MHC expression on B cells, inhibits T_H1 effects primarily through inhibiting IFN-γ production, inhibits cytokine release from macrophages, and stimulates mast cell growth. IL-10-deficient mice often have inflammatory bowel disease.

The mechanism by which tumor cells evade recognition by the immune system may include IL-10. Lung cancer cells, for example, induce T lymphocytes to produce IL-10 *in vitro*. In the Lewis lung murine model, tumors were found to be more aggressive in IL-10 transgenic mice, and that transfer of lymphocytes from transgenic mice transferred enhanced tumor growth. Defects in antigen-presenting cell function were implicated in the explanation for these observations. IL-10 has been shown to induce a long-term antigen-specific anergic state for human CD4$^+$ T cells. Also, IL-10 causes immature dendritic cells to become tolerant as antigen-presenting cells, with marked decreased production of IL-2 and IFN-γ. Such anergy has been demonstrated to be antigen specific, as exemplified in an *in vitro* melanoma model against tyrosinase. The ability of dendritic cells to reverse this antigen-specific unresponsiveness is dependent on the concentration of IL-10 that the T cells have been exposed to and the degree of dendritic cell maturation. While direct use of IL-10 in the clinical setting is more complicated, understanding its immunosuppressive biology and effects on antigen presentation will improve our abilities to vaccinate patients with antigen-specific dendritic cells and improve the efficacy of other immunotherapies against cancer.

J. Other Interleukins

A number of other interleukins may ultimately have clinical applications. IL-15 and IL-2 have similar functions in stimulating T-cell proliferation. Evidence from receptor signaling studies suggests that these interleukins are involved in distinct pathways of primary T-cell expansion. IL-15 is ubiquitously expressed and has profound proliferative effects on a number of hematologic cell types, including adult T-cell leukemia and B-cell chronic lymphocytic leukemia. The opportunities for use of IL-15 in clinical investigations against cancer are currently being explored.

Trials are currently underway using several interleukins in attempts to improve outcomes after bone marrow transplantation. One of these is IL-7 (pre-B-cell growth factor), which is involved in T-cell growth and activation, proliferation of LAK, B cells, and NK cells, as well as activating macrophages. It is being evaluated in the postbone marrow transplantation setting to accelerate T-cell recovery. Other potentially active cytokines include IL-8 (monocyte-derived neutrophil chemotactic factor), which attracts neutrophils, basophils, and T cells; IL-9, which assists in T-cell proliferation; IL-13, which is similar to IL-4 and synergistically acts with IL-2 in regulating IFN-γ production; and IL-14 (high molecular weight B-cell growth factor), which is produced by T cells that selectively expand certain B-cell populations.

The number of identified interleukins has risen to 23. The specific functions and receptor-binding motifs of these molecules are still being defined. Many do have influences on T_H1 and T_H2 function and may be synergistic with previously described cytokines. Their particular roles in cancer pathogenesis and treatment have yet to be determined.

III. CONCLUSION

We are just beginning to learn the function and clinical applications for the interleukins. What is evident thus far is a complex interplay of cytokines in their biologic effects. Early trials have demonstrated their immunostimulatory effects, as well as their use as hematopoietic factors. The therapeutic index for these interleukins is often quite narrow. We still do not know the best means to utilize these agents in the clinic, but it is likely that as we gain experience, we will be better able to determine what their clinical role should be.

See Also the Following Articles

CYTOKINE GENE THERAPY • CYTOKINES: HEMATOPOIETIC GROWTH FACTORS • INTERFERONS: CELLULAR AND MOLECULAR BIOLOGY OF THEIR ACTIONS • T CELLS, FUNCTION OF • TUMOR NECROSIS FACTORS

Bibliography

Akdis, C., Blesken, T., Akdis, M., *et al.* (1998). Role of interleukin 10 in specific immunotherapy. *J. Clin. Invest.* **102,** 98–106.

Aoki, Y., Jones, K., and Tosato, G. (2000). Kaposi's sarcoma-associated herpesvirus-encoded interleukin-6. *J. Hematother. Stem Cell Res.* **9,** 137–145.

Arai, K., Lee, F., Miyajima, A., *et al.* (1990). Cytokines: Coordinators of immune and inflammatory responses. *Annu. Rev. Biochem.* **59,** 783.

Atkins, M. (1998). Immunotherapy and experimental approaches for metastatic melanoma. *Hematol. Oncol. Clin. North Am.* **12,** 877–902.

Atkins, M., Lotze, M., Dutcher, J., *et al.* (1999). High-dose recombinant interleukin 2 therapy for patients with metastatic melanoma: Analysis of 270 patients treated between 1985 and 1993. *J. Clin. Oncol.* **17,** 2105.

Atkins, M., O'Boyle, K., Sosman, J., *et al.* (1994). Multiinstitutional phase II trial of intensive combination chemoimmunotherapy for metastatic melanoma. *J. Clin. Oncol.* **12,** 1553–1560.

Atkins, M., Robertson, M., Gordon, M., *et al.* (1997). Phase I evaluation of intravenous recombinant human interleukin 12 in patients with advanced malignancies. *Clin. Cancer Res.* **3,** 409–417.

Banchereau, J., Bazan, F., Blanchard, D., *et al.* (1994). The CD40 antigen and its ligand. *Annu. Rev. Immunol.* **12,** 881–922.

Baron, C., Scholl, S., Bausinger, H., *et al.* (1999). Two distinct cell populations are obtained from human blood monocytes cultured with M-CSF, GM-CSF, and IL-4. *Eur. J. Cancer* **35**(Suppl. 3), S39–S40.

Barth, J., Bock, S., Mule, J., *et al.* (1990). Unique murine tumor-associated antigens identified by tumor infiltrating lymphocytes. *J. Immunol.* **144,** 1531–1537.

Biesma, B., Pokorny, R., Kovarik, J., *et al.* (1993). Pharmacokinetics of recombinant human interleukin 3 administered subcutaneously and by continuous intravenous infusion in patients after chemotherapy for ovarian cancer. *Cancer Res.* **53,** 5915–5919.

Braunschweiger, P., Basrur, V., Santos, O., *et al.* (1993). Synergistic antitumor activity of cisplatin and interleukin 1 in sensitive and resistant solid tumors. *Cancer Res.* **53,** 1091–1097.

Brouwer, R., Vellenga, E., Zwinderman, K., *et al.* (1999). Phase III efficacy study of interleukin-3 after autologous bone marrow transplantation in patients with malignant lymphoma. *Br. J. Haematol.* **106.**

Brown, M., and Hural, J. (1997). Functions of IL-4 and control of its expression. *Crit. Rev. Immunol.* **17,** 1–32.

Caliguiri, M., Murray, C., Robertson, M., *et al.* (1993). Selective modulation of human natural killer cells in vivo after prolonged infusion of low dose interleukin2. *J. Clin. Invest.* **91,** 123–132.

Cavallo, F., Signorelli, P., Giovarelli, M., *et al.* (1997). Antitumor efficacy of adenocarcinoma cells engineered to produce interleukin 12 (IL-12) or other cytokines compared with exogenous IL-12. *J. Natl. Cancer Inst.* **89,** 1049–1058.

Chen, M., Wang, F., Lee, P., *et al.* (2001). Interleukin-10-induced T cell unresponsiveness can be reversed by dendritic cell stimulation. *Immunol. Lett.* **75,** 91–96.

Clark, J., Gaynor, E., Martone, B., *et al.* (1999). Daily subcutaneous ultra-low-dose interleukin 2 with daily low-dose interferon-alpha in patients with advanced renal cell carcinoma. *Clin. Cancer Res.* **5,** 2374–2380.

Coughlin, C., Salhany, K., Wysocka, M., *et al.* (1998). Interleukin-12 and interleukin-18 synergistically induce murine tumor regression which involves inhibition of angiogenesis. *J. Clin. Invest.* **101,** 1441–1452.

Davis, S., Aldrich, T., Stahl, N., *et al.* (1993). LIFR and gp 130 as heterodimerizing signal transducers of the tripartite CNTF receptor. *Science* **260,** 1805–1808.

Dillman, R. (1994). The clinical experience with interleukin-2 in cancer therapy. *Cancer Biother.* **9,** 183–209.

Dillman, R. (1999). What to do with IL-2? *Cancer Biother. Radiopharm.* **14,** 423–434.

Dinarello, C. (1996). Biologic basis for interleukin-1 in disease. *Blood* **87,** 2095–2147.

Dinarello, C. (1999). Interleukin-18. *Methods* **19,** 121–132.

Douillard, J., Bennouna, J., Vavasseur, F., *et al.* (2000). Phase I trial of interleukin-2 and high-dose arginine butyrate in metastatic colorectal cancer. *Cancer Immunol. Immunother.* **49,** 56–61.

Dranoff, G., Jaffee, E., Lazenby, A., *et al.* (1993). Vaccination with irradiated tumor cells engineered to secrete murine granulocyte-macrophage colony-stimulating factor stimulates potent, specific, and long-lasting anti-tumor immunity. *Proc. Natl. Acad. Sci. USA* **90,** 3539–3543.

Du, X., and Williams, D. (1994). Interleukin-11: A multifunctional growth factor derived from the hematopoietic microenvironment. *Blood* **83,** 2023–2030.

Du, X., and Williams, D. (1997). Interleukin-11: Review of molecular, cell biology, and clinical use. *Blood* **89,** 3897–3908.

Dutcher, J., Logan, T., Gordon, M., *et al.* (2000). Phase II trial of interleukin 2, interferon alpha, and 5-fluorouracil in metastatic renal cell cancer: A cytokine working group study. *Clin. Cancer Res.* **6,** 3442–3450.

Figlin, R., Thompson, J., Bukowski, R., *et al.* (1999). Multicenter, randomized, phase III trial of CD8(+) tumor-infiltrating lymphocytes in combination with recombinant interleukin-2 in metastatic renal cell carcinoma. *J. Clin. Oncol.* **17,** 2521–2529.

Flaherty, L., Redman, B., Chabot, G., *et al.* (1990). A phase II study of dacarbazine in combination with outpatient interleukin-2 in metastatic malignant melanoma. *Cancer* **65,** 2471–2477.

Frankel, A., Ramage, J., Kiser, M., *et al.* (2000). Characterization of diphtheria fusion proteins targeted to the human interleukin-3 receptor. *Protein Eng.* **13,** 575–581.

Gado, K., Domjan, G., Hegyesi, H., *et al.* (2000). Role of interleukin-6 in the pathogenesis of multiple myeloma. *Cell. Biol. Int.* **24**, 195–209.

Ganser, A., Lindemann, A., Seipelt, G., *et al.* (1990). Effects of recombinant human interleukin-3 in aplastic anemia. *Blood* **76**, 1287–1292.

Gillespie, M., and Horwood, N. (1998). Interleukin-18: Perspectives on the newest interleukin. *Cytokine Growth Factor Rev.* **9**, 109–116.

Golab, J. (2000). Interleukin-18—interferon gamma inducing factor: A novel player in tumour immunotherapy? *Cytokine* **12**, 332–338.

Gollob, J., Murphy, E., Mahajan, S., *et al.* (1998). Altered interleukin 12 responsiveness in Th1 and Th2 cells is associated with the differential activation of STAT 5 and STAT 1. *Blood* **91**, 1341–1354.

Gollob, J., Schnipper, C., Orsini, E., *et al.* (1998). Characterization of a novel subset of CD8(+) T cells that expands in patients receiving interleukin-12. *J. Clin. Invest.* **102**, 561–575.

Groux, H., Bigler, M., Vries, J. D., *et al.* (1996). Interleukin-10 induces a long-term antigen-specific anergic state in human CD4$^+$ T cells. *J. Exp. Med.* **184**, 19–29.

Hajek, R., and Butch, A. (2000). Dendritic cell biology and the application of dendritic cells to immunotherapy of multiple myeloma. *Med. Oncol.* **17**, 2–15.

Hempel, L., Korholz, D., Bonig, H., *et al.* (1995). Interleukin-10 directly inhibits the interleukin-6 production in T-cells. *Scand. J. Immunol.* **41**, 462–466.

Holmberg, L. (2000). The biology and currently approved uses of interleukin-11. *From Research to Practice* **2**, 4–10.

Janeway, C., Travers, P., Walport, M., *et al.* (1999). "Immunobiology: The Immune System in Health and Disease," 4th Ed. Garland, New York.

Jordan, C., Upchurch, D., Szilvassy, S., *et al.* (2000). The interleukin-3 receptor alpha chain is a unique marker for acute myelogenous leukemia stem cells. *Leukemia* **14**, 1777–1784.

Kilian, P., Kaffka, K., Biondi, D., *et al.* (1991). Antiproliferative effect of interleukin-1 on human ovarian carcinoma cell line (NIH:OVCAR-3). *Cancer Res.* **51**, 1823–1828.

Kuhn, R., Rajewsky, K., and Muller, W. (1991). Generation and analysis of interleukin-4 deficient mice. *Science* **254**, 707–710.

Kurzrock, R., Kantarjian, H., Wetzler, M., *et al.* (1993). Ubiquitous expression of cytokines in diverse leukemias of lymphoid and myeloid lineage. *Exp. Hematol.* **21**, 80–85.

Lafreniere, R., and Rosenberg, S. (1985). Successful immunotherapy of murine experimental hepatic metastases with lymphokine-activated killer cells and recombinant interleukin 2. *Cancer Res.* **45**, 3735–3741.

Lafreniere, R., and Rosenberg, S. (1985). Adoptive immunotherapy of murine hepatic metastases with lymphokine activated killer (LAK) cells and recombinant interleukin 2 (RIL2) can mediate the regression of both immunogenic

and nonimmunogenic sarcomas and an adenocarcinoma. *J. Immunol.* **135**, 4273–4280.

Lebel-Binay, S., Berger, A., Zinzindohoue, F., *et al.* (2000). Interleukin-18: Biological properties and clinical applications. *Eur. Cytokine Netw.* **11**, 15–26.

Legha, S., Ring, S., Eton, O., *et al.* (1997). Development and results of biochemotherapy in metastatic melanoma: The University of Texas M.D. Anderson Cancer Center Experience. *Cancer J. Sci. Am.* **3**, S9–S15.

Leonard, J., Sherman, M., Fisher, G., *et al.* (1997). Effects of single-dose interleukin-12 exposure on interleukin-12-associated toxicity and interferon-gamma production. *Blood* **90**, 2541–2548.

Li, X., Demirci, G., Ferrari-Lacraz, S., *et al.* (2001). IL-15 and IL-2: A matter of life and death for T cells in vivo. *Nature Med.* **7**, 114–118.

Lissoni, P. (1997). Effects of low-dose recombinant interleukin-2 in human malignancies. *Cancer J. Sci. Am.* **3**(Suppl. 1), 115–120.

Maas, R., Dullens, H., and Otter, W. D. (1993). Interleukin-2 in cancer treatment: disappointing or (still) promising? *Cancer Immunol. Immunother.* **36**, 141–148.

Mangi, M., and Newland, A. (1999). Interleukin-3 in hematology and oncology: Current state of knowledge and future directions. *Cytokines Cell Mol. Ther.* **5**, 87–95.

Margolin, K. (2000). Interleukin-2 in the treatment of renal cancer. *Semin. Oncol.* **27**, 194–203.

Mckenzie, R., Park, E., Brown, W., *et al.* (1994). Effect of ultraviolet-inducible cytokines on melanoma growth in vivo: Stimulation of melanoma growth by interleukin-1 and -6. *Photodermatol. Photoimmunol. Photomed.* **10**, 74–79.

Mckenzie, R., Saunder, D., and Dinarello, C. (1993). Inhibition of B16 melanoma growth in vivo after treatment with interleukin-1 receptor antagonist. *Clin. Res.* **41**, 465.

Micallef, M., Tanimoto, T., Kohno, K., *et al.* (1997). Interleukin 18 induces the sequential activation of natural killer cells and cytotoxic T lymphocytes to protect syngeneic mice from transplantation with Meth A sarcoma. *Cancer Res.* **57**, 4557–4563.

Minami, Y., Kono, T., Miyazaki, T., *et al.* (1993). The IL-2 receptor complex: Its structure, function, and target genes. *Annu. Rev. Immunol.* **11**, 245–267.

Moreau, P., Harousseau, J., Wijdenes, J., *et al.* (2000). A combination of anti-interleukin 6 murine monoclonal antibody with dexamethasone and high-dose melphalan induces high complete response rates in advanced multiple myeloma. *Br. J. Haematol.* **109**, 661–664.

Mosmann, T., Coffman, R. (1989). TH1 and TH2 cells: Different patterns of lymphokine secretion lead to different functional properties. *Annu. Rev. Immunol.* **7**, 145–173.

Mu, J., Zou, J., Yamamoto, N., *et al.* (1995). Administration of recombinant interleukin 12 prevents outgrowth of tumor cells metastasizing spontaneously to lung and lymph nodes. *Cancer Res.* **55**, 4404–4408.

Nastala, C., Edington, H., McKinney, T., *et al.* (1994).

Recombinant IL-12 administration induces tumor regression in association with IFN-gamma production. *J. Immunol.* **153,** 1697–1703.

Negrier, S., Caty, A., Lesimple, T., *et al.* (2000). Treatment of patients with metastatic renal carcinoma with a combination of subcutaneous interleukin-2 and interferon alfa with or without fluorouracil. Groupe Francais d'Immunotherapie, Federation Nationale des Centres de Lutte Contre le Cancer. *J. Clin. Oncol.* **18,** 4009–4015.

Neta, R., Sztein, M., Oppenheim, J., *et al.* (1987). The in vivo effects of interleukin 1. I. Bone marrow cells are induced to cycle after administration of interleukin 1. *J. Immunol.* **139,** 1861–1866.

Neta, R., Vogel, S., Plocinski, J., *et al.* (1990). In vivo modulation with antiinterleukin-1 (IL-1) receptor (p80) antibody 35F5 of the response to IL-1: The relationship of radioprotection, colony-stimulating factor, and IL-6. *Blood* **76,** 57–62.

O'Day, S., Gammon, G., Boasberg, P., *et al.* (1999). Advantages of concurrent biochemotherapy modified by decrescendo interleukin-2, granulocyte colony-stimulating factor, and tamoxifen for patients with metastatic melanoma. *J. Clin. Oncol.* **17,** 2752–2761.

Palmeri, S., Leonardi, V., Danova, M., *et al.* (1999). Prospective, randomized trial of sequential interleukin-3 and granulocyte-macrophage colony-stimulating factor after standard-dose chemotherapy in cancer patients. *Haematologica* **84,** 1016–1023.

Panelli, M., Wunderlich, J., Jeffries, J., *et al.* (2000). Phase 1 study in patients with metastatic melanoma of immunization with dendritic cells presenting epitopes derived from the melanoma-associated antigens MART-1 and gp100. *J. Immunother.* **23,** 487–498.

Pappo, I., Tahara, H., Robbins, P., *et al.* (1995). Administration of systemic or local interleukin-2 enhances the antitumor effects of interleukin-12 gene therapy. *J. Surg. Res.* **58,** 218–226.

Qin, Z., Noffz, G., Mohaupt, M., *et al.* (1997). Interleukin-10 prevents dendritic cell accumulation and vaccination with granulocyte-macrophage colony-stimulating factor gene-modified tumor cells. *J. Immunol.* **159,** 770–776.

Rao, J., Chamberlain, R., Bronte, V., *et al.* (1996). IL-12 is an effective adjuvant to recombinant vaccinia virus-based tumor vaccines: enhancement by simultaneous B7-1 expression. *J. Immunol.* **156,** 3357–3365.

Rinehart, J., Margolin, K., Triozzi, P., *et al.* (1995). Phase I trial of recombinant interleukin 3 before and after carboplatin/etoposide chemotherapy in patients with solid tumors: a southwest oncology group study. *Clin. Cancer Res.* **1,** 1139–1144.

Rodolfo, M., and Colombo, M. (1999). Interleukin-12 as an adjuvant for cancer immunotherapy. *Methods* **19,** 114–120.

Rodolfo, M., Melani, C., Zilocchi, C., *et al.* (1998). IgG2a induced by interleukin (IL) 12-producing tumor cell vaccines but not IgG1 induced by IL-4 vaccine is associated with the eradication of experimental metastases. *Cancer Res.* **58,** 5812–5817.

Rodolfo, M., Zilocchi, C., Melani, C., *et al.* (1996). Immunotherapy of experimental metastases by vaccination with interleukin gene-transduced adenocarcinoma cells sharing tumor-associated antigens: Comparison between IL-12 and IL-2 gene-transduced tumor cell vaccines. *J. Immunol.* **157,** 5536–5552.

Rosenberg, S., Lotze, M., Muul, L., *et al.* (1985). Observations on the systemic administration of autologous lymphokine-activated killer cells and recombinant interleukin-2 to patietns with metastatic cancer. *N. Engl. J. Med.* **313,** 1485–1492.

Rosenberg, S., Lotze, M., Muul, L., *et al.* (1987). A progress report on the treatment of 157 patients with advanced cancer using lymphokine-activated killer cells and interleukin-2 or high-dose interleukin-2 alone. *N. Engl. J. Med.* **316,** 889–987.

Rosenberg, S., Lotze, M., Yang, J., *et al.* (1989). Experience with the use of high-dose interleukin-2 in the treatment of 652 cancer patients. *Ann Surg.* **210,** 474–484.

Rosenberg, S., Mule, J., Speiss, P., *et al.* (1985). Regression of established pulmonary metastases and subcutaneous tumor mediated by the systemic administration of high-dose recombinant interleukin 2. *J. Exp. Med.* **161,** 1169–1188.

Rosenberg, S., Spiess, P., and Lafreniere, R. (1986). A new approach to the adoptive immunotherapy of cancer with tumor-infiltrating lymphocytes. *Science* **233,** 1318–1321.

Rosenberg, S., Yang, J., Schwartzentruber, D., *et al.* (1998). Immunologic and therapeutic evaluation of a synthetic peptide vaccine for the treatment of patients with metastatic melanoma. *Nature Med.* **4,** 321–327.

Rosenberg, S., Yang, J., Topalian, S., *et al.* (1994). Treatment of 283 consecutive patients with metastatic melanoma or renal cell cancer using high-dose bolus interleukin 2. *JAMA* **271,** 907–913.

Rosenberg, S., Yannelli, J., Yang, J., *et al.* (1994). Treatment of patients with metastatic melanoma with autologous tumor-infiltrating lymphocytes and interleukin 2. *J. Natl. Cancer Inst.* **86,** 1159–1166.

Salazar-Onfray, F. (1999). Interleukin-10: a cytokine used by tumors to escape immunosurveillance. *Med. Oncol.* **16,** 86–94.

Schmidinger, M., Steger, G., Wenzel, C., *et al.* (2000). Sequential administration of interferon gamma and interleukin-2 in metastatic renal cell carcinoma: Results of a phase II trial. Austrian Renal Cell Carcinoma Study Group. *Cancer Immunol. Immunother.* **49,** 395–400.

Sharma, S., Stolina, M., Lin, Y., *et al.* (1999). T cell derived IL-10 promotes lung cancer growth by suppressing both T cell and APC function. *J. Immunol.* **163,** 5020–5028.

Soiffer, R., Murray, C., Cochran, K., *et al.* (1992). Clinical and immunologic effects of prolonged infusion of low-dose recombinant interleukin-2 after autologous and T-cell depleted allogeneic bone marrow transplantation. *Blood* **79,** 517–526.

Soiffer, R., Murray, C., Gonin, R., et al. (1994). Effect of low-dose interleukin-2 on disease relapse after T-cell depleted allogeneic bone marrow transplantation. *Blood* **84**, 964–971.

Steinbrink, K., Jonuleit, H., Muller, G., et al. (1999). Interleukin-10-treated human dendritic cells induce a melanoma-antigen-specific anergy in CD8(+) T cells resulting in a failure to lyse tumor cells. *Blood* **93**, 1634–1642.

Steinbrink, K., Wolfl, M., Jonuleit, H., et al. (1997). Induction of tolerance by IL-10-treated dendritic cells. *J. Immunol.* **159**, 4772–4780.

Sun, Y., Jurgovsky, K., Moller, P., et al. (1998). Vaccination with IL-12 gene-modified autologous melanoma cells: Preclinical results and a first clinical phase I study. *Gene Ther.* **5**, 481–490.

Tahara, H., Lotze, M., Robbins, P., et al. (1995). IL-12 gene therapy using direct injection of tumors with genetically engineered autologous fibroblasts. *Hum. Gene Ther.* **6**, 1607–1624.

Tahara, H., Zitvogel, L., Storkus, W., et al. (1995). Effective eradication of established murine tumors with IL-12 gene therapy using a polycistronic retroviral vector. *J. Immunol.* **154**, 6466–6472.

Taniguchi, M., Nagaoka, K., Kunikata, T., et al. (1997). Characterization of anti-human interleukin-18 (IL-18)/interferon-gamma-inducing factor (IGIF) monoclonal antibodies and their application in the measurement of human IL-18 by ELISA. *J. Immunol. Methods* **206**, 107–113.

Teramura, M., Kobayashi, S., Hoshino, S., et al. (1992). Interleukin-11 enhances human megakaryocytopoiesis. *Blood* **79**, 327–331.

Terheyden, P., Becker, J., Kampgen, E., et al. (2000). Sequential interferon-alpha2b, interleukin-2 and fotemustine for patients with metastatic melanoma. *Melanoma Res.* **10**, 475–482.

Tester, W., Kim, K., Krigel, R., et al. (1999). A randomized phase II study of interleukin-2 with and without beta-interferon for patients with advanced non-small cell lung cancer: An Eastern Cooperative Oncology Group study (PZ586). *Lung Cancer* **25**, 199–206.

Topalian, S., Solomon, D., Avis, F., et al. (1988). Immunotherapy of patients with advanced cancer using tumor-infiltrating lymphocytes and recombinant interleukin-2: A pilot study. *J. Clin. Oncol.* **6**, 839–853.

Topalian, S., Solomon, D., and Rosenberg, S. (1989). Tumor-specific cytolytis by lymphocytes infiltrating human melanomas. *J. Immunol.* **142**, 3714–3725.

Trentin, L., Zambello, R., Facco, M., et al. (1997). Interleukin-15: A novel cytokine with regulatory properties on normal and neoplastic B lymphocytes. *Leukocyte Lymphoma* **27**, 35–42.

Trinchieri, G. (1998). Proinflammatory and immunoregulatory function of interleukin-12. *Int. Rev. Immunol.* **16**, 365–396.

Vries, J. D. (1995). Immunosuppressive and anti-inflammatory properties of interleukin-10. *Ann. Med.* **27**, 537–541.

Wakkach, A., Cottrez, F., and Groux, H. (2000). Can interleukin-10 be used as a true immunoregulatory cytokine? *Eur. Cytokine Netw.* **11**, 153–160.

Wang, J., Homer, R., Hong, L., et al. (2000). IL-11 selectively inhibits aeroallergen-induced pulmonary eosinophilia and Th2 cytokine production. *J. Immunol.* **165**, 2222–2231.

Weisdorf, D., Katsanis, E., Verfaillie, C., et al. (1994). Interleukin-1 alpha administered after autologous transplantation: A phase I/II clinical trial. *Blood* **84**, 2044–2049.

Wolf, S., Temple, P., Kobayashi, M., et al. (1991). Cloning of cDNA for natural killer cell stimulatory factor, a heterodimeric cytokine with multiple biologic effects on T and natural killer cells. *J. Immunol.* **146**, 3074–3081.

Wu, S., Meeker, W., Wiener, J., et al. (1994). Transfection of ovarian cancer cells with tumor necrosis factor-alpha (TNF-alpha) antisense mRNA abolishes the proliferative response to interleukin-1 (IL-1) but not TNF-alpha. *Gynecol. Oncol.* **53**, 59–63.

Wu, Y., Hong, J., Huang, H., et al. (2000). Mechanisms mediating the effects of IL-3 gene expression on tumor growth. *J. Leukocyte Biol.* **68**, 890–896.

Yamada, Y., and Kamihira, S. (1999). Pathological roles of interleukin-15 in adult T-cell leukemia. *Leukocyte Lymphoma* **35**, 37–45.

Yamamoto, K., Yajima, A., Terashima, Y., et al. (1999). Phase II clinical study on the effects of recombinant human interleukin-3 on thrombocytopenia after chemotherapy for advanced ovarian cancer. *J. Immunother.* **22**, 539–545.

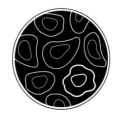

Jak/STAT Pathway

Michael David

University of California, San Diego

I. Signaling via the Jak/STAT Pathway
II. Animal Models in the Jak/STAT Pathway
III. The Jak/STAT Pathway and Cancer

GLOSSARY

signaling pathway The molecular mechanism by which an extracellular condition, such as the attachment of a growth factor to its receptor, is translated into a change in gene expression through a series of molecular interactions, often involving protein kinase activities and alterations in transcription factors.

signal transducing activator of transcription A protein classification.

T he combination of genetic and biochemical approaches has led to the elucidation of a novel signaling pathway whose key components are the Janus tyrosine kinases (Jak) and the signal transducers and activators of transcription (STAT). Although initially identified as the signal transduction system that triggers the activation of immediate early genes in response to interferons (IFN), it has become increasingly clear that the Jak/STAT pathway fulfills a central role in the biologic responses of numerous cytokines and growth factors. This article outlines the components of the Jak/STAT pathway, describes their mechanisms of activation and attenuation, and discusses the contributions of the Jak/STAT pathway to cancer etiology.

I. SIGNALING VIA THE JAK/STAT PATHWAY

Many cytokines and growth factors exert their pleiotropic biological effects by binding to specific cell surface receptors, leading to the activation of latent cytoplasmic proteins, which subsequently transmit the signals to the cell nucleus. One of the newer additions to this diverse group of signaling cascades is the Jak/STAT pathway, whose discovery is due to the quest for the mechanism by which interferons activate immediate early response genes.

A. Jak/STAT Family Members

The first STAT proteins were identified as the regulatory components of the type I interferon-induced transcription factor complex, ISGF3. STAT1 and STAT2, in conjunction with the DNA-binding subunit p48, were found to bind the interferon-stimulated response element (ISRE) enhancer as a heterodimer in response to IFNα/β. Alternatively, STAT1 homodimers activated via the IFNγ receptor can bind a distinct element termed GAS (IFNγ-activated sequence). Shortly after cloning of STAT1 and STAT2, numerous other cytokines and growth factors were reported to activate DNA-binding proteins with STAT-like characteristics (summarized in Table I). Efforts to identify these proteins resulted in the cloning of five additional mammalian STAT genes (STAT3, STAT4, STAT5A, STAT5B, STAT6), which, in analogy to the interferon-signaling model, bind to GAS-like elements. Several of the STAT proteins are represented by various splice variants; however, STAT5A and STAT5B are encoded by two distinct genes. In contrast to the more restricted expression of STAT4 in spleen, heart, brain, peripheral blood cells, and testis, most STAT proteins are found ubiquitous. All seven STAT proteins share several conserved structural and functional domains (Fig. 1). A carboxy-terminal tyrosine residue, which serves as the target for ligand-induced phosphorylation, is crucial for dimerization, nuclear translocation, and DNA binding of STAT molecules. The src-homology 2 (SH2) domain of STAT proteins facilitates homo- or heterodimerization via reciprocal interaction with the phosphorylated tyrosine residue. In addition, the SH2 domain

TABLE I

Receptor family	Tyk2	Jak1	Jak2	Jak3	STAT1	STAT2	STAT3	STAT4	STAT5	STAT6
IFN										
IFNα/β	+	+	−	−	+	+	+	+	+	+
IFNγ	−	+	+	−	+	−	−	−	+	−
gp130										
LIF	+	+	+	−	+	−	+	−	−	−
G-CSF	−	+	−	−	+	−	+	−	+	−
IL-6	+	+	+	−	+	−	+	−	+	−
IL-11	−	+	−	−	+	−	+	−	−	−
IL-12	+	−	+	−	−	−	+	+	−	−
CNTF	+	+	+	−	+	−	+	−	−	−
OSM	+	+	+	−	+	−	+	−	−	−
Common γ chain										
IL-2	−	+	−	+	+	−	+	−	+	−
IL-4	−	+	−	+	+	−	+	−	−	+
IL-7	−	+	−	+	−	−	−	−	+	−
IL-9	−	+	−	+	−	−	−	−	+	−
IL-13	−	+	−	−	?	?	?	?	?	?
IL-15	−	+	−	+	−	−	−	−	+	−
Common β chain										
IL-3	−	−	+	−	−	−	−	−	+	−
IL-5	−	−	+	−	−	−	−	−	+	−
GM-CSF	−	−	+	−	−	−	−	−	+	−
Single chain										
EPO	−	−	+	−	−	−	−	−	+	−
GH	−	+	+	−	+	−	+	−	+	−
PRL	+	+	+	−	+	−	−	−	+	−
TPO	+	+	−	−	+	−	+	−	+	−
Growth factors										
EGF	−	+	+	−	+	−	+	−	−	−
PDGF	+	+	+	−	+	−	+	−	−	+
CSF-1	−	+	+	−	+	−	+	−	−	−

NH2-TERM DOMAIN	**COILED-COIL DOMAIN**	DNA BINDING	**LINKER DOMAIN**	**SH2 DOMAIN**	pTyr	(pSer)

FIGURE 1 Shared conserved structural and functional domains of STAT proteins.

accounts for the specific interaction of STAT molecules with activated, tyrosine phosphorylated cytokine and growth factor receptors, as well as Jak tyrosine kinases. Dimerization of STAT proteins allows the centrally located DNA-binding domains to interact with consensus palindromic sequences that differ only in their core nucleotide sequence. Interestingly, STAT2 is unable to bind DNA in such a manner, rather its function as a transcriptional activator appears to be restricted to its participation in the multimeric ISGF3 complex. The more divergent region carboxy-terminal to the tyrosine phosphorylation site harbors the transactivation domain (TAD). Posttranslational modification of several STAT members through serine phosphorylation, presumably by members of the ERK/SAPK kinase family, accounts for the regulated interaction of the STAT-TAD domains with transcriptional coactivators such as CBP/p300 or MCM5. Intriguingly, naturally occurring carboxy-terminal truncations created by RNA splicing can act as dominant-negative mutants when artificially overexpressed; however, no evidence exists for such function of these proteins at endogenous levels.

It was again the paradigm of the interferon signaling cascade that led to the discovery of the participation of the Janus tyrosine kinases in STAT-mediated gene transcription. The demonstration that mutagenically ablated expression of Tyk2 or Jak1 results in IFNα/β unresponsive cells, while similar abrogation of Jak1 and Jak2 expression resulted in the loss of IFNγ responsiveness, provided the basis for understanding the function of these tyrosine kinases and the identity of this novel signaling pathway. Contrary to the ubiquitous expression of these kinases, a fourth family member, Jak3, was identified whose expression is restricted to cells of hematopoietic origin. The most striking feature in the structure of Jak family members is the presence of a kinase-like domain of thus far unclear function in addition to the true kinase domain. Also noteworthy is the absence of any SH2- or SH3-like structures that are commonly found in cytoplasmic tyrosine kinases. The relatively large (120–140

kDa) Jak kinases are constitutively associated with many cytokine and growth factor receptors; nevertheless, this association can be increased after cytokine stimulation.

B. Mechanism of Activation

The general outline of the sequential events that lead to STAT-mediated gene transcription has been derived mostly from evidence gathered from the interferon-signaling paradigm. It is believed that the engagement of ligands to their respective receptors results in an increased local concentration of Jak proteins due to receptor aggregation and increased affinity of the receptors for Jak kinases. Subsequent cross-phosphorylation of Jaks results in the activation of their kinase activity, such that they can phosphorylate tyrosine residues in the receptor chains. These phosphotyrosine moieties provide docking sites for the STAT proteins via their SH2 domains, leading to their tyrosine phosphorylation, dimerization, and nuclear translocation. Parallel signaling events, presumably involving ERK/SAPK family members, are responsible for further phosphorylation of the serine residues in the carboxy terminus of the STAT proteins (Fig. 2), which are required for efficient transcriptional response. In the case of growth factor receptors, the intrinsic tyrosine kinase activity of the receptors is required for the tyrosine phosphorylation of STAT proteins, rather than the presence of Jak kinases.

C. Cross Talk with Other Signaling Pathways

In addition to the association with the transcriptional coactivator CBP, which has been observed with several of the STAT proteins, other interactions of STAT molecules that link to distinct signaling pathways have been described. STAT3 and STAT5A/B interact with the glucocorticoid receptor, and STAT3

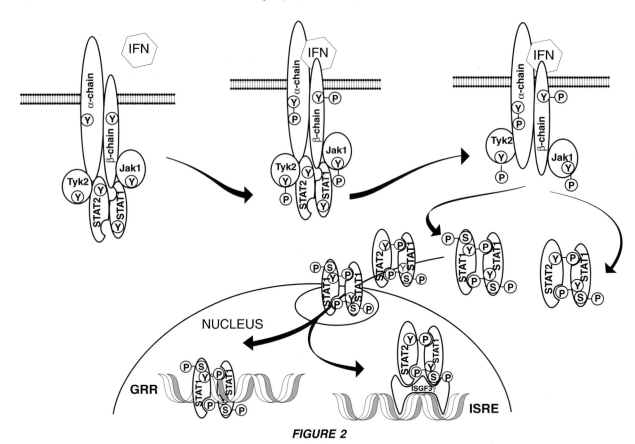

FIGURE 2

associates with c-Jun as well. STAT1 interactions have been described for Sp1 and BRCA1, and all but STAT2 interact with Nmi. Further examples of STAT participation in complex signaling networks are evidenced by the requirement of STAT1 for efficient caspase expression and TNFα-induced apoptosis, or by the inhibition of TGFβ signaling through induction of the inhibitory SMAD7 by IFNγ.

D. Attenuation of Jak/STAT Signaling

Of equal importance to the activation of a signaling pathway is its spatially and temporally coordinated attenuation. Several independent mechanism are responsible for the negative regulatory control over the Jak/STAT pathway. The tyrosine phosphatase SHP1 acts on activated receptors and the Jak kinases, whereas an unidentified nuclear tyrosine phosphatase dephosphorylates STAT proteins. SH2 domain-containing SOCS proteins have been identified as a family of cytokine-inducible inhibitors of Jak kinase

activity, thus acting in a classical negative feedback loop. In contrast, the constitutively expressed PIAS proteins do not prevent the phosphorylation of STAT proteins, but exert their negative regulatory role by association with tyrosine-phosphorylated STAT dimers and preventing them from binding DNA.

II. ANIMAL MODELS IN THE JAK/STAT PATHWAY

As is the case with other signaling pathways, much of our understanding of the diverse functions of Jak and STAT proteins *in vivo* has been revealed through the generation of knockout mice. With the exception of STAT2 and Tyk2, all members of the Jak/STAT pathway have been subjected to gene targeting to elucidate their biological function (Table II). STAT1-deficient mice display dramatically increased sensitivity toward viral and microbial pathogens, presumably due to their inability to respond to interferons. Inter-

TABLE II

Major Phenotypes of Jak and Stat-Deficient Mice

Jak1	Defective lymphocyte development due to impaired IL-7 signaling; loss of certain gp130-mediated responses, defective IFNα/β and IFNγ signaling
Jak2	Impaired erythropoiesis; defective response to IL-3, GM-CSF, IL-5, TPO, and IFNγ
Jak3	Severe combined immunodeficiency due to impaired IL-2, IL-4, and IL-7 signaling
Tyk2	Impaired IFNα and IFNγ response; loss of IL-12-induced IFNγ production in splenocytes
Stat1	Defective response to type I and type II IFNs; highly susceptible to microbial and viral infections
Stat2	Loss of type I IFN-induced antiviral and antiproliferative response
Stat3	Embryonic lethal; conditional knockout: lack of IL-6 response (T cells), defective wound healing (skin), highly susceptible to endotoxic shock (macrophage)
Stat4	Disrupted IL-12 signaling; defective Th1 development
Stat5A	Defective breast development and lactation
Stat5B	Defective IL-2-induced IL-2Rα expression in splenic T cells, loss of sexual dimorphism of body growth rates and liver gene expression
Stat6	Disrupted IL-4 signaling; defective Th2 cell function

estingly, despite the broad spectrum of cytokines and growth factors that lead to STAT1 activation, these mice respond normally to other cytokines and show no apparent defects in development. In contrast, disruption of the STAT3 gene results in early embryonic lethality, and only the use of conditional gene targeting revealed an essential role for STAT3 in T cell and macrophage function. As predicted by the restricted activation of STAT4 by IL-12, Th1 cell development is severely impaired by the disruption of the STAT4 gene. STAT5a and STAT5b share over 90% sequence homology, thus it is not surprising to find both redundant and nonredundant functions for these proteins. Consistent with the activation of STAT5 by prolactin, STAT5a-deficient mice fail to lactate; in contrast, the absence of STAT5b causes failure to respond to growth hormone. Both knockout mice exhibit defects in T and natural killer (NK) cell proliferation and/or function, with the loss of STAT5b being more severe. STAT5a/STAT5b double knockout mice totally lack NK cells; furthermore, their T cells fail to respond to anti-CD3 stimulation. The role of STAT6 in IL-4 signaling was confirmed by the impairment of Th2 development, lack of IgE class switching, and defective antigen-induced airway reactivity in the absence of STAT6. Jak1-deficient mice fail to nurse, display severely impaired lymphocyte development, and die perinatally. The function of Jak2 in erythropoietin signaling is evidenced by embryonic lethality due to defective erythropoiesis in

its absence. Of particular interest are results obtained from Jak3-deficient mice, as mutations in Jak3 have also been identified in humans. Jak3 interacts with the common cytokine receptor γ chain, a component of the receptors for IL-2, IL-4, IL-7, IL-9, and IL-15, and mutation of which is responsible for X-SCID. Similarly, Jak3 deficiency in mice or mutations of Jak3 in humans cause SCID-like phenotypes. However, the effects of impaired signaling though Jak3 in B cells are less severe in humans, presumably because the requirement for IL-7 as a pre-B-cell growth factor exists only in mice but not in humans.

III. THE JAK/STAT PATHWAY AND CANCER

Considering the extent to which cytokines and growth factors that activate the Jak/STAT pathway contribute to the regulation of cell growth, differentiation, and apoptosis, it is not surprising to find a role for members of this signaling cascade in oncogenesis. No mutations have been identified in any component of the Jak/STAT pathway that result in malignant transformation; however, the loss of components of the Jak/STAT pathway has been recognized as the cause for interferon resistance of certain tumors, particularly melanomas. Inversely, the constitutive tyrosine phosphorylation of several STAT proteins has been described as a result of transformation by tyrosine kinases such as v-src, v-Abl, or Bcr/Abl or as a result of viral transformation by HTLV or EBV. Furthermore, constitutive serine phosphorylation of STAT proteins was reported in several cases of hematopoietic malignancies. The extent to which the STAT proteins contribute to the transformation process is still largely unclear. While conditionally activated STAT3 displays oncogenic potential in its own right, its ability to support anchorage-independent growth is only 10% of that observed in v-src-transformed cells. Additional contributions of STAT proteins to oncogenesis might be through their participation in the regulation of apoptosis, either by induction of the antiapoptotic factors bcl-2 and bcl-x or by accounting for the constitutive expression of several caspases.

We have just begun to elucidate the contributions of the Jak/STAT pathway to physiological and pathological processes. Further studies on the role of the Jak/STAT pathway in the etiology and progression of malignant transformation should provide the necessary basis for new therapeutic approaches against cancer.

See Also the Following Articles

Cytokines: Hematopoietic Growth Factors • Interferons: Cellular and Molecular Biology of Their Actions

Bibliography

Akira, S. (1999). Functional roles of STAT family proteins: Lessons from knockout mice. *Stem Cells* **17,** 138–146.

Hilton, D. J. (1999). Negative regulators of cytokine signal transduction. *Cell Mol. Life Sci.* **55,** 1568–1577.

Hoey, T., and Schindler, U. (1998). STAT structure and function in signaling. *Curr. Opin. Genet. Dev.* **8,** 582–587.

Imada, K., and Leonard, W. J. (2000). The Jak-STAT pathway. *Mol. Immunol.* **37,** 1–11.

Leonard, W. J., and O'Shea, J. J. (1998). Jaks and STATs: Biological implications. *Annu. Rev. Immunol.* **16,** 293–322.

Liu, K. D., Gaffen, S. L., and Goldsmith, M. A. (1998). JAK/STAT signaling by cytokine receptors. *Curr. Opin. Immunol.* **10,** 271–278.

McCubrey, J. A., May, W. S., Duronio, V., and Mufson, A. (2000). Serine/threonine phosphorylation in cytokine signal transduction. *Leukemia* **14,** 9–21.

Miyajima, A., Ito, Y., and Kinoshita, T. (1999). Cytokine signaling for proliferation, survival, and death in hematopoietic cells. *Int. J. Hematol.* **69,** 137–146.

Schindler, C., and Brutsaert, S. (1999). Interferons as a paradigm for cytokine signal transduction. *Cell Mol. Life Sci.* **55,** 1509–1522.

Schindler, C., and Darnell, J. E., Jr. (1995). Transcriptional responses to polypeptide ligands: the JAK-STAT pathway. *Annu. Rev. Biochem.* **64,** 621–651.

Touw, I. P., De Koning, J. P., Ward, A. C., and Hermans, M. H. (2000). Signaling mechanisms of cytokine receptors and their perturbances in disease. *Mol. Cell. Endocrinol.* **160,** 1–9.

Weber-Nordt, R. M., Mertelsmann, R., and Finke, J. (1998). The JAK-STAT pathway: Signal transduction involved in proliferation, differentiation and transformation. *Leuk. Lymphoma* **28,** 459–467.

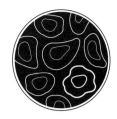

Kidney, Epidemiology

Joseph P. Grande
The Mayo Foundation, Rochester, Minnesota

I. Introduction
II. Cytogenetic Alterations in Renal Cell Carcinoma
III. Cytogenetic Alterations in Inherited
    Cancer Syndromes
IV. Progression of Renal Cell Carcinoma
V. Summary and Conclusions

GLOSSARY

hemangioblastoma Highly vascular benign neoplasms that arise within the central nervous system (cerebellum, spinal cord, and brain stem) of patients with von Hippel–Lindau syndrome.

hepatocyte growth factor The ligand for the MET protooncogene.

MET protooncogene A membrane-bound protein with tyrosine kinase activity. Missense mutations located within the tyrosine kinase domain of this gene are thought to be associated with the development of hereditary papillary renal cell carcinoma.

pheochromocytoma A tumor arising from chromaffin cells of the adrenal medulla. Some forms of hereditary pheochromocytomas are associated with specific mutations in the VHL gene.

pVHL The protein product of the von Hippel–Lindau disease gene.

Von Hippel–Lindau disease A hereditary syndrome characterized by the development of clear cell renal cell carcinoma and a number of extrarenal tumors, including retinal hemangiomas and central nervous system hemangioblastomas.

Familial forms of renal cell carcinoma are relatively uncommon, accounting for less than 5% of all renal cancers. However, analysis of families with inherited renal cell carcinoma syndromes has led to the development of powerful tools to identify the genes involved in the pathogenesis of both familial and sporadic forms of renal cell carcinoma. The identification of characteristic cytogenetic alterations in histologically distinct forms of renal cell carcinoma has prompted a refinement of the histologic classification of renal tumors. Analysis of structure–function relationships of genes altered in renal cell carcinoma will continue to provide important insights into renal tumorigenesis and may lead to the identification of novel targets for the treatment of patients with renal cell carcinoma.

I. INTRODUCTION

Renal cell carcinomas account for approximately 2–3% of all malignant neoplasms in adults. The incidence of renal cell carcinoma increases with age; the peak incidence is in the sixth decade of life. A variety of environmental factors have been implicated in the pathogenesis of renal cell carcinoma, the most important of which is exposure to tobacco smoke.

The vast majority of renal cell carcinomas are not associated with an inherited cancer syndrome. However, several clinical features should prompt investigation for a possible hereditary cancer syndrome, including early age at onset, the development of multicentric or bilateral tumors, or the presence of one of several characteristic extrarenal tumors. In general, familial renal cell carcinoma syndromes are inherited in an autosomal-dominant manner, with incomplete penetrance.

Both familial and sporadic forms of renal cell carcinoma have been shown to have recurrent, nonrandom chromosomal abnormalities that are characteristic of particular histologic variants of renal tumors. These chromosomal abnormalities are now being considered in the histopathologic classification of renal tumors and may provide important diagnostic and prognostic information.

II. CYTOGENETIC ALTERATIONS IN RENAL CELL CARCINOMA

The classification of renal tumors is based on architecture, growth pattern, cytoplasmic features, and nu-clear grade. A summary of the characteristic cytogenetic abnormalities in subtypes of renal tumors is shown in Table I. By definition, renal adenomas have no capacity to metastasize. Nevertheless, papillary renal cell adenomas contain some of the cytogenetic alterations—loss of the Y chromosome, trisomy 7, and trisomy 17—that are observed in papillary renal cell carcinomas. Frequent cytogenetic alterations in oncocytomas include loss of chromosomes 1p, 14q, and the Y chromosome, and translocations among t11, q13, and other chromosomes. Rearrangement of mitochondrial DNA is also noted in oncocytomas.

In nonpapillary renal cell carcinoma, there is loss of chromosome 3p13pter in a majority of tumors. The VHL gene is located on 3p25.3 (see later). In VHL-associated renal cell carcinoma, a mutated VHL gene is inherited; in sporadic cases, this allele is inactivated by a somatic mutation. The second allele is inactivated by subsequent mutation or by hypermethylation in at least 65% of cases. Evidence indicates the presence of another tumor suppressor gene, called the RCC gene, at chromosome 3p, proximal to the VHL locus. It is possible that homozygous expression of the mutated VHL gene is responsible for renal cyst development, and inactivation of both alleles of the RCC gene on chromosome 3p is required for the development of both sporadic and VHL-associated tumors. Partial trisomy of 5q is the second most frequent alteration in renal cell carcinoma. This may occur, in some cases, by a nonhomologous recombination between the 3p breakpoint regions and 5q22, resulting in monosomy 3p and partial trisomy of 5q22-qter. Whereas alterations of genes at 3p and 5q are associated with tumor development, alterations of 6q, 8p, 9, and 14q are associated with aggressive behavior of nonpapillary renal cell carcinoma during tumor progression. The most common cytogenetic alteration

TABLE I

Cytogenetic Classifications of Renal Neoplasms

Tumor histology	Cytogenetic alterations
Papillary renal cell adenoma	+7, +17, −y
Oncocytoma	−1p, −14q, −y, t(11q13)
Renal cell carcinoma, clear cell variant	3p−, +5q22, −6q, −8p, −9p, −14q
Papillary renal cell carcinoma	+3q, +7, +8, +12, +16, +17, +18, +20, −y
Chromophobe renal cell carcinoma	−1, −2, −6, −10, −10, −13, −17, −21

in papillary renal cell carcinoma is trisomy of chromosome 7.

The MET protooncogene has been localized to chromosome 7 and appears to be involved in the pathogenesis of hereditary and sporadic papillary renal cell carcinoma. Other common cytogenetic abnormalities in papillary renal cell carcinoma are loss of the Y chromosome and trisomy 17. In chromophobe renal cell carcinoma, there is a loss of chromosomes 1, 2, 6, 10, 13, 17, and 21 in 76–100% of cases, and a frequent loss of the Y chromosome. At least five to seven chromosomes are lost before a chromophobe renal cell carcinoma develops. These tumors also demonstrate a gross rearrangement of mitochondrial DNA.

III. CYTOGENETIC ALTERATIONS IN INHERITED CANCER SYNDROMES

Although histologic variants of renal cell carcinoma are associated with recurrent, nonrandom chromosomal abnormalities, most tumors are thought to arise from somatic mutations in affected patients. However, a minority of patients that develop clear cell renal cell carcinoma or papillary renal cell carcinoma have an inherited predisposition to develop these tumors. Studies of these patients and their families have led to the characterization of genes that are involved in the pathogenesis of both familial and sporadic renal cell carcinoma. Two of the most completely described familial renal cancer syndromes include von Hippel–Lindau disease, which is associated with the development of clear cell renal carcinoma, and familial papillary renal cell carcinoma, which is associated with mutations of the MET protooncogene. The syndromes will be described in detail, with an emphasis on cytogenetic structure–function relationships.

A. von Hippel–Lindau Syndrome

Von Hippel–Lindau syndrome is a familial multiple cancer syndrome in which there is a predisposition to a variety of neoplasms (Table II). Von Hippel–Lindau syndrome affects 1 in 36,000 individuals and is inherited in an autosomal-dominant fashion with a vari-

TABLE II

Incidence of Tumors in Patients with von Hippel–Lindau Syndrome[a]

Lesion	Incidence (%)
Retinal angioma	57
Cerebellar hemangioblastoma	55
Spinal cord hemangioblastoma	14
Renal cell carcinoma	24
Pheochromocytoma	19

[a]Adapted from Richards et al. (1998).

able but high degree of penetrance. In addition to renal cell carcinoma, patients with von Hippel–Lindau syndrome frequently develop retinal and central nervous system hemangioblastomas, pheochromocytomas, pancreatic islet cell tumors, and endolymphatic sac tumors. Tumors associated with von Hippel–Lindau syndrome tend to be highly vascular.

Hemangioblastomas may be early clinical manifestations of von Hippel–Lindau syndrome and affect both retina and central nervous systems. Central nervous system hemangioblastomas are most frequently found within the cerebellum, followed by the spinal cord and brain stem. Hemangioblastomas are well-demarcated neoplasms containing both cystic and solid components (Fig. 1A). The solid component consists of cells with abundant pink cytoplasm traversed by numerous thin-walled vascular channels (Fig. 1B). In approximately 20% of cases, the tumor cells secrete erythropoietin and induce polycythemia.

Pheochromocytomas are also vascular neoplasms that are associated with von Hippel–Lindau syndrome in up to 20% of cases. Pheochromocytomas are tumors of chromaffin cells of the adrenal medulla that secrete catecholamines. Grossly, pheochromocytomas are encapsulated, spongy, reddish masses with prominent central scars. The tumors frequently contain foci of cystic degeneration and hemorrhage. Microscopically, the tumor cells are polyhedral to fusiform and contain a granular amphophilic or basophilic cytoplasm and vesicular nuclei (Fig. 2B). Nuclei are frequently enlarged, hyperchromatic, and pleomorphic. The tumor is traversed by numerous capillaries. The incidence of pheochromocytoma in von Hippel–Lindau syndrome is greatly influenced by the specific mutation of the VHL gene; missense mutations

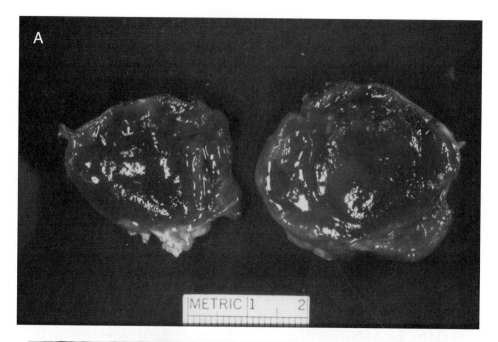

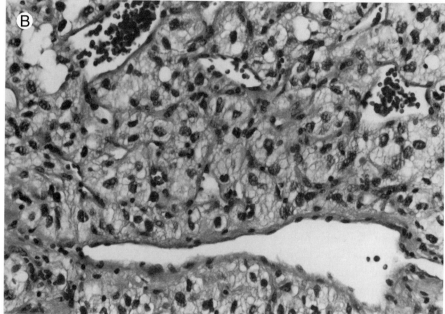

FIGURE 1 (A) Hemangioblastoma, gross appearance. The tumor is well circumscribed and contains a large cystic region with hemorrhage. (B) Hemangioblastoma, microscopic appearance. The tumor is composed of cells with an abundant pink cytoplasm and is traversed by numerous thin-walled vascular channels lined by endothelial cells.

are associated with the much higher incidence of pheochromocytoma than are large deletions or truncations (see later).

Pancreatic cysts, which frequently occur in patients with von Hippel–Lindau syndrome, are usually of no clinical significance. However, patients may develop nonsecretory islet cell tumors, which are frequently malignant. Up to 10% of patients with von Hippel–Lindau syndrome may develop endolymphatic sac tumors. These are low-grade papillary adenocarcino-

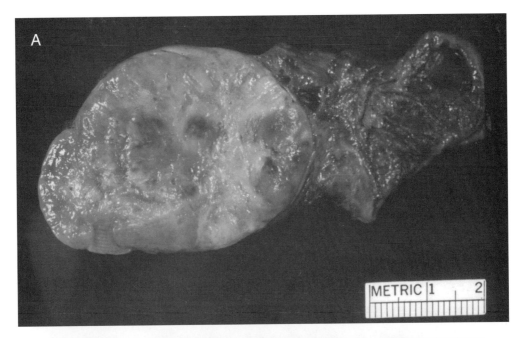

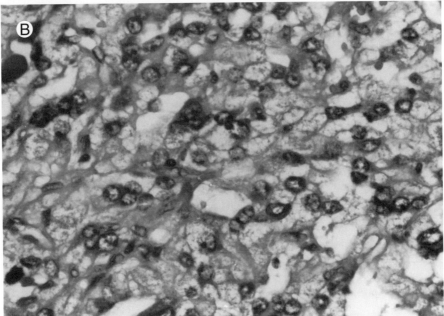

FIGURE 2 (A) Pheochromocytoma, gross appearance. The tumor arises from the adrenal medulla and is sharply circumscribed. An uninvolved adrenal gland is shown on the right side. (B) Pheochromocytoma, microscopic appearance. The tumor consists of anastomosing cords of cells. Cells are polygonal, with a finely granular cytoplasm; considerable nuclear pleomorphism is present.

mas, which may be bilateral. Many of these tumors are asymptomatic.

Renal cysts develop in 50–70% of patients with von Hippel–Lindau syndrome. The renal neoplasm characteristically associated with von Hippel–Lindau syndrome is clear cell carcinoma. These tumors consist of sheets or acini of round cells with abundant clear cytoplasm (Fig. 3). The lifetime risk of developing renal cell carcinoma is greater than 70%. Renal cell carcinoma is the most common cause of death in

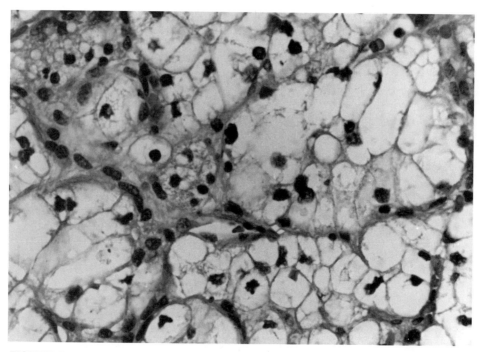

FIGURE 3 Renal cell carcinoma, microscopic appearance. The tumor cells are round to polygonal with an abundant clear cytoplasm.

patients with von Hippel–Lindau syndrome. Studies of patients with this syndrome have led to the identification of a region within chromosome 3 (3p25-26), which is frequently deleted or altered.

The von Hippel–Lindau gene was cloned by Latif and colleagues in 1993. The gene consists of three exons (Fig. 4); the mRNA encodes a protein of 213 amino acid residues with an apparent molecular mass of 30 kDa (pVHL-L). A second form of VHL (pVHL-S) with an apparent molecular mass of 19 kDa is generated by translation initiation at an internal ATG codon at residue 54. In addition, two isoforms of VHL mRNA are generated through alternative splicing. In

isoform 1, exons 1, 2, and 3 are present. In isoform 2, exon 2 is deleted. Some VHL patients contain a germline deletion of exon 2, resulting in the expression of isoform 2 only. Because these patients develop VHL syndrome, it is unlikely that isoform 2 encodes a fully functional gene product.

In situ hybridization analysis for VHL mRNA shows widespread expression throughout all three germ layers during development, with strongest expression in the central nervous system, kidney, testis, and lung. Within the kidney, the developing collecting ducts, proximal tubule, and loop of Henle show the strongest expression. The primary sequence of pVHL is not

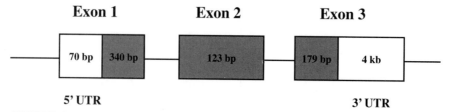

FIGURE 4 Structure of the von Hippel–Lindau (VHL) gene. The VHL coding sequence is contained within three exons (boxes). Exon 1 contains 70 bp of a 5′-untranslated sequence (clear box) and 340 bp of a coding sequence (shaded box). Exon 2 contains 123 bp of a coding sequence (shaded box). Exon 3 encodes 179 bp of a coding sequence (shaded box) and 4 kb of a 3′-untranslated sequence (white box).

highly similar to that of any known protein. pVHL becomes phosphorylated on serine residues. Kinases that phosphorylate pVHL are unknown, as are the functional consequences of pVHL phosphorylation. The VHL protein is a cytoplasmic protein, which may shuttle between the cytoplasm and nucleus in a cell density-dependent manner. A fraction of pVHL is found within cell membranes, including the Golgi and endoplasmic reticulum. The physiologic relevance of this is not clear. Homozygous deletion of pVHL in mouse embryos is lethal during embryogenesis. In these embryos, vascularization of the placenta is defective.

Because the primary sequence of pVHL is not similar to that of any known protein and therefore does not provide any clues regarding possible function, initial studies to determine the role of pVHL in renal carcinogenesis have focused on the identification of pVHL-binding proteins. These studies have uncovered at least four potential functions of pVHL (Table III).

In vitro studies have shown that pVHL interacts with a transcriptional elongation complex called elongin or SIII. This elongation complex suppresses transient pausing during transcription. SIII, or elongin, is a heterotrimer composed of elongin A, B, and C. Elongin A is a 110-kDa protein that contains transcriptional elongation activity. Elongin C is a 15-kDa protein that directly binds elongin A and increases its activity. Elongin B is an 18-kDa protein and participates in transcriptional elongation by stabilizing the elongin complex. Loss of VHL function leads to an increased expression of genes regulated by this pathway. *In vitro*, pVHL competes with elongin A for binding to elongin B and C, thereby inhibiting elongin activity. However, most pVHL appears to reside in the cytoplasm rather than in the nucleus, as would be expected for a transcriptional regulator. Elongin B and C are also present within the cytoplasm. There is no direct evidence that pVHL inhibits elongin/SIII *in vivo* or that elongin plays a specific as opposed to a general role in transcriptional regulation. Therefore, cytoplasmic elongin/pVHL complexes may have other roles than that of transcriptional regulation.

Along these lines, studies have shown that Cullin 2 (Cul2), a member of the Cullin family of proteins, binds pVHL/elongin B/elongin C complexes. Cullins are believed to target certain cellular proteins for covalent linkage to a ubiquitin. Ubiquitinated proteins are rapidly degraded. Cul2 shares similarity with the yeast Cdc53 that targets proteins for ubiquitin-dependent proteolysis. Targets of Cdc53 are proteins involved in the cell cycle control and adaptation to nutritional deprivation. Evidence suggests that complexes containing pVHL, elongin B, elongin C, and Cul2 earmark certain proteins for degradation.

Potential targets for the pVHL–elongin–Cul2 complex stems from clinical pathologic observations that many tumors associated with VHL disease are highly vascular and are associated with paraneoplastic erythrocytosis. The hypervascular nature of tumors is linked to the overproduction of vascular endothelial growth factor (VEGF), whereas paraneoplastic erythrocytosis is linked to the ectopic production of erythropoietin by tumor cells. Both of these gene products are induced by hypoxia to augment delivery of oxyhemoglobin to cells. These genes are induced both through transcriptional activation and increased mRNA stability. Renal cell carcinomas lacking pVHL produce a high level of hypoxia-inducible mRNAs such as VEGF under both hypoxic and normoxic conditions. The VHL protein has been shown to inhibit the accumulation of hypoxia-inducible mRNAs under normoxic conditions. It is hypothesized that pVHL/elongin/Cul2 regulates the stability of hypoxia-induced genes, perhaps by regulating the stability of various RNA-binding proteins. However, the precise mechanism by which the VHL protein alters VEGF or other hypoxia-induced genes stability awaits clarification. Furthermore, some pVHL mutants retain the ability to bind elongin/Cul2. This suggests that biochemical activities unrelated to elongin/Cul2 binding contribute to tumor suppression by pVHL.

One such activity may be related to the interaction of VHL with fibronectin. VHL interacts with fibronectin in association with the endoplasmic reticulum and Golgi apparatus. Every pVHL mutant

TABLE III
Functions of pVHL

Regulates transcriptional elongation
Regulates protein ubiquitination
Interacts with fibronectin
Regulates hypoxia-inducible genes

examined to date, including those that interact with elongin/Cul2, has lost the ability to bind fibronectin. Fibronectin may contribute to the ability of pVHL to suppress tumor cell growth. Malignant cells typically produce low levels of fibronectin. Fibronectin and integrin signaling can, in some experimental settings, suppress malignant behavior. VHL null tumors, as well as cells from VHL knockout cells, fail to assemble a fibronectin matrix. The role of pVHL–fibronectin interactions in regulation of renal cell carcinogenesis awaits clarification.

Mutations in the VHL gene have been identified in 75% of VHL patients. Tumor development in these patients is associated with somatic loss or inactivation of the remaining wild-type VHL allele, consistent with a notion that the VHL gene functions as a tumor suppressor. Over 75% of patients with sporadic renal cell carcinoma and over 50% of patients with sporadic cerebellar hemangioblastomas contain inactivation of both VHL alleles. Mutation of the VHL gene, with loss of the remaining VHL allele, has also been documented in early premalignant lesions of the kidney, including atypical cysts and microscopic renal cell carcinoma *in situ*. Therefore, inactivation of VHL function appears to be an early step in the pathogenesis of both hereditary and sporadic renal cell carcinoma.

A variety of VHL mutations have been identified, including large deletions, microdeletions, insertions, frameshift point mutations, and nonsense mutations. The risk of developing pheochromocytoma varies widely in different families with VHL; this has been associated with characteristic mutations in the VHL gene (Table IV). Patients with large deletions and mutations predicted to cause a truncated protein are associated with a lower risk of pheochromocytoma (type I patients). Patients with one of several charac-

teristic missense mutations are at a high risk of developing pheochromocytoma (risk of up to 80%; type II patients, Table IV). Other missense mutations are associated with a high risk for pheochromocytoma and a low risk of renal cell carcinoma (type IIa).

B. Hereditary Papillary Renal Cell Carcinoma

Affected patients tend to develop multiple, bilateral renal tumors with a papillary histology (Figure 5). Unlike the von Hippel–Lindau syndrome, the major neoplastic manifestations of hereditary papillary renal cell carcinoma appear to be confined to the kidney, although sporadic reports of other tumors of the pancreas, breast, colon, and other organs have been described. The most consistent cytogenetic finding in sporadic and inherited papillary renal cell carcinoma is trisomy 7, suggesting that a gene on this chromosome is involved in the pathogenesis of papillary renal cell carcinoma. Mutational analysis has subsequently identified the MET protooncogene to be involved in hereditary papillary renal cell carcinoma. The MET protooncogene is a membrane-bound protein with tyrosine kinase activity. Patients with hereditary papillary renal cell carcinomas have missense mutations located within the tyrosine kinase domain of the MET gene.

In contrast to the von Hippel–Lindau syndrome, wherein many of the germline and somatic mutations are predicted to inactivate the protein product, in hereditary papillary renal cell carcinoma, all mutations of the MET gene are of the missense type. In hereditary papillary renal cell carcinoma syndromes, the mutations are localized in a small region of the gene. No frameshift mutations or large deletions that are likely to produce an inactive MET protein have been identified in papillary renal cell cancer. These observations suggest that mutations in the tyrosine kinase domain of the MET protooncogene produce a gain of function.

The ligand for the MET protooncogene is hepatocyte growth factor (HGF), also known as scatter factor. HGF is a mesenchymal cytokine that triggers a variety of pathways, including proliferation, survival, motility, invasion of matrix, and induction of polarity. During embryogenesis, HGF promotes the forma-

---

TABLE IV
VHL Phenotypes

Type I	No pheochromocytoma
Type II	Pheochromocytoma present
Type IIa	No renal cell carcinoma
Type IIb	Renal cell carcinoma
Type IIc	Pheochromocytoma present but no other tumors

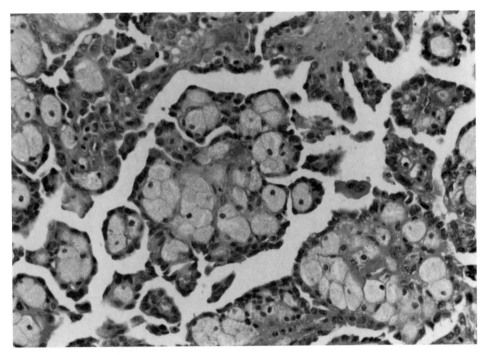

FIGURE 5 Papillary renal cell carcinoma, microscopic appearance. Papillary renal cell carcinomas are associated with sporadic or germline mutations of the MET protooncogene on chromosome 7. The tumor consists of a single layer of cuboidal cells lining a fibrovascular stalk. The fibrovascular core contains numerous lipid-laden macrophages.

tion of tubular structures in epithelial organs. During development, the coordinated control of invasive growth by HGF or its receptor, MET, is essential. Knockouts of ligand or receptor are embryonic lethal due to liver and placental defects. HGF treatment of responsive cells activates a number of pathways via phosphorylation of the cytoplasmic domain of MET. The phosphorylated MET leads to cytoplasmic activation of the tyrosine kinase pp60 SRC, phospholipase Cγ, and MAP kinase. Using specific mutants, studies have demonstrated that coupling of the receptor to the Ras pathway is essential and sufficient for proliferation, whereas activation of PI3 kinase alone is sufficient to induce cellular motility. Concomitant activation of both Ras and PI3K is necessary and sufficient for HGF/MET-mediated invasion and metastasis.

Mutations in the MET protooncogene have been found, so far, in only a small proportion of sporadic papillary renal cell carcinomas (approximately 5%). Either the mutations in the MET protooncogene in sporadic papillary renal cell carcinoma have not yet been identified or the MET oncogene may play a role in the pathogenesis of only a small proportion of sporadic renal cell carcinomas. In sporadic papillary carcinoma, there may be somatic mutations in other genes on chromosome 7, perhaps the hepatocyte growth factor/scatter factor (the ligand for the MET protooncogene) or yet another receptor tyrosine kinase located on chromosome 7. Alternatively, sporadic papillary renal cell carcinoma may be associated with overexpression of the MET protein and its ligand, without mutation, associated with a trisomy of chromosome 7. Somatic (X;1)(p11;q21) translocations have been identified in a subset of papillary renal cell carcinoma, occasionally as a sole abnormality. This translocation results in a fusion of the transcription factor TFE3 on the X chromosome to a novel gene, designated PPRC on chromosome 1 (papillary renal cell carcinoma). Both of the reciprocal translocation products are expressed in papillary renal cell carcinomas. This translocation produces a papillary renal cell carcinoma with distinct clear cell features.

In summary, there are at least three gene products that predispose to the development of papillary renal cell carcinoma: the MET protooncogene on chromosome 7, TFE3 on the X chromosome, and PPRC on chromosome 1. Further studies are needed to determine the mutation frequency of MET, TFE3, and PPRC in sporadic cases of papillary renal cell carcinoma.

IV. PROGRESSION OF RENAL CELL CARCINOMA

In accord with multistep models of carcinogenesis, the progression of renal cell cancers is associated with an accumulation of multiple cytogenetic abnormalities. As previously discussed, angiogenic growth factors such as basic fibroblast growth factor and vascular endothelial cell growth factor are highly expressed in the clear cell variant of renal cell carcinomas. Elevated levels of the myc oncogene are found in a large proportion of sporadic renal cell cancers, but this finding does not appear to have prognostic significance. The p53 gene, located on chromosome 17p, is one of the most frequently altered genes in cancer. However, less than 10% of primary renal cell carcinomas contain mutations of the p53 gene, indicating that this gene plays a minor role in the progression of renal cell carcinoma. Analysis of the 9p21-22 and MTS1/cdkN2/p16 locus demonstrates loss of heterozygosity in 50% of primary renal cell carcinomas associated with metastases, but only 13% of primary renal cell carcinomas without metastases. Renal cell carcinomas with metastatic potential also express VLA-4 (very late antigen-4). VLA-4 expression increases the adhesion of renal cell carcinoma cells to endothelial cells *in vitro*. Loss of the retinoblastoma protein does not appear to contribute significantly to malignant transformation or progression of renal cell carcinoma. Overexpression of epidermal growth factor receptor and/or its ligand (TGF-α) has been observed in renal cell carcinoma. Overexpression of insulin-like growth factor receptors has also been reported.

V. SUMMARY AND CONCLUSIONS

A variety of histologically distinct carcinomas may arise from renal tubular epithelium, which have char-

acteristic cytogenetic alterations. Although the vast majority of renal cell carcinomas are sporadic, analysis of familial cancer syndromes has led to the identification of genes involved in the pathogenesis of both hereditary and sporadic renal cell carcinomas. In patients with VHL, the identification of specific mutations may provide important information regarding the risk for developing extrarenal tumors, pheochromocytoma in particular. Whereas the majority of patients with familial papillary renal cell carcinoma have gain-of-function mutations involving the MET oncogene, the specific abnormalities in patients with sporadic papillary renal cell carcinoma await clarification. Through further studies to define structure–function relationships between cytogenetic alterations and signaling pathways involved in renal carcinogenesis, it may be possible to identify potential targets for therapeutic intervention.

See Also the Following Articles

BLADDER CANCER: EPIDEMIOLOGY • LIVER CANCER: ETIOLOGY AND PREVENTION • PANCREATIC CANCER, CELLULAR AND MOLECULAR MECHANISMS • RENAL CELL CANCER • THYROID CANCER • TOBACCO CARCINOGENESIS

Bibliography

Bardelli, A., Pugliese, L., and Comoglio, P. (1997). "Invasive-growth" signaling by the *Met/HGF* receptor: The hereditary renal carcinoma connection. *Biochim. Biophys. Acta* **1333**, M41–M51.

Fleming, S. (1997). Genetics of renal tumors. *Cancer Metastasis Rev.* **16**, 127–140.

Iliopoulos, O., and Kaelin, W. (1997). The molecular basis of von Hippel–Lindau Disease. *Mol. Med.* **3**, 289–293.

Kaelin, W. J., and Maher, E. (1998). The VHL tumour-suppressor gene paradigm. *Trends Genet.* **14**, 423–426.

Kovacs, G., Akhtar, M., Beckwith, B., *et al.* (1997). The Heidelberg classification of renal cell tumours. *J. Pathol.* **183**, 131–133.

Latif, F., Tory, K., Gnarra, J., *et al.* (1993). Identification of the von Hippel-Lindau disease tumor suppressor gene. *Science* **260**, 1317–1320.

Maher, E., and Kaelin, W. (1997). von Hippel-Lindau disease. *Medicine* **76**, 381–391.

Neumann, H., and Zbar, B. (1997). Renal cysts, renal cancer and von Hippel-Lindau disease. *Kidney Int.* **51**, 16–26.

Richards, F., Webster, A., McMahon, R., Woodward, E., Rose, S., and Maher, E. (1998). Molecular genetic analysis of von Hippel-Lindau disease. *J. Intern. Med.* **243**, 527–533.

Zbar, B., and Lerman, M. (1998). Inherited carcinomas of the kidney. *Adv Cancer Res.* **75**, 163–201.

Kinase-Regulated Signal Transduction Pathways

Peter Blume-Jensen
Serono Reproductive Biology Institute

Tony Hunter
The Salk Institute

GLOSSARY

amplification The phenomenon that activation of one molecule in a signaling pathway leads to activation of several molecules at the next level within the pathway. Amplification is supposedly a common theme in kinase cascades (see "signaling cascade").

cross talk Mechanisms whereby activated signaling molecules in a primary signal transduction pathway can regulate signaling molecules in another primary signal transduction pathway.

feedback regulation Mechanisms by which activated signaling molecules can regulate upstream components within the same signal transduction pathway.

functional redundancy Indicates that certain molecules or signaling pathways have overlapping functions, such that they can (in part) substitute for each other.

growth factor A molecule, in most cases a polypeptide, that binds specifically to a cell membrane receptor, thereby regulating cell growth and differentiation.

kinase An enzyme that catalyzes phosphorylation of a protein, lipid, or carbohydrate. A majority of protein kinases are specific for either tyrosine residues or for serine/threonine residues.

oncogene A gene whose protein product can cause malignant transformation.

phosphatase An enzyme that catalyzes dephosphorylation of a protein, lipid, or carbohydrate. A majority of protein phosphatases are specific for either phosphotyrosine residues or for phosphoserine/phosphothreonine residues.

protooncogene The normal cellular counterpart of an oncogene. Protooncogenes can become oncogenes upon structural alterations.

receptor protein tyrosine kinase A subgroup of tyrosine-specific protein kinases that is composed of transmembrane receptors for growth factors and have intrinsic, ligand-stimulatable tyrosine kinase activity in their cytoplasmic parts.

signaling cascade A signal transduction pathway where activation of one molecule, often a protein kinase, is linked to the activation of, often several, molecules immediately downstream in the pathway. Consequently, amplification is part of the signaling mechanism (see "amplification").

signal transduction Molecular events that take place in response to extracellular biological stimuli to elicit specific cellular responses.

The cells in growing and adult multicellular organisms respond to a plethora of extracellular stimuli that initiate a number of biochemical signal transduction pathways within the cells. Signal transduction is the intracellular molecular events that convey extracellular stimuli into specific cellular responses. Thus, at each given moment within a multicellular organism, multiple signaling pathways are active inside a single cell. It has become clear that two intracellular enzymes, phosphoinositide 3'-kinase (PI 3'-K) and the mammalian target of rapamycin (mTOR), are central for orchestrating and regulating numerous protein kinase signaling pathways that mediate cell survival, growth, proliferation, protein synthesis, and metabolism.

Cell growth (increase in cell mass), cell proliferation (increase in cell number), and cell survival are distinct processes, but yet coupled through the combined actions of both PI 3'-K and mTOR. PI 3'-K is a dual-specificity protein serine/threonine (S/T) and lipid kinase, whereas mTOR exhibits only protein S/T kinase activity, despite the presence of a C-terminal PI kinase (PIK) homology domain in mTOR. While PI 3'-K and one of the major targets for mTOR, the p70 ribosomal S6 kinase, are activated by almost all known growth factors that stimulate receptor protein tyrosine kinases (RPTKs), the upstream regulation of mTOR itself is more unclear. It was recently shown that phosphatidic acid directly binds, and partially activates, mTOR. This provides a direct link between growth factor stimulation of cells and subsequent activation of mTOR through formation of phosphatidic acid. Mutations of several proteins within the PI 3'-K- and mTOR-regulated signaling pathways, causing deregulated activity of these pathways, have been identified in humans. Such mutations result in perturbed cell growth and ultimately malignant cell transformation and cancer. This shows the importance of tight and proper regulation of PI 3'-K and mTOR signaling pathways, including negative

mechanisms to prevent hyperactivity of each of these pathways. Such regulation is achieved by several means. Thus, the amplitude and duration of the activated signaling pathways need to be carefully balanced and coordinated. This coordination occurs by biochemical interactions between signaling molecules in the different primary signal transduction pathways. By means of reversible protein phosphorylation, the pathways can monitor and regulate each other by cross talk, branching and feedback regulation. It is clear that the regulatory interactions between the same two signaling pathways will differ in different cell types, depending on the expression pattern of intracellular proteins that mediate the cross talk and regulation. This also constitutes the basis for cell-type specificity in the responses elicited by one and the same pathway, and why deregulation of specific signaling molecules only gives rise to cancer in selected tissues. This article describes the PI 3'-K- and mTOR/ribosomal S6 kinase-regulated signaling pathways and what is known about their regulation.

I. INTRODUCTION

In response to extracellular stimuli, intracellular signaling molecules become modified and organize into signaling pathways by means of specific protein–protein interactions. The mechanisms regulating these protein–protein interactions have been described elsewhere and include reversible protein phosphorylation, modular interactions, and binding proteins regulating subcellular localization and compartmentalization. One of the most well-studied intracellular signaling molecules is PI 3'-K, which is activated in response to almost all extracellular stimuli. It was known for a long time that agonist-stimulated PI 3'-Ks phosphorylate the 3'-OH position of the inositol ring in inositol phospholipids, generating 3'-phosphoinositides, and that the 3'-PIs mediate many of the cellular effects of PI 3'-K signals, but the mechanim(s) remained elusive until recently. Identification of the pleckstrin homology (PH) domain as a specialized lipid-binding domain provided a breakthrough in understanding the mechanisms by which 3'-PIs convey PI 3'-K signals to the cytosol. It also led to the identification of several PH domain-containing targets for PI 3'-K, including the protein S/T kinase

3′-phosphoinositide dependent kinase-1 (PDK-1) and protein kinase B (PKB), also known as Akt, itself a substrate for PDK-1. Many of the effects mediated by PI 3′-K downstream of the insulin and insulin-like growth factor-1 (IGF-1) receptors include changes in glucose metabolism, protein synthesis, and cell growth. These effects overlap with those mediated by the protein S/T kinase "mammalian target of rapamycin" (mTOR; also known as FRAP or RAFT) and its targets, including the protein S/T kinase ribosomal S6 kinase. Accordingly, several mTOR targets depend on PI 3′-K for full activation. This link between PI 3′-K signaling and mTOR/ribosomal S6-kinase signaling is in part explained by the finding that p70 ribosomal S6-kinase serves as a substrate for PDK-1, which phosphorylates a threonine residue in the activation loop of S6-kinase, whereas mTOR is a direct substrate for Akt. It has since turned out that PDK-1 phosphorylates numerous members of the so-called AGC protein kinase family, which includes protein kinase A (PKA), PKG, and PKC, on a homologous conserved site in the activation loop of these kinases. However, only a subset of these are physiological substrates (see later). The regulation of these and other proteins by phosphorylation enables interaction between components within and between the PI 3′-K and mTOR pathways as well as with other signal transduction pathways. Some of the known cross talk between these different signal pathways will be discussed throughout the text. Feedback and cross talk regulation are clearly important means to balance all simultaneously active signaling pathways within a cell.

II. PHOSPHOINOSITIDE 3′-KINASE SIGNALING

There are multiple mammalian isoforms of PI 3′-Ks that fall into three classes: I, II, and III. The catalytic subunits of all PI 3′-Ks share a conserved region that consists of an N-terminal PI kinase homology domain of unknown function followed by the core part of the catalytic domain, which is structurally related to catalytic domains of members in the protein kinase superfamily. However, the main defining feature of PI 3′-Ks is their ability to phosphorylate the 3′-OH position of the inositol ring in inositol phospholipids

(Fig. 1). Such lipids consist of a diacylglycerol with an inositol-1′-phosphate group attached at position 3 of the glycerol backbone. If the inositol ring contains no additional phosphate groups, this phospholipid is called phosphatidylinositol (PtdIns). In cells, all the inositol OH groups, except for those at positions 2 and 6, can become phosphorylated singly or in combination. Such phosphorylated PtdIns derivatives are called phosphoinositides (PIs). Several class I and III, but not II, PI 3′-K members are dual-specificity kinases and also possess protein serine/threonine kinase activity *in vitro* (see later). Class I PI 3′-Ks are heterodimers made up of a ~110-kDa catalytic subunit (p110) and an adaptor/regulatory subunit. This class, which is further discussed later, is subdivided into the RPTK-activated subclass IA and the heterotrimeric G protein-coupled receptor-activated subclass IB of PI 3′-Ks. Class II PI 3′-Ks are ≥170-kDa molecules with a phospholipid-binding C2 domain in their C terminus. Their substrate preference *in vitro* is different from that of classes I and III, they preferentially phosphorylate PtdIns over PtdIns(4)P, which again is preferred over PtdIns(4,5)P_2. Several growth factors, including insulin, platelet-derived growth factor (PDGF), and epidermal growth factor (EGF), activate class II PI 3′-Ks through as yet an unknown mechanism(s). Class III PI 3′-Ks are the mammalian homologues of the yeast vesicular protein-sorting protein Vps34p. They can only use PtdIns as a substrate and probably generate the majority of cellular PtdIns(3)P in cells. This is the most abundant PI in mammalian cells, and its levels remain rather constant, indicating that class III PI 3′-Ks are not acutely activated by cellular stimulation. They are probably important for intracellular vesicular transport and membrane trafficking.

A. Phosphoinositide 3′-Kinase: Structure and Function

Although class I PI 3′-Ks can utilize PtdIns, PtdIns(4)P, and PtdIns(4,5)P_2 as substrates *in vitro*, their preferred substrate in the intact cell appears to be PtdIns(4,5)P_2. The resulting PtdIns(3,4,5)P_3 then acts as a substrate for the slightly delayed generation of PtdIns(3,4)P_2 through the action of 5′-inositol lipid phosphatases. Accordingly, the usually very low intracellular levels of PtdIns(3,4,5)P_3 and

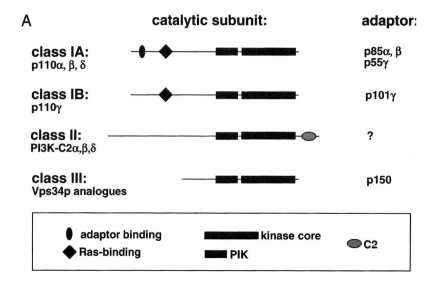

A   **catalytic subunit:**   **adaptor:**

class IA:
p110α, β, δ   p85α, β
p55γ

class IB:
p110γ   p101γ

class II:
PI3K-C2α,β,δ   ?

class III:
Vps34p analogues   p150

| ● adaptor binding | ▬▬▬ kinase core | ● C2 |
| ◆ Ras-binding | ▬ PIK | |

B

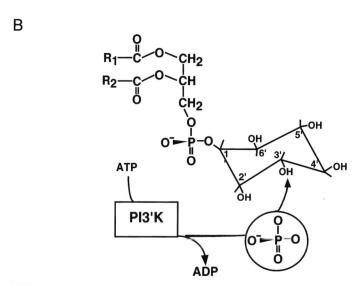

FIGURE 1 PI 3′-kinase structure and function. (A) Structure of the catalytic subunits from class IA, IB, II, and III PI 3′-Ks. (B) All PI 3′-Ks phosphorylate the 3′-OH group of the inositol ring in inositol phospholipids. See text for details.

PtdIns(3,4)P$_2$ rise several fold within seconds after agonist stimulation in a biphasic manner. All mammalian class I PI 3′-Ks, and the formation of PtdIns(3,4,5)P$_3$ and PtdIns(3,4)P$_2$, can be inhibited both *in vitro* and in the intact cell by each of two unrelated, small molecule compounds: wortmannin (IC$_{50}$ *in vitro* ≈5 nM) and LY294002 (IC$_{50}$ *in vitro* ≈1 μM).

Several members of the class IA PI 3′-Ks have been identified in mammals. The three isoforms of the p110

catalytic subunit, p110α, β, and δ, are each encoded by a distinct gene. They have a similar overall structure, consisting of, most N-terminally, an adaptor-binding domain followed by a Ras-binding domain in front of the PIK and catalytic domains. Seven adaptor proteins have been identified so far, and they are generated by expression and alternative splicing of three different genes: p85α, p85β, and p55γ. From the N toward the C terminus, p85α and β contain an SH3 domain, a region with homology to the C terminus of Bcr, and two SH2 domains. The C terminus of Bcr has GAP activity toward p21rac, but such Rho-GAP activity has not been demonstrated for p85. In the N terminus are also two proline-rich regions, each of which binds to SH3 domains in Src family kinases. This leads to PI 3'-kinase activation. The inter-SH2 domain contains the binding site for p110, which is bound via its N terminus. The p55γ subunit contains a unique N terminus, a proline-rich region, and two SH2 domains, but no SH3 or Rho-GAP domain.

Almost all ligand-stimulated RPTKs directly bind and activate PI 3'-K, with noticeable exceptions, including the EGF and ErbB2 receptors. However, these receptors induce activation indirectly, through heterodimerization with ErbB3, which bind PI 3'-K upon tyrosine phosphorylation by its kinase-active receptor partners. The two SH2 domains of p85 and p55 mediate the binding of PI 3'-kinase to RPTKs through the consensus recognition motif Y-M/V-X-M, where Y is phosphorylated. However, there are exceptions to this, for instance the activated Met/hepatocyte growth factor receptor binds to p85 through a distinct motif. *In vitro*, the C-terminal SH2 domain is responsible for the high-affinity interaction with several RPTKs. The binding has two functions: it translocates PI 3'-kinase to the membrane in close proximity to its substrates and it leads to a conformational change in p85, which is transferred to the catalytic domain, leading to PI 3'-kinase activation. p85 is tyrosine phosphorylated upon binding to some RPTKs. Tyrosine phosphorylation of p85 might be involved in the allosteric activation of PI 3'-kinase; simultaneous binding of GTP-bound Ras to the p110 catalytic subunit is involved in the activation of PI 3'-K (Fig. 2). As mentioned earlier, class IA PI 3'-Ks also exhibit protein serine/threonine kinase activity. Hence, the p85/p110 heterodimer is negatively regulated by p110-mediated serine phosphorylation of serine 608 in the inter SH2 domain of p85 *in vitro*. In addition, p110δ is phosphorylated in intact cells upon stimulation in a PI 3'-K-dependent manner. IRS-1 is another potential substrate for p110 serine kinase activity. However, both wortmannin and rapamycin, inhibitors of PI 3'-kinase and mTOR, respectively, can prevent insulin-stimulated serine phosphorylation of IRS-1 *in vivo*, and mTOR, p70 ribosomal S6 kinase, and PKCζ have

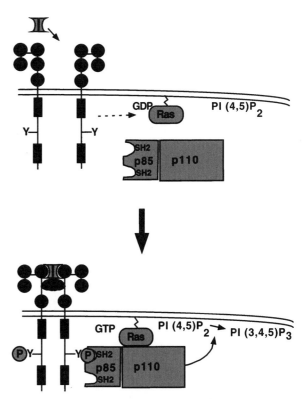

FIGURE 2 Schematic illustration of receptor protein tyrosine kinase-initiated activation of class IA PI 3'-Ks as described in the text. Growth factor stimulation leads to receptor dimerization and kinase activation, resulting in tyrosine autophosphorylation. Specific phosphorylated tyrosine residues in the activated RPTK recruit and bind the SH2 domains of the p85 and/or p55 adaptor subunit of PI 3'-K. This results in allosteric transactivation of the catalytic p110 subunit, resulting in the production of PtdIns(3,4)P_2 and PtdIns(3,4,5)P_3. Note that Ras•GTP in the membrane might cooperate in activating p110 by binding to its N terminus.

all been reported to phosphorylate IRS-1 as well. Finally, TNF-α treatment and chronic hyperinsulinemia associated with insulin resistance result in increased serine/threonine phosphorylation and decreased tyrosine phosphorylation of IRS-1 and IRS-2, and decreased insulin receptor association. Consistently in all these cases, serine phosphorylation of IRS-1 is involved in the negative regulation of insulin receptor signaling and correlates with the degradation of IRS-1 by the proteasome.

The normal physiological roles of PI 3'-K are numerous and cell type specific. It is clearly involved in RPTK-induced processes, including cell migration, proliferation, cell survival, and insulin-induced glucose metabolism and protein synthesis. The effects of

PIs in cells are mediated through the specific binding to at least two lipid-binding protein domains: the FYVE and pleckstrin homology (PH) domain. FYVE domains bind selectively to PtdIns(3)P, whereas a subgroup of PH domains bind PtdIns(3,4)P$_2$ and PtdIns(3,4,5)P$_3$. Accordingly, the latter group of proteins is important in mediating the effects of class IA PI 3'-Ks. PI-binding PH domains are found in a variety of proteins, including certain AGC protein kinases, discussed in more detail later, the Tec family of tyrosine kinases, including Bruton's tyrosine kinase (Btk), phospholipase C- (PLC-) γ2, GTP/GDP exchange factors (GEFs) for Rac and ARF GTPases, and, finally, GTPase-activating proteins (GAPs). For instance, the cytoplasmic tyrosine kinase Btk is required for normal B-cell development and function. Accordingly, germline mutations in Btk cause immunodeficiency, and several of these mutations have been found to reside in the PH domain of Btk. These mutations prevent PtdIns(3,4,5)P$_3$ binding, and subsequent Btk membrane translocation. This interferes with the activation of Btk, which depends on Tyr and Ser phosphorylation at the membrane, most likely by Src family and PDK-1-like protein kinases, respectively. In addition, it interferes with the proper activation of PLC-γ2, which is also recruited to the membrane by PtdIns(3,4,5)P$_3$ binding to its PH domain, and is a supposed substrate for Btk. The relevance of this is reflected in the phenotype of mice with targeted disruptions of the first exon of the p85α gene, causing disappearance of p85α and p55αi, whereas p55α and p50α are still expressed. These mice develop a B-cell immunodeficiency, reminiscent of the immunodeficiency seen in patients with mutations in the PH domain of Btk.

Binding of PtdIns(3,4,5)P$_3$ to Rho family GEFs seems important for mediating RPTK-induced membrane ruffling and chemotaxis. These motility responses depend on Rac, and there is an increased level of Rac•GTP in response to RPTK-induced PI 3'-K activation. This might be mediated in part through the 3'-PI-stimulated activation of Vav, a GEF for Rac, through binding to the PH domain of Vav. GEFs for the ARF family of small GTPases are translocated to the membrane in response to PI 3'-K activation and, again, this is stimulated by the binding of PtdIns(3,4,5)P$_3$ to their PH domain. They stimulate active ARF•GTP formation. Activated ARFs play a role in vesicular membrane trafficking and induce the docking of vesicle coat proteins. The role of 3'-PI binding to PH domains of GAPs is less clear.

Deregulated PI 3'-K activity is involved in malignant cell transformation as well. Originally, PI 3'-kinase activity was observed as an enzymatic activity associated with middle T antigen, the transforming protein of polyomavirus. In addition to polyoma middle T, PI 3'-kinase also associates with numerous other retroviral oncogene products, and it was long known that there is a strong correlation between their transforming activity and the ability to bind PI 3'-kinase and increase the level of 3'-PIs in the cell. Based on a wealth of recent *in vitro* and *in vivo* studies, it has become clear that most, if not all, cases of deregulated PI 3'-K activity cause tumorigenesis through deregulated PDK-1 and Akt activity. However, the deregulated activity of other downstream targets is likely to be involved secondarily in the pathogenesis as well.

B. Phosphoinositide-Dependent Kinase-1 (PDK-1) and Protein Kinase B/Akt

As mentioned, most of the effects of class I PI 3'-K are thought to be mediated by the binding of the resulting lipids, PtdIns(3,4,5)P$_3$ and PtdIns(3,4)P$_2$, to specific pleckstrin homology (PH) domains contained in numerous intracellular signaling proteins. PH domains are independently folded protein modules of ~100 amino acids, some of which bind phospholipids with high affinity. A subset of PH domains preferentially bind the PIs PtdIns(3,4,5)P$_3$ and PtdIns(3,4)P$_2$. The binding motif, which resides in the N terminus of PH domains, is K-X(7-13)-R/K-X-R, where X is any amino acid. The inositol phosphate groups interact with the basic amino acid residues in this motif, and PtdIns(3,4,5)P$_3$ in general binds with higher affinity than PtdIns(3,4)P$_2$. Two PH domain-containing signaling molecules, the protein serine/threonine kinases 3'-phosphoinositide-dependent kinase-1 (PDK-1) and protein kinase B (PKB)/Akt, are central mediators of class I PI 3'-K signaling.

PKB/Akt was originally identified as the cellular homologue of the transforming viral oncogene product v-Akt. The name PKB refers to its high homology with PKA and PKC. Three mammalian isoforms have been identified—PKBα, PKBβ, and PKBγ—each encoded by a separate gene. All three isoforms are widely expressed, but the α isoform is the most studied. All PKBs are ~56-kDa molecules consisting of an N-terminal PH domain, a central kinase domain, and a C-terminal regulatory tail with a hydrophobic motif containing a conserved, regulatory serine phosphorylation site (Fig. 3). Its PH domain binds preferentially PtdIns(3,4,5)P$_3$ over PtdIns(3,4)P$_2$. PKB/Akt is mainly cytosolic in unstimulated cells, while it is translocated to the membrane to become activated upon PI 3'-K stimulation. Some of the activated Akt molecules subsequently translocate to the nucleus where several of its substrates are located.

PDK-1 was identified as a Thr308-PKB-kinase, which phosphorylates Akt in a 3'-PI-dependent manner, reflected in its name. So far, only one mammalian isoform has been identified. It is a ~63-kDa, ubiquitously expressed serine/threonine kinase consisting of an N-terminal kinase domain and a C-terminal PH domain (Fig. 3). The PH domain in PDK-1 binds the same phospholipids as the PH domain in Akt, but with ~10-fold higher affinity. A significant fraction of PDK-1 is bound to the plasma membrane even in unstimulated cells, which might be explained by the ability of its PH domain to also bind PtdIns(4,5)P$_2$,

at least *in vitro*. Accordingly, a PH domain-deleted version of PDK-1 is unable to associate with the cell membrane. PDK-1 was originally suggested to exist in a constitutively active, phosphorylated state under basal conditions, refractive to further stimulation. This viewpoint has been challenged by a report suggesting that a C-terminal region of PKC-related kinase 2 (PRK2) can interact with, and allosterically regulate, PDK-1 so that it can undergo a three- to fivefold increased activity in response to binding of PtdIns(3,4,5)P$_3$. However, the physiological relevance of these findings remains to be proven. PDK-1 is excluded from the nucleus of both resting and stimulated cells.

C. Activation of PDK-1 and Akt

Numerous *in vitro* studies have addressed the mechanism of activation of Akt, and these have for the most part been supported by studies in cells and tissues. This has led to the following model for activation, where amino acid numbering in Akt refers to the α isoform: Activation of class IA and IB PI 3'-Ks by RPTKs and serpentine family G protein-coupled receptors, respectively, leads to the formation of PtdIns(3,4,5)P$_3$ and PtdIns(3,4)P$_2$ at the plasma

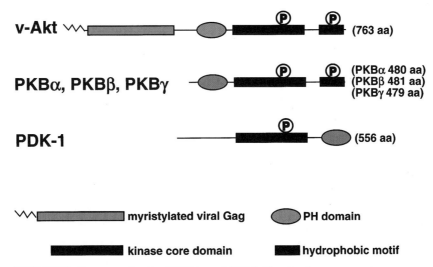

FIGURE 3 Structures of v-Akt, PKB/Akt, and PDK-1. Phosphorylation sites in the activation loop of the kinase core domains and in the hydrophobic motifs are illustrated by P in a circle. Numbers in parentheses after the structures indicate their size in amino acids (aa) for the human sequence. Figure not drawn to scale.

membrane. PKB interacts through its PH domain with these phospholipids, causing its translocation to the inner leaflet of the membrane, where PI-bound, constitutively active PDK-1 is prelocated. The interaction of the Akt PH domain with 3′ PIs causes a conformational change of Akt, exposing its two phosphorylation sites: Thr308 in the activation loop of the kinase domain and Ser476 in the hydrophobic C-terminal motif. Phosphorylation of both these sites is required for the full activation of PKB. While it is clear that the Thr308 kinase is PDK-1, it has been postulated that an as yet unidentified serine/threonine kinase PDK-2 phosphorylates Ser476. An alternative model suggests that Ser476 is an Akt autophosphorylation site. Accordingly, studies using PDK-1 −/− embryonic stem cells have established that PDK-1 is required for the activation of PKB, p70 ribosomal S6 kinase (see later), and p90RSK, and also that protein kinases other than PDK-1 can mediate phosphorylation of the hydrophobic motif Ser476 in Akt. The true identity of the Ser476-Akt kinase awaits further studies. It is likely in this activation model that the proximity of Akt and PDK-1 is in part mediated by dimerization between their PI-bound PH domains. As mentioned, PDK-1 might be constitutively active and able to induce phosphorylation of Akt once Akt is recruited to the vicinity of PDK-1 in the membrane.

D. Downstream of PDK-1: AGC Superfamily Protein Kinase Signaling Pathways

Thr308 and Ser476 in PKBα are surrounded by amino acid sequences conserved in other AGC serine/threonine protein kinase family members. These include PKA, PKG, and PKC isoforms, the original AGC family members, as well as p70 ribosomal S6 kinases, serum- and glucocorticoid-induced protein kinases (SGKs), mitogen- and stress-activated protein kinases (MSKs), the Rac effector p21-activated protein kinase (PAK), and the PKC-related kinase 2 (PRK2). The Thr308 equivalent in these kinases lies in a region of the kinase domain between subdomains VII and VIII, known as the activation loop or T loop. The consensus motif is T/S-F/L-C-G-T-X-X-Y-X-A-P-E/D, where T/S indicates the phosphorylated T or

S residue and X is any amino acid. Phosphorylation of this site is a prerequisite for kinase activation, and PDK-1 is centrally involved in activating many AGC kinase members. PDK-1 has been shown to phosphorylate the equivalent residue to Thr308 in PKC isoforms, SGK isoforms, and PKA. Results obtained using PDK-1-/- embryonic stem cells suggest that only a subset of AGC kinases, including Akt, the p70 isoform of ribosomal S6 kinase, and the protein S/T kinase Rsk, are physiological substrates of PDK-1. In contrast, PDK-1 is not required for the phosphorylation of PKA, the mitogen- and stress-activated protein kinase 1 (MSK1), and the AMP-activated protein kinase (AMPK). PDK-1, which is itself an AGC kinase, also requires phosphorylation of its Thr308 equivalent, Ser241, to become activated, which occurs by autophosphorylation.

The hydrophobic consensus motif in AGC kinases is F-X-X-F/Y-S/T-Y/F, where S or T is the phosphorylated residue and X is any amino acid. It is possible that PDK-1 might phosphorylate the equivalent residue in the hydrophobic motif of p70 ribosomal S6 kinase. This is supported by findings showing that kinase-negative mutants of PKB and p70 S6 kinase are still phosphorylated at this residue in intact cells in response to agonists that activate PI 3′-K and by the lack of IGF-1-induced phosphorylation at this p70 S6 kinase site in PDK-1 -/- cells. In PKC members, the equivalent site seems to be autophosphorylated, and kinase-inactive PKC mutants are not phosphorylated at the hydrophobic motif when transfected into cells. So far, most evidence indicates that the activity of PDK-1 is not directly regulated. Rather, it has been suggested that PDK-1 has constitutive kinase activity and is able to phosphorylate many of its substrates upon agonist-induced conformational changes in these. For instance, PKB is converted into an efficient PDK-1 substrate upon binding of PtdIns(3,4,5)P$_3$ to its PH domain, and many PKC members become converted into PDK-1 substrates upon binding of phorbol esters, diacylglycerol, phosphatidylserine, phosphatidylcholine, or PtdIns(3,4,5) P3 to their regulatory domain. P70 ribosomal S6 kinase and SGK seem to become converted into PDK-1 substrates upon their phosphorylation at the hydrophobic motif (see later), and PRK1 and PRK2 are converted into PDK-1 substrates upon their binding to Rho•GTP. In all cases the regulated event seems to be the induced conformational change of the PDK-1 substrate. In some cases, these conformational changes may allow direct binding to PDK-1.

E. Downstream of Akt: Cell Survival, Proliferation, Protein Synthesis, and Oncogenesis

At least 12 PKB/Akt substrates have been identified in mammalian cells to date. The majority fall into two major classes: proteins that are mainly involved in mediating cell survival through suppression of apoptosis and proteins mainly involved in mediating (IGF and insulin-induced) cellular metabolic functions, including protein synthesis and glycogen metabolism, respectively. Through a wealth of in vitro phosphorylation studies, an optimal, minimal sequence motif for phosphorylation by PKB has been identified: R-X-R-X-X-S/T, where S or T is the phosphorylated residue, and the immediate C-terminal residue to the phosphorylation site tends to be a bulky hydrophobic residue, like Phe or Leu. In all the identified substrates, this is the motif phosphorylated by Akt in intact cells. However, similar sequences with an Arg at position −3 and −5 of a Ser are also consensus motifs for p70 S6 kinase and MAPKAP kinase-1, and so phosphorylation of a consensus motif for Akt in vitro does not necessarily mean that it is a substrate for Akt in vivo. A good example is provided by 6-phosphofructo-2-kinase (PFK-2), which is phosphorylated at two Ser residues within Akt consensus motifs in vitro, and was originally suggested to be an Akt substrate in vivo. Based on the use of dominant-negative constructs, it turns out that phosphorylation at these two sites in vivo is dependent on PDK-1, but not Akt, and is most likely mediated by a PDK-1-regulated kinase other than Akt. In most cases, identification of physiological Akt substrates has been achieved using PI 3′-K inhibitors, dominant-negative versions of Akt or overexpression of Akt, and mapping of the phosphorylation sites by mutagenesis studies and using phospho-specific antibodies. The substrates involved in cell death regulation include Forkhead (FH) transcription factors, the proapoptotic Bcl-2 family member Bad, and the cyclic AMP response element-binding protein (CREB), and,

although unclear at the moment, possibly human caspase-9 and IκB kinase. PKB substrates involved in mediating protein and glycogen synthesis, in particular in response to insulin and IGF-1, include glycogen synthase kinase-3 (GSK-3), phosphodiesterase-3B, the mammalian target of rapamycin (mTOR), insulin receptor substrate-1 (IRS-1), and the FH transcription factor member FKHR. Finally, phosphorylation of the substrates Raf-1, endothelial nitric oxide synthase (eNOS), and breast cancer susceptibility gene 1 (BRCA-1) regulate diverse aspects of cell proliferation, angiogenesis, and transcription and DNA repair, respectively. For an illustration of the main PDK-1 and Akt targets, see Fig. 4.

A lot of attention has been paid to the role of Akt/PKB in promoting cell survival. This activity has been suggested as the main tumorigenic mechanism for deregulated Akt activity. PKB phosphorylation of molecules involved in cell death regulation prevents their death function (Bad and caspase-9), prevents transcription of pro-apoptotic genes, such as FAS ligand (FH transcription factors), or promotes the transcription of antiapoptotic genes (CREB and IκB kinase). PKBα is overexpressed in pancreatic and ovarian carcinomas. In addition, numerous human malignancies, including breast cancer, glioblastoma, and germ cell tumors, are associated with inactivating mutations in a tumor suppressor gene called PTEN, leading to a deregulated hyperactivity of Akt. PTEN is a 3′-PI phosphatase, which dephosphorylates the 3′-OH position of the inositol ring in PtdIns(3,4,5)P$_3$ and PtdIns(3,4)P$_2$. Consequently, PTEN inactivation leads to increased levels of 3′-PIs, causing enhanced Akt activity and cellular transformation. PKB also activates the transcription factor E2F and upregulates cyclin D1 levels, which might cause cell cycle progression and be part of the transforming mechanism of deregulated Akt activity.

The role of Akt in phosphorylating and inactivating Bad is very well established. Activated Akt phosphorylates Bad directly in vitro and in vivo on Ser136, leading to its dissociation from the antiapoptotic protein Bcl-X$_L$, and its subsequent sequestration and inactivation in the cytosol by binding to 14-3-3 proteins. An additional site, Ser155, is phosphorylated by PKA and seems important for completely abolishing the proapoptotic function of Bad. However, the

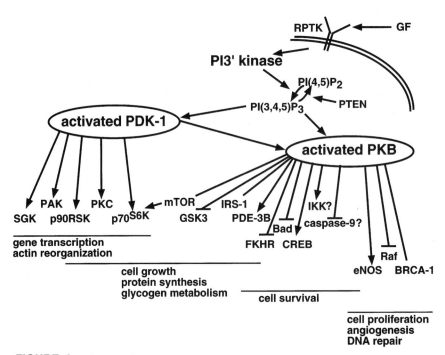

FIGURE 4 Schematic illustration of PDK-1- and PKB/Akt-regulated signaling pathways. GF, growth factor; RPTK, receptor protein tyrosine kinase; PDE-3B, phosphodiesterase-3B. For other abbreviations, see text. Arrows indicate a stimulatory effect, a solid line with a bar indicates an inhibitory effect, whereas a solid line indicates that the effect of the phosphorylation is currently unknown. See text for further details.

tissue expression of Bad is very limited, and so it is unclear whether this is a general mechanism for apoptosis suppression. Phosphorylation of human caspase-9 by Akt, an initiator protease in the proteolytic cascade involved in promoting apoptosis, causes its inhibition. However, this mechanism for Akt-mediated cell survival is not evolutionary conserved, as the inactivating phosphorylation site in human caspase-9 is not conserved in mouse, rat, and monkey caspase-9. Because PKB, in addition, seems to promote cell survival by intervening with the apoptotic cascade before the step of cytochrome c release, this is probably not a major antiapoptotic mechanism even in humans. The FH transcription factors, FKHR, FKHRL1, and AFX, are more likely to be important antiapoptotic targets for Akt. Activated Akt is thought to dissociate from the membrane and translocate to the nucleus, causing the phosphorylation of nuclear targets. Among these are the FH transcription factors, which are directly phosphorylated on three residues by PKB. This inhibits their transcriptional activity and promotes their export to the cy-

tosol, where binding to the scaffold protein 14-3-3 sequesters the phosphorylated transcription factors. This prevents expression of FAS ligand, among others, a proapoptotic molecule that acts through paracrine or autocrine stimulation in many tissues. Another nuclear target for Akt is the transcription factor CREB, which is phosphorylated at a single Ser residue. Phosphorylation at this residue, Ser133, leads to recruitment of the transcriptional cofactor, CREB-binding protein (CBP), and Akt/PKB-stimulated target gene expression via CREB is dependent on phosphorylation at this site. Among target genes for CREB is the antiapoptotic Bcl-2 family member mcl-1, which is upregulated in response to several growth factors and cytokines. This occurs through binding of the CREB–CBP complex to a CRE-2 promoter site in the mcl-1 gene. The role of Akt-mediated phosphorylated of IκB kinase (IKK), finally, is controversial. Activated Akt/PKB has been reported to associate with and phoshorylate IKKα, causing its activation and subsequent phosphorylation of IκB. This leads to IκB degradation through the proteasome and allows

NF-κB to translocate to the nucleus where it activates transcription of the inhibitor of apoptosis (IAP) genes, c-IAP1 and c-IAP2. However, the predicted phosphorylation site in IκBα kinase does not lie within an optimal consensus sequence for PKB and, importantly, there is no evidence for its phosphorylation in intact cells in response to PI 3'-K activation. Finally, *in vivo* only IKKβ, not IKKα, is required for TNF-α-induced IκB degradation by the proteasome. In conclusion, the role of IKK in Akt-promoted cell survival is doubtful.

PI 3'-K inhibitors prevent most insulin- and IGF-1-induced cellular effects, including cell growth, protein and glycogen synthesis, among others, and it is thought that PKB mediates most of these effects of insulin. The first described substrate for Akt, GSK-3, is inhibited by PKB phosphorylation. This prevents its inhibition of glycogen synthase, resulting in stimulated glycogen synthesis. Phosphorylation of GSK-3 by Akt also abolishes phosphorylation of the cytoplasmic signaling molecule β-catenin. This results in stabilization of β-catenin, which translocates to the nucleus and associates with T-cell factor/lymphocyte enhancer-binding factor-1 (TCF/LEF-1) to form an activated transcription factor. The β-catenin–TCF/LEF-1 complex induces the transcription of several genes, including cyclin D1. Cyclin D1, which is important for the progression in G1 of the cell cycle, is also stabilized as a result of the Akt-induced inhibition of GSK-3, as this results in decreased phosphorylation at a GSK-3 site in cyclin D1, which promotes cyclin D1 proteolytic turnover. Finally, phosphorylation of GSK-3 by Akt also prevents its inhibitory effect on the GTP/GDP exchange factor elongation initiation factor 2B (eIF2B), which is involved in eIF2-directed methionyl-tRNA binding to the 40S ribosome. Phosphorylation of the Akt substrate phosphodiesterase-3B results in enhanced cAMP production, involved in the activation of PKA. The effect of mTOR phosphorylation by PKB is unclear. It was originally suggested that this causes activation of the mTOR targets p70 ribosomal S6 kinase and 4E-BP1, both of which are involved in protein synthesis regulation (see later). However, later studies showed that mutation of the Akt phosphorylation site in mTOR has no effect.

Finally, the roles of phosphorylation of Raf, eNOS, and BRCA-1 by Akt are still being explored. It has been suggested that phosphorylation of Ser259 in Raf-1, a serine/threonine protein kinase in the Ras-MAPK cascade, by Akt causes its sequestration and inactivation by 14-3-3. This might inhibit the Ras-Raf-MAPK cascade under some conditions, depending on the differentiation stage of the cells, and allow PI 3'-K to exert a survival function, e.g., in differentiated skeletal muscle myotubes, without concomitant ERK-induced cell proliferation. In response to VEGF or shear stress of endothelial capillary cells, PKB becomes activated and phosphorylate eNOS, which is expressed in the local endothelial cells. This causes its activation, leading to NO production by the endothelial cells. NO is important for angiogenesis and gene regulation so it has been suggested that PKB-mediated NO production might be a mechanism by which tumor-produced VEGF stimulates tumor angiogenesis. Phosphorylation of BRCA-1 by Akt, finally, might cause exclusion of BRCA-1 from the nucleus and prevent its DNA repair and transcriptional functions of importance for its tumor suppressive role(s). Another possibility is that phosphorylation by Akt promotes BRCA-1 degradation.

III. mTOR AND RIBOSOMAL S6 KINASE SIGNALING

The p70 ribosomal S6 kinase and its upstream regulator mammalian target of rapamycin (mTOR) were for a long time known to be activated in a PI 3'-K-dependent fashion. The identification of PDK-1 as a kinase that phosphorylates p70 ribosomal S6 kinase and of Akt as a kinase that phosphorylates mTOR for the first time revealed a biochemical link between PI 3'-K, mTOR/ribosomal S6 kinases, and cell growth. Cell growth, defined as increase in cell mass, is controlled by mTOR and ribosomal S6 kinase in a variety of ways.

A. mTOR (Target of Rapamycin): Structure and Regulation

The protein encoded by the mammalian TOR gene belongs to an evolutionary conserved family of proteins, including TOR1, TOR2, MEC1, TEL1 and

RAD3 in budding yeast, MEI-41 in *Drosphila* and DNA-dependent protein kinase (DNA-PK), ataxia-telangiectasia-mutated (ATM), ATM-related (ATR), transformation/transcription domain-associated protein (TRRAP), and mTOR in mammals. mTOR is also called FK506-binding protein (FKBP)-rapamycin-associated protein (FRAP) in humans, and rapamycin and FKBP12 target-1 (RAFT-1) in rats, based on the ability of the FKBP–rapamycin complex to bind and inhibit mTOR. Proteins in the mTOR family belong to the class IV PI 3′-K-related kinases based on the presence of a C-terminal kinase domain with homology to the kinase core domain of PI 3′-Ks and PI 4-Ks. However, all evidence indicates that these so-called PI kinase (PIK-)-related proteins exhibit serine/threonine protein kinase activity rather than lipid kinase activity. The PIK family of kinases is involved in the regulation of cell growth, cell cycle progression, DNA damage check points, and maintenance of chromosome telomere length. Mutations in these proteins are involved in immunodeficiencies, developmental and neurological disorders, and several cancers in humans.

TOR was originally identified in temperature-sensitive yeast mutants, as a protein required for macromolecular synthesis, including RNA and protein synthesis. When mutated, it conferred resistance to the growth-inhibitory properties of the immunophilin-immunosuppressant complex (FKBP)–rapamycin. The mTOR counterpart was identified by its ability to bind FKBP–rapamycin and is structurally and functionally conserved. mTOR is a ~270- to 290-kDa protein, which, going from the N toward the C terminus, consists of two clusters of ~20 random repeats called HEAT motifs, a ~500 amino acid FAT domain, an FKBP–rapamycin-binding (FRB) domain, the kinase domain, and, most C-terminally, a ~35 amino acid FATC domain (Fig. 5). Each HEAT motif is a ~40 amino acid antiparallel α-helical protein–protein interaction motif involved in the formation of multiprotein complexes. The FAT domain, unique to members of the PIK family, might serve a role in causing interaction with other proteins or lipids. The FRB domain adjacent to the kinase domain provides the binding site for the inhibitory FKBP–rapamycin complex. The FATC domain is thought to regulate the kinase activity of mTOR by an allosteric mechanism.

Almost nothing is known about the physiological mechanisms involved in the regulation of mTOR activity. However, both amino acids and growth factors are involved in regulating mTOR activity. Insulin-induced activation of PI 3′-K results in direct phosphorylation of mTOR at two C-terminal sites by Akt/PKB within optimal consensus sequences, but only one of these is a major site for phosphorylation by Akt *in vivo*. However, this phosphorylation is not required for the ability of mTOR to phosphorylate two of its substrates, eukaryotic initiation factor-4E (eIF-4E) binding protein, PHAS-1, and p70 ribosomal S6 kinase (see later). However, deletion of the mTOR C terminus containing the two phosphorylation sites results in increased kinase activity of mTOR, suggesting a suppressor function of the C-terminal domain. It has been suggested that mTOR is constitutively active and that this enables a basal level of phosphorylation of one substrate, translation inhibitor protein 4E-BP1 (see later). This phosphorylation is a prerequisite for further growth factor-induced phosphorylation of 4E-BP1, which is dependent on PI 3′-K and PKB activity. The exact details await further studies, but mTOR is activated by nutrients rich in amino acids and growth factors under physiological conditions. mTOR is shuttled back and forth between the cytoplasm and the nucleus of growth factor-stimulated cells, and this is required for the normal function of mTOR. The regulation of mTOR localization is unknown at present.

B. Downstream of mTOR: Cell Growth Regulation, Proliferation, and Cancer

Based on results obtained by inhibiting mTOR with the immunosuppressant and antibiotic rapamycin, more is known about mTOR targets and their functions. Thus, mTOR regulates translation initiation in response to nutrients, ribosome biogenesis, transcription, and PKC signaling. Finally, mTOR is involved in cancers, including pancreatic cancer, through its upregulation of Myc levels and activation of signal transducer and activator of transcription 3 (STAT3), among others.

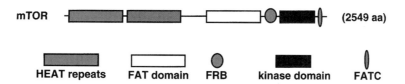

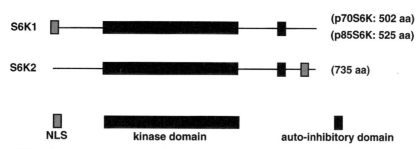

FIGURE 5 Structures of mTOR and the ribosomal S6 kinases, S6K1 and S6K2. The two isoforms of S6K1, p70 S6K and p85 S6K, are produced by use of alternative translation initiation sites in the same transcript. The only difference is the presence of an additional 23 amino acid nuclear localization signal (NLS) in p85 S6K, which is the isoform illustrated. Numbers in parentheses after the structures indicate their size in amino acids (aa) for the human sequence. Figure not drawn to scale.

Two mTOR targets, p70 ribosomal S6 kinase (see later) and the translation initiation inhibitor 4E-BP1, are central in mediating the effects of mTOR on translation initiation. Although three phosphorylation sites in p70 ribosomal S6 kinase are sensitive to rapamycin, probably only one of these, Thr389 in the C-terminal regulatory domain, is critically regulated by mTOR. Phosphorylation of this mTOR-dependent site, which also depends on PI 3′-K activity, is an essential part of the activation mechanism of p70 ribosomal S6 kinase, which concludes with PDK-1-mediated phosphorylation of the activation loop phosphorylation site in S6 kinase. Once activated, p70 S6 kinase phosphorylates the 40S ribosomal protein subunit S6 and ultimately drives the translation of 5′ terminal oligopyrimidine-rich tract (5′-TOP) mRNAs. Although there are only a few hundred of these mRNAs, they constitute up to 20% of total cellular mRNA and encode primarily ribosomal proteins and other protein components of the translation machinery. Thus, under favorable growth conditions, mTOR becomes activated, resulting in an increased expression of proteins that mediate protein translation. The 4E-BP1 protein exists in a complex with the translation initiation factor eIF4E in serum-starved cells. The binding of 4E-BP1 inhibits the activity of eIF4E, which is involved in cap-dependent translation through binding to (m7G(5′)ppp(5′)N) present at the 5′ termini of mRNAs. Upon growth factor stimulation, 4E-BP1 becomes phosphorylated directly by mTOR, resulting in the dissociation of eIF4E, enabling the latter to induce cap-dependent translation. Thus, mTOR is also important for eIF4E-mediated activation, which is particularly important for the translation of mRNAs with a highly structured 5′-untranslated region, such as the transcripts encoding c-Myc, cyclin D1, and other genes involved in cell cycle progression. The mTOR kinase also controls the synthesis of rRNAs. In addition, RNA polymerase I and III activity is positively controlled by mTOR, possibly through rapamycin-sensitive phosphorylation and inactivation of Rb, as active Rb inhibits RNA polymerase I and III transcription.

STAT3 becomes phosphorylated in response to stimulation with numerous growth factors and cytokines, causing its nuclear translocation and transcriptional activation. Both tyrosine and serine phosphorylation of STAT3 are required for its maximal activation. While both RPTKs and JAK family kinases can phosphorylate STAT3 on tyrosine, serine phosphorylation of STAT3 is rapamycin sensitive. It is possible that mTOR phosphorylates Ser727 in STAT3 directly, a site that is also phosphorylated by ERK/MAPK. This might, under some circumstances, serve an important oncogenic mechanism, as overactive STAT3 has been implicated in the tumorigenesis of mammalian cells.

As mentioned earlier, activation of PKC members, as of other AGC kinases, involves phosphorylation of the phosphorylaton site central in the conserved activation loop, as well as phosphorylaton of a hydrophobic C-terminal site. Phosphorylation of the latter site in the classical PKC isoform PKCα and in the novel PKCδ is dependent on rapamycin, just like Thr389 in p70 ribosomal S6 kinase. However, the phosphorylation of this site might also be mediated by atypical PKCs, which are, in turn, either directly regulated by mTOR or by an associated phosphatase, which is inhibited by mTOR. PKC isoforms are involved in the regulation of numerous processes, including cell proliferation, differentiation, migration, and survival, so they provide an important link to the regulation of several cellular processes by mTOR. Based on findings described earlier, only a minimal mTOR phosphorylation site consensus motif, S/T-P, where S/T is the phosphorylated residue, has been derived. See Fig. 6 for an illustration of mTOR-regulated molecules.

C. Ribosomal S6 Kinase: Structure and Regulation

S6 kinases, S6K1 and S6K2, are the key mediators of the regulation of cell growth by mTOR through their control of biosynthesis of the protein translational apparatus, in particular ribosomal proteins. Two isoforms of S6K1, denoted p70[S6K] and p85[S6K], are pro-

duced through the use of alternative translation start sites from the same transcript. Most of our current knowledge about S6 kinase signaling is derived from studies of the shorter p70 form, which is largely cytoplasmic. In contrast, the larger form is exclusively nuclear due to the presence of a nuclear localization signal in the additional 23 residues residing at the N terminus. The S6K2 protein is 70% identical to p70[S6K]. It was identified more recently through studies of S6K1 knockout mice as an upregulated gene product, which, in part, compensates for the S6K1 deficiency. S6 kinases contain a highly acidic domain in the N terminus, followed by a serine/threonine kinase domain, and a regulatory C terminus (Fig. 5). Within the C-terminal tail is an autoinhibitory region of high homology to the region of phosphorylation in the 40S ribosomal S6 protein. There are four S/T-P phosphorylation sites in this region, and they were the first regulatory phosphorylation sites identified in p70 ribosomal S6 kinase. There are three additional phosphorylation sites in the C terminus of p70 ribosomal S6 kinase, one of which, Thr389, is the equivalent of the site in the hydrophobic motif of AGC kinase members. Finally, there is a phosphorylation site in the kinase activation loop. This site resides in a highly conserved region, and its phosphorylation is required for full activation of all AGC kinases.

Numerous studies have led to a hierarchical model of ribosomal S6 kinase activiation. The first step of kinase activation is mediated by phosphorylation of the S/T-P sites in the autoinhibitory domain. While these sites fulfill the criteria for phosphorylation by ERK/MAPK, and ERK/MAPK is able to phosphorylate these in vitro, it is still debatable which protein kinase phosphorylates these sites. One site, Ser411, is phosphorylated by Cdk1/cyclin B in vitro; however, its in vivo relevance is doubtful. Phosphorylation of the autoinhibitory sites is thought to change the conformation of S6 kinase, enabling substrate access to the active site. This is a prerequisite for further kinase activation. The next step is phosphorylation of Thr389, a site that is conserved in the C-terminal hydrophobic motif of AGC kinases. This site is located just N-terminal to the autoinhibitory phosphorylation sites. Phosphorylation of Thr389 is important for disrupting the interaction between N and the C ter-

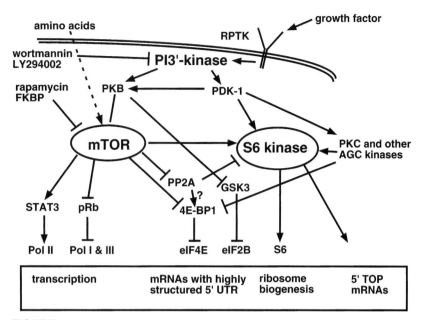

FIGURE 6 Schematic illustration of mTOR- and ribosomal S6 kinase-regulated signaling pathways. RPTK, receptor protein tyrosine kinase. For other abbreviations, see text. Arrows indicate a stimulatory effect, a solid line with a bar indicates an inhibitory effect, whereas a solid line indicates that the effect of the phosphorylation is currently unknown. The broken line with an arrowhead indicates that it is currently unclear how amino acids stimulate mTOR activity. See text for details.

mini of p70 ribosomal S6 kinase. This phosphorylation is both rapamycin and wortmannin sensitive, indicating a role for both mTOR and PI 3'-K in this step. It has been shown that mTOR can phosphorylate p70 ribosomal S6 kinase directly at this site *in vitro*, but the physiological role of this is unclear. Rather, it has been suggested that mTOR might inhibit a ribosomal S6 kinase-directed serine/threonine protein phosphatase, and PP2A is a strong candidate. Thus, PP2A has been shown to associate directly with and dephosphorylate S6 kinase, and PP2A is inhibited by insulin stimulation in a rapamycin- and wortmannin-sensitive manner. In addition, mTOR phosphorylates PP2A *in vitro*. It remains to be shown that this phosphorylation is inhibitory for PP2A. As mentioned previously, it is also possible that PDK-1 is able to phosphorylate the hydrophobic site in the C terminus of p70 ribosomal S6 kinase under some physiological conditions. Consistent with this, in PDK-1 -/- embryonic stem cells, the hydrophobic Thr389 site in p70S6K is not phosphorylated in response to IGF-1, indicating that PDK-1 phosphory-

lates this site directly or activates a protein kinase and/or inhibits a phosphatase responsible for this. In conclusion, it is likely that both mTOR and PDK-1 are involved in phosphorylation of this site under physiological conditions. The third and final step in S6 kinase activation is the direct phosphorylation of Thr229 in the activation loop ("T loop") by PDK-1. This is enabled by the phosphorylation of Thr389, which disrupts the interaction between the N and the C terminus of S6 kinase, and hence makes the activation loop Thr229 accessible for phosphorylation. Finally, it should be noted that Ser404 and Ser371 are additional sites regulated in a wortmannin- and rapamycin-sensitive manner and that phosphorylation of either of these regulates S6 kinase activity. Some sites in S6 kinase are phosphorylated by atypical PKCs *in vitro*, and they have been shown to associate with p70 ribosomal S6 kinase *in vivo*. As mentioned earlier, atypical PKCs are in part regulated by PDK-1, and some of them are regulated in a rapamycin-sensitive manner. The regulation of S6 kinase is complex, and more studies are needed to fully address this issue.

D. Downstream of Ribosomal S6 Kinase: Protein Translation and Ribosome Biogenesis

The effects of mTOR on protein translation, including ribosome biogenesis and translation of 5′ TOP mRNAs, which encode components of the protein synthetic apparatus, are mediated by ribosomal S6 kinase. Consistent with this, S6K1-deficient mice are very small, despite the compensatory effect of upregulated S6K2. The regulation of 5′ TOP mRNA translation has already been discussed.

Additional roles for S6 kinase includes enhanced transcriptional activity of E2F, which is important for the transcription of genes involved in cell cycle progression. Thus, rapamycin- and wortmannin-sensitive phosphorylation of the inhibitory E2F-binding proteins Rb and p107 by cyclin/cdk complexes causes their dissociation from E2F. S6 kinase has also been implicated in insulin-induced PI 3′-K-dependent insulin gene expression in pancreatic β cells. Overexpression of S6 kinase directly enhances insulin gene transcription in a rapamycin-sensitive manner, as measured using an insulin promoter reporter construct, and expression of a rapamycin-resistant S6 kinase rescued the inhibitory effect. It is still a possibility, though, that the regulation of E2F and insulin gene promoter activity is exerted at the level of translation.

IV. CONCLUDING REMARKS AND PERSPECTIVES

Over the past few years it has become clear that the PI 3′-K- and mTOR/ribosomal S6 kinase-regulated signaling pathways control a variety of cellular processes, ultimately governing cell growth and cell proliferation. In addition, studies of these pathways have revealed a crucial role in the pathogenesis of human diseases, including numerous highly malignant tumors. Carcinogenesis is a multistep process, where accumulated mutations result in a multitude of effects all geared toward deregulated cell proliferation and enhanced cell survival. Even a single mutation in each of several proteins individually can cause the deregulation of PI 3′-K-regulated signaling pathways. It is intriguing to speculate that through the resulting multiple effects of enhanced cell survival, deregulated cell proliferation and activation of many oncogenes through cross talk induced by such a mutation, it would circumvent the need for additional mutations in the oncogenic process. Accordingly, there are indications that deregulated PI 3′-K signaling is associated with human malignancies without concomitant secondary genetic changes. It will be interesting to await the development of animal models with inducible single genomic point mutations. Most human cancers are due to a single or a few amino acid changes in a few gene products, and so the development of mouse models that could mimic the human disease more closely would be important for shedding light on the pathogenesis of malignancies in humans. It seems that the PI 3′-K pathway would provide an obvious target for such attempts of genetic manipulations. In support of the idea that carcinogenesis might, at least initially, require only one genetic point mutation is the fact that inactivating mutations in the tumor suppressor PTEN, a negative regulator of PI 3′-K, often seem to occur without any other noticeable genetic alterations. PTEN is among the most frequently mutated genes associated with human malignancies, being targeted as frequently as the tumor suppressor p53 and more frequently than the oncogene Ras.

Acknowledgments

P. B.-J. is a Special Fellow of the Leukemia and Lymphoma Society of America and T. H. is a Frank and Else Schilling American Cancer Society Professor.

See Also the Following Articles

MAP KINASE MODULES IN SIGNALING • PROTEIN KINASE INHIBITORS • SIGNAL TRANSDUCTION MECHANISMS INITIATED BY RECEPTOR TYROSINE KINASES

Bibliography

Alessi, D. R., and Cohen, P. (1998). Mechanism of activation and function of protein kinase B. *Curr. Opin. Genet. Dev.* **8,** 55–62.

Chan, T. O., Rittenhouse, S. E., and Tsichlis, P. N. (1999). AKT/PKB and other D3 phosphoinositide-regulated kinases: Kinase activation by phosphoinositide-dependent phosphorylation. *Annu. Rev. Biochem.* **68,** 965–1014.

Chin, L., and DePinho, R. A. (2000). Flipping the oncogene switch: Illumination of tumor maintenance and regression. *Trends Genet.* **16,** 147–150.

Hunter, T. (2000). Signaling: 2000 and beyond. *Cell* **100,** 113–127.

Scheid, M. P., and Woodgett, J. R. (2000). Protein kinases: Six degrees of separation? *Curr. Biol.* **10,** R191–R194.

Schmelzle, T., and Hall, M. N. (2000). TOR, a central controller of cell growth. *Cell* **103,** 253–262.

Stocker, H., and Hafen, E. (2000). Genetic control of cell size. *Curr. Opin. Genet. Dev.* **10,** 529–535.

Toker, A. (2000). Protein kinases as mediators of phosphoinositide 3-kinase signaling. *Mol. Pharm.* **57,** 652–658.

Toker, A., and Newton, A. C. (2000). Cellular signaling: Pivoting around PDK-1. *Cell* **103,** 185–188.

Vanhaesebroeck, B., and Waterfield, M. D. (1999). Signaling by distinct classes of phosphoinositide 3-kinases. *Exp. Cell Res.* **253,** 239–254.

Volarevic, S., Stewart, M. J., Ledermann, B., Zilberman, F., Terracciano, L., Montini, E., Grompe, M., Kozma, S. C., and Thomas, G. (2000). Proliferation, but not growth, blocked by conditional deletion of 40S ribosomal protein S6. *Science* **288,** 2045–2047.

Weinkove, D., and Leevers, S. J. (2000). The genetic control of organ growth: Insights from Drosophila. *Curr. Opin. Genet. Dev.* **10,** 75–80.

ISBN 0-12-227557-8

90038

9 780122 275579